Common childhood rashes

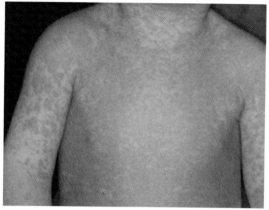

Plate 1 Measles—typical morbilliform rash.

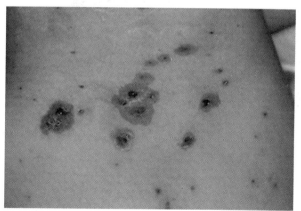

Plate 2 Varicella—widespread vesicles.

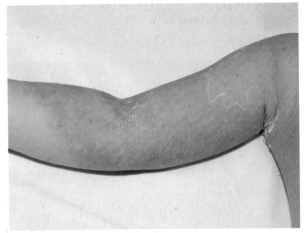

Plate 3 Scarlet fever with desquamation.

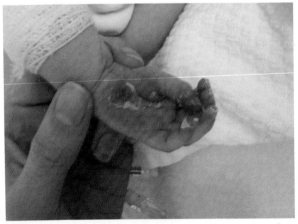

Plate 4 Syphilis with palmar desquamation.

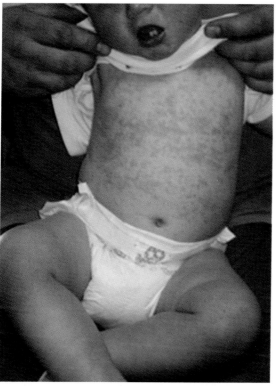

Plate 5 A typical viral rash.

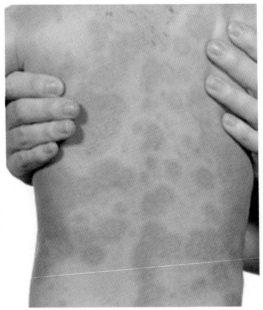

Plate 6 Erythema multiforme.

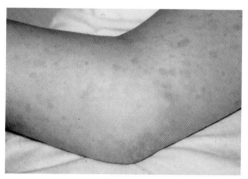

Plate 7 Rash of Juvenile idiopathic arthritis.

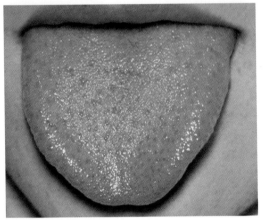

Plate 8 Strawbery tongue.

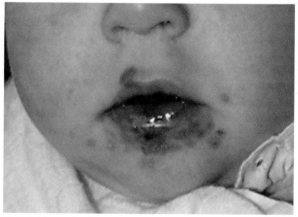

Plate 9 Herpes simplex virus stomatitis.

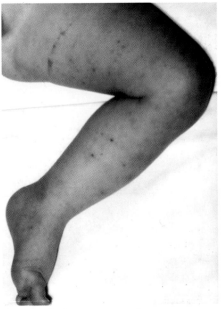

Plate 10 Pupuric rash of meningococcaemia.

Manual of
Childhood
Infections

Manual of Childhood Infections

Third edition

Chief Editor
Mike Sharland

Professor of Paediatric Infectious Diseases,
St George's Hospital, London, UK

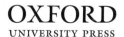
OXFORD
UNIVERSITY PRESS

OXFORD
UNIVERSITY PRESS

Great Clarendon Street, Oxford OX2 6DP.

Oxford University Press is a department of the University of Oxford.
It furthers the University's objective of excellence in research, scholarship,
and education by publishing worldwide in

Oxford New York

Auckland Cape Town Dar es Salaam Hong Kong Karachi
Kuala Lumpur Madrid Melbourne Mexico City Nairobi
New Delhi Shanghai Taipei Toronto

With offices in

Argentina Austria Brazil Chile Czech Republic France Greece
Guatemala Hungary Italy Japan Poland Portugal Singapore
South Korea Switzerland Thailand Turkey Ukraine Vietnam

Oxford is a registered trade mark of Oxford University Press
in the UK and in certain other countries

Published in the United States
by Oxford University Press Inc., New York

British Library Cataloguing in Publication Data
Data available

Library of Congress Cataloging-in-Publication-Data
Data available

Typeset by Glyph International, Bangalore, India
Printed in Great Britain
on acid-free paper through
Ashford Colour Press Ltd, Gosport, Hampshire

ISBN 978–0–19–957358–5

10 9 8 7 6 5 4 3 2 1

Foreword by Professor Terrence Stephenson

President of The Royal College of Paediatrics and Child Health, United Kingdom

I am delighted to write a foreword for the third edition of *The Manual of Childhood Infections*. The last edition was ten years ago. This new edition has been completely re-written and updated. The aim of the book is to provide a practical, evidence-based handbook approach to the management of both common and unusual infections in children. The editorial board found nearly two hundred authors to write the one hundred and twenty chapters of this new edition. The book has been written by paediatricians, microbiologists and a wide range of international experts in paediatric infectious diseases. The book is aimed at both trainee and practising hospital and community based paediatricians, nursing and other medical staff caring for children in the United Kingdom, Europe and internationally. It provides an up-to-date reference guide, including common differential diagnoses, practical management hints and information for over one hundred drugs. The overall aim of the book is to improve the evidence-base for the management of childhood infections.

In the United Kingdom, a recent confidential enquiry into maternal and child health notes infection still to be the largest single cause of death in children dying of an acute illness. Overall, infection was a contributory cause in at least twenty per cent of all childhood deaths, and this was over one quarter of all deaths in children between one and four years of age. Despite the success of recent immunisation campaigns, nearly two thirds of these deaths are still due to bacterial infection. Prompt diagnosis of serious bacterial infections remains a major challenge in paediatrics globally. In both healthy children and in those with underlying medical conditions, still too many children die of unrecognised infections, particularly children with long-term medical conditions, including prematurity. There is still much to be done to prevent nosocomial and opportunistic infections.

Paediatricians also have a duty in not over-treating or over-managing children with minor, self-limiting infectious illness. There has been a rise of around forty per cent of short stay admissions to hospital of less than two days in England in the last decade. The majority of these are for minor illnesses, particularly infections that could be managed more appropriately in the community. Antibiotics remain a precious and finite resource. The rise of antimicrobial resistance is now recognised by the UK Departments of Health, the European CDC and World Health Organization as a major threat to human health in the future. The antibiotic 'pipeline' particularly for agents acting against gram negative infections, is worryingly sparse. Gram negative resistance is becoming increasingly common in hospital acquired infection and the optimal use of our current antibiotics becomes ever more important. Prudent use of antibiotics and antibiotic stewardship are ever more necessary now. Imported infections and new global pandemics will remain a continued threat, so the Manual also highlights the early recognition and prompt management of less common infections.

The new edition has been produced in collaboration with the European Society for Paediatric Infectious Diseases (ESPID) and the Royal College welcomes the development of collaborative educational initiatives between the United Kingdom and Europe.

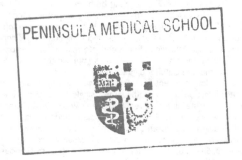

Foreword by Professor Ulrich Heininger

President of the European Society for Paediatric Infectious Diseases (ESPID)

The European Society for Paediatric Infectious Diseases is delighted to be working in partnership with the Royal College of Paediatrics and Child Health in this third edition of the Manual of Childhood Infections – the *Blue Book*. This edition has a strong European and global focus and has tried to define the evidence-base for the management of common childhood infectious diseases. There is still much variation in the practice and management of childhood infections across Europe today. ESPID accepts and welcomes this diversity of care, much of which reflects cultural differences in child care across Europe. Moreover, there are variations in the prevalence of specific infectious diseases and variations in antimicrobial resistance patterns across Europe. Clearly evidence-based guidelines will continue to vary across European countries for many years to come.

This manual has therefore attempted to be a synthesis of the published evidence, collating wherever possible, Cochrane and other systematic reviews, and has as its core an up to date evidence base. It does *not* aim to replace local, regional or country-specific guidance for either the hospital or office-based paediatrician but rather has been produced as a teaching tool for trainees across Europe, and for practising paediatricians. It should be used as a source to check, look up or think about the management plan, the differential diagnosis or recent epidemiology. In many cases, chapters define clearly what we do not know, and authors have tried to outline areas of important research for the future. ESPID hopes to be taking forward some of these ideas through its new research committee.

The *Blue Book* also recognises that antimicrobial dosing varies considerably across Europe. The drug, the dose and the duration of treatment are often poorly evidence-based in paediatrics, especially in neonatal medicine. The *Blue Book* formulary again, does not replace local guidelines, but is designed to be a short, easy to use, pragmatic and reasonable summary of the published evidence for each drug. It is hoped that further work in defining variations in guidelines, drug dosing and indication, can be fed into initiatives such as the European Medicines Agency's Priority Drug List. Collaborative research projects across Europe will hopefully in time improve the evidence-base for both old and new antimicrobials used in children.

The *Blue Book* is part of ESPID's mission, aiming at improving the education of paediatricians and the optimal management of infectious diseases. We recognise that not everyone will agree with everything written in this edition and we encourage your comments, suggestions for improvements and contributions for the next edition. The *Blue Book* is still a relatively new venture (on its third edition whereas the *Red Book* is on its twenty seventh edition) but I am confident that over time it will become a core part of the management of paediatric infectious diseases across Europe.

Contents

Section 1 **Clinical syndromes**

Section 2 Specific infections

Appendices

Section editors

Andrew Cant
Consultant in Paediatric
Immunology and Infectious
Diseases, Great North Children's
Hospital, Newcastle, UK

Graham Davies
Consultant Paediatric
Immunologist, Great Ormond
Street Hospital for Children,
London, UK

David Elliman
Consultant in Paediatrics,
Great Ormond Street Hospital
for Children, London, UK

Susanna Esposito
Director of the Pediatric Infectious
Diseases Unit, Università degli
Studi di Milano, Fondazione IRCCS
Ca' Granda Ospedale Maggiore
Policlinico, Milan, Italy

Adam Finn
David Baum Professor of
Paediatrics; Head, Unit of Child
Health, Department of Clinical
Sciences, University of Bristol;
Director, South West Medicines
for Children Local Research
Network; Honorary Consultant
Paediatrician, Bristol Royal
Hospital for Children, UK

Jim Gray
Consultant Medical
Microbiologist, Birmingham
Children's Hospital
NHS Foundation Trust and
Birmingham Women's
NHS Foundation Trust, UK

Paul T. Heath
Reader and Honorary Consultant
in Paediatric Infectious Diseases,
St George's, University of London,
London, UK

Hermione Lyall
Consultant Paediatrician,
Infectious Diseases, Chief of
Service for Paediatrics, Imperial
College Healthcare NHS Trust, UK

Andrew J. Pollard
Professor of Paediatric
Infection and Immunity,
University of Oxford and
Honorary Consultant Paediatrician,
Oxford Children's Hospital,
Oxford, UK

Mary Ramsay
Consultant Epidemiologist and
Head, Immunisation, Hepatitis and
Blood Safety Department,
Health Protection Agency Centre
for Infections,
London, UK

Andrew Riordan
Consultant in Paediatric Infectious
Diseases and Immunology,
Alder Hey Children's NHS
Foundation Trust, Liverpool, UK

Delane Shingadia
Consultant in Paediatric Infectious
Diseases, Great Ormond Street
Hospital for Children,
London, UK

Contributors

Mario Abinun

Consultant in Paediatric
Immunology & Infectious Diseases,
Newcastle upon Tyne Hospitals
NHS Trust,
Newcastle upon Tyne, UK

Alasdair Bamford

NIHR Research Training Fellow,
Imperial College,
London, UK

Jolanta Bernatoniene

Consultant Paediatrician,
Paediatric Infectious Disease and
Immunology Department,
Bristol Royal Hospital for Children,
Bristol, UK

Jan Bonhoeffer

Consultant,
Paediatric Infectious Diseases
and Vaccines,
University Children's Hospital
Basel, Switzerland

Paul A Brogan

Senior Lecturer in Paediatric
Vasculitis, and Honorary
Consultant Paediatric
Rheumatologist,
Department of Rheumatology,
UCL Institute of Child Health,
and Great Ormond Street Hospital
NHS Trust,
London, UK

Penelope A Bryant

Consultant in Paediatric Infectious
Diseases, Royal Children's
Hospital; and Monash
Medical Centre,
Melbourne, Australia

Jim Buttery

Infectious Diseases Physician,
Paediatric Infectious Diseases,
Monash & Royal Children's
Hospitals, Murdoch Children's
Research Institute,
Department of Paediatrics,
Monash University
Melbourne, Australia

Anuradha Chawla

Consultant Medical Virologist
and Honorary
Senior Lecturer,
The Royal Liverpool and
Broadgreen University
Hospitals NHS Trust,
Liverpool, UK

Hsin Chi

Senior Attending Physician of
Division of Infectious
Diseases,
Department of Pediatrics,
Mackay Memorial Hospital,
Taipei, Taiwan

Nan-Chang Chiu

Chief,
Division of Pediatric
Infectious Diseases,
Department of Pediatrics,
Mackay Memorial Hospital,
Taipei, Taiwan

Georgi Christov

Clinical Fellow in Paediatric
Cardiology, Great Ormond
Street Hospital for Children,
London, UK

Ed Clark

Academic Clinical Lecturer in
Paediatrics,
Institute of Child Life
and Health,
University Hospitals Bristol
Education Centre,
Bristol, UK

Julia Clark

Consultant in Paediatric
Immunology & Infectious
Diseases,
Newcastle General Hospital,
Newcastle, UK

David Cliff

Childhood Empyema Research
Fellow
Newcastle University,
Newcastle, UK

Theresa Cole

Specialist Registrar in Paediatric
Immunology & Infectious Diseases,
Newcastle upon Tyne Hospitals
NHS Trust,
Newcastle, UK

Nigel Curtis

Professor of Paediatric
Infectious Diseases, Department
of Paediatrics,
The University of Melbourne;
Head of Infectious Diseases Unit,
Department of General Medicine,
The Royal Children's Hospital
Melbourne;
Leader, Infectious Diseases &
Microbiology Group,
Murdoch Children's Research
Institute,
Parkville, Victoria, Australia

Graham Davies

Consultant Paediatric
Immunologist,
Immunology Department,
Great Ormond Street Hospital
for Children,
London, UK

Garth LJ Dixon

Consultant Medical Microbiology,
Great Ormond Street Hospital for
Children;
Honorary Senior Lecturer,
Infectious Disease and
Microbiology Unit,
Institute of Child Health at UCL,
London, UK

Simon Dobson

Clinical Associate Professor,
University of British Columbia,
Vancouver, Canada;
Canada Attending Physician,
Pediatric Infectious Diseases,
British Columbia Children's Hospital,
Vancouver, BC, Canada

Katja M Doerholt

Consultant, Paediatric Infectious
Diseases,
St George's Healthcare NHS Trust,
London, UK

Geoffrey Edwards

Senior Lecturer in Pharmacology,
School of Biomedical Sciences,
The University of Liverpool,
Liverpool, UK

Mohamed Elemraid

Paediatric Registrar/Research
Fellow
Newcastle upon Tyne Hospitals
NHS Trust,
Newcastle upon Tyne, UK

Alyson Elliman

Consultant in Sexual and
Reproductive Healthcare,
Croydon Community Provider
Services,
Croydon, UK

David AC Elliman

Consultant in Community
Child Health,
Great Ormond Street Hospital
for Children,
London, UK

Matthew Ellis
Senior Clinical Lecturer,
Centre for Child and Adolescent Health,
University of Bristol,
Bristol, UK

Susanna Esposito
Director of the Pediatric Infectious Diseases Unit,
Università degli Studi di Milano,
Fondazione IRCCS, Ca' Granda
Ospedale Maggiore Policlinico,
Milan, Italy

Saul N Faust
Senior Lecturer in Paediatric Immunology & Infectious Diseases,
University of Southampton;
Director, Wellcome Trust Clinical Research Facility,
Southampton, UK

Susanna Felsenstein
Paediatric Registrar,
Royal Alexandra Children's Hospital,
Brighton, UK

Terry J Flood
Consultant in Paediatric Immunology & Infectious Diseases
Newcastle upon Tyne Hospitals NHS Trust,
Newcastle, UK

Helen R Freeman
Specialist Registrar in Paediatrics,
Bristol Royal Hospital for Children,
Bristol, UK

Eva Galiza
Clinical Research Fellow,
St. George's Vaccine Institute,
St. George's University of London,
London, UK

Roger I Glass
Director,
Fogarty International Center,
National Institutes of Health,
Bethesda, USA

Jim Gray
Consultant Medical Microbiologist,
Birmingham Children's Hospital
NHS Foundation Trust
and Birmingham Women's NHS Foundation Trust,
Birmingham, UK

Scott J Hackett
Consultant in Paediatric
Infectious Diseases, Immunology and Allergy,
Birmingham Heartlands Hospital,
Birmingham, UK

Jennifer Handforth
Consultant Paediatrician,
Croydon University Hospital,
Croydon, UK

Catherine A Harwood
Clinical Senior Lecturer and Consultant Dermatologist,
Centre for Cutaneous Research,
Blizard Institute of Cell and Molecular Science,
Barts and the London School of Medicine and Dentistry,
Queen Mary University of London,
London UK

Paul T Heath
Reader and Honorary Consultant in Paediatric Infectious Diseases,
St George's Hospital, and
University of London,
London, UK

Rowan Heath
Consultant Paediatrician,
Kingston Hospital,
Kingston upon Thames, UK

Terho Heikkinen
Assistant Professor of Paediatrics,
University of Turku,
Turku, Finland

Ulrich Heininger
President,
ESPID

Jethro Herberg
Clinical Lecturer in Paediatric
Infectious Disease,
Imperial College,
London, UK

David R Hill
Director,
The National Travel Health
Network and Centre;
Honorary Professor,
London School of Hygiene and
Tropical Medicine,
London, UK

Peter Hotez
Distinguished Research Professor,
George Washington University;
President, Sabin Vaccine Institute
Washington D.C., USA

David Isaacs
Senior Staff Specialist,
Department of Infectious Diseases,
The Children's Hospital at
Westmead, and Clinical Professor
in Paediatric Infectious Disease,
University of Sydney,
Sydney, Australia

Lyda P Jadresić
Consultant Paediatrician,
Department of Paediatrics,
Gloucestershire Royal Hospital,
Gloucester, UK

Heath Kelly
Head, Epidemiology Unit,
Victorian Infectious Diseases
Reference Laboratory;
Associate Professor,
School of Population Health,
University of Melbourne,
Melbourne, Australia

Alison M Kesson
Head of Infectious Diseases and
Microbiology,
Children's Hospital at Westmead;
Conjoint Associate Professor of
Paediatrics and Child Health,
Sydney Medical School,
University of Sydney,
Sydney, Australia

Julia M Kenny
Senior Clinical Research Fellow,
Institute of Child Health,
University College London,
London, UK

Nigel Klein
Professor and Consultant in
Paediatric Infectious Diseases and
Immunology,
Great Ormond Street Hospital for
Children,
London, UK

Shamez Ladhani
Consultant in Paediatric Infectious
Diseases,
Health Protection Agency Centre
for Infections, and Paediatric
Infectious Diseases Unit,
St. George's Healthcare NHS
Trust,
London, UK

Susan Liebeschuetz
Consultant Paediatrician,
Newham University Hospital,
London, UK

Samantha Lissauer
Paediatric Specialist Trainee,
Heartlands Hospital,
Birmingham, UK

Suzanne Luck

Consultant Paediatrician,
Kingston Hospital NHS Trust;
Research Fellow,
University College London,
London, UK

Ian Maconochie

Consultant in Paediatric A&E,
St Mary's Hospital,
London, UK

Richard Malley

Associate Professor of Pediatrics,
Harvard Medical School;
Kenneth McIntosh Chair in
Pediatric Infectious Diseases,
Children's Hospital Boston,
Boston, USA

Nuria Martinez-Alier

Consultant in Paediatric Infectious
Diseases, Immunology and General
Paediatrics,
Evelina Children's Hospital,
St Thomas' Hospital,
London, UK

Janet McCulloch

Regional Health Protection
Nurse,
Health Protection Agency, UK

Esse N Menson

Consultant in Paediatric Infectious
Diseases & Immunology,
Evelina Children's Hospital,
St Thomas' Hospital, London, UK

Mike Millar

Consultant Microbiologist,
Barts and the London NHS Trust,
London, UK

Anita Modhi

Locum Consultant in Paediatrics,
Department of Paediatrics,
Luton and Dunstable Hospital,
Luton, UK

Andrew Morgan

Professor of Virology,
University of Bristol,
Bristol, UK

Dilys Morgan

Head of Department,
Gastrointestinal, Emerging and
Zoonotic Infections,
Health Protection Agency Centre
for Infections,
London, UK

Karyn Lee Moshal

Consultant and Specialty Lead,
Department of Infectious Diseases,
Great Ormond Street Hospital for
Children,
London, UK

Eleni Nastouli

Consultant Virologist,
University College London
Hospitals NHS Trust;
Honorary Consultant in Paediatric
Infectious Diseases,
Great Ormond Street Hospital for
Children NHS Trust,
London, UK

Olaf Neth

Head of the Department of
Paediatric Infectious Diseases and
Immunodeficiencies,
University Hospital
Virgen del Rocio,
Seville, Spain

Vas Novelli

Consultant in Paediatric Infectious
Diseases,
Great Ormond Street Hospital for
Children,
London, UK

Ursula Nusgen

Consultant Microbiologist,
Birmingham Children's Hospital,
Birmingham, UK

Ita O'Connor
Vascular Access Device Nurse,
Barts and the London NHS Trust,
London, UK

Milos Ognjanovic
Consultant Paediatric
Nephrologist,
Newcastle upon Tyne Hospitals
NHS Trust,
Newcastle upon Tyne, UK

Peter Olbrich
Specialist Registrar in Paediatrics,
Department of Paediatric
Infectious Diseases and
Immunodeficiencies,
University Hospital
Virgen del Rocio,
Seville, Spain

Marta Palusinska-Szysz
Senior Lecturer,
Maria Curie-Sklodowska
University,
Department of Genetics and
Microbiology,
Institute of Microbiology and
Biotechnology,
Lublin, Poland

Christopher M Parry
Senior Clinical Research Fellow,
Oxford University Clinical
Research Unit
Oxford, UK;
Hospital for Tropical Diseases,
Ho Chi Minh City, Vietnam

Manish Patel
Epidemiologist,
Viral Gastroenteritis Team,
Division of Viral Diseases,
Centers for Disease Control and
Prevention,
Atlanta, USA

Mitul Patel
Consultant Microbiologist,
Birmingham Children's Hospital,
Birmingham, UK

Sanjay Patel
Specialist Registrar in Paediatric
Immunology & Infectious Diseases,
Newcastle-upon-Tyne Hospitals
NHS Trust,
Newcastle, UK

Stéphane Paulus
Consultant in Paediatric Infectious
Diseases,
Alder Hey Children's Hospital,
Liverpool, UK

Stanley A Plotkin
Emeritus Professor of Pediatrics,
University of Pennsylvania,
Philadelphia, USA;
Adjunct Professor,
Johns Hopkins School of
Public Health,
Baltimore, USA;
Principal,
Vaxconsult.com

Andrew J Pollard
Professor of Paediatric Infection
and Immunity,
University of Oxford, and
Honorary Consultant Paediatrician,
Oxford Children's Hospital,
Oxford, UK

Andrew Prendergast
Academic Clinical Lecturer,
Department of Paediatrics,
University of Oxford,
Oxford, UK

Nicola Principi
Director of the Pediatric
Department,
Università degli Studi di Milano,
Fondazione IRCCS, Ca'
Granda Ospedale Maggiore
Policlinico,
Milan, Italy

A V Ramanan

Lead Consultant Paediatric
Rheumatologist,
Bristol Royal Hospital for
Children & Royal
National Hospital for
Rheumatic Diseases;
Honorary Reader,
University of Bristol,
Bristol, UK

Martin Richardson

Consultant Paediatrician,
Department of Paediatrics,
Peterborough District Hospital,
Peterborough, UK

Andrew Riordan

Consultant in Paediatric Infectious
Diseases and Immunology,
Alder Hey Children's
NHS Foundation Trust,
Liverpool, UK

Valerie Rogers

Specialist Registrar in
Paediatric Rheumatology and
General Paediatrics,
Bristol Royal Hospital for Children,
Bristol, UK

Peter T Rudd

Consultant Paediatrician,
Children's Centre,
Royal United Hospital,
Bath, UK

Manish Sadarangani

Clinical Research Fellow,
Department of Paediatrics,
University of Oxford;
Honorary Specialist Registrar in
Paediatrics,
Children's Hospital,
Oxford, UK

Rebecca Salter

Consultant in Paediatric A&E,
St Marys Hospital,
London, UK

Shelley Segal

Consultant Paediatrician,
Honorary Senior Lecturer,
University of Oxford,
Oxford, UK

Paul Shears

Consultant Microbiologist/
Director of Infection Prevention
and Control,
Wirral University Teaching
Hospital,
Microbiology Department,
Clatterbridge Hospital,
Wirral, UK

Delane Shingadia

Consultant in Paediatric Infectious
Diseases,
Great Ormond Street Hospital for
Children,
London, UK

Hilary J Simons

Senior Specialist Nurse
(Travel Health),
The National Travel Health
Network and Centre,
Liverpool School of Tropical
Medicine,
Liverpool, UK

Mary Slatter

Associate Specialist in Paediatric
Bone Marrow Transplantation,
Newcastle General Hospital,
Newcastle upon Tyne, UK

Mary PE Slack

Consultant Medical
Microbiologist,
Respiratory & Systemic Infection
Laboratory,
Health Protection Agency
Microbiology Services Division,
London, UK

Nikos P Spyridis

Lecturer in Paediatric Infectious Diseases,
Aglaia Kyriakou Children's Hospital
University of Athens,
Athens, Greece

Andrew C Steer

Pediatric Infectious Diseases Fellow,
University of British Columbia,
Vancouver, Canada;
Paediatrician,
Centre for International Child Health,
University of Melbourne,
Melbourne, Australia

Marc Tebruegge

Department of Paediatrics,
The University of Melbourne;
Infectious Diseases Unit,
Department of General Medicine, Royal Children's Hospital Melbourne;
Murdoch Children's Research Institute,
Parkville, Victoria, Australia

Julian E Thomas

Consultant Paediatric Gastroenterologist
Newcastle upon Tyne Hospitals NHS Trust,
Newcastle upon Tyne, UK

Alistair Thomson

Consultant Paediatrician,
Department of Paediatrics,
Leighton Hospital,
Crewe, UK

Bruce Thorley

Head, Polio Reference Laboratory,
Victorian Infectious Diseases Reference Laboratory,
Melbourne, Australia

Stephen Tomlin

Principal Paediatric Pharmacist,
Guy's and St Thomas' NHS Trust,
London, UK

Pat A Tookey

Senior Lecturer,
MRC Centre of Epidemiology for Child Health,
UCL Institute of Child Health,
London, UK

Yinsent Tse

Specialist Registrar in Paediatric Nephrology,
Newcastle upon Tyne Hospitals NHS Trust,
Newcastle upon Tyne, UK

Jim Wai-Tim

Paediatric ICU Attending Physician,
Tamshui Branch,
Mackay Memorial Hospital,
Taipei, Taiwan

Amanda L Walsh

Senior Scientist,
Gastrointestinal, Emerging and Zoonotic Infections Department,
Health Protection Agency
Centre for Infections
London, UK

Steve Welch

Consultant in Paediatric Infectious Diseases,
Heartlands Hospital,
Birmingham, UK

Elizabeth Whittaker

Wellcome Trust Research Training Fellow, Department of Academic Paediatrics,
Imperial College,
London, UK

Lalith P M Wijedoru

Clinical Lecturer (Paediatrics),
Child and Reproductive
Health Group,
Liverpool School of
Tropical Medicine,
Liverpool, UK

Bhanu Williams

Specialist Registrar in Paediatric
Infectious Diseases,
Great Ormond
Street Hospital,
London, UK

Eleri Williams

Specialist Registrar in Paediatric
Immunology & Infectious Diseases,
Newcastle upon Tyne Hospitals
NHS Trust,
Newcastle upon Tyne, UK

Lucinda C Winckworth

ST4 Paediatrics,
The Whittington Hospital NHS
Trust,
London, UK

Abbreviations and symbols

5-FC	5-fluorocytosine
γ-GG	γ-glutamyl transferase
AAP	American Academy of Pediatrics
ABCD	amphotericin B colloidal dispersion
ABLC	amphotericin B lipid complex
ABPA	allergic bronchopulmonary aspergillosis
ADA	adenosine deaminase
ADH	antidiuretic hormone
AHC	acute haemorrhagic conjunctivitis
AIDS	acquired immune deficiency syndrome
ALA	amoebic liver abscess
ALP	alkaline phosphatase
ALT	alanine aminotransferase
ANA	antinuclear antibody
ANCA	antineutrophilic cytoplasmic antibody
AOM	acute otitis media
ARDS	acute respiratory distress syndrome
ARF	acute rheumatic fever
ART	antiretroviral therapy
ARV	antiretroviral
ASOT	antistreptolysin O titre
AST	aspartate aminotransferase
AUC	area under the curve
BAAF	British Association for Adoption and Fostering
BAL	bronchoalveolar lavage
BCG	bacille Calmette Guérin
BMT	bone marrow transplantation
BNFC	*British National Formulary for Children*
BPSU	British Paediatric Surveillance Unit
BSE	bovine spongiform encephalopathy
CCHF	Crimean-Congo haemorrhagic fever
CDC	Centers for Disease Control and Prevention
CFS	chronic fatigue syndrome
CFU	colony forming units
CGD	chronic granulomatous disease
CJD	Creutzfeldt–Jakob disease
CL	cutaneous leishmaniasis

C_{max}	maximal drug concentration
CMV	cytomegalovirus
CNPA	chronic necrotizing pulmonary aspergillosis
CNS	central nervous system
CONS	coagulase-negative staphylococci
CRMO	chronic recurrent multifocal osteomyelitis
CRP	C-reactive protein
CRS	congenital rubella syndrome
CSF	cerebrospinal fluid
CT	computed tomography
CVC	central venous catheter
CVL	central venous line
CVP	central venous pressure
CVS	congenital varicella syndrome
CYP	cytochrome P-450
CXR	chest X-ray
DFA	direct fluorescent antibody (staining)
DGS	DiGeorge's syndrome
DHF	dengue haemorrhagic fever
DIC	disseminated intravascular coagulopathy
DPT	diphtheria/pertussis/tetanus
EBV	Epstein–Barr virus
ECHO virus	enteric cytopathic human orphan virus
ECMO	extracorporeal membrane oxygenation
EDTA	ethylenediaminetetraacetic acid
EEG	electroencephalogram
EHEC	enterohaemorrhagic *Escherichia coli*
EIA	enzyme immunoassays
ELBW	extremely low birthweight
ELISA	enzyme-linked immunosorbent assay
ERCP	endoscopic retrograde cholangiopancreatography
ESR	erythrocyte sedimentation rate
FBC	full blood count
FDA	Food and Drug Administration
IFI	invasive fungal infection
FiO_2	fraction of inspired oxygen
FITC	fluorescein isothiocyanate
FNA	fine needle aspiration
G6PD	glucose-6-phosphate dehydrogenase
GABA	γ-aminobutyric acid
GABHS	Lancefield group A β-haemolytic streptococcus

GAS	group A streptococcus
GBS	group B streptococcus
GCS	Glasgow Coma Scale
G-CSF	granulocyte colony-stimulating factor
GFR	glomerular filtration rate
GT	genotype
GT	glutaryl transferase
GVHD	graft versus host disease
HACEK	*Haemophilus* species (*H. influenzae*, *H. parainfluenzae*), *Aggregatibacter actinomycetemcomitans*, *Aggregatibacter aphrophilus*, *Cardiobacter hominis*, *Eikenella corrodens*, *Kingella kingae*
HAdV	human adenoviruses
HBcAg	hepatitis B core antigen
HBeAg	hepatitis B envelope antigen
HBsAg	hepatitis B surface antigen
HBV	hepatitis B virus
HCAI	healthcare-associated infection
HCC	hepatocellular carcinoma
HCV	hepatitis C virus
HDU	high-dependency unit
HFRS	haemorrhagic fever with renal syndrome
HHV	human herpesvirus
HIDA	hepatobiliary iminodiacetic acid
Hib	*Haemophilus influenzae* type b
HIV	human immunodeficiency virus
HLA	human leucocyte antigen
HLH	haemophagocytic lymphohistiocytosis
HPA	Health Protection Agency
HPU	health protection unit
HPV	human papillomavirus
HRCT	high-resolution computed tomography
HSCT	haematopoietic stem cell transplantation
HSV	herpes simplex virus
HTLV	human T cell lymphotropic virus
HUS	haemolytic–uraemic syndrome
ICD	implantable cardioverter-defibrillator
ICD	International Classification of Diseases
ICP	intracranial pressure
ICVP	International Certificate of Vaccination or Prophylaxis
IE	infective endocarditis
IFA	immunofluorescent antibody/assay

IFI	invasive fungal infection
IGRA	interferon-γ release assay
IL	interleukin
IM	intramuscular
INF	interferon
INR	international normalized ratio
IPA	invasive pulmonary aspergillosis
IPV	inactivated poliovirus vaccine
IUGR	intrauterine growth retardation
IV	intravenous
IVIG	intravenous immunoglobulin
JIA	juvenile idiopathic arthritis
KD	Kawasaki disease
L-amB	liposomal amphotericin B
LDH	lactate dehydrogenase
LFT	liver function test
LGV	lymphogranuloma venereum
LIP	lymphocytic interstitial pneumonitis
LN	lymph node
LP	lumbar puncture
LRTI	lower respiratory tract infection
LTBI	latent tuberculosis infection
M-CSF	macrophage-colony stimulating factor
MIC	minimum inhibitory concentration
MIF	microimmunofluorescence
ML	mucocutaneous leishmaniasis
MMR	measles, mumps, and rubella
MRCP	magnetic resonance cholangiopancreatography
MRI	magnetic resonance imaging
MRSA	meticillin-resistant *Staphylococcus aureus*
MSMD	mendelian susceptibility to mycobacterial diseases
MSSA	meticillin-sensitive *Staphylococcus aureus*
MTB	mycobacterial tuberculosis
NAAT	nucleic acid amplification test
NEC	necrotizing enterocolitis
NEMO	nuclear factor-κB essential modifier
NICE	National Institute for Health and Clinical Excellence
NICU	neonatal intensive care unit
NPA	nasopharyngeal aspirate
NPV	negative predictive value
NSAID	non-steroidal anti-inflammatory drug

NT Pro-BNP	N-terminal pro-brain natriuretic peptide
NTM	non-tuberculous mycobacteria
OAI	osteoarticular infection
OM	osteomyelitis
OPV	oral polio vaccine
ORS	oral rehydration solution
$PaCO_2$	arterial carbon dioxide tension
PcP	*Pneumocystis* pneumonia
PCR	polymerase chain reaction
PCV	pneumococcal conjugate vaccine
PICU	paediatric intensive care unit
PID	pelvic inflammatory disease
PK-PD	pharmacokinetics-pharmacodynamics
PML	progressive multifocal leucoencephalopathy
PNP	purine nucleoside phosphorylase
PPE	personal protective equipment
PPV	positive predictive value
PSGN	post-streptococcal glomerulonephritis
PT	prothrombin time
PTT	partial thromboplastin time
PTLD	post-transplant lymphoproliferative disorder
PUO	pyrexia of unknown origin
PVL	Panton-valentine leucocidin
RADT	rapid antigen detection test
RAST	radioallergosorbent test
RCT	randomized controlled trial
RPR	rapid-plasma-reagin
RSV	respiratory syncytial virus
RT-PCR	reverse transcriptase polymerase chain reaction
SA	septic arthritis
SARS	severe acute respiratory syndrome
SCID	severe combined immunodeficiency syndrome
SCT	stem cell transplantation
SHT	*Shigella* toxin
SIADH	syndrome of inappropriate antidiuretic hormone secretion
SIRS	systemic inflammatory response syndrome
SLE	systemic lupus erythematosus
SNHL	sensorineural hearing loss
SSPE	subacute sclerosing pan encephalitis
STI	sexually transmitted infection

SVR	sustained viral response
TB	tuberculosis
TBE	tickborne encephalitis
TBI	total body irradiation
TNF	tumour necrosis factor
TP	tonsillo-pharyngitis
TPN	total parenteral nutrition
TPPA	*Treponema pallidum* particle agglutination
TRAPS	TNF receptor-associated periodic syndrome
TSE	transmissible spongiform encephalopathies
TSH	thyroid-stimulating hormone
TSS	toxic shock syndrome
TST	tuberculin skin test
TTG	tissue transglutaminase
TTP	thrombotic thrombocytopenic purpura
U&E	urea and electrolytes
UPEC	uropathogenic *Escherichia coli*
URTI	upper respiratory tract infection
UTI	urinary tract infection
VAPP	vaccine-associated paralytic poliomyelitis
VCT	verocytotoxin
V_d	volume of distribution
VDPV	vaccine-derived polioviruses
VDRL	Venereal Disease Research Laboratory
VGCV	valganciclovir
VHF	viral haemorrhagic fever
VL	visceral leishmaniasis
VLBW	very low birthweight
VRE	vancomycin-resistant enterococci
VTEC	verocytotoxigenic *Escherichia coli*
VUR	vesicoureteric reflux
VZIG	varicella zoster immunoglobulin
VZV	varicella zoster virus
WBC	white blood cell count
WHO	World Health Organization

Symbols

📖	cross reference
✍	online resource/web address
↑	increase
↓	decrease

Clinical syndromes

Antibiotics and resistance

📖 see also Chapters 5, 6, 8, 14, 15, 16, 17, 20, 22, 27, 28, 29, 30, 36, 38, 43, 44

Basic principles in the use of antibiotics

- Antimicrobial agents target sites or pathways that are unique to the bacterium in order to achieve maximum toxicity for the microorganisms and minimal toxicity to humans.
- All antibiotics produce human toxicity to varying degrees and the therapeutic index (maximal tolerated dose divided by the minimum effective dose) provides a numerical expression of this. Some antibiotics, such as penicillins, are very safe and thus have a very high therapeutic index. Others, e.g. gentamicin, have a low maximum tolerated dose and thus a therapeutic index that is low.
- Antimicrobials alter the host's normal flora (e.g. ampicillin or amoxicillin/clavulanate are re-excreted into the gastrointestinal tract) and affect the predominantly anaerobic flora of the large bowel resulting in antibiotic-associated diarrhoea or promoting colonization by *Clostridium difficile*.
- 'Use it and lose it!' Use and misuse of antibiotics contribute to development of antimicrobial resistance. There is reasonably good evidence that rational use of antibiotics can prevent or decrease the development of resistance.
- Choosing the right antibiotic for therapy of a given infection is more challenging than ever and following the key steps listed below will allow for a systematic approach to antibiotic selection:
  - What is (are) the most likely causative pathogen(s) for the diagnosed clinical syndrome?
  - What is the probable susceptibility of the isolated (or suspected) pathogen based on lab results or local epidemiological parameters?
  - What is the appropriate dose and duration of therapy according to the host and the site of infection?
- Presumptive and empirical therapy:
  - Initial choice of antibiotic is usually based on a clinical syndrome and anatomical site of infection. The initial antibiotic choice can often later be changed to the most narrow-spectrum, yet effective, antibiotic with activity against the identified organism.
  - For suspected (unproven) infections presumptive therapy may be considered.

- Information about current local resistance should be readily available and considered in choosing antibiotics especially for infections on high-risk units, e.g. neonatal intensive care or oncology wards.
- 24–48 hours after initial administration of antibiotics, always review antimicrobial chemotherapy with microbiology results and stop or rationalize wherever possible.
- Wherever possible, switch from intravenous (IV) antibiotics to oral at 48 hours and stop at 5 days.

- Pharmacokinetics-pharmacodynamics (PK-PD): Consider the PK-PD properties of the antibiotic that are predictive of efficacy in relationship to the infection site. The three most important PK-PD measures are:
  - Duration of time a drug concentration remains above the minimum inhibitory concentration (MIC) (T>MIC).
  - Ratio of the maximal drug concentration over the MIC (C_{max}:MIC).
  - Ratio of the area under the concentration time curve at 24 hours over the MIC (AUC_{0-24}:MIC).

- Drug distribution: While serum levels of antibiotics are used to predict responses, the knowledge of the distribution of a drug is often important. For example:
  - Passive diffusion to tissue such as lung or skin and skin structure.
  - Blood–brain barrier penetration into the cerebrospinal fluid (CSF) (may require higher than standard dosages of antibiotics).
  - Poorly vascularized spaces such as abscesses depend on passive diffusion of antibiotics for killing of bacteria. Surgical intervention to drain or debride infected tissue is frequently required for good clinical outcome.
  - Intracellular accumulation allows for effective treatment of intracellular organisms (e.g. azithromycin).
  - Changes in volume of distribution (V_d) and elimination of antibiotics or hepatic and renal impairment may require adjustments of dosing as well as redosing.
  - Protein binding may be relevant, e.g. in neonates in whom ceftriaxone should be avoided because it is highly protein bound and may replace bilirubin from albumin binding sites.

- An antibiotic may be bactericidal (actively killing bacteria) or bacteriostatic (preventing bacteria from dividing) depending on the circumstances, such as infection site and dosing.
- Postantibiotic effect describes the phenomenon of an extended period of time of inhibition of bacterial growth even after antibiotic concentrations drop below the MIC (e.g. with aminoglycosides, which allows less frequent dosing).
- Duration of antibiotic therapy is the least evidence-based part of antibiotic prescribing and is usually decided on the notoriously unreliable expert opinion. The shortest duration should be used wherever possible. Every antibiotic prescription should have a clear stop date.

- Host factors should always be considered when choosing an antibiotic.
  - The most likely aetiology of infections is typically age dependent (e.g. need to cover *Listeria* in all neonates with meningitis, but not in older immunocompetent children with meningitis).
  - The prior use of antibiotics in a patient is critical information because this may represent failure of treatment (and may thus provide clues to aetiology) and in some cases, it may have caused selective pressure on the patient's flora, making subsequent infection with resistant bacteria more likely.
  - Choice of route of administration is influenced by the host. Questions to ask include the patient's ability to take antibiotics orally (palatability is part of this!) as well as enteric absorption. Oral antibiotics should be used wherever possible. The need for IV antibiotics over 48 hours should always be questioned.
  - Underlying conditions may be associated with a large number of host factors, most importantly this includes impaired defence mechanisms (e.g. immune deficiency, medical devices), abnormal flora, interactions with the patient's regular medications, and impaired clearance in some—if an underlying condition is known it will inform about typical causative pathogens.
  - Abnormal renal or hepatic function require dose adjustments according to estimated change in function (e.g. calculated creatinine clearance).
  - Age-related changes in physiology lead to significant pharmacokinetic changes; this needs to be reflected when dosing antibiotics (e.g. neonates).
  - Allergies to drugs and antibiotics need to be asked about routinely and the type of reaction should be documented in detail. Specific allergy testing may be required for those drugs where it is available, especially if the risk of anaphylactic reactions cannot be clearly assessed based on history. In some situations, desensitization is an option.
- **If a patient is not getting better on a regimen, a careful review of all microbiological and host factors is mandatory and frequently reveals potential causes of failure.**
- Prophylactic use:
  - There are few absolute indications for the prophylactic use of antimicrobials and this is one area where misuse is common.
  - An example of appropriate prophylaxis would be rifampicin or ciprofloxacin for close contacts of cases of meningococcal or *Haemophilus influenzae* type b disease.
  - Evidence supporting indications and dosing recommendations is lacking.
  - Surgical prophylaxis should be as a single dose wherever possible. Prolonged surgical prophylaxis is one of the commoner causes of serious misuse of antibiotics.

Antibiotic resistance

- Microorganism fitness depends on their capacity to adapt to changing environmental conditions.
- Antimicrobial agents exert a strong selective pressure on bacterial populations, favouring those that have the ability to resist them.
- The main driver for the development of resistance is the inappropriate use of antibiotics, especially for infections of the upper respiratory tract. New antibiotic production has slowed markedly—especially for resistant Gram-negative organisms—leading to increasing anxiety when selecting an antibiotic. The pipeline for new antibiotics under development is strikingly empty!

Useful definitions

- **Antibiotic sensitivity**: In laboratory testing it is usual to test the organism in drug concentrations that can be easily achieved in body fluids. Organisms susceptible to this or lower concentration are regarded as sensitive.
- **Antibiotic resistance:** Organisms able to grow under those drug concentrations *in vitro* are considered resistant.
- **Minimum inhibitory concentration:** This is the lowest concentration of the agent that prevents the development of visible growth of the test organism during overnight incubation.
- **Minimum bactericidal concentration**: This is the lowest concentration able to reduce the original inoculum by a factor of a thousand.

Predictable and variable sensitivity

- The susceptibility of common pathogens may change over time, although for some of them the sensitivity is often predictable. Once the organism is known and while waiting for sensitivity testing, the most likely effective antibiotic treatment can be chosen based on the particular characteristics of the pathogen and local epidemiology. Table 1.1 describes the most common pathogens encountered in clinical practice and useful sensitivity characteristics.

Table 1.1 Bacterial targets and examples of typical sensitivities for commonly encountered organisms

Organism	Bacterial targets	Usually sensitive[a,b]	Usually resistant[a]
β-haemolytic streptococci	Cell wall replication	Penicillin	
	Translation	Erythromycin, clindamycin	Aminoglycosides
Streptococcus pneumoniae	Cell wall replication	Penicillin,[e] vancomycin	Penicillin[e]
	Translation	Erythromycin[e]	Aminoglycosides
Enterococcus	Cell wall replication	Ampicillin, vancomycin	Ceftriaxone
	Translation	Quinupristin/ dalfopristin, linezolid	Aminoglycosides
Staphylococcus aureus (meticillin sensitive; MSSA)	Cell wall replication[c]	Flucloxacillin, 1st generation cephalosporins, amoxicillin/ clavulanate	Most penicillins
	Translation	Clindamycin	
	Transcription	Rifampicin	
S. aureus (meticillin resistant; MRSA)	Cell wall replication	Vancomycin	All β-lactam antibiotics
	Translation[d]	Quinupristin/ dalfopristin, linezolid	Aminoglycosides
	Cell membrane	Daptomycin	
Coagulase-negative staphylococci	Cell wall replication	Vancomycin	Most penicillins
Listeria monocytogenes	Cell wall replication	Penicillin, ampicillin	Cephalosporins
Neisseria meningitidis	Cell wall replication	Penicillin	
Escherichia coli	Cell wall replication	Extended-spectrum penicillins, 2nd and 3rd generation cephalosporins, co-trimoxazole	Penicillin, vancomycin
	DNA replication	Ciprofloxacin	
	Translation	Gentamicin, tigecycline	Metronidazole

(Continued)

Table 1.1 (Contd.)

Organism	Bacterial targets	Usually sensitive[a,b]	Usually resistant[a]
Proteus mirabilis	Cell wall replication	Extended-spectrum penicillins, 2nd and 3rd generation cepholosporins, co-trimoxazole	Penicillin, vancomycin
	Translation	Gentamicin, tigecycline	
	DNA replication	Ciprofloxacin	Metronidazole
Klebsiella	Cell wall replication	Extended-spectrum penicillins, 2nd and 3rd generation cephalosporins, co-trimoxazole	Penicillin, vancomycin
	Translation	Gentamicin	Metronidazole
	DNA replication	Ciprofloxacin	
Pseudomonas	Cell wall replication	Extended-spectrum penicillins, ceftazidime, cefepime, meropenem	Penicillin, 1st–3rd generation cephalosporins
	Translation	Gentamicin	Metronidazole
	DNA replication	Ciprofloxacin	Co-trimoxazole
Anaerobes	Cell wall replication	Piperacillin/ tazobactam, cefotetan, carbapenems	
	Translation	Metronidazole	
Treponema pallidum	Cell wall replication	Penicillin	
Mycoplasma, chlamydia	Translation	Macrolides, tetracyclines	

[a]These common susceptibility patterns vary significantly depending on local epidemiology (for both community and healthcare-associated infections) and are quite dynamic; they should be reviewed regularly.

[b]Representative antibiotics from different drug classes are listed; bacteria may also be sensitive to other agents from the same class.

[c]While MSSA is susceptible to vancomycin, this antibiotic should be reserved for cases where MRSA is suspected to avoid overuse and also because of poor bactericidal activity for *S. aureus* compared with β-lactam antibiotics.

[d]Depending on the epidemiology and origin of MRSA strains they are frequently susceptible to the following antibiotics: ciprofloxacin, tetracyclines, clindamycin, co-trimoxazole.

[e]Rates for penicillin intermediate and fully resistant *S. pneumoniae* vary from <5% to 50% within Europe; alteration of penicillin-binding proteins results in decreased activity of β-lactam antibiotics; intermediate resistance can be overcome by high doses of β-lactams.

Control of resistance

Antibiotic prescribing habits of clinicians and general practitioners are largely responsible for the emergence of resistant pathogens. The unnecessary use of antibiotics acts as a strong selective tool for the emergence of resistant microorganisms, and restriction of use should lead to the opposite effect (although this is more difficult to demonstrate outside controlled environments) Reducing antibiotic prescribing is far from easy and a combined effort is mandatory. Adherence to prescribing guidelines (for hospital and community prescribing) and restriction policies that reduce use of certain antibiotics (for hospital prescribing) may lead to the reduction in antibiotic overuse and resistance. All children's hospitals should develop an antimicrobial stewardship programme.

New agents and conservation of old drugs

There is a marked shortage of new antibiotics under development by pharmaceutical companies, especially for multidrug-resistant Gram-negative infections. Clinicians should generally reserve new antibiotics for third line use. Improved incentives to invest in new antimicrobial agents are underway in both the European Union and the USA.

Improved stewardship of current agents should be based on a better understanding of current resistance rates in children across Europe. Point prevalence surveys can be standardized to produce comparative prescribing data between and within countries.

Further reading

Boucher HW, Talbot GH, Bradley JS, *et al.* Bad bugs, no drugs; no ESKAPE! An update from the IDSA. *Clin Infect Dis* 2009;**48**:1–12.

Goossens H. Antibiotic consumption and link to resistance. *Clin Microbiol Infect* 2009;**15** Suppl 3:12–15.

Antifungal drugs

📖 see also Chapters 6, 8, 15, 17, 20, 22, 23, 28, 29, 30, 51, 55, 110

Introduction

Conventional amphotericin B deoxycholate, fluconazole, and 5-fluorocytosine (5-FC) have until recently been the mainstay of antifungal therapy in invasive fungal infection (IFI). Lipid amphotericin preparations are less toxic than conventional preparations, and along with azole antifungal agents, increase the options for treating invasive fungal diseases. With the advent of novel azoles, such as voriconazole and posaconazole, along with echinocandin drugs such as caspofungin, treatment can be tailored to the fungus species isolated and its drug sensitivity, as well as the degree of risk from immunosuppression. However, there is a paucity of high-quality data evaluating the efficacy of antifungal drugs in children, and paediatric pharmacokinetic data for the older and the newer antifungal agents are limited, making research in this field a key priority. For all drug doses, 📖 see Appendix 5.

Fungal classification

Yeasts:
- *Candida*
- *Cryptococcus*

Moulds:
- Non-septate hyphae
  - Zygomycetes
- Septate hyphae
  - *Aspergillus*
  - *Fusarium*
  - *Scedosporium*

Dimorphic fungi (can exist as a mould or yeast):
- *Blastomyces dermatitiditis*
- *Coccidioides immitis*
- *Histoplasma capsulatum*
- *Paracoccidioides brasiliensis*

Classes of antifungal drugs

Polyenes:
- Nystatin, conventional amphotericin B deoxycholate, lipid amphotericin preparations
- Act on the ergosterol component of the fungal cell wall, causing cell membrane lysis (Fig. 2.1).

Pyrimidine analogues:
- 5-FC
- Converted to 5-fluorouracil within susceptible fungal cells, which inhibits fungal DNA synthesis and protein synthesis.

Azoles
- Fluconazole, itraconazole, voriconazole, posaconazole
- Inhibit fungal cytochrome P-450, which is involved in ergosterol synthesis.

Echinocandins
- Caspofungin, micafungin, anidulafungin
- Inhibit β-1,3-glucan synthase, an enzyme present in fungal but not mammalian cells, causing impaired cell wall synthesis.

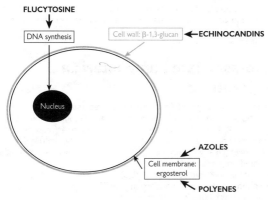

Fig. 2.1 Sites of action of antifungal drugs.

Fungicidal versus fungistatic action

The differing mechanisms of action of the antifungal drugs lead to varying fungicidal and fungistatic activity (Table 2.1). Fungicidal agents are probably better for treating invasive fungal infection in the neutropenic patient.

Table 2.1 Fungicidal versus fungistatic action of antifungal drugs against different fungi

Antifungal agent	*Aspergillus*	*Candida*	*Cryptococcus*
Amphotericin B	Cidal	Cidal	Cidal
Fluconazole	Nil	Static	Static
Itraconazole	Cidal	Static	Static
Voriconazole	Cidal	Static	Static
Posaconazole	Cidal	Static	Static
Caspofungin	Static	Cidal	Nil

Spectrum of action and dosing

The pharmacology of antifungal drugs often differs considerably between children and adults. This has significant implications for optimal dosing in children and is discussed in more detail below.

Lipid-associated amphotericin B preparations

The major advantage of lipid-associated preparations compared with conventional amphotericin B is their significantly reduced nephrotoxicity (12% vs. 52%). Lipid-preparations are also thought to have better reticuloendothelial penetration (liver, spleen, and lung), although this difference has not been clearly confirmed in efficacy studies. There are three lipid-associated preparations:

- Amphotericin B lipid complex (ABLC)
- Amphotericin B colloidal dispersion (ABCD)
- Liposomal amphotericin B (L-amB).

Pharmacology

- Distribution into the cerebrospinal fluid (CSF) is poor, cerebrospinal fluid (CSF) concentrations reaching 2–4% of serum concentrations, making these drugs a poor choice for fungal meningitis.
- Fungicidal activity is concentration dependent, requiring high drug concentrations at the site of infection. Antifungal activity continues when concentrations are below the MIC (post-antifungal effect). Thus once-daily dosing is effective.

- Elimination is via the kidneys, but dose adjustment is not usually necessary even in patients with pre-existing renal impairment.
- Pharmacokinetic data in neonates are very limited, but appear to be similar to older children. Therefore, similar dosing strategies can be used.

Efficacy

- Although large randomized controlled trial (RCT) data are lacking, small RCTs in children do not suggest that lipid-associated amphotericin B preparations are more effective than conventional amphotericin B.
- Good paediatric dosing studies are lacking, but an adult RCT comparing standard dose 3mg/kg/d and high dose 10mg/kg/d also showed no difference in efficacy but increased nephrotoxicity at the higher doses.
- A large study addressing the efficacy of ABLC in immunocompromised children showed response rates (cured + improved) of 58% (101 of 174) in patients with proven *Candida* infections and 39% (27 of 69) in patients with proven *Aspergillus* infection.[1]
- Neonates: There are few published studies using lipid preparations, but one study of 40 neonates with candidiasis reported a success rate of 70%, with other smaller studies reporting even higher success rates.[2]

Toxicity

- Toxicity occurs because amphotericin B binds not only to ergosterol in fungal cells but also to cholesterol in human cells, e.g. the kidney. Binding to cholesterol is reduced by the lipids in lipid preparations, leading to reduced toxicity.
- The three lipid-associated preparations vary in their rates of toxicity, with L-amB associated with the lowest rates of discontinuation. Rates of fever, chills, and nephrotoxicity are all significantly lower with L-amB.
- Children can tolerate higher doses of L-amB for longer periods than adults. Rates of nephrotoxicity are lower, but tubular toxicity such as hypokalaemia can still be severe.
- Risk factors for nephrotoxicity include pre-existing renal impairment, hyponatraemia, hypovolaemia, and the concurrent use of nephrotoxic drugs.

5-Fluorocytosine

5-FC is used mainly for cryptococcal meningitis, which is far less common since the introduction of effective antiretroviral regimens for childhood human immunodeficiency virus (HIV) infections. If used as monotherapy, antifungal resistance develops rapidly, thus it should only be used as part of combination therapy. It probably enhances antifungal activity of amphotericin B at sites where amphotericin B has poor penetration, such as the CSF and heart valves.

Pharmacology
- 5-FC has good oral bioavailability.
- Distribution is good because of its small size and lack of protein binding, resulting in good penetration into CSF, heart valves, and inflamed joints.
- Neonates have slower clearance than older children/adults; therefore neonatal dosing is every 12–24 hours compared with 6 hourly in older children.

Efficacy
- Adult data have shown 5-FC + amphotericin B to be more effective in treating cryptococcal meningitis than amphotericin B alone.[3]
- Longer treatment courses are required in immunocompromised patients compared with immunocompetent patients (6 weeks vs. 4 weeks).

Toxicity
- Trough levels of >100µg/ml are associated with bone marrow aplasia. Aim to maintain levels between 40µg/ml and 80µg/ml.

Fluconazole

Although fluconazole is commonly used for fungal prophylaxis, it has no activity against *Aspergillus*. It has activity against most *Candida* species except *Candida krusei*, which is inherently resistant to fluconazole, and *Candida glabrata*, which maybe susceptible with dose escalation.

Pharmacology
- Fluconazole has 90% oral bioavailability.
- Distribution is good because of its low protein binding, resulting in CSF/vitreous concentrations of 80% of blood concentrations.
- Excreted by the kidney. Urinary concentrations are 10–20 times that of the blood, making it a very effective treatment for fungal urinary tract infections.
- Paediatric and adult pharmacokinetics differ. Clearance is more rapid in children, leading to a shorter half-life (t½), necessitating higher drug doses in children. Pharmacokinetic modelling show that 12mg/kg/d is required to achieve comparable plasma concentrations to adults receiving 400mg/d.
- Neonates have a higher volume of distribution but slower clearance. Therefore, higher dosing but reduced frequency is required—dosing is recommended every 72 hours in babies aged 0–2 weeks and every 48 hours in babies aged 2–4 weeks.

Efficacy
- Adult data suggest equivalence between fluconazole and amphotericin B in treating invasive candidiasis.
- Two small studies of neonates/infants with invasive candidiasis report success rates of between 80% and 97%.

- Adult RCTs evaluating the role of fluconazole as antifungal prophylaxis following bone marrow transplantation showed protection against disseminated candidal infections and improved mortality. However, concerns exist about its lack of anti-*Aspergillus* activity.
- Fluconazole prophylaxis in selected low birthweight infants reduces the development of invasive fungal infections.[4]

Toxicity

- Fluconazole causes less cytochrome P–450 (CYP) inhibition than most other azoles.
- Hepatotoxicity does occur, but is rare (2/24 in one study); the most common side effect is nausea and vomiting.

Itraconazole

Itraconazole is not only active against *Candida*, but also against *Aspergillus*, making it a more attractive prophylactic agent compared with fluconazole. However, its unpredictable bioavailability and frequent drug interactions limits its role in the treatment of IFI.

Pharmacology

- Itraconazole has unpredictable oral absorption. Absorption is increased in acid environments, such as when taken with food or acidic drinks. H2 blockers reduce absorption.
- Absorption varies with the drug formulation; capsules are better absorbed with food while the suspension is better absorbed on an empty stomach. The suspension has a 30% better bioavailability but this is reduced when it is given via a nasogastric tube.
- Itraconazole is highly protein bound in the blood and has very poor CSF penetration.
- Hepatic elimination, therefore dose adjustment is not required in renal impairment.
- A higher volume of distribution in children results in lower serum concentrations. Therefore, children require a twice-daily regimen, compared with once daily in adults.
- Measurement of trough levels is necessary to ensure that adequate drug levels are achieved at the start of therapy, especially because drug interactions can affect blood levels. Aim for >0.5mg/l if the high-performance liquid chromatography assay is used. There is a different target level if a bioassay is used; consult the laboratory for clarification.

Efficacy

- There is a paucity of paediatric data comparing itraconazole with other antifungal agents in the treatment of invasive fungal disease. A small RCT involving 43 children with invasive candidiasis showed equivalence between itraconazole and fluconazole.[5]
- No paediatric RCTs have been performed comparing itraconazole with other prophylactic antifungal agents. A large adult RCT showed itraconazole to be superior to fluconazole in preventing fungal infections.

Toxicity
- Causes significant CYP inhibition, resulting in frequent drug interactions (rifampicin, carbamazepine, macrolides, warfarin, sirolimus, ciclosporin A, etc.).
- Beware of high ciclosporin A and tacrolimus levels.

Voriconazole

Similar spectrum of activity to itraconazole but has less erratic oral bio-availability.

Pharmacology
- Excellent oral bioavailability in adults (96%) but paediatric bioavailability is only about 45%, due to higher first-pass metabolism, and is markedly reduced when taken with food.
- Excellent CNS penetration.
- Metabolized in the liver. Liver metabolism varies widely between individuals, correlating with the CYP2C19 genotype. Poor metabolizers (5–7% Caucasians and 20% non-Indian Asians), have far higher voriconazole levels.
- Complex pharmacokinetics in children, resulting in weight-based IV dosing and fixed dose oral dosing, to achieve equivalent of adult 4mg/kg twice daily.
  - Treatment should initially be given IV to achieve therapeutic levels before changing to the oral route. IV loading doses are required in children >12 years.
- Measurement of trough levels is necessary to ensure that adequate drug levels are achieved. Aim for >2mg/l. Levels may need to be rechecked when the route of administration is changed or if the patient is clinically unstable. Target levels may vary if different assays are used—always consult the laboratory for clarification.

Efficacy
- A landmark study compared voriconazole and amphotericin B for the treatment of adults with invasive aspergillosis.[6] Voriconazole was found to be superior, with a complete or partial response in 50% of patients, compared with 30% in the amphotericin B arm.
- Effective treatment against *Candida*, with studies demonstrating equivalence with amphotericin B in treating invasive candidiasis.
- Paucity of paediatric data.
- No neonatal data because of concerns about its effect on the developing retina.

Toxicity
- Causes CYP inhibition, but less than itraconazole. Sirolimus contraindicated because of markedly elevated levels.
- Reversible dose-dependent visual disturbance (especially blurred vision and increased brightness) can occur.
- Skin rash (10–20%), including photosensitive rashes (5%), and elevated liver enzymes (10–20%), especially with increasing doses.

Posaconazole

Posaconazole has a wide spectrum of action, including *Aspergillus*, *Candida* and Zygomycetes. Its action against Zygomycetes gives it a potential advantage over voriconazole in the empirical treatment of invasive fungal infection.

Pharmacology

- Paucity of pharmacokinetic data in children. Children >8 years appear to have similar pharmacokinetics to adults.
- Divided oral doses are thought to result in higher bioavailability in children.
- Less CNS penetration than voriconazole, but has been used successfully to treat CNS fungal infection.
- Currently only available as an oral formulation.
- Drug monitoring is recommended but difficult—discuss with mycology reference laboratory for recommended trough levels.

Efficacy

- Paucity of paediatric and adult data.
- A complete response was noted in 6/7 children given posaconazole as salvage therapy after failure with other antifungal drugs.[7]

Toxicity

- Less CYP inhibition compared with other triazoles.
- Generally milder side effects than other triazoles.

Caspofungin

The echinocandins have a wide spectrum of activity, including *Candida* and *Aspergillus*. Caspofungin is fungicidal against *Candida* but fungistatic against *Aspergillus*, and has no action against Zygomycetes. Its main advantage over amphotericin B is its lack of nephrotoxicity, but it is more expensive.

Pharmacology

- Oral bioavailability is limited, therefore only available IV.
- Highly protein bound with slow generalized distribution, which explains its poor CNS penetration.
- Metabolized by the liver, necessitating dose reduction in hepatic, but not renal, insufficiency.
- To achieve similar drug levels to adults, paediatric dosing is based on body surface area.
- Some *Candida* species, such as *Candida parapsilosis* and *Candida lusitaniae*, tend to display higher MICs to caspofungin, compared with other *Candida* species. Risk of inadequate treatment or the development of resistance.

Efficacy

- Most efficacy data are limited to caspofungin used as part of combination therapy.
- Paucity of high-quality data in children, with no RCTs comparing caspofungin with other antifungal drugs. An open-labelled study

in immunocompromised children suggests a 50% efficacy against *Aspergillus* and 80% efficacy in invasive candidiasis.
- Data suggest equivalence to amphotericin B in treating children with persistent febrile neutropenia.
- Initial neonatal data are encouraging; 10 babies with persistent candidaemia despite amphotericin B treatment, cleared their infection after receiving caspofungin.

Toxicity
- Minimal toxicity because echinocandins target β-1,3-glucan, which is not present in mammalian cells.
- Interactions with tacrolimus and ciclosporin A. Monitor liver function tests when used with ciclosporin A.
- Rifampicin, nevirapine, and efavirenz lead to increased clearance, necessitating an increase in the caspofungin dose.

Micafungin

Like caspofungin, micafungin has fungicidal activity against *Candida* and fungistatic activity against *Aspergillus*.

Pharmacology
- Very little pharmacokinetic data beyond phase I studies.
- Good penetration to lungs and abdominal organs, but very poor CSF penetration.
- Licensed for use in neonates.
- Shorter t½ in younger children necessitates higher doses, but currently no approved dosing for children.

Efficacy
- Paucity of paediatric data comparing micafungin with other antifungal drugs. Most data are limited to micafungin used as part of combination therapy.
- One RCT comparing micafungin and amphotericin B for the treatment of invasive candidiasis showed equivalent treatment responses, with fewer adverse events seen with micafungin.[8]

Anidulafungin

Anidulafungin has a similar spectrum of activity to other echinocandins.

Pharmacology
- Excellent lung and liver penetration.
- Very little paediatric pharmacokinetic data to guide dosing.

Efficacy
- There are no paediatric efficacy data for anidulafungin.

Toxicity
- Minimal drug interactions.
- Can be used in patients with liver failure, unlike caspofungin, which should be used with caution.
- NOTE: contains 24% alcohol.

Future research

A number of paediatric antifungal studies are currently recruiting in the USA and Europe. Data on clinical trials can be found on the International Paediatric Fungal Network website, 📖 see Further reading.

There is an urgent need to better define dosing regimens in both neonates and older children and to develop an improved evidence base for salvage and combination therapy.

Key references

1 Wiley JM, Seibel NL, Walsh TJ. Efficacy and safety of amphotericin B lipid complex in 548 children and adolescents with invasive fungal infections. *Pediatr Infect Dis J* 2005;**24**:167–74.
2 Scarcella A, Pasquariello MB, Giugliano B, Vendemmia M, de Lucia A. Liposomal amphotericin B treatment for neonatal fungal infections. *Pediatr Infect Dis J* 1998;**17**:146–8.
3 Bennett JE, Dismukes WE, Duma RJ, Medoff G, Sande M A, Gallis H, *et al.* A comparison of amphotericin B alone and combined with flucytosine in the treatment of cryptococcal meningitis. *N Engl J Med* 1979;**301**:126–8.
4 Kaufman D, Boyle R, Hazen KC, Patrie JT, Robinson M, Donowitz LG, *et al.* Fluconazole prophylaxis against fungal colonization and infection in preterm infants. *N Engl J Med* 2001;**345**:1660–6.
5 Mondal RK, Singhi SC, Chakrabarti AMJ. Randomized comparison between fluconazole and itraconazole for the treatment of candidemia in a pediatric intensive care unit: a preliminary study. *Pediatr Crit Care Med* 2004;**5**:561–5.
6 Herbrecht R, Denning DW, Patterson TF, Bennett JE, Greene RE, Oestmann JW, *et al.* Voriconazole versus amphotericin B for primary therapy of invasive aspergillosis. *N Engl J Med* 2002;**347**:408–15.
7 Segal BH, Barnhart LA, Anderson VL, Walsh TJ, Malech HL, Holland SM. Posaconazole as salvage therapy in patients with chronic granulomatous disease and invasive filamentous fungal infection. *Clin Infect Dis* 2005;**40**:1684–8.
8 Queiroz-Telles F, Berezin E, Leverger G, Freire A, van der Vyver A, Chotpitayasunondh T, *et al.* Micafungin versus liposomal amphotericin B for pediatric patients with invasive candidiasis: substudy of a randomized double-blind trial. Micafungin Invasive Candidiasis Study Group. *Pediatr Infect Dis J* 2008;**27**:820–6.

Further reading

Chowdhry R, Marshall WL. Antifungal therapies in the intensive care unit. *J Intensive Care Med* 2008;**23**:151–8.

International Pediatric Fungal Network. Available at: 🔗 http://pfn.pediatrics.duke.edu (accessed 1 February 2011). This reference library offers free access to important fungal articles.

Steinbach WJ, Walsh TJ. Mycoses in pediatric patients. *Infect Dis Clin North Am* 2006;**20**:663–78.

Steinbach WJ, Dvorak CC. Antifungal drugs. In: Long SS, Pickering LK, Prober CG, eds. *Principles and Practice of Pediatric Infectious Diseases.* Philadelphia, PA: Churchill Livingstone, 2008:1452–60.

Chapter 3

Antiparasitics

📖 see also Chapters 47, 50, 61, 67, 74, 82, 85, 96, 103, 109, 111, 112

Introduction

- Antiparasitic agents are medications indicated for the treatment of parasitic diseases. Such infections may broadly be divided into those caused by single-celled protozoa and those caused by helminths (worms), which are multicellular organisms.
- Antiparasitic agents may be used in disease prevention (i.e. prophylaxis), control, and treatment, notably against malaria.
- Protozoal diseases include amoebiasis and malaria. Diseases caused by worms may be due to gastrointestinal (e.g. roundworms and tapeworms) or systemic parasites (e.g. filaria and schistosomes).
- While there are numerous antimalarial agents in clinical use or under development, the same tends not to be true for anthelmintics as diseases caused by worms attract relatively less attention, often to the point of neglect.
- However, there are a number of broad-spectrum agents effective against gastrointestinal nematodes. Three of the most widely used are albendazole/mebendazole, ivermectin, and praziquantel.
- Life cycles of helminths are complex, but most do not reproduce within the human host. This means that each individual parasite is the result of a separately acquired infection.
- Children are particularly susceptible to gastrointestinal infections caused by parasites and this chapter will focus principally on treatments for such diseases. However, it should be remembered that treatment recommendations are often empirical or merely extrapolated from observations in adults.
- The prevalence and intensity of infection with soil-transmitted helminths tends to be low in children aged <24 months, but there is accumulating evidence that severe and recurrent infections may have a detrimental effect on growth and development.
- The World Health Organization (WHO) recommends that children as young as 12 months, originally excluded from deworming programmes, should be treated, bearing in mind the relatively low toxicity of many of the available drugs and the positive outcome of risk–benefit analyses. For young children with intestinal worms, the health benefits of treating geohelminthic infections include reduced likelihood of growth stunting and improved nutritional and cognitive outcomes.

Anthelmintic drugs

- Anthelmintics can be divided into a variety of classes based on their chemistry and pharmacology. There are three broad-spectrum drugs in routine use: albendazole (a benzimidazole), ivermectin (a macrocyclic lactone and one of the avermectins), and praziquantel (a pyrazinoisoquinolone).
- Recent interest has focused on nitazoxanide, an analogue of metronidazole. This drug has a wide spectrum of activity against parasites (both protozoa and helminths) and viruses and presents an exciting new development in an area where there have been relatively few breakthroughs.
- Note that the doses given in Appendix 5 (p. 810) refer to those recommended for children except when there is no information available. However, in these cases, the drug in question has proved safe with minimal toxicity.

Benzimidazoles

Note:
Drugs marked with a superscript 'a' are unlicensed in the UK and only available from 'special-order' manufacturers or specialist importing companies (see the *British National Formulary for Children* (BNFC)).
  Drugs marked with a superscript 'b' are unlicensed in the UK and only available from the manufacturer (see the BNFC).

- Thiabendazole was the first drug in this class to be described and subsequently other benzimidazoles were introduced, notably mebendazole and albendazole.
- There is an extensive clinical literature on these compounds emphasizing their utility in a variety of gastrointestinal and systemic diseases.
- Their anthelmintic efficacy relates to their ability to interfere with the functions of the cytoskeleton through a highly selective interaction with parasitic β-tubulin.

Albendazole[a]

- Albendazole is the most important and clinically useful member of the benzimidazole class. Originally a veterinary product, it was first approved for human use in 1982.
- A single oral dose is usually recommended for clearance of gastrointestinal nematodes (i.e. *Ascaris*, *Trichuris*, hookworm (*Ancylostoma* and *Necator*) and *Enterobius*) from children >2 years of age. Fasting or purging is not required.
- Additional or more frequent dosage may be necessary in certain conditions, e.g. those caused by *Taenia* spp., and systemic infections caused by, e.g. *Strongyloides* and *Echinococcus*. This may relate to the relatively low bioavailability and rapid metabolism of albendazole.

In children >2 years, albendazole can be given once or twice daily for 3 days and repeated after 3 weeks if necessary. In *Echinococcus* infections, albendazole is given to children for 28 days followed by a 14-day break and then repeated for up to 2–3 cycles.

- Albendazole seems to be the drug of choice for *Toxocara*, although the evidence for this recommendation is marginal. The optimal dose and duration of therapy remains to be established, but a single daily dose for 14 days has been recommended.
- Although albendazole has not been fully evaluated in children <2 years of age, no adverse effects or biochemical abnormalities have been noted in children aged 9–23 months. No routine blood testing is required.

Mebendazole

- Mebendazole is used mainly in treatment of intestinal parasite infections. Its main therapeutic indications are threadworms, roundworms and whipworms.
- Tablets may be chewed, swallowed, or crushed and mixed with food. Additional or more frequent dosing may be advised in certain conditions and fasting or purging is unnecessary.
- At therapeutic doses, the bioavailability of mebendazole tablets is only 1–2%. The low bioavailability is due to both the poor solubility of this formulation, and extensive first-pass metabolism in the liver.
- Mebendazole has not been fully evaluated in children and is unlicensed but well tolerated in children <2 years of age. Adverse effects were no higher in the week following treatment than in a placebo group in children.

Diethylcarbamazine[a]

- Diethylcarbamazine was shown to be an effective chemotherapeutic agent in 1947, yet its mechanism of action still remains to be elucidated.
- Although diethylcarbamazine is the drug of choice for treatment of lymphatic filariasis and loiasis, it is no longer indicated in onchocerciasis (river blindness) due to a potentially fatal post-treatment reaction, and the availability of ivermectin.
- In filariasis, to minimize reactions to treatment in children >1 month, treatment is started with a low dose of diethylcarbamazine citrate on the first day and increased gradually over 3 days. Length of treatment varies according to infection. Heavy infection may lead to febrile reaction and in loiasis there is a tiny risk of encephalopathy.
- It should be noted that single dose therapy is effective in community-based therapy of lymphatic filariasis and is as effective as previously used higher multiple doses. While such regimens may not result in total or rapid clearance of microfilaraemia, levels of microfilariae and prevalence of infection are similar 12 months post dose.

Other anthelmintic agents

Ivermectin[a]

- Ivermectin (22–23 dihydroavermectin) is a semi-synthetic derivative of a family of macrocyclic lactones called avermectins originally isolated from the soil-dwelling actinomycete, *Streptomyces avermitilis*. Its main therapeutic indications are onchocerciasis and strongyloidiasis.
- Ivermectin is active against most nematodes, including onchocerciasis and strongyloidiasis. It can also be used in combination with diethylcarbamazine or albendazole for the treatment of lymphatic filariasis.
- Ivermectin causes an influx of Cl⁻ ions through the cell membrane of invertebrates by activation of specific ivermectin-sensitive ion channels with resultant hyperpolarization muscle paralysis.
- In children >5 years ivermectin is generally administered as a single dose for the treatment of human filariasis, with re-treatment at 6–12 months, dependent on symptoms.
- Ivermectin given to children >5 years in a higher single daily dose for 2 days may be the most effective treatment for chronic strongyloidiasis.

Praziquantel[b]

- Praziquantel shows broad-spectrum activity against all trematodes except *Fasciola*. Its main therapeutic indication is schistosomiasis, where it is active against all major species.
- The exact mechanism of action of praziquantel is unknown but an antiparasitic antibody response is required. Resistance to praziquantel is the subject of intense debate. For liver, lung and intestinal flukes, there are no specific recommendations for children. For infections with *Schistosoma haematobium* and *Schistosoma mansoni* the suggested dose for children >4 years is a single dose initially followed 4–6 hours later by another single dose.
- Praziquantel is considered safe in children >2 years. It should be taken with food and plenty of water to prevent gagging or vomiting due to its bitter taste. The tablets can be divided but should not be chewed.

Levamisole[a]

- Levamisole is a useful alternative to the benzimidazoles in roundworm infections, i.e. *Ascaris*.
- A single oral dose is used both for individual treatment (1–18 years of age) and in community-based campaigns. In severe hookworm infection, a second dose may be given after 1 week.

Niclosamide[a]

- Niclosamide is highly effective against various tapeworm infections such as those caused by *Taenia saginata* (beef tapeworm), *Taenia solium* (pork tapeworm), *Diphyllobothrium latum* (fish tapeworm), and *Hymenolepis nana* (dwarf tapeworm).

- Niclosamide acts as an oxidative phosphorylation uncoupler thereby blocking the uptake of glucose by intestinal tapeworms, resulting in their death.
- Niclosamide is given as a single oral dose.
- Niclosamide is not active against the larval form (cysticerci) of *T. solium* infection. For *H. nana* infection, treatment should be continued for 7 days.
- Niclosamide is considered safe with minor gastrointestinal upset being the only side effect.

Piperazine

- The anthelmintic activity of piperazine is restricted to *Ascaris* and *Enterobius*. Its main use is for threadworms in younger infants (3–6 months).
- Piperazine causes flaccid paralysis of *Ascaris lumbricoides*. It is an agonist at extrasynaptic γ-aminobutyric acid (GABA) receptors, causing an influx of Cl^- ions.
- Piperazine is available as a hydrate. It is available with sennosides (laxatives) as an oral powder sachet stirred into milk or water. In children 3 months to 1 year, a single level spoonful is given as a single dose in the morning and repeated after 2 weeks. For children 1–6 years, a level 5 ml spoonful should be given. In children 6–18 years, one sachet is given as a single dose, repeated after 2 weeks.
- Dosages for *Ascaris* infections are the same as for *Enterobius* infections but may be repeated monthly for up to 3 months if the infection reoccurs.

Further reading

Drugs for Parasitic Infections. Available at: ℗ http://secure.medicalletter.org/para/ (accessed September 2010).

Yu VL, Edwards G, McKinnon PS, Peloquin C, Morse GD, eds. *Antimicrobial Therapy and Vaccines, Volume II, Antimicrobial Agents*, 2nd edn. Pittsburgh, PA: ESun Technologies, 2005. Available at: ℗ www.antimicrobe.org (accessed 1 February 2011).

Antivirals

📖 see also Chapters 14, 19, 46, 57, 62, 64, 75, 76, 77, 80, 99

Introduction

Development of antiviral compounds has followed increased understanding of the processes of viral replication as well as host—virus interactions. This knowledge has aided drug development by identifying viral or host specific targets for antivirals at all time points of the viral life cycle: entry, uncoating, genome replication, protein synthesis, assembly, and maturation. The number of antiviral compounds available has greatly increased over the past 25 years, concurrent with significant developments in virology and genomic amplification techniques, and driven by an increased population of immunosuppressed patients, highly susceptible to viral infections. In particular, those infected with HIV and those iatrogenically immunosuppressed for treatment of malignancy or other conditions.

Host—virus interactions in the normal and immunocompromised host

Viruses can only replicate by using the host cell machinery. Thus eradication of the viral infection may also lead to loss of the infected cell. Many viral infections are trivial or completely asymptomatic in the immunocompetent, but can be devastating in those with immunodeficiency, e.g. cytomegalovirus (CMV) infections. Other viral infections are usually symptomatic, but in most hosts cause minor symptoms which are self-limiting, e.g. infections caused by rhinoviruses. Viruses that establish latency within the host after primary infection, such as the herpesviruses, may only later cause symptoms, e.g. if they reactivate during a subsequent period of host immunosuppression. Families of viruses such as the hepatitis viruses, may be rapidly cleared from some hosts after initial infection, but in others go onto cause chronic infections that lead to long-term organ damage and even malignancy (e.g. hepatocellular carcinoma with hepatitis B). Slow virus infections, e.g. with retroviruses such as HIV, may only cause clinical symptoms after many years of viral replication that eventually lead to dysfunction of the host immune system and susceptibility to opportunistic infections.

Antiviral strategies appropriate for all these different types of infection are constantly being refined. More than one antiviral agent, acting at different points in the replicative life cycle, may be required to completely suppress viral replication (e.g. triple therapy for HIV), or the antiviral agent may require to be supported by immune modulation with antibody or cytokine therapy (e.g. ribavirin with interferon for hepatitis C).

Randomized controlled trial data confirming treatment efficacy are available for the most common treatment scenarios, but for rare infections clinical case series data may be all that are available.

Mechanisms of antiviral action

Antiviral compounds may act at many different stages along the viral replication cycle. Some require chemical activation by viral enzymes and others by host cell enzymes. Thus many antivirals can have significant side effects on host cells. The schema in Figure 4.1 is an 'over all' model of antiviral actions that can be adapted for each virus, its host cell, and its antiviral treatments.

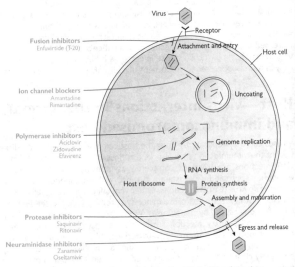

Fig. 4.1 A composite picture of potential sites of antiviral action along the replicative pathway of different viruses in an infected host cell.

(Kindly reproduced with permission, Fig. 14.1 from Knipe DM, Howley PM, Griffin DE, Lamb RA, Martin MA, Roizman B, eds. *Fields' Virology*, 5th edn. Philadelphia, PA: Lippincott Williams & Wilkins, 2007).

Sites of antiviral action

Prevention of viral entry, absorption, penetration

- **Maraviroc** blocks the CD4 cell surface CCR5 co-receptor for HIV, thus inhibiting viral entry to the cell.
- **Enfuvirtide** (T20) inhibits viral cell fusion, mimicking a homologous region in gp41, the HIV surface glycoprotein responsible for the fusion event.
- **Amantadine/rimantadine** block the influenza A M2 protein. The M2 protein is a viral transmembrane protein that functions as an ion channel, enabling the process of viral uncoating so that viral nucleic acid can be transported to the host cell nucleus.
- **Pleconaril** binds to a pocket of the capsid (coating) of enteroviruses and rhinoviruses, and prevents virus attachment and uncoating.

Inhibition of viral genome replication

- **Aciclovir** is a guanine nucleoside analogue which is mono-phosphorylated by the thymidine kinase encoded by herpes simplex virus (HSV) and varicella zoster virus (VZV), and then di and tri phosphorylated by host cellular kinases. The active compound, aciclovir-triphosphate, competes with the natural nucleoside guanine to bind to the viral DNA polymerase, and this terminates elongation of the viral DNA – aciclovir is an obligate 'DNA chain terminator'.
- **Ganciclovir** is another guanine nucleoside analogue with activity against CMV. It is activated to the triphosphate GCV-TP form by HSV thymidine kinases and CMV protein kinases encoded by the viral UL97 gene as well as cellular kinases. It is both a substrate and a competitive inhibitor of the viral polymerase. However, ganciclovir is not an obligate 'chain terminator' like aciclovir and can inhibit cellular polymerases as well as the CMV polymerase. It is not as selective as aciclovir and therefore more toxic (📖 see Antiviral drug toxicity, p. 35).
- **Cidofovir** is a phosphonate-containing cytosine analogue, so does not require the initial viral phosphorylation step, but depends on cellular kinases to convert it to its active form. Although cidofovir can be taken up by both infected and non-infected cells, the viral DNA polymerase has a 25–50 × greater affinity for the molecule compared with the host cell enzyme. Cidofovir is not a DNA 'chain terminator' but rather slows elongation of the chain. It is effective against all the herpesviruses as well as other DNA viruses such as poxviruses.
- **Zidovudine, lamivudine, abacavir** (and others) are nucleoside analogues that are phosphorylated by cellular kinases and inhibit the reverse transcriptase enzyme of HIV. Lamivudine and the closely related drug emtricitabine are also effective against hepatitis B virus.
- **Foscarnet** directly inhibits the DNA polymerase of all herpesviruses by binding to the site occupied by pyrophosphate. It is about 100 × more active against viral than host cell DNA polymerase. It is also effective against HIV reverse transcriptase.
- **Nevirapine and efavirenz** are non-nucleoside molecules that inhibit the reverse transcriptase of HIV.

- **Ribavirin** is a guanosine nucleotide analogue; it is phosphorylated to its active forms by cellular kinases. The mechanism of action is not well understood. Ribavirin has a wide spectrum of antiviral activity against both RNA and DNA viruses (see below).

Prevention of integration with host cell genome

- **Raltegravir** blocks the HIV integrase, the enzyme integrating viral linear DNA to the host cell genome. It therefore inhibits provirus formation.

Prevention of viral assembly, release or deaggregation

- **Lopinavir, ritonavir, darunavir** (and others) are protease inhibitors that disrupt maturation, an essential step for production of infectious HIV virions.
- **Zanamivir and oseltamivir** are neuraminidase inhibitors that target the neuraminidase enzyme of influenza A and B. Inhibition of this enzyme prevents sialic acid cleavage and release of the viral particles from the cell membrane.

Combined antiviral effects

- **Type 1 interferons (INFs)** (alpha and beta) are secreted by all nucleated cells after viral infection. INF beta is produced mainly by white blood cells, and INF alpha by fibroblasts. RNA viruses are more susceptible to INFs than DNA viruses. The cellular effects of INFs are mediated indirectly by more than 20 effector proteins. All elements of the viral replication cycle can be blocked including: cell entry, uncoating, mRNA synthesis, viral protein translation, assembly, and release. The main effects differ according to the virus and the viral families.

Families of viruses, and their most appropriate treatments

Specific antiviral treatments exist for some but not all infections; these may also be augmented by additional interventions, e.g. intravenous immunoglobulin. See Tables 4.1 and 4.2 for the most effective recommended treatments for infections with DNA and RNA viruses. For more details on individual conditions see the specific infection chapters listed at the start of the chapter.

Treatment dose recommendations of many antiviral drugs for neonates, infants, and children are often based on very small cohorts of treated individuals. With the considerable changes in renal, hepatic, and gut function during growth and development the doses are not always adequately optimized, especially those for infants. Maximizing doses is important for antiviral effect, but this must be balanced with the need to minimize potential toxic effects. The most up-to-date dosing schedules should be used (📖 see the BNFC or the drug information leaflet), and if appropriate drug levels may also be measured, e.g. for aciclovir or ganciclovir. Caution is required in interpreting serum levels of drugs that act principally at the intracellular level. Drug level monitoring is also an essential part in follow-up of combination therapy, e.g. in HIV infections to ensure adherence, safety, and efficacy.

Table 4.1 DNA viruses and recommended treatments

Virus family	Antiviral drugs	Other treatments
Variola (small pox)	Limited data—no human studies Cidofovir may be effective	Urgent vaccination of contacts may prevent or modify disease
Molluscum contagiosum	Topical or systemic cidofovir	Physical disruption (e.g. cryotherapy)
		Chemical disruption (e.g. topical podophyllin)
		Immune modulation (e.g. topical imiquimod)
Vaccinia virus	Limited data—no human studies Cidofovir may be effective	
HSV 1 and 2	Aciclovir/valaciclovir Famciclovir/penciclovir Foscarnet Cidofovir	
VZV	Aciclovir/valaciclovir Famciclovir/penciclovir Foscarnet Cidofovir	Varicella zoster immunoglobulin
Cytomegalovirus	Ganciclovir/valganciclovir Foscarnet Cidofovir	
Epstein–Barr virus (EBV)	Ganciclovir/valganciclovir Foscarnet Cidofovir	Rituximab as anti-B cell treatment or anti-EBV cytotoxic T cell infusions for post-transplant lymphoproliferative disorder
Human herpesvirus 6 and 7	Ganciclovir/valganciclovir Foscarnet Cidofovir	
Human herpesvirus 8	Ganciclovir/valganciclovir Foscarnet Cidofovir	Augmentation of immunity (e.g. treating concurrent HIV infection) Chemotherapy for Kaposi's sarcoma

(Continued)

Table 4.1 (Contd.)

Virus family	Antiviral drugs	Other treatments
Adenoviruses	Cidofovir	IVIG[a]
	Ribavirin	
Human papillomaviruses		Excision/laser/cryotherapy/electrocautery
		Chemical disruption (e.g. topical podophyllin)
		Immune modulation (e.g. topical imiquimod)
		Intralesional interferon
JC and BK viruses		Augmentation of immunity (e.g. treating concurrent HIV infection) or reducing immunosuppression
Hepatitis B virus (HBV)	Lamivudine[b]	Interferon alfa
	Adefovir/tenofovir[b]	
	Entecavir	
Human parvovirus		IVIG[a]

[a] IVIG, intravenous immunoglobulin.

[b] May be used for those infected with HIV + HBV.

Table 4.2 RNA viruses and recommended treatments

Virus family	Antiviral drugs	Other treatments
Rotaviruses		IVIG
Togaviridae, e.g. Chikungunya virus		Avoid mosquito exposure
Yellow fever virus		Interferon
		IVIG
West Nile virus	Ribavirin	Interferon
		IVIG
Hepatitis C virus	Ribavirin,	Interferon alfa
	New protease and polymerase inhibitors in clinical trials	

Table 4.2 (*Contd.*)

Virus family	Antiviral drugs	Other treatments
Rubella virus		
Coronaviridae, e.g. SARS	Ribavirin Lopinavir/ritonavir	Interferon
Parainfluenza viruses	Ribavirin	
Mumps virus		
Respiratory syncytial virus	Ribavirin	Palivizumab—passive monoclonal antibody protection for specific vulnerable hosts (e.g. premature infants born <26 weeks)
Human metapneumovirus	Ribavirin	
Measles	Ribavirin	Vitamin A (in countries with morbidity/mortality from measles) IMIG, IVIG
Subacute sclerosing pan encephalitis (SSPE)		SSPE—interferon, isoprinosine
Rabies virus		Postexposure prophylaxis vaccine Human rabies immune globulin
Influenza viruses	Oseltamivir Zanamivir Amantadine (only effective against influenza A)	
Ebola and Marburg		
Lassa virus	Ribavirin	
Lymphocytic choriomeningitis virus	? Ribavirin	
Human T cell lymphotrophic viruses	Nucleoside analogue reverse transcriptase inhibitors Protease inhibitors	

(*Continued*)

Table 4.2 (Contd.)

Virus family	Antiviral drugs	Other treatments
Human immunodeficiency virus	Nucleoside analogue reverse transcriptase inhibitors	
	Non-nucleoside reverse transcriptase inhibitors	
	Protease inhibitors	
	Integrase inhibitors	
	Fusion inhibitors	
	Co-receptor inhibitors	
Polioviruses	Pleconaril (n/a)	IVIG
Enteroviruses	Pleconaril (n/a)	IVIG
Hepatitis A virus		Vaccine for post exposure prophylaxis
Rhinoviruses	Pleconaril (n/a)	Interferon alpha
Caliciviruses, e.g. noroviruses		
Hepatitis E virus		

Development of resistance to antiviral agents

Ongoing viral replication in the presence of antivirals promotes emergence of mutant viruses that are less sensitive to the drug treatment. Therefore treatment must be optimized to achieve maximal viral suppression. Drug resistance is most problematic in relation to long-term treatment of persistent infections including herpes viruses, HIV, and hepatitis. This is particularly a problem for infections caused by HIV and hepatitis C viruses, both RNA viruses exhibiting high turnover of infectious particles, with viral polymerases that lack proofreading ability with a consequent significant spontaneous mutation rate. Effective therapy of HIV depends on combination antiretroviral (ARV) therapy from different classes. Inadequate treatment with sequential exposure to different drugs leads to complex drug resistance patterns. Molecular assays as well as phenotypic and gene sequence databases have been developed to aid interpretation of ARV resistance provided by expert clinical virologists (e.g. the Stanford HIV Drug Resistance Database, ℘ http://hivdbostanford.edu/pages/algs/HIVdb.html).

Drug resistance should always be suspected when there is lack of virological response with good adherence/absorption or evidence of viral rebound. Poor adherence to treatment makes development of resistance more likely. Table 4.3 lists the patterns of viral drug resistance and alternative treatments.

Table 4.3 Patterns of viral drug resistance and alternative treatments

Antiviral drug	Mechanism of resistance	Clinical manifestation of resistance	Possible alternative treatments
Aciclovir/ valaciclovir Famciclovir/ penciclovir	Usually due to mutations in the HSV/ VZV thymidine kinase gene, which lead to loss of enzyme activity so that the active drug form is not produced. Rarely due to mutations in the viral DNA polymerase gene	Usually occurs in immunosuppressed patients on long-term suppressive therapy (e.g. post BMT or those with AIDS). They may get more frequent HSV or VZV, recurrences often with increased severity, e.g. in the central nervous system	Foscarnet Ganciclovir Cidofovir
Ganciclovir/ valganciclovir	Reduced intracellular phosphorylation due to mutation of the CMV *UL97* gene, or due to mutations in the viral polymerase (*Pol*) *UL54* gene	Usually occurs in immunosuppressed patients on long-term suppressive therapy (e.g. post BMT or those with AIDS). They get more frequent CMV recurrences, often with increased severity, e.g. in the eye	Foscarnet Cidofovir *Pol* mutants are resistant to famciclovir/ cidofovir *UL97* mutants are not
Cidofovir	Mutations in the viral DNA polymerase gene	Only very rarely reported	
Foscarnet	Mutations in the viral DNA polymerase gene	Only very rarely reported	
Amantadine	Mutations in the influenza A ion channel M2 gene Does not work for influenza B	May be found in treated individuals within 48 hours— uncertain clinical relevance	Oseltamivir Zanamivir
Oseltamivir	Neuraminidase mutations may occurred after 4 days of treatment	Primary infection with oseltamivir-resistant strains has occurred— clinically similar to wild-type infection	The guidance varies depending on susceptibility of seasonal/ epidemic strains Amantadine (for influenza A)

(Continued)

Table 4.3 (Contd.)

Antiviral drug	Mechanism of resistance	Clinical manifestation of resistance	Possible alternative treatments
Zanamivir	Neuraminidase and/or haemagglutinin mutations may cause reduced sensitivity	Occurs in immunosuppressed patient on >2 weeks of treatment with persistent viral shedding	The guidance varies depending on susceptibility of seasonal/epidemic strains Amantadine (for influenza A)
Lamivudine (for treatment of HBV) (should not be given as monotherapy for HBV due to high risk of resistance) (Can be used as part of combination ARV for patients with HIV + HBV)	Most common mutations affect the YMDD motif in the catalytic domain of the HBV polymerase (common mutations: rtM204I and rtM204V)	Occur in 42–70% of individuals treated for 2–5 years with lamivudine monotherapy Associated with HBV rebound	Adefovir Tenofovir Entecavir (not preferred for lamivudine-treated patients, unless necessary and no mutations) Patients already on lamivudine should receive add-on therapy with adefovir or tenofovir, not switch
Entecavir (for treatment of HBV) (Must not be used for patients with HIV + HBV)		Rare in naïve patients, but may occur in individuals who already have lamivudine mutations (requires 3 mutations) Resistance occurs in 0% and 1.2% at year 1 and 5, respectively	Tenofovir
Adefovir (for treatment of HBV) (Must not be used for patients with HIV + HBV)	Common polymerase mutations: rtN236T, rtA181T, rtA181V	Resistance occurs in 0%, 3%, 11%, 18%, and 29% at year 1, 2, 3, 4, and 5, respectively	Usually as add-on for patients already on lamivudine Entecavir

Table 4.3 (Contd.)

Antiviral drug	Mechanism of resistance	Clinical manifestation of resistance	Possible alternative treatments
Tenofovir (for treatment of HBV)	Common polymerase mutations : rtA194T	No resistance seen at 2 years	Entecavir
(Can be used as part of combination ARV for patients with HIV+HBV)			
Ribavirin		Clinically significant viral resistance has not been observed	
Antiretrovirals (ARVs)		Complex patterns of ARV class-related resistance develop when full HIV suppression is not achieved	

AIDS, acquired immune deficiency syndrome; BMT, bone marrow transplant.

Antiviral drug toxicity

The serious side effects of some antiviral treatments mean that often these drugs are only used in critical situations, such as to treat severely immunosuppressed patients. Over time, it is hoped that less host toxic drugs with equal or greater antiviral effect will emerge.

- **Aciclovir, valaciclovir** (prodrug of aciclovir with increased oral absorption): intravenous (IV) aciclovir may cause reversible renal toxicity when administered to patients who are poorly hydrated. Accumulation of aciclovir in such patients may also cause reversible neurotoxicity. High-dose IV aciclovir used to treat neonates may cause reversible neutropenia. Oral aciclovir may cause mild gastrointestinal upset. To date, aciclovir has not been found to be teratogenic in humans.
- **Ganciclovir, valganciclovir** (prodrug of ganciclovir with increased oral absorption): IV ganciclovir causes reversible myelosuppression, with neutropenia in up to 40% of patients who receive the drug. This effect can be mitigated by the use of granulocyte colony-stimulating factor. Toxicity tests have demonstrated that ganciclovir is mutagenic, carcinogenic, and teratogenic in animals, so it is treated as a cytotoxic drug within the clinical setting. Close monitoring for such toxicities in humans is essential, and this drug should only be used when it is considered that benefits outweigh these potential risks. Oral

valganciclovir is now also available for children and may be used as continuation after IV use or as prophylaxis for CMV infection in the severely immunocompromised.

- **Cidofovir**: IV cidofovir has a long intracellular half-life and can be dosed weekly. Cidofovir is highly concentrated in the renal tubules, with a significant risk of nephrotoxicity, so treatment must be preceded by hyper-hydration and the dose titrated to renal function. Carcinogenic and teratogenic effects as well as hypospermia have been demonstrated in animal studies.
- **Foscarnet**: This causes severe but reversible nephrotoxicity in up to half of patients; the dose must be titrated to renal function. Renal toxicity is often associated with other metabolic derangements of calcium, magnesium, and phosphate; this is aggravated by concomitant treatment with other nephrotoxic agents (e.g. amphotericin and aminoglycosides). CNS side effects and bone marrow suppression may also occur.
- **Ribavirin**: In low doses, ribavirin may cause haemolytic anaemia, and in high doses anaemia due to bone marrow suppression. These effects do not occur with aerosolized treatment (e.g. for respiratory syncytial virus (RSV) bronchiolitis). Ribavirin has been demonstrated to be teratogenic and embryo-lethal in animals, so is contraindicated for pregnant women.
- **Oseltamivir**: This may cause gastrointestinal upset which is usually mild.
- **Zanamivir**: This may cause bronchospasm when administered by inhalation.
- **Pleconaril**: This has minimal side effects.
- **Interferon**: Side effects are dose related. Immediately after administration flu-like symptoms with fever, myalgia, and headache are very common. In the longer term, after several weeks of therapy, depression or other neuropsychiatric effects as well as bone marrow suppression may occur. When used in combination with ribavirin, bone marrow toxicity must be monitored very closely. Pegylated interferon has a longer half-life and can be dosed less frequently; it also has less severe side effects.
- **Antiretrovirals**: The different families of ARVs have numerous side effects and interactions with each other and other classes of drugs; these are important as the ARVs must always be used in combination with each other to achieve sufficient potency for full HIV suppression. More details of side effects, toxicity and interactions can be found at the Penta website (www.pentatrials.org).

Future research

- Improved antiviral formulae for children, especially for better absorbed oral preparations.
- Development of treatment for severe manifestations of enterovirus infection (e.g. neonatal infection, myocarditis, encephalitis).
- Development of less toxic treatments for herpesvirus infections.

- Better understanding of host genetics (including metabolism and immune function) and how they affect responses to viruses as well as antiviral treatments.

Further reading

Knipe DM, Howley PM, Griffin DE, Lamb RA, Martin MA, Roizman B, eds. *Fields Virology*, 5th edn. Philadelphia, PA: Lippincott Williams & Wilkins, 2007.

Chapter 5

Bone and joint infections

📖 see also Chapters 38, 40, 105, 106

Introduction

Empirical treatment of osteoarticular infection depends on the age of the child and the likely pathogen.

Pathophysiology

Osteomyelitis and septic arthritis

- Usually arises by haematogenous spread of bacteria, most commonly in the metaphyseal region of a larger bone.
- May be secondary to contiguous infection or due to direct inoculation.
- Acute septic arthritis (SA) may be an extension of osteomyelitis (OM) or by haematogenous spread seeding directly to the joint space without bone involvement.
- In neonates, bone infection affects the growth plate or joint in 76%.
- Discitis is an infection of the intervertebral disc space.

Osteomyelitis

- Haematogenous infection is the most common, acute or subacute.
- Long bones are most often affected in children.
- Most unifocal, 5–20% multifocal.
- In neonates, OM is often multifocal with associated SA.

Septic arthritis

- Usually secondary to bacteraemia.
- The epiphyseal growth plate can be affected in young children.
- Permanent joint destruction can occur if treatment is not prompt.

Chronic recurrent multifocal osteomyelitis

- Rare inflammatory condition.
- Recurrent, sterile, lytic lesions.
- Often in the clavicle, humerus, and tubular bones.

Incidence

- Estimate: 5–12 cases per 100 000 children per year.
- Half of the children with acute OM are <5 years old.
- Boys are 1.2–3.7 times more likely to be affected by OM or SA than girls.

Aetiology

Neonates

- Group B streptococcus (GBS), Methicillin sensitive *Staphylococcus aureus* (MSSA), *Escherichia coli*/Gram-negatives, *Candida albicans*

<2 years

- MSSA, *Kingella kingae*, *Streptococcus pneumoniae*, non-typeable *Haemophilus* spp., *E. coli*, MSSA PVL (uncommon in the UK), MRSA PVL (very rare in the UK)

2–5 years

- MSSA, *K. kingae*, group A streptococcus (GAS), *S. pneumoniae*, non-typeable *Haemophilus* spp., MSSA PVL (uncommon in the UK), MRSA PVL (very rare in the UK)

>5 years

- MSSA, MSSA PVL (uncommon in the UK), MRSA PVL (very rare in the UK)

Other much rarer organisms (consider in immunosuppressed children or other risk factors)

- *H. influenzae* type b (unimmunized), coagulase-negative *Staphylococcus* (subacute), *Pseudomonas* spp., *Neisseria gonorrhoeae*, *Neisseria meningitidis*, *Mycobacterium tuberculosis*, *Salmonella* spp. (sickle cell disease), *Bartonella henselae*, non-tuberculous mycobacteria, *Klebsiella* spp., *Fusobacterium* (often multifocal), *Aspergillus*, *Candida albicans*

Clinical features

Neonates

- Irritability, ± fever, widespread pain often difficult to localize on examination.
- Pseudoparalysis, erythema, bone or limb swelling. Several sites may be involved. (Note pseudoparalysis of arm may be mistaken for delayed onset of Erb's Palsy in late-onset GBS OM of humeral head.)

- May be no focal signs, but unexplained sepsis or positive blood culture should warrant consideration of bone or joint infection.

Child
- Usually short history, with an ill child in pain.
- Fever frequent, but may be absent.
- Refusal to move the limb or to weight bear, limp, erythema, bone or limb swelling, local tenderness.
- In SA there is a unifocal hot, immobile, tender peripheral joint, with pain on passive joint movement.
- May have no focal signs.

Subacute or chronic osteomyelitis
- Longer history, maybe weeks, with no systemic symptoms.
- Often no fever.
- Less acute local signs with limp, refusal to move the limb or weight bear, local bony swelling or tenderness.

Discitis
- Insidious onset, no systemic illness, fever uncommon.
- Back pain, refusal to sit, stand or walk.
- Refusal to flex the spine, local tenderness.
- Constipation or abdominal pain.

Chronic recurrent multifocal osteomyelitis
- Initially indistinguishable from acute/subacute OM.
- Histology non-specific.
- Pain may be severe, persistent and debilitating.

Risk factors
- Trauma, sickle cell disease, immunodeficiency, penetrating wounds, bone fixators or plates, varicella infection (GAS).

Differential diagnosis
- Trauma including non-accidental injury, malignancy (osteosarcoma, leukaemia, neuroblastoma), reactive arthritis, haemarthrosis, Henoch–Schönlein purpura, juvenile idiopathic arthritis, tuberculosis.

Investigations and diagnosis

Blood tests
- C-reactive protein (CRP) and erythrocyte sedimentation rate (ESR) are more reliably increased than white cell count but normal values do not absolutely exclude OM or SA (although osteoarticular infection is less likely if CRP and ESR are normal).

- Microbiological culture of blood (all cases), joint fluid (from aspiration), periosteal pus or bone biopsy.
- Difficult cases may require molecular diagnostic techniques (e.g. 16S rDNA polymerase chain reaction (PCR), targeted multiplex PCR).

Imaging

- Plain radiographs are often unhelpful in acute presentations as osteolytic changes/periosteal elevation occur 10–21 days after the onset of symptoms. They are important as a baseline assessment, to exclude trauma and in subacute presentations.
- Ultrasonography is useful for identifying deep effusions in SA and subperiosteal collections in OM.
- Magnetic resonance imaging with enhancement has best diagnostic sensitivity and specificity.
- Technetium radionuclide bone scan (^{99m}Tc):
  - High sensitivity and specificity but used less often due to the radiation burden
  - May give false-negative results in infancy.

Management

- Multidisciplinary including paediatricians, orthopaedic surgeons, radiologists and microbiologists.
- Little high quality evidence to guide therapy, but established, consistent practice.

Surgical

- Often not required in OM with early radiographic signs.
- Surgical drainage in acute OM is indicated if no response to antibiotics after 48–72 hours or if radiological evidence of a substantial pus collection.
- Urgent wash-out and drainage of SA in hip, aspiration and irrigation in other joints, to reduce pressure on growth plate.
- More aggressive surgical management if PVL MSSA or MRSA suspected or confirmed.
- Immobilize any surgically treated limb or focus of infection.

Medical

- Start empirical intravenous antibiotics on clinical diagnosis of acute OM or SA.
- In SA, start antibiotics following surgery unless delay of >4 hours anticipated.
- **Use high doses:**
  - Neonates to <3 months: intravenous cefotaxime ± amoxicillin as in suspected sepsis/meningitis
  - ≥ 3 months to ≤5 years: intravenous cefuroxime monotherapy
  - ≥ 6 years: intravenous flucloxacillin or clindamycin monotherapy.
- Optimize antimicrobial treatment if organism is identified.

- In *simple unifocal disease* a rapid switch to oral therapy may be appropriate:
  - Neonates to <3 months: consider intravenous to oral switch after 14–21 days if:
    > Afebrile + pain-free for at least 24 hours
    > *and*
    > CRP <20 mg/L or CRP decreased by ≥2/3 of highest value.
  - Child ≥3 months: consider intravenous to oral switch after 48–72 hours if :
    > Afebrile + pain-free for at least 24 hours
    > *and*
    > CRP <20 mg/L or CRP decreased by ≥2/3 of highest value.
- When switching to oral antibiotics, dose, administration frequency, and palatability must be considered.
- Suggested pragmatic empirical oral antibiotic choices where organism remains unknown. Use high doses:
  - **Neonatal**: Co-amoxiclav suspension three times daily
  - **1–2 months**: Co-amoxiclav suspension three times daily
  - **2 month – 2 years**: Co-amoxiclav suspension three times daily
  - **2–5 years**: Co-amoxiclav suspension three times daily
  - **6–8 years**: Co-amoxiclav suspension three times daily or flucloxacillin four times daily (only if child can take tablets)
  - **9–18 years**: Flucloxacillin four times daily or clindamycin four times daily
- Antibiotic therapy is continued for a total of 3–4 weeks in SA and 4–6 weeks in OM.
- Complex disease (multifocal, significant bone destruction, resistant/unusual pathogen, immunosuppressed, sepsis, or shock) requires prolonged intravenous antibiotic therapy and the total length of antibiotic course may need to exceed 6 weeks. Treatment of complex disease should be managed in conjunction with experts in bone and joint infection.
- Prolonged intravenous therapy can be given in the community in some cases.
- If confirmed PVL-positive disease use the latest guidelines from the Health Protection Agency (HPA; ℘ www.hpa.org.uk).
- *Discitis*: Antibiotics appear to speed resolution, length of therapy is usually 4–6 weeks.
- *Chronic recurrent multifocal osteomyelitis*: Use simple analgesia and non-steroidal anti-inflammatory drugs (NSAIDs); refer to paediatric rheumatologist if alternative or experimental therapies are considered necessary.

Outcome

- Most children with simple disease are discharged without long-term care or further assessment of growth or function.
- Significant risk of deep venous thrombosis and thromboembolism in children with OM.
- In severe diseases, risk of joint stiffness, limb shortening, dislocation (acutely neonates), and avascular necrosis of affected epiphysis.

Future research

- The optimal duration of therapy is unknown and shorter treatment courses should be studied in randomized clinical trials.
- The safety of early oral switching in OM and SA should be further investigated in randomized clinical trials.

Further reading

Krogstad P. Osteomyelitis and septic arthritis. In: Feigin RD, ed. *Textbook of Pediatric Infectious Diseases.* Philadelphia: WB Saunders, 2004:713–36.

Yagupsky P. Kingella kingae: from medical rarity to an emerging paediatric pathogen. *Lancet Infect Dis* 2004;**4**:358–67.

Zaoutis T, Localio AR, Leckerman K, Saddlemire S, Bertoch D, Keren R. Prolonged intravenous therapy versus early transition to oral antimicrobial therapy for acute osteomyelitis in children. *Pediatrics* 2009;**123**:636–42.

Chapter 6

Cardiac infections: endocarditis

📖 see also Chapters 8, 105, 106

Introduction and definitions

There are three distinct forms of cardiac infection: endocarditis, myocarditis, and pericarditis. The latter two often occur together and are considered in Chapter 7 (📖 p. 54).

Infective endocarditis (**IE**) is an infection of the endocardium, valves, or related structures of the heart.

Infective endarteritis is similar to IE. May involve: patent ductus arteriosus, shunts (native and constructed), aneurysms, stents, collateral closing devices, neonatal umbilical lines, damaged arterial walls.

Classification

There are several recognized subtypes of IE (Table 6.1).

Table 6.1 Classification of IE

According to localization and presence/absence of intracardiac material		
Left-sided native valve IE		
Left-sided prosthetic valve IE	Early	<1 year after replacement
	Late	>1 year after replacement
Right-sided IE		
Device-related IE[a]	Permanent	Pacemaker, ICD
According to mode of acquisition		
Healthcare-associated IE	Nosocomial	Hospitalized >48 h prior to onset of symptoms
	Non-nosocomial	Hospitalized <48 h prior to onset of symptoms
Community-acquired IE		Onset of symptoms out of hospital or <48 h after hospitalization if criteria for healthcare associated not fulfilled
IV drug abuse-associated IE		IE in active injection drug user without alternative source of infection

Table 6.1 (Contd.)

Active IE
IE with persistent fever or positive blood culture
Active signs of inflammation at surgery
Still on antibiotic therapy
Histopathological evidence of active IE

Recurrence of IE	
Relapse	Repeat episode with same microorganism <6 months after the initial episode
Reinfection	Repeat episode with same microorganism >6 months after the initial episode
	Infection with different microorganism

ªRelated also to central venous lines as well as closure devices (atrial septal defect/ventricular septal defect/patent ductus arteriosus closing) before endothelialization.
ICD, implantable cardioverter-defibrillator.
Adapted from the European Society of Cardiology (ESC) guidelines (2009).[1]

Epidemiology

- Overall incidence of IE in the general population varies between 3 and 10 cases/100 000 person-years.
- No controlled studies in the paediatric age group and the exact incidence is unknown.
- Likely to be less than in the adult population.
- A significant proportion (>50%) of paediatric patients with IE have had previous procedures.
- Infective endarteritis in children is very rare.

Predisposing factors for IE

- Prosthetic valve or prosthetic material.
- Structural congenital heart disease (cyanotic, small or residual defects).
- Previous IE.
- Hypertrophic cardiomyopathy.
- Intracardiac devices (permanent pacemakers, ICDs, long-term catheters).
- IV drug abuse.
- Acquired valvular heart disease with stenosis or regurgitation.

Changing profile of IE in developed countries

Changing predisposing factors:
- ↓ Acquired rheumatic heart disease
- ↑ Device/prosthesis usage
- ↑ IV drug abuse
- ↑ Previous infective endocarditis (recurrence, reinfection).

Changing microbiology:
- ↑ Staphylococcal
- ↓ Streptococcal
- ↑ Blood-culture positive (>85%) (improved diagnosis: techniques, fastidious organisms)
- ↑ Intracellular organisms (improved diagnosis: sensitive serology, PCR from vegetations).

Changing mode of acquisition:
- ↓ Community acquired
- ↑ Healthcare associated
- ↑ Recurrent IE.

Changing localization of lesions:
- ↑ Multiple-site (neighbouring and non-neighbouring)
- ↑ Right-sided.

Clinical presentation and diagnosis

Diagnosis is often a challenge due to the heterogeneous clinical manifestations and often multiorgan involvement. Symptoms and signs may be atypical in very young children. Presentations may be:
- Classic subacute presentation (over weeks and sometimes months), characteristic of infections caused by oral streptococci, is seen less often than previously.
- Acute presentation due to infection with staphylococci has become more common.
- Prolonged indolent course of IE due to intracellular organisms (such as *Bartonella* and *Coxiella burnetii*).

Clinical features are related to:
- **Infection**: Fever (>90%), positive markers of inflammation (elevated ESR/CRP, anaemia normocytic or microcytic with low serum iron and normal or high ferritin, leucocytosis with neutrophilia), positive blood culture (>85%).
- **Destruction** (>90%): New cardiac murmur, heart failure (30–60%), conduction abnormality.
  - New murmur may be difficult to differentiate from pre-existing murmurs.
  - Heart failure caused by acute severe aortic or mitral insufficiency or intracardiac fistulae or, rarely, by valvular obstruction.
  - Conduction abnormality (right/left bundle branch block or complete heart block) is due to spread of infection to the conduction system.
- **Embolism** (20–50%): systemic (brain, spleen, kidney, peripheral) or pulmonary.
- **Immunological phenomena** (positive antinuclear antibody (ANA) and rheumatoid factor, low C3/C4).
  - **Haematuria**: May be related both to immune complex deposition or small renal emboli.

See also Table 6.2.

Table 6.2 Revised Dukes' clinical diagnostic criteria for infective endocarditis

Major criteria	Minor criteria
Positive blood culture with typical IE microorganism, defined as one of the following:	Predisposing factor
Typical microorganism consistent with IE from 2 separate blood cultures, as noted below:	
• Viridans-group streptococci, S. bovis, or HACEK group, or	• Fever >38°C
• Community-acquired S. aureus or enterococci, in the absence of a primary focus	• Evidence of embolism
Microorganisms consistent with IE from persistently positive blood cultures defined as:	
• Two positive cultures of blood samples drawn >12 hours apart, or	• Immunological problems
• All of 3 or a majority of 4 separate cultures of blood (with first and last sample drawn 1 hour apart)	• Positive blood culture (that doesn't meet a major criterion)
• Positive echocardiography findings (vegetation, new or worsening regurgitation, partial dehiscence of prosthetic valve, abscess, aneurysm or pseudoaneurysm)	• Positive echocardiogram (that doesn't meet a major criterion)

Definite clinical diagnosis: 2 major criteria or 1 major and 3 minor criteria or 5 minor criteria.
Possible clinical diagnosis: 1 major and 1 minor criteria or 3 minor criteria.
Source: Adapted from Li et al.[2]

Differential diagnosis
- Other chronic infections.
- Rheumatological and autoimmune diseases.
- Malignancy with systemic features. Cardiac myxomas can manifest with low-grade fever, immunological phenomena, and positive markers of inflammation.

Neonatal IE
- Most often related to intravascular catheters.
- Systemic hypotension.
- Signs of generalized sepsis.
- Particularly prone to septic embolization (focal neurological signs) and development of satellite infections (meningitis, osteomyelitis).
- Candidal endocarditis is relatively more common.

When to suspect IE

- New regurgitant heart murmur
- Embolic events of unknown origin
- Sepsis of unknown origin (especially if associated with IE causative organism)
- Fever associated with:
  - Intracardiac prosthetic material (e.g. prosthetic valve, pacemaker, ICD, surgical baffle/conduit)
  - Previous history of IE
  - Previous valvular or congenital heart disease
  - Other predisposition for IE (e.g. immunocompromised, intravenous drug user)
  - Predisposition and recent cardiac intervention with associated bacteraemia
  - Evidence of congestive heart failure
  - New conduction disturbance
  - Positive blood culture with typical IE causative organism or positive serology for Q-fever (microbiological findings may precede cardiological manifestations)
  - Vascular or immunologic phenomena: embolic event, Roth spots, splinter haemorrhages, Janeway lesions, Osler's nodes
  - Focal or non-specific neurological symptoms and signs
  - Evidence of pulmonary embolism/infiltration (right-sided IE)
  - Peripheral abscesses (renal, splenic, cerebral, vertebral) of unknown cause.

Adapted from the ESC guidelines (2009).[1]

Investigations

Cardiological investigations

- Echocardiography to look for: vegetations, regurgitation, valvular perforation, chordal rupture, fistula formation, prosthetic device dehiscence, abscesses, aneurysms, or pseudoaneurysms. Transthoracic images have high diagnostic yield in children. Transoesophageal echocardiography may be indicated in prosthetic valves, chest wall deformity, obesity. If negative and suspicion remains high, it should be repeated.
- Electrocardiography to look for conduction disturbances and arrhythmias.
- Computed tomography (CT), and magnetic resonance imaging (MRI), may be useful for visualization of embolic phenomena.

Microbiological diagnosis of IE

Blood culture still remains the cornerstone of the diagnosis of IE and a major criterion for Dukes' classification. It is **imperative** that in cases of suspected IE, a sufficient number of correctly taken blood cultures are drawn. It is essential that the request indicates that IE is suspected as the laboratory will prolong the incubation period accordingly.

In children the following volumes and frequency are recommended:
- Volumes:
  - Infants and young children 1–3ml per bottle
  - Older children 5–7ml per bottle (up to 30ml blood/day).
- Frequency:
  - Three sets of separate venepunctures over 24 hours, ideally with one set 12 hours apart, but with at least the first and last set 1 hour apart
  - If patient is unstable and presentation acute, take **two** blood cultures at separate sites immediately and a third at least 1 hour later and commence empirical therapy **without delay**.

Additional investigations

Serological testing
Serological testing can be very useful (and can sometimes be only method available) for diagnosing IE caused by *Coxiella* (Q fever), *Bartonella*, *Legionella*, *Chlamydia*, and *Brucella* species.

Molecular methods
- Molecular tests should be used as an adjunctive test to culture methods.
- Can be applied to both blood samples and infected lesions removed at surgery.
- Include broad range (16S ribosomal sequencing) or specific real time (*Staphylococcus aureus*, *Streptococcus pyogenes*, etc.).

Histological diagnosis
Still remains a major criterion if an organism can be demonstrated by appropriate staining methods in the resected lesion.

Table 6.3 Causative agents of bacterial IE

	Approximate frequency (%)
Viridans group streptococci	40
S. aureus	30
Coagulase-negative staphylococci	8
S. pneumoniae	6
HACEK[a]	5
Enterococci	5
Culture negative (see section)	6

The most common causative agents of IE in very low birthweight (VLBW) neonates are *S. aureus*, coagulase-negative staphylococci and *Candida* species, usually with long-term indwelling venous catheters.

[a]HACEK organisms grow slowly and can be difficult to identify. Sensitivity testing can be difficult, and delayed. They include: *Haemophilus* species (*H. influenzae*, *parainfluenzae*), *Aggregatibacter actinomycetemcomitans*, *Aggregatibacter aphrophilus*, *Cardiobacter hominis*, *Eikenella corrodens*, *Kingella kingae*.

Culture-negative IE

Applies to cases in which there is clinical and radiological evidence of IE but blood cultures are persistently negative. Causes include prior antibiotic therapy or infections due to fastidious organisms (particularly HACEK group or nutritionally dependent organisms such as *Abiotrophia*). Sometimes, the organism can be cultured from vegetations.

Treatment

Management of IE requires close collaboration between paediatricians, cardiologists, and infectious disease/microbiology specialists. IE in children with implanted prosthetic material should be managed in centres with access to cardiothoracic surgeons as revision surgery, whether immediate or delayed, is usually necessary.

Antimicrobial treatment

The determinants of choice of antibiotic regimen and length of therapy are:
- The identity of the pathogen
- Its antimicrobial sensitivity profile
- The nature of the infective lesion, i.e. native or surgically implanted prosthetic material
- Presence of septic embolic phenomena.

In IE, microbial pathogens are embedded in fibrin platelet matrix, with associated biofilm. Organisms in biofilms tend to be metabolically inactive and less susceptible to cell wall active agents such as B-lactams and glycopeptides. For this reason doses of these agents tend to be high and the duration of therapy long.

The general principles of antimicrobial therapy in IE are:
- Use at least one agent that is bactericidal for the organism concerned
- A cell wall active agent (B-lactam or glycopeptide) combined with aminoglycoside often provides synergy.

Tables 6.4–6.6 summarize the drugs recommended in IE, depending on the presentation and causative organisms.

Table 6.4 Empirical antibiotic therapy based on clinical presentation

Acute presentation (native valve)	Flucloxacillin
	Gentamicin
Subacute presentation (native valve)	Penicillin + ceftriaxone
	Gentamicin
Penicillin allergy	
Presence of intracardiac prosthetic material	Vancomycin + rifampicin + gentamicin
Suspicion/risk of MRSA	

Table 6.5 Empiric antibiotic therapy based on organism

Organism and site	Antimicrobial agent	Duration
Staphylococcal:		
Native valve	Flucloxacillin	6 weeks
Meticillin-sensitive	plus	
	Gentamicin	3–5 days
β-lactam allergic or meticillin resistant organism	Vancomycin	6 weeks
	plus	
	Gentamicin and/or	3–5 days
	Rifampicin	6 weeks
Staphylococcal with prosthetic material	Flucloxacillin or vancomycin	≥6 weeks
	plus	
	Rifampicin	≥6 weeks
	plus	
	Gentamicin	2 weeks

Treatment of culture-negative IE

In most instances therapy should be directed against streptococci, staphylococci, and HACEK group organisms.
In subcute cases (patient stable) use ceftriaxone and gentamicin.
Acute presentation or a patient with prosthetic material requires staphylococcal cover—use vancomycin/teicoplanin plus gentamicin.
If known exposure history to *Coxiella* or *Bartonella* infection, treatment options are additionally directed against those pathogens.
Usually 6 weeks therapy is warranted for culture-negative IE (with exceptions, *Coxiella* IE requires 2–3 years therapy).

Treatment of fungal endocarditis

Less common in children than adults.
Neonates (mainly pre-term) with disseminated candidaemia may have cardiac involvement such as valvular lesions or infected mural thrombi.
Cardiac involvement should be excluded in all neonatal candidaemia.
Infected prosthetic valves almost always require surgical revision.
Most authorities recommend a combination of amphotericin and flucytosine. Echinocandins (e.g. caspofungin) and azoles (e.g. fluconazole) are alternatives. Duration is at least 6 weeks.
In non-operable prosthetic material endocarditis lifelong therapy may be warranted.

Table 6.6 Duaration of antibiotic therapy by organism

Organism	Antimicrobial agent	Duration
Viridans (A-haemolytic streptococci and S. bovis)	Penicillin G or ceftriaxone	2–4 weeks
	plus gentamicin	2 weeks
		4 weeks
MIC penicillin >16 or	Vancomycin	4 weeks
β-lactam allergic	plus gentamicin	2 weeks
Nutritionally variant streptococci (e.g. *Abiotrophia* species)	Penicillin G plus gentamicin	4–6 weeks
Enterococcal species:	Ampicillin	
Ampicillin susceptible	plus gentamicin	4–6 weeks
Ampicillin resistant or β-lactam allergic	Vancomycin plus gentamicin	4–6 weeks
HACEK group	Ceftriaxone	4 weeks
	plus	
	gentamicin	2 weeks
Coliforms and other Gram-negatives *Escherichia coli, Klebsiella, Pseudomonas* species	Cephalosporin or piperacillin/tazobactam or carbapenem plus aminoglycoside	6+ weeks

- IE due to filamentous fungi such as *Aspergillus spp.* is usually only seen in highly immunocompromised patients and occasionally in patients with prosthetic valves. These cases are extremely difficult to diagnose (blood cultures rarely positive) and are often detected at post-mortem or after surgery. Treatment of filamentous fungal IE is rarely successful without surgical intervention. Both voriconazole and amphotericin are useful agents.

Surgical treatment
Surgery is indicated for most of the cases of IE. In some cases there might be urgent indications:

Risk of emboli (systemic or pulmonary)
- Anterior mitral leaflet vegetation with significant size (>10mm)
- One or more embolic events during first 2 weeks of antimicrobial therapy
- Increase of vegetation size after 4 weeks of antimicrobial therapy.

Intractable heart failure
- Acute insufficiency (especially mitral and aortic) with signs of ventricular dysfunction
- Valve rupture or significant perforation.

Perivalvular extension
- Valvular dehiscence, rupture or fistula
- New heart block
- Large abscess or extension of abscess despite therapy.

Antithrombotic therapy

There is no indication for the initiation of antithrombotic drugs (thrombolytic, anticoagulant, or antiplatelet) in patients with active IE.

Outcomes

Outcome is significantly improved, with mortality in developed countries decreased to as low as 10%. There is no accurate recent study on the paediatric population.

Prophylaxis

Recommendations for antibiotic prophylaxis against IE have changed in the recent years, with the lack of scientific evidence for its efficacy being widely accepted.

In the UK, the National Institute of Health and Clinical Excellence (NICE) guidelines for prophylaxis against IE published in March 2008[3] state that antibiotic prophylaxis solely to prevent IE should *not* be given to people at risk of IE undergoing dental and non-dental procedures.

The recommendations in the 2009 ESC guidelines[1] are similar but suggest that prophylaxis is still recommended for a small group of high-risk patients.

Key references

1 Guidelines on the prevention, diagnosis, and treatment of infective endocarditis (new version 2009). The Task Force on the Prevention, Diagnosis, and Treatment of Infective Endocarditis of the European Society of Cardiology (ESC). Endorsed by the European Society of Clinical Microbiology and Infectious Diseases (ESCMID) and by the International Society of Chemotherapy (ISC) for Infection and cancer. *Eur Heart J* 2009;**30**:2369–413. Available at: ℘ http://www.escardio.org/guidelines-surveys/esc-guidelines/GuidelinesDocuments/guidelines-IE-FT.pdf (accessed October 2010).

2 Li JS, Sexton DJ, Mick N, *et al.* Proposed modifications to the Duke criteria for the diagnosis of infective endocarditis. *Clin Infect Dis* 2000;**30**:633–8.

3 Richey R, Wray D, Stokes T. Prophylaxis against infective endocarditis: summary of NICE guidance. *BMJ* 2008;**336**:770–1. Available at: ℘ http://www.nice.org.uk/nicemedia/pdf/CG64NICEguidance.pdf; ℘ http://www.nice.org.uk/nicemedia/pdf/CG64PIEQRG.pdf (accessed October 2010).

Further reading

Ferrieri P, Gewitz MH, Gerber MA, *et al.* Unique features of infective endocarditis in children. *Circulation* 2002;**105**:2115–26.

Chapter 7

Cardiac infections: myocarditis and pericarditis

📖 see also Chapter 64

Definitions

Myocarditis is characterized by inflammatory infiltrate in the cardiac muscle with or without necrosis of myocytes (see Table 7.1).

Table 7.1 What is myocarditis?

Histopathology	Immunohistochemistry	Magnetic resonance imaging features
Cellular infiltrate (>14 leucocytes/mm²)	T lymphocytes (CD3)	Tissue oedema
Myocyte necrosis	Monocytes/macrophages/natural killer (CD68)	Capillary leakage
	Antigen-presenting cells (human leucocyte antigen (HLA) class II DRA)	Necrosis/fibrosis

Pericarditis is inflammation of the epicardium and/or the pericardium that leads to accumulation of excessive fluid in the pericardial sac (pericardial effusion). Not all pericardial effusions are due to inflammation. Non-inflammatory causes of effusions include congestive heart failure (hydropericardium), haemopericardium, and chylopericardium.

Constrictive pericarditis is a rigid non-compliant pericardium due to fibrosis and calcification. There is usually small or absent pericardial effusion with the exception of the effusive-constrictive subtype. The pericardium may not be thickened in up to 30%.

Acute pericarditis is of <1 month duration.

Chronic pericarditis is of >3 months duration.

Recurrent pericarditis is of:
- Intermittent type: symptom-free intervals without therapy
- Incessant type: discontinuation of therapy leads to relapse.

Aetiology

Many infections can cause both myocarditis and pericarditis. Viral causes are listed in Table 7.2. Coxsackie virus predominates in the newborn period whereas in older children adenovirus is the commonest cause. Non-viral causes are listed in Table 7.3.

The detection of viral genomes by PCR appears to be of aetiopathogenic importance only in the presence of an immunohistologically proven reactive inflammatory infiltrate. In patients without inflammation, the finding may represent latent viral genome persistence.

Table 7.2 Viral causes of myocarditis and pericarditis

Enteroviruses	Influenza A
Coxsackie A	RSV
Coxsackie B	Mumps
ECHOvirus	Measles
Poliovirus	Rubella
Adenovirus	Rabies
Parvovirus B19	Hepatitis B, C
HHV-6	HIV
EBV	
CMV	
HSV	
VZV	

Table 7.3 Non-viral causes of myocarditis and pericarditis

Infectious	
Bacterial	*Staphylococcus aureus, Haemophilus influenzae* type B, *Streptococcus pyogenes* and *pneumoniae, Neisseria meningitides* and *gonorrhoeae, Salmonella* sp., *Pseudomonas aeruginosa, Escherichia coli, Mycobacterium tuberculosis, Borrelia* (Lyme disease), *Corynebacterium diphtheriae*
Fungal	*Candida, Coccidioides, Histoplasma*
Protozoa and helminths	*Entamoeba histolytica, Trypanosoma, Schistosoma, Trichinella, Toxocara*

(Continued)

Table 7.3 Non-viral causes of myocarditis and pericarditis

Non-infectious	
Systemic inflammatory	Kawasaki disease, systemic lupus erythematosus and lupus-like, juvenile idiopathic arthritis, scleroderma, inflammatory bowel disease.
Toxic for myocarditis	Scorpion sting, snake venom, drug-induced
Other for pericardial effusion	Post radiation, uraemia, hypothyroidism, tumours (lymphoma, metastatic), post cardiotomy syndrome.

Myocarditis

Epidemiology

Myocarditis is an underdiagnosed condition and its true incidence is unknown. The reported incidence and prevalence largely depends on how strictly and which diagnostic criteria are applied. Up to 9% of paediatric dilated cardiomyopathy may be a consequence of myocarditis.

Clinical manifestations

The presence and severity of clinical signs as well as the course of disease vary hugely (Table 7.4). A significant proportion of myocarditis probably remains undiagnosed (see Table 7.5) and patients recover spontaneously. However, there may be rapid worsening leading to haemodynamic compromise or death. In a proportion of patients there is a chronic course with dilated cardiomyopathy that may worsen or recover in months to years.

Table 7.4 The course of myocarditis

Preceding	Course	Outcome
Viral infection	Mild	Recovery
	Acute	Death
	Fulminant	Dilated cardiomyopathy
	Chronic	Transplant

Table 7.5 When to suspect myocarditis

Clinical features	Cause
Sudden death	Ventricular tachycardia/fibrillation
Syncope, cardiac collapse	Complete atrioventricular block
	Atrioventricular block grade II
	Atrial fibrillation
New-onset heart failure in the absence of previous structural heart disease	Left ventricular dysfunction
	Biventricular dysfunction
Palpitations	Compensatory sinus tachycardia, premature beats, supraventricular tachycardia
Chest pain	Concomitant pericarditis
	Coronary artery spasm
Chronic heart failure	Dilated cardiomyopathy

In children, clinical manifestations are more often acute and severe; in neonates they are often fulminant. Preceding viral symptoms such as respiratory illness are often not apparent.

Myocarditis is a difficult clinical diagnosis at onset:

- Up to 30% may have respiratory symptoms, 30% cardiac symptoms, and 6% gastrointestinal symptoms
- Heart failure in infants is atypical with decreased appetite, profuse sweating on feeding and crying, tachypnoea, cough on strain, poor perfusion with mottled skin. Systemic venous congestion may cause hepatomegaly and consequently abdominal distension, pain and vomiting; neck vein distension and peripheral oedema are characteristic of later age
- Chest pain is the rarest symptom and raises the suspicion only if some of the other symptoms is present
- Chest X-ray and electrocardiography (ECG) have a combined high sensitivity.

Investigations

Table 7.6 Investigations for myocarditis

Investigation	Findings
Chest X-ray	Cardiomegaly
	Pulmonary venous congestion
Electrocardiography	Sinus tachycardia
	Low voltage QRS
	Inverted/flat T-waves in left precordial leads
	Myocardial infarction pattern (localized wide Q, ST segment depression/elevation)
	Axis deviation
	Pericarditis pattern (wide spread ST segment elevation)
	Conduction abnormalities (AV block, LBBB)
	Arrhythmias (VT, SVT)
Echocardiography	Hypocontractile left or both ventricles with variable dilation[a]. Mitral regurgitation (papillary dysfunction). Global or less frequently segmental myocardial deformation abnormalities. Intracavitary thrombi. Concomitant pericardial effusion
Laboratory biomarkers	Cardiac myocytolysis: cardiac troponin I, creatine kinase-MB isoform
	Heart failure: NT Pro-BNP
cMRI	Global or regional
	Oedema (increased intensity on T2-weighted)
	Capillary leak (gadolinium early enhancement)
	Necrosis/scarring (gadolinium late enhancement)

Table 7.6 (*Contd.*)

Investigation	Findings
Endomyocardial biopsy	Focal inflammatory infiltration with/without necrosis
	Immunohistology (anti-CD3, CD4, CD8, CD20, CD68, HLA class II)
PCR/RT-PCR	Viral DNA/RNA[b]
Serology and immunology	For *Borrelia*
	IgM or rising titre IgG antiviral antibodies
	Antimyosin antibodies

[a]The more acute forms have less significant dilation; right ventricular dysfunction is a sign of severity and bad prognosis.

[b]Highly specific; lower sensitivity in blood, higher sensitivity in tissue samples.

AV, atrioventricular; LBBB, left bundle branch block; HLA, human leucocyte antigen; NT Pro-BNP, N-terminal pro-brain natriuretic peptide; SVT, supraventricular tachycardia.

Echocardiography remains the cornerstone of diagnosis.
- Ventricular diameter is reported as absolute value as well as a z-score (number of standard deviations from the mean i.e. $Z > +2.0$ suggests dilation).
- Systolic function of the left ventricle is assessed by the indices of pump function and a hypocontractile left ventricle has fractional shortening (FS) <30% and ejection fraction (EF) <55%.

Laboratory biomarkers are important in the acute phase.
- Transaminases, especially aspartate aminotransferase (AST), are highly sensitive but of very low specificity.
- Troponin T and I are highly sensitive and specific markers which persist up to a week.

Magnetic resonance imaging (MRI) may visualize affected areas but is not validated in paediatric patients:
- Tissue oedema, which may result in an elevated T2 signal
- Capillary leakage, which is speculated to be associated with an increased signal on early gadolinium enhancement T1-weighted spin-echo images after gadolinium administration (elevated global relative enhancement)
- Myocardial necrosis or scarring as indicated by the presence of late gadolinium enhancement.

Endomyocardial biopsy with conventionally stained heart-tissue samples has been abandoned from the routine panel of the diagnostic work-up because of low sensitivity (about 10%).

There is increasing interest in investigating older patients as the rate of complication falls.

When is endomyocardial biopsy necessary?

Acute or fulminant heart failure of unknown aetiology:
- Rapid deterioration
- Ventricular arrhythmias
- Atrioventricular block
- No response to conventional heart failure therapy

Suspected fulminant myocarditis:
- Unexplained new-onset heart failure of <2 weeks
- Haemodynamic compromise
- Normal size or dilated left ventricle

Suspected giant cell myocarditis
- Unexplained new-onset heart failure of 2 weeks to 3 months duration
- Ventricular arrhythmias and atrioventricular block grade II (Mobitz type II), complete heart block
- No response to conventional heart failure therapy with progressive worsening

---

Establishing the cause of myocarditis may be difficult:
- The development of highly sensitive and specific PCR assays that can detect viral DNA/RNA in both blood and tissue has improved diagnostic yield, especially in the acute phase of enterovirus myocarditis.
- This enhanced capacity to detect viral genome is not without controversy, as the detection of viral genome even on myocardial biopsy does not necessarily imply that this is the aetiologic agent. This is particularly so when parvovirus is detected by PCR.
- Serological studies for viral infections can also be useful, either detectable IgM antibodies for recent infection or rising titre of IgG. Serology is still the mainstay of diagnosis of myocarditis due to *Borrelia*, especially in the presence of conduction disturbances.
- Protozoal and parasitic diseases (such as trypanosomiasis) should be considered if there is good epidemiological history.
- Diphtheria is now very rare in most of Europe/USA, however, it should be considered in any patient with appropriate signs who is from an endemic region.

Treatment

Specific antimicrobial treatment is of limited use because of the significant period between the infection and the myocarditis. Interferon has been used with variable success.

The use of immunosuppressive and anti-inflammatory treatments (corticosteroids, ciclosporin, IVIG) is controversial and not proven.

Management of heart failure

- Drugs: Diuretics, inodilators (PDE3 inhibitors: milrinone), inotropes (cathecholamines), vasodilators, calcium sensitizers (levosimendan).
- Mechanical circulatory support: extracorporeal membrane oxygenation (ECMO) or ventricular assist devices.
- Treatments aimed at providing a bridge to recovery or to allow time for cardiac transplantation.

Management of arrhythmias

- Should be treated immediately.
- Sustained ventricular tachycardia often leads to haemodynamic compromise and may require DC cardioversion.
- Amiodarone infusion is often effective.
- Oral amiodarone should be used for several months.

Outcome

- There is no validated set of criteria to predict which patients will recover, die, or be chronically ill with dilated cardiomyopathy requiring possible later transplantation.
- Fulminant lymphocytic myocarditis, with a distinct onset within 2 weeks of viral infection, has a favourable prognosis with aggressive support.
- Acute lymphocytic myocarditis, with an unclear onset and a more indolent course, more often has a poor outcome. Acute myocarditis in newborns has a poor prognosis with a mortality rate of up to 75% with most of the deaths occurring very soon after onset of disease.
- In older infants, mortality varies between 10% and 25%.
- Availability of mechanical support and transplantation significantly improves outcome.

Predictors of unfavourable outcome

- Neonatal age
- Pathologic Q-waves
- Left bundle branch block
- Right ventricular dysfunction
- High serum interluekin-10 and Fas-ligand*
- Giant cell myocarditis

Future research

The use of immunohistochemistry and MRI will allow more specific epidemiological studies in the future. The use of quantitative PCR and assessment of replicative viral intermediates is needed to differentiate between replicative viral infection and viral latency.

New and validated biomarkers for prognostic purposes are needed.

Pericarditis

In developed countries, idiopathic pericarditis comprises about 80% of all cases. These cases are presumed to be viral; as patients recover no further investigations are required and the aetiology remains unconfirmed. Pathogenesis involves both direct infection and an indirect associated immune/inflammatory response.

Epidemiology

No good population studies are available in UK. In a study in Italy published in 2008, an incidence of 27.7 cases per 100 000 of the population per year was found.

- Tuberculous pericarditis is rare in developed countries.
- Up to 5% of HIV-infected patients may have pericarditis in the absence of additional infection.
- Bacterial purulent pericarditis is a rare isolated disease and immune deficiency should be ruled out. It is more often part of a generalized infection (sepsis, osteomyelitis) or spread from a neighbouring organ (lungs, mediastinum).
- Parasitic causes should be considered when eosinophils predominate in the pericardial fluid.
- Recurrent pericarditis is most probably an autoimmune disease.
- The incidence of paediatric constrictive pericarditis has fallen in developed countries with the waning of tuberculosis and improved management of purulent pericarditis.

Clinical manifestations and course

> **When to suspect pericarditis**
>
> - Chest pain
> - General infection (pyrexia, malaise)
> - Tachypnoea, breathlessness, often without crackles
> - Systemic venous congestion (jugular venous distension, hepatomegaly, abdominal pain, vomiting, oedema)
> - Pericardial rub
> - Muffled heart sounds
> - Pulsus paradoxus (reduced volume pulse on inspiration)
> - Reduced cardiac output (tachycardia, high capillary refill time, hypotension, bradycardia)

- **Chest pain** is a highly sensitive symptom but is nonspecific and can be reported only in older children. Pericardial rub is specific but is less pronounced in bigger effusions and in those containing less fibrin.
- Children often present with respiratory or abdominal symptoms.
- Large effusions that develop slowly can be asymptomatic while smaller effusions that accumulate rapidly can present with tamponade.

Investigations

Table 7.7 Investigations for pericarditis

Chest X-ray	Cardiomegaly (normal to water bottle shadow)
	Additional pulmonary/mediastinal pathology
ECG	Early:
	Widespread concave ST-segment elevation (J-point elevated >25% of T, may be anterior + inferior only)
	PR segment deviation opposite to P
	Late:
	T-flattening and depression
Echocardiography	Pericardial effusion
	Size (small, moderate, large)
	Distribution (even, collections)
	Characteristics (streaks of fibrin, roughness of epicardial surface)
	Pretamponade, tamponade
Plasma biomarkers	Inflammation (high CRP, ESR, fibrinogen, WBC)
	Cardiac myocytolysis (cTnT/I, CK-MB, AST, ALT, LDH)
Pericardial fluid	Microscopy and culture (including for tuberculosis)
	Cell count (blood cells, unusual cells)
	Protein, albumin, triglycerides
	For tuberculosis: adenosine deaminase (ADA) >50U/l, IFN, pericardial lysozyme, PCR
Aetiology specific	PCR/RT-PCR blood/fluid for viral and bacterial causes
	Serology for IgM or rising titre of IgG antibodies
CT chest	Adjacent organs and tissues
MRI	Pericardial thickening (>4 mm in 70% of constrictive pericarditis)

ALT, alanine aminotransferase; CK, creatine kinase; LDH, lactate dehydrogenase; WBC, white blood cell.

Echocardiography (Fig. 7.1) is the mainstay of diagnosis and impacts management.

- Pericardial effusion is seen on two-dimensional sections as echolucent areas around the heart.
- Size is assessed by measuring the separation in diastole: for adults and big children small = <10 mm, moderate = 10–20 mm, and large = >20 mm; for infants and small children these values are halved i.e. small = 5 mm, moderate = 5–10 mm, large = >10 mm.
- Predominant location and presence of collections is very important to guide the decision about type of pericardiocentesis.

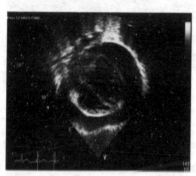

Fig. 7.1 Echocardiogram demonstrating pericardial effusion

Echocardiography signs of tamponade

- Freely floating 'swinging' heart
- Diastolic collapse of the right ventricle/atrium, less frequently left atrium and least frequently left ventricle
- Respiratory variation of inflow >25% (inspiratory increase on right and decrease on left)

These usually coincide with clinical signs:
- Worsening tachypnoea, breathlessness (often without crackles)
- Worsening tachycardia
- Low cardiac output
- Hypotension and bradycardia signal a life-threatening stage

Table 7.8 Differential diagnosis of specific forms of pericarditis

	Viral	Bacterial	Tuberculosis	Autoimmune
Aetiological evidence	PCR	Gram stain	Ziehl–Nielsen	Ig binding to epi/pericardium
		Bacterial culture	PCR	Negative viral PCR
		16S PCR	Culture	
		PCR for *Borrelia* and *Chlamydia*		
Clinical	Mild	Severe	Chronic	Chronic
		Fulminant		
Tamponade	Infrequent	80%	Frequent	Infrequent
Fluid Macroscopic	Serous/ serosanguinous	Purulent	Serosanguinous	Serous
Leucocyte count	>5000/ml	>10 000/ml	8000–10 000/ml	<5000/ml
Protein	>30g/l	High	Intermediate	Intermediate
Additional	Activated lym/ macro (sparse)	Neu/macro	ADA >40U/l	Activated lym/ macro
			PCR positive for *M. tuberculosis*	
Pericardial biopsy	Lymphocytic	Neutrophilic	Caseous granulomata, PCR	Lymphocytic
Recurrence	30–50 %	Rare	Frequent	Frequent
Mortality if left untreated	Low, depends on agent	100%	85%	25% in untreated tamponade
Constriction	Rare	Frequent	30–50%	Rare

Treatment

- Treatment of acute viral pericarditis aims to relieve symptoms, and prevent relapses. Anti-inflammatory drugs are the mainstay of therapy of acute non-purulent pericarditis.

- NSAIDs: Ibuprofen or diclofenac as well as nimesulide (selective cyclo-oxygenase-2 inhibitor) are preferred and should be continued for a minimum of 2 weeks or at least 1 week after effusion and symptoms resolve
- Corticosteroids (necessary in autoimmune diseases, usually not needed in viral).
- Percutaneous pericardiocentesis is indicated in tamponade, pretamponade and ineffective conservative management of large effusions. It is echo/fluoroscopy guided unless in emergency and a pigtail catheter may be left in situ usually for 24 hours or until drainage is less than 25ml/day or 1ml/kg/day.
- Purulent bacterial pericarditis is fatal if left untreated (Table 7.9).

Table 7.9 Treatment of purulent pericarditis

Surgical drainage of pericardium	Local antibiotics	Systemic antibiotics	Pericardiectomy
Investigate the cause	Intrapericardial helpful but not sufficient	Start with flucloxacillin (vancomycin if reason to suspect MRSA) and cefotaxime/ceftriaxone tailored to the culture results Duration: 4 weeks	Late in some cases with dense adhesions.

- Fungal pericarditis should be treated with the appropriate antifungal agent for at least 4 weeks. Tuberculosis is treated with quadruple antituberculous regimen (📖 see Chapter 113, Tuberculosis, p. 753) for 12 months. Most centres use additional adjunctive corticosteroids for the initial 1–2 months.
- In chronic pericarditis treatment should be aimed at eradicating the cause. Pericardiocentesis and anti-inflammatory drugs are supportive treatment. Pleuropericardial window or pericardectomy may be considered.
- Recurrent pericarditis should be treated with corticosteroids with a starting dose of 1.0–1.5 mg/kg/day for at least 1 month, then tapering slowly over 3 months. If relapse occurs, the last effective dose should be used for at least 3 months. NSAIDs should then be started. Colchicine is reported as being helpful.
- Chronic constrictive pericarditis requires pericardectomy, which is usually a safe and effective procedure. However, it may be difficult and risky if adhesions between the epicardium and myocardium are present.

Outcome

- The majority of viral pericarditis resolves uneventfully and quickly. Recurrence may occur in up to 30% of cases and after first relapse there is a 50% chance of this continuing.

- Purulent pericarditis still carries a mortality risk although reduced from the previously reported 25%. It may evolve into constrictive pericarditis.
- Recurrent pericarditis although difficult to manage has a favourable prognosis and usually resolves eventually.

Key reference

1 Towbin JA, Myocarditis. In: Allen HD, Driscoll DJ, Shaddy RE, Feltes TF, eds. *Moss and Adams' Heart Disease in Infants, Children, and Adolescents: Including the Fetus and Young Adults.* Lippincott Williams & Wilkins, 2007:1207–25.

Further reading

Myocarditis

Cooper LT. Myocarditis. *N Engl J Med* 2009;**360**:1526–38.

Freedman SB, Haladyn JK, Floh A, Kirsh JA, Taylor G, Thull-Freedman J. Pediatric myocarditis: emergency department clinical findings and diagnostic evaluation. *Pediatrics* 2007;**120**:1278–85.

Matthias G, Sechtem U, Schulz-Menger J, et al. for the International Consensus Group on cardiovascular magnetic resonance in Myocarditis. Cardiovascular magnetic resonance in myocarditis: A JACC white paper. *J Am Coll Cardiol* 2009;**53**:1475–87.

Towbin JA, Myocarditis. In: Allen HD, Driscoll DJ, Shaddy RE, Feltes TF, eds. Moss and Adams' Heart Disease in Infants, Children, and Adolescents: Including the Fetus and Young Adults. Lippincott Williams & Wilkins, 2007:1207–25.

Pericarditis

Imazio M, Brucato A, Trinchero R, Adler Y. Diagnosis and management of pericardial diseases. *Nat Rev Cardiol* 2009;**6**:743–51.

Maisch B, Seferovic' PM, Ristic' AD, et al. Task Force on the diagnosis and management of pericardial diseases of the European Society of Cardiology. Guideline on the diagnosis and management of pericardial diseases. *Eur Heart J* 2004;**25**:587–610.

Chapter 8

Central venous catheter infections

📖 see also Chapters 105,106

Background

Intravenous catheters are widely used to support administration of drugs, fluids, electrolytes, blood products, feeding solutions, and for haemo-dynamic monitoring.

Definition of a central venous catheter

A central venous catheter (CVC) is a catheter that is passed through a vein to end up in the thoracic (chest) portion of the vena cava (the large vein returning blood to the heart) or in the right atrium of the heart.

Types of CVC

Types of CVC include:
- Tunnelled—those placed through a subcutaneous tunnel (such as Broviac, Hickmann, Groshong). These have a Dacron cuff, which anchors the catheter and which may become enmeshed in fibrous tissue.
- Port—subcutaneous port accessed as required using a transdermal needle.
- Peripherally inserted central catheter—those placed through a peripheral vein.
- Untunnelled.
- Single or multi-lumen.
- Materials used include plastics, metals, silicone, and polyurethane.
- Antimicrobial CVCs and heparin bonded CVCs.

Advantages of CVC over peripheral cannula
- Painless and convenient vascular access.
- Reduced chance of phlebitis.
- Potential for multiple access channels.
- Large bore.
- Delivery of high concentration drugs too irritating for peripheral veins including high osmolality drugs.
- Can remain in place for months or years (if tunnelled or port).

Disadvantages
- Significant mechanical and infective complications.

Complications associated with central venous catheters
- Attributable mortality associated with severe complications may exceed 25%.
- *Mechanical*:
  - Bleeding, thrombosis, haemothorax, pneumothorax, catheter occlusion, cardiac arrhythmias, cardiac tamponade, air embolism, haematoma, local tissue damage associated with reaction to device components or extravascular leakage of infusate.
- *Infective*:
  - CVCs are the most frequent risk factor associated with hospital acquired blood stream infection, endocarditis, septic emboli, septic shock, exit site infection, phlebitis.

Frequency of infection
- Usually measured as rate/numbers of days at risk (device days): <1 to >15/1000 CVC days.
- Rates of infection vary with patient population and associated risk factors (see below).

Risk factors for CVC-associated infection
- Site of insertion: Risk lowest for subclavian, highest for femoral.
- Numbers of lumens: Increased numbers of lumens increases risk.
- Type of CVC:
  - Port probably lower risk than tunnelled CVC
  - Antimicrobial CVCs lower risk than non-antimicrobial.
- Prematurity.
- Skin disease.
- Infections at other sites.
- IV feeding.
- Co-morbidities that compromise immunity or predispose to translocation.
- Poor compliance with insertion and postinsertion 'best practice'.

Routes of CVC colonization
- Contamination at the time of insertion.
- Migration of bacteria from contaminated connections.
- Migration from the skin surface.
- Haematogenous or contiguous spread.
- Contaminated infusates.
- Early infections (within 2 weeks of implantation) more likely to result from outer surface contamination and late infections from intra-luminal contamination.

Microbiology of CVC-associated infection
- Most commonly bacteria, less commonly fungi.
- Usually skin commensals such as coagulase-negative staphylococci.
- A wide range of opportunistic pathogens have been described.
- Causative agent is an important consideration in treatment decisions.

Diagnosis

Clinical signs suggestive of CVC-associated infection

- Inflammation, induration, discharge at exit site or along tunnel.
- Exit site infection usually has local induration only of 0.5–1cm around CVC skin exit site.
- Tunnel infection has pain and induration >2cm from the skin exit site.
- Fever and/or rigors and/or hypotension associated with device manipulations.
- Septic shock or persistent fevers with a CVC in place and without alternative explanation.
- Evidence of septic emboli.
- Vomiting, limb pains and rigors in immunocompromised children with a CVC and fever is associated with a high probability of blood stream infection.

Laboratory indicators

- Raised inflammatory markers (CRP, white cell count, procalcitonin) without other explanation.
- Isolation of microbes from blood cultures.

More specific microbiological indicators

- Isolation of skin bacteria from two or more blood cultures (multisite or multisample) collected within a 48-hour period.
- Isolation of indistinguishable bacteria from the CVC tip *and* blood cultures.
- Quantitative blood cultures:
  - Blood from CVC with >1000 colony forming units (CFU)/ml
  - Difference >5-fold in CFU between blood collected from CVC and peripheral sample or between blood samples from different lumens of a CVC
  - Differential time to positivity between blood collected from CVC and periphery of >2 hours.
- Isolation or visualization of microbes on the CVC post removal.
- Presence of bacteria in blood drawn through the CVC detected by microscopy (e.g. acridine orange leucocyte cytospin (AOLC) test).
- Quantitative molecular detection of bacterial components (16SrDNA).
- Semi-quantitative CVC tip culture with >15 CFU from a 2cm segment rolled on an agar plate.

Good blood culture collection technique is very important

- Ensure an adequate blood volume is collected (depends on the size of the patient).
- Try to collect before the initiation of antibiotic therapy.
- Decontaminate skin or hubs with 2% chlorhexidine in 70% IPA (isopropyl alcohol) and allow to dry before sampling.
- Decontaminate the top of the blood culture bottles with 2% chlorhexidine in 70% IPA after removing the caps.
- Use aseptic non-touch technique when sampling blood.
- Ideally collect blood from the periphery and CVC.
- Collect blood from all CVC lumens.

Treatment

- Depends on agent of infection.
- Approximately 80% of CVC associated infections caused by coagulase-negative staphylococci (CONS) can be treated without CVC removal
- Consider the criteria for CVC removal (📖 see Criteria for CVC removal for infection).
- Antimicrobials must be administered through the CVC.
- Consider antimicrobial locks that may reduce the risk of recurrent infection (📖 see Prevention, p.72) and possibly duration of fever.
- Port-associated infection (particularly if it involves the subcutaneous pocket) may be harder to eradicate without CVC removal than infection associated with a tunnelled CVC.
- Empirical treatment in patients with suspected CVC associated infection should include a glycopeptide (such as vancomycin) and an agent active against Gram-negative bacteria.
- Consider empirical use of anti-fungals in patients at risk of fungal infection (immunocompromised, following use of broad-spectrum antibiotics, those with femoral CVCs, and those with multisite *Candida* colonization).

Antibiotic treatment duration

- Duration of therapy is defined as starting from the time that the blood cultures become negative.
- Optimum duration unknown.
- Uncomplicated infection with CONS duration 7–14 days.
- Prolonged durations may be required when bacteraemia/fungaemia persists despite CVC removal.
- Prolonged durations may be required with *Staphylococcus aureus* infection, unless the patient is immunocompetent, the CVC is removed promptly and there is no evidence of complications, in which case 1–2 weeks may be sufficient.

Some antimicrobial lock solutions

- Vancomycin 2.5 mg/ml or 5.0 mg/ml with heparin 2500 or 5000 IU/ml
- Gentamicin 1.0 mg/ml with heparin 2500 IU/ml
- Ethanol 70%

Criteria for CVC removal for infection

When:
- The CVC is the suspected source of infection and is no longer critically required or relatively straightforward to replace
- Clinical evidence of infection persists despite appropriate antibiotic treatment
- There is tunnel infection (extending >2cm from exit site)
- There is evidence of serious complications (suppurative thrombophlebitis, septic shock, endocarditis, septic emboli)
- There is persistent fever, bacteraemia, or fungaemia despite appropriate antibiotic treatment
- There is CVC infection with *S. aureus* (high risk of endocarditis etc.), antibiotic-resistant species (e.g. *Pseudomonas* spp., *Stenotrophomonas*

spp., *Mycobacterium* spp., *Acinetobacter* spp., *Corynebacteria*), Candida or other fungi.

Prevention

There is considerable evidence from quality improvement programmes that many CVC associated infections can be prevented by:

- Specific training with respect to both insertion technique and post insertion care
- The use of maximal sterile barrier precautions at the time of CVC insertion
- Chlorhexidine in 70% isopropyl alcohol-based skin disinfection (2% probably better than 0.5%)
- Good hand hygiene every time pre and post care
- Standardization of equipment and techniques (CVC insertion pack/trolley)
- Use of needle-less injectable hubs on all ports, decontaminated with 2% chlorhexidine in 70% IPA prior to accessing
- Aseptic non-touch technique for drug administration and blood sampling
- Limit disconnections and reconnections to essential only
- Tunnelled or port CVCs for longer-term CVCs
- Slow-release chlorhexidine dressing at the exit site probably reduces the risk of infection, particularly with short-term CVCs
- Antimicrobial CVCs reduce the risk of infection with short-term CVCs
- Antibiotic impregnated and heparin benzalkonium-bonded probably more effective at preventing infection than silver-based CVCs—a trial is underway
- Considerable evidence that antimicrobial locks can prevent >50% of CVC-associated infections.

Further research

- Role of antibiotic- and heparin-bonded lines in children and neonates.

Further reading

Mermel LA, Allon M, Bouza E, *et al.* Clinical practice guidelines for the diagnosis and management of intravscular catheter-related infection: 2009 Update by the Infectious Diseases Society of America. *Clin Infect Dis* 2009;**49**:1–45.

Pittiruti M, Hamilton H, Biffi R, MacFie J, Pertkiewicz M. ESPEN guidelines on parenteral nutrition: central venous catheters (access, care, diagnosis and therapy of complications). *Clin Nutr* 2009;**28**:365–77.

Raad I, Hanna H, Maki D. Intravascular catheter-related infections: advances in diagnosis, prevention, and management. *Lancet Infect Dis* 2007;**7**:645–7.

Chronic fatigue syndrome

📖 see also Chapter 65

Introduction

The aetiology of chronic fatigue syndrome (CFS) is unclear and it is likely that a number of factors are involved. There is limited evidence that infective, immunological, family, and psychological factors all have some part in the causation of CFS.

Causative organism/evidence of infection

- A subgroup of children with apparent chronic fatigue will describe a viral infection at the onset of symptoms.
- When there is laboratory evidence of such an infection then the diagnosis of postviral fatigue can be made.
- These cases form a minority of cases of chronic fatigue.
- In a study from Australia involving adults (16 years and over) chronic fatigue followed infection with *Coxiella burnetii* (Q fever), EBV (glandular) fever, and Ross river virus (epidemic polyarthritis) in 28/253 (11%) of patients assessed 6 months after infection.
- There is no evidence that minor upper respiratory or gastrointestinal infections lead to postviral fatigue.

Epidemiology

- A UK-based general practitioner (GP) survey of medically unexplained fatigue for >3 months suggested a prevalence of 62/100 000.
- Surveys from elsewhere have suggested a wide range of prevalence in teenagers from 2.7 to 48/100 000.
- The mean range of onset when just children and young adults are considered tends to be 12–14 years.
- There appears to be a female preponderance.

Clinical presentation and differential diagnosis

- The most commonly reported symptom is severe fatigue (mental and/ or physical) exacerbated by exercise, activity, or intercurrent infection.
- Often associated features include: severe malaise; headache; sleep disturbance; depressed mood; myalgia; muscle pain at rest and on exercise; nausea; sore throat; tender lymph nodes; abdominal pain and arthralgia.
- The patients seen in primary care reported a mean of three symptoms at presentation but those seen attending a tertiary clinic, who had been ill for longer, reported eight symptoms.
- Some children have symptoms or diagnosis of depression and anxiety. Others also exhibit school phobia, somatization, and social withdrawal.
- A number of specific diagnostic criteria have been proposed (☐ see Evidence Based Guideline for the Management of CFS/ME (Chronic Fatigue Syndrome/Myalgic Encephalopathy[1]).
- The main symptom in these criteria is disabling, disruptive fatigue that is persistent; and a diagnosis is made when other causes of fatigue have been excluded by clinical examination and laboratory tests.
- A diagnosis of postviral fatigue can be made in a subgroup of children with apparent fatigue who give a history of a virus infection at the onset of symptoms with confirmed laboratory evidence of this.
- The main differential diagnosis is with psychiatric symptoms, such as depression.
- Other diagnoses that need to be considered include: anaemia (which may be dietary, or the result of other causes such as chronic renal failure and leukaemia); chronic infections, such as recurrent tonsillitis, EBV infection; gastrointestinal conditions such as Crohn's and coeliac disease. Endocrine conditions such as hypothyroidism and Addison's disease should also be considered.
- Rarely, in some of the more persistent cases in which no improvement occurs over a long period, or parents seem unwilling to comply with treatment, child abuse should be considered.
- A full physical examination is important. This should include: measurement of height and weight; assessment of anaemia; neurological examination including that of the fundi and assessment of muscle wasting; assessment of lymph nodes including spleen; palpation of the sinuses to identify chronic sinusitis; measurement of blood pressure; and examination of the neck to exclude a goitre and abdomen for signs of inflammatory bowel disease. In children with CFS there are very rarely any objective clinical signs, despite many clinical symptoms.

Investigations

- As one would expect there is no specific diagnostic test but investigations are required to exclude conditions within the differential diagnosis.
- Even if the clinical picture makes anything other than CFS unlikely, parents often find it reassuring for investigations to be performed.

Recommended blood tests for CFS
- Full blood count and film
- Ferritin
- Viscosity or ESR
- CRP
- Blood glucose
- Urea and electrolytes
- Creatinine kinase
- Thyroid function
- Liver function
- Viral serology—for EBV IgM and IgG, and EBNA (EBV nuclear antigen)
- Screening test for coeliac disease (tissue transglutaminase (TTG) or antiendomysial antibodies)

Treatment

Part of the treatment is a clear clinical diagnosis of CFS, and a thorough explanation of the diagnosis and outcome.

- Although there are claims made for the effectiveness of many different types of treatment including anti-infective agents—antibiotics; immunoglobulins; complementary therapy (acupuncture, aromatherapy to name but a few) these are not based on any supportive evidence.
- The recommended treatment involves activity management—establishing a baseline of activity level and gradual increases as appropriate; clear psychological support giving advice and symptomatic treatment as required and a regular clinical review of progress. It helps families to see the same person with regular planned appointments every few months, with a thorough clinical examination every time. It is not usually necessary to repeat blood tests.
- In children with a more severe and prolonged illness, a multidisciplinary team approach is recommended, including a paediatrician, physiotherapist, occupational therapist and psychologist.
- The outcome overall is good, with most studies reporting 75–90% improvement over 2–3 years. There are often periods of relapse associated with intercurrent viral upper respiratory infections, especially in the winter. Children with CFS are usually better in the summer periods. Families should be encouraged towards slow but steady progress over time, recognizing that relapses and set backs will occur. Continued attendance at school (even if only for a few mornings a week) is very important, as is social contact with friends. A positive attitude towards eventual recovery is realistic based on the literature.

Key reference

1 Evidence Based Guideline for the Management of CFS/ME (Chronic Fatigue Syndrome/Myalgic Encephalopathy) in Children and Young People. London:Royal College of Paediatrics and Child Health, 2004; Available at: ℛ www.rcpch.ac.uk (accessed 1 February 2011).

Further reading

Davenport T, Wakefield D, et al. Post-infective and chronic fatigue syndromes precipitated by viral and non-viral pathogens: prospective cohort study. BMJ 2006;**333**:575–8.

Congenital infections

📖 see also Chapters 30, 57, 58, 62, 64, 77, 93, 101, 107, 112

Introduction

- Congenital infections include those acquired by the infant during gestation. They may be divided according to the timing of acquisition: intrauterine (first, second, or third trimester), perinatal, or even postnatal.
- The timing of transmission during gestation may significantly affect the outcome in the infant. The ability of organisms to cross to the fetus changes according to the maturity of the placenta.
- The effects of the organism on the fetus also vary during gestation (e.g. with toxoplasmosis, transplacental infection is much more likely to occur during the third trimester, however, when first trimester transmission does occur severe fetal organ damage is more likely).
- It is important to know what proportion of maternal infections transmit to the fetus, as this is by no means inevitable (e.g. for CMV overall only 40% of maternal infections will transmit to the fetus).
- Congenital infections may be caused by a new or primary infection in the mother, which may be symptomatic or asymptomatic (e.g. rubella, CMV, syphilis, toxoplasmosis); primary infections are more likely to have severe manifestations in the fetus.
- Congenital infections may also be caused by reactivation of a latent maternal infection (e.g. CMV, syphilis, HSV), these tend to have less frequent or less severe manifestations as there is some degree of maternal immunity that may be passed to the fetus.
- The usual lack of significant maternal illness means that screening for congenital infections is often the only way to diagnose that they have occurred.
- Screening programmes also have to consider the frequency of the infection: the sensitivity and specificity of the tests used (high rates of false-positive tests are not acceptable in this setting); and the availability of effective interventions to prevent transmission.
- In the UK the following serological pregnancy screening tests are routinely undertaken at booking: rubella, syphilis, HIV, HBV. In other countries, depending on seroprevalence, regional or national programmes of serological screening for CMV, hepatitis C (HCV), and toxoplasmosis are also undertaken.
- Antenatal screening may identify women at risk of: acquiring infection in pregnancy (e.g. those with no antibodies to rubella); transmitting persistent bloodborne infections (e.g. HIV, HBV, HCV); or transmitting acquired and treatable infections (e.g. syphilis).
- Table 10.1 lists important microorganisms causing congenital infections.

Transplacental infections

These may occur at different times during gestation, and the organisms often have a predilection for infection of placental tissue.

- Bacteria: *Listeria*, syphilis, tuberculosis
- Protozoa: *Toxoplasma*, malaria
- Viruses: rubella, CMV, parvovirus B19, HSV, varicella, enteroviruses

Perinatal infections

These may be transmitted late in pregnancy via the placenta, via birth canal exposure, or early familial/nosocomial exposure.

- Bacteria (including atypicals): gonococcus, *chlamydia*, *Mycoplasma*, GBS, MRSA
- Viruses: HIV 1 and 2, HBV, HCV, human papillomavirus (HPV), HSV 1 and 2, CMV, EBV, human herpesvirus-6 (HHV-6), VZV, enteroviruses

Postnatal infections

These may be transmitted via breast milk or early family/nosocomial exposure.

- Viruses: HIV 1 and 2, human T cell lymphotropic virus 1 (HTLV-1), HBV, CMV, varicella, enteroviruses

Table 10.1 Microorganisms and vertical transmission

	Intrauterine	Perinatal
Bacteria	*Listeria*	Gonococcus
	Tryponema pallidum	*Chlamydia*
	Mycobacterium tuberculosis	*Mycoplasma*
Protozoa	*Toxoplasma*	
	Plasmodium	
Viruses	Rubella	HIV 1 and 2
	Cytomegalovirus	Hepatitis B, C
	Parvovirus B 19	Human papilloma virus
	Herpes simplex virus <———>	Herpes simplex virus
	Varicella <·········>	Varicella
	Enterovirus <·········>	Enterovirus

Clinical presentation

After intrauterine transmission the infant may present at delivery with signs of fetal infection and organ damage. In addition, infants apparently normal at birth may subsequently develop manifestations of disease.

The **neonate with severe symptomatic infection** may present with multisystem disease and may be severely unwell; the differential diagnosis includes: sepsis, metabolic disorders, and malignancy (Fig. 10.1).

- **Skin/mucous membranes**: Petechial rash of thrombocytopenia; 'blueberry muffin' ecchymotic rash of intradermal haematopoiesis; ulcerating/blistering lesions from herpetic or syphilitic infection.
- **CNS**: Signs of long-term and ongoing damage with microcephaly, calcification, hydrocephalus, migration defects, microphthalmia, cataracts, retinitis, hearing loss.
- **Reticuloendothelial system**: Lymphadenopathy, hepatosplenomegaly, bone marrow failure with cytopenias.
- **Lungs**: Pneumonitis.
- **Heart**: Multiple structural defects.
- **Gut**: Hepatitis, jaundice, luminal strictures, malabsorption.
- **Bones**: Osteochondritis in syphilis.

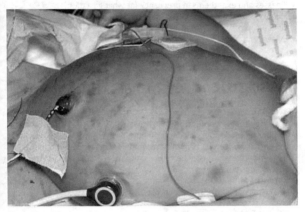

Fig. 10.1 'Blueberry muffin baby'—a sick neonate with a congenital infection, but which one?

(Thanks to Dr Rodney Rivers for this image).

Approach

- Diagnosis of suspected congenital infection *in utero* depends on investigation of mother and fetus; diagnosis after birth depends on investigation of the mother, neonate, and placenta.
- Serology is rarely sufficient and, especially in symptomatic neonates, the immature immune system may not have mounted a timely serological response.
- Absence of infection-specific fetal IgM is common at birth and the antibodies may only be produced after several months, if at all.
- Every effort should be made to specifically detect the infection whether by culture or PCR.

- When samples are taken from a symptomatic infant after birth this should be as soon as possible, as the yield will be greater.
- This multipronged investigational approach should replace the old fashioned serological 'TORCH' screen. The blood test 'TORCH screen' should never be ordered any more!
- Always discuss these cases with your microbiologist/virologist.

Maternal history

- Prior immunization history
- Occupational history (works in childcare—CMV; healthcare—MRSA)
- Contact with animals (*Toxoplasma*)
- Travel history (malaria, tuberculosis, West Nile)
- Vegetarian or eats rare/cured meats (*Toxoplasma*, *Listeria*)
- Illnesses and exanthems in pregnancy (at what gestation?)
- History of sexually transmitted infections
- Illnesses in other children
- Evidence of poor *in utero* growth
- Labour history and duration of rupture of membranes.

Investigations

Maternal

- **Serology for new infections**: High avidity IiG (more mature immune response—more sticky/avid IgG) implies previous infection; low avidity IgG and presence of IgM implies recent infection, usually within the last 6 months, which may be relevant to fetal transmission (e.g. for *Toxoplasma*, parvovirus or CMV).
- **Persistent infections**: Serological tests are undertaken as part of screening, risk of transmission is usually related to maternal burden of disease so plasma viral load testing is also required (e.g. HIV 1, 2, HBV, HCV, HTLV-1).

Fetus

Serial ultrasound scanning, amniocentesis with amniotic fluid sampling, and fetal blood sampling, may all be used to identify transmission of infection, and severity of fetal organ damage. Serology, culture, and PCR on samples may be undertaken. Fetal MRI is an increasingly used modality, although care should be taken with interpretation.

Neonate

- **Cultures and/or PCR**: Specimens should be collected from skin, mucous membranes, any vesicular lesions, blood, urine, CSF. Dark ground microscopy of ulcerated skin or mucosal lesions may give a rapid diagnosis of syphilis. Diagnosis of congenital as opposed to perinatally acquired CMV depends on a positive urine result (by PCR, culture or DEAFF test) within the first 21 days of life. This demonstrates how important it is to get the neonatal samples as soon as possible after birth, ideally within 24 hours. But do not use cord blood as it may be contaminated.

- **Paired serology at birth**, from mother and newborn may identify significantly raised titres in the infant or presence of fetal IgM (e.g. for syphilis).

Placenta

This can be very helpful in achieving the diagnosis, by histology, culture, or PCR (e.g. for *Listeria*, tuberculosis, or syphilis).

Specific congenital infections to consider

Cytomegalovirus

Virus characteristics: HHV-5, double-stranded DNA virus. Infection of the host leads to establishment of viral latency with the risk of later reactivation. The majority of severe congenital infections are caused by primary infections in pregnancy rather than reactivation of latent infection.

Epidemiology: Primary CMV infection in pregnancy occurs in around 0.5% of seronegative women. Antenatal seropositivity depends on previous early life exposure (Caucasian—50%; Asian/African Caribbean—95%). Mothers at risk of infection include: adolescents; mothers with other children <2 years of age; and mothers who work in children's nurseries. The UK incidence of congenital CMV is around 0.5–1/1000 livebirths.

Transmission and incubation period: Most infections in children and adults are asymptomatic, but a febrile, mononucleosis-like illness with rash may occur. Women who have been diagnosed with a primary CMV infection are advised not to get pregnant for the next year to reduce the risk of fetal transmission.

- *Fetus:* Transmission is not inevitable, only 40% of infants born to a mother with CMV infection during pregnancy are CMV infected. Where the fetus has early *in utero* evidence of CNS damage (e.g. calcification, hydrocephalus, microcephaly, etc.) the long-term prognosis is poor. Echogenic bowel on fetal ultrasound scan can be a sign of congenital CMV infection.
- *Infant:* At birth, 5–10% of CMV infected infants present with multisystem disease (see above), the remainder are clinically asymptomatic. CMV plasma viral load at birth is highest in the most symptomatic infants, but it is a poor predictor of outcome. The main CMV related problem that may manifest later is sensory neural deafness; this may be detected on newborn hearing screening, but can develop at any time in the first 5 years of life. The incidence of significant sensory neural hearing loss due to congenital CMV infection is 0.2–0.4/1000 livebirths.

Perinatal CMV infection from the birth canal or breast milk is common and usually asymptomatic. To distinguish between perinatal and congenital infection neonatal samples should be taken as soon as possible after birth.

Congenitally and perinatally infected infants may asymptomatically excrete high levels of CMV in the urine for months or even years, this is why seronegative women working in daycare are at increased risk of infection.

Diagnosis:
- *Mother:* Seroconversion, with low avidity IgG and IgM.
- *Fetus:* Ultrasound scans; amniotic fluid CMV PCR; fetal blood CMV PCR.
- *Neonate:* Blood, urine, CSF—CMV PCR; antigen detection; culture; seroconversion not reliable, may only produce IgM many months after birth.

Management: antenatally, for the severely affected fetus, early termination of pregnancy may be offered. Antenatally, anti-CMV treatment to the mother is not recommended, but trials of immunoglobulin and valaciclovir are under way.

The symptomatic neonate may be treated with 6 weeks of iv ganciclovir; especially if there is evidence of CNS disease, severe hepatitis, pneumonitis, retinitis, bone marrow suppression, etc. Treatment will also reduce the risk of progression of deafness. A randomized controlled trial of 6 weeks versus 6 months of oral valganciclovir in neonates with all symptomatic CMV disease has started.

Prevention: Increased public awareness of CMV infection; good hygiene procedures in children's nurseries. A vaccine for seronegative women is in development.

Rubella

Congenital rubella syndrome was the first congenital infection identified; the syndrome was recognized before the virus was discovered.

Virus characteristics: Rubella is an RNA togavirus. The virus particle is 70 nm in diameter with nucleocapsid containing genomic RNA and lipid envelope. Humans are the only known hosts.

Epidemiology: Prior to widespread availability of rubella vaccine, 200–300 babies per year were born with congenital rubella syndrome (CRS) in the UK. Due to widespread vaccination CRS is very rare now in the UK; 8 of the 11 cases of CRS in England and Wales reported between 2000 and 2007 were infected abroad.

Transmission and incubation period: Incubation period is 13–20 days. Transplacental spread occurs during periods of viraemia.
- *Adults:* there may be prodromal symptoms including low-grade fever, headache, coryza, cough, sore throat, malaise, and conjunctivitis lasting 1–5 days prior to rash becoming visible. There may be an erythematous pinpoint rash seen on the soft palate. The rubella rash appears after an average incubation period of 14 days (range 12–21 days). Lymphadenopathy is classically suboccipital but may be generalized.

- *Fetus*: The outcome is predominantly dependent on fetal gestation at acquisition of maternal infection. At 8–10 weeks of gestation up to 90% of surviving fetuses may be damaged. The risk of damage thereafter falls greatly to less than 20% between 11 and 16 weeks. Deafness may result from infection prior to 20 weeks' gestation, although severe fetal damage is rare after 16 weeks.
- *Neonates* with congenital rubella syndrome may be born with intrauterine growth retardation, microcephaly, structural cardiac anomalies, cataracts, deafness and focal inflammatory damage in the bone marrow, liver, lungs, and brain.

Asymptomatic neonates may later develop abnormal neurology, and haematological and immunological dysfunction.

Diagnosis: Laboratory diagnosis may be made by rubella PCR on a range of samples including EDTA blood, nasopharyngeal aspirate (NPA), urine, and CSF. Rubella IgM is not a reliable marker. Chorionic villous sampling can be used to identify infection in the first trimester.

Management: Symptomatic and supportive.

Prevention: Vaccination (but current poor uptake of the measles, mumps, and rubella (MMR) vaccine in certain areas may put young mothers at increased risk in the future).

Parvovirus B19

Virus characteristics: Small non-enveloped DNA virus. Bone marrow erythroid precursors are preferentially infected.

Transmission: Host range limited to humans, spread by respiratory secretions.

- *Adults:* Parvovirus causes slapped cheek or fifth disease in children, adults may develop an exanthematous rash accompanied by arthralgias, but infections are often asymptomatic. Most women infected with parvovirus B19 infection during pregnancy have healthy babies. However, in around 5–10% hydrops fetalis and even fetal death may rarely occur secondary to viral replication in the bone marrow and possibly also the fetal myocardium. Spontaneous recovery of hydropic fetuses may occur with subsequent delivery of a normal infant.
- *Fetus:* Infection without fetal loss or hydrops is common. There is no evidence of B19-associated congenital abnormality in the newborn or developmental abnormalities appearing later in childhood.

Diagnosis: Maternal infection with B19 virus elicits prompt IgM and IgG-peaks within 30 days. IgG persists for years. IgM falls 30–60 days after onset of illness and may reach undetectable levels by 60–90 days.

Management: Maternal serum should be collected as soon after contact as possible and submitted to the laboratory with full clinical and epidemiological details:

- On diagnosis of parvovirus B19 infection, ultrasound scanning of the fetus is started 4 weeks post onset of illness or date of seroconversion, and then at 1–2 weekly intervals until 30 weeks' gestation.
- If findings suggestive of hydrops fetalis, or its development, are found, the patient should be referred to a regional unit for fetal medicine for consideration of fetal blood sampling and intrauterine blood transfusion. Doppler assessment of the middle cerebral artery for anaemia and parvovirus B19 genome detection in amniotic fluid may also be undertaken.

Varicella zoster virus

Virus characteristics: HHV-3, DNA virus. Early infection in pregnancy may lead to the very rare **congenital varicella syndrome**. Perinatal exposure around the time of delivery may lead to severe **neonatal varicella syndrome**.

Epidemiology: 90% of adults are VZV-seropositive, primary maternal infection occurs in 5/10 000 pregnancies.

Transmission and incubation period: Respiratory droplet spread, 10–20 days.

Congenital varicella syndrome

Risk of CVS if pregnant woman gets chicken pox:
- <1% prior to 13 weeks' gestation
- 2% between 13 and 20 weeks.

Clinical features:
- Cataracts and chorioretinitis
- Limb hypoplasia
- Cortical and muscular atrophy
- Low birthweight
- Dermatomal skin scarring—unique to VZV.

Neonatal varicella syndrome:
If chicken pox occurs in pregnant woman up to 1 week before or 1 week after delivery a severe or fatal infection may occur in the neonate due to disseminated VZV.

All such neonates should receive varicella zoster immunoglobulin (VZIG). If any symptoms develop, despite VZIG, high-dose IV aciclovir treatment should be started as soon as possible. Most neonatologist give prophylactic IV aciclovir in neonates whose mothers develop varicella from 4 days before to 3 days after delivery (these babies are at highest risk of fatal outcome despite VZIG prophylaxis).

Diagnosis:
- *Maternal:* Mothers who are in contact with VZV in pregnancy and do not have a good clinical history of chicken pox should be tested for IgG; if negative they should be offered VZIG.

- *Neonate*: VZV immunofluorescence and PCR of vesicle fluid, CSF (if available) and EDTA blood.

Treatment:
- Supportive management
- High dose IV aciclovir
- Exposed: VZIG

Syphilis

Bacterial characteristics: Spirochaete, *Treponema pallidum*.

Epidemiology: In the UK in 2004 there were 2254 cases of syphilis (a rise of 30% on the preceding year), and in 2005 there were 36 cases of congenital syphilis. An HPA/ British Paediatric Surveillance Unit (BPSU) UK prospective study of congenital syphilis is currently underway.

Transmission and incubation period: Infants are much more likely to be infected if mother has primary (100%) or secondary syphilis during pregnancy than if she acquired syphilis months or years before conception.

Clinical features:
- *Fetal:* 30–40% fetuses with congenital syphilis are stillborn. Infection of the fetus occurs most commonly in the second/third trimesters.
- *Neonatal:* Two-thirds of infected infants are asymptomatic at birth but present with symptoms within the first 5 weeks.

Congenital syphilis may present with: Hepatosplenomegaly (nearly always present), prematurity, intrauterine growth retardation (IUGR), generalized lymphadenopathy, osteochondritis, mucocutaneous, renal, CNS, and ocular manifestations.

If a neonate has unexplained prematurity, failure to thrive, persistent rhinitis, jaundice, or low platelets and no other explanation, consider syphilis. Neonatal syphilis may follow contact with maternal primary lesions in the birth canal during delivery.

Late disease after 2 years: multisystem involvement of brain, bones, joints, teeth, skin and eyes. Interstitial keratitis may present after 5 years of age and deafness may present only in adulthood.

Diagnosis: all infants born to mothers with positive syphilis serology should be assessed for congenital infection:
- Dark ground microscopy for presence of *T. pallidum* in mucocutaneous lesions (but negative result does not exclude infection).
- Presence of treponemal specific IgM is diagnostic but of low sensitivity.
- Greater than fourfold rise in Venereal Disease Research Laboratory (VDRL)/rapid plasma reagin (RPR) or *Treponema pallidum* particle agglutination (TPPA) titres compared to maternal titres.
- Test at birth, 6 weeks, 3, 6, and 12 months or until passive maternal antibody lost.
- CSF—antibodies with VDRL test and Treponemal PCR.
- Radiological examination of long bones and ribs.
- Placenta—examine directly for organisms, by PCR and by immunohistochemistry.

Management:
- *Maternal:* Liaise with adult genitourinary medicine team to ascertain whether the mother has had a documented complete course of treatment. There is still a risk of neonatal infection if the mother is treated for syphilis within 1 month of delivery, if erythromycin or other non-penicillin containing treatment regimen is used or if the mother shows poor serological response to therapy.
- *Infant:*
  - Treatment: Aqueous crystalline penicillin G for 10–14 days (IV or intramuscular (IM))
  - After treatment 70% should be VDRL negative by 1 year
  - All should have a negative treponemal antibody test at 15–18 months.

Which infants should be treated for congenital syphilis?
Treat if:
- Clinical signs and VDRL positive
- No signs but infant VDRL titre 4× higher than maternal titre
- Any abnormal investigation and VDRL positive.

Consider treating if:
- No signs, no abnormal investigations + VDRL positive but mother unlikely to return for follow-up.

Follow closely if:
- No signs, no abnormal investigations and VDRL positive
- Mother possible inadequate treatment
- Late gestation infection
- Previously undiagnosed mother develops secondary or tertiary disease within a few years of birth.

Prevention:
- Effective antenatal serological screening and treatment
- In outbreaks screen women infected in the third trimester as well as in the first.

Toxoplasma

Protozoal characteristics: *Toxoplasma gondii* is an obligate intracellular protozoan that causes widespread zoonosis. Although the cat is the definitive host, most human infections are from eating undercooked or cured meat (lamb, beef).

Epidemiology: USA 0.08/1000 livebirths; Paris, Vienna, 3/1000 livebirths.

Transmission and incubation period: Risk of fetal infection increases with gestation but the severity of infection is correspondingly reduced:
- Infections in first and second trimester most harmful to fetus
- Infection in third trimester usually subclinical with infected baby appearing normal.

Clinical features:
Congenital infection: Almost exclusively due to primary maternal infection in pregnancy. Most maternal infections asymptomatic or mild. The classical infant triad of hydrocephalus, cerebral calcification,

and chorioretinitis is rarely seen. Features vary widely and include: hydrocephalus, cerebral calcification, microcephaly, microphthalmia, chorioretinitis, hepatosplenomegaly, and jaundice.

Up to 85% congenitally infected babies seem normal at birth but may later develop retinitis, epilepsy, and learning difficulties. (Note: a similar picture can be seen very rarely with congenital lymphocytic choriomeningitis virus; check if hydrocephalus and *Toxoplasma* serology is all negative)

Diagnosis:
- *Mother:* Seroconversion (IgG, IgA, IgM)
- *Fetus:* Amniotic fluid, fetal blood, seroconversion and/or *Toxoplasma* PCR. Ultrasound may show cerebral ventricular dilatation, intracranial calcifications, placental thickening, and an enlarged, echogenic liver
- *Placenta:* PCR, histopathology
- *Infant:* Seroconversion (IgG, IgA, IgM); CSF—*Toxoplasma* PCR, or IgA, IgM

Treatment:
This is controversial, potentially toxic, and should be discussed with an infectious diseases team.

In pregnancy:
- Before 32 weeks gestation, use spiramycin; after 32 weeks, use pyrimethamine and sulfadiazine.

In neonate:
- Before starting treatment in the neonate a full examination of all the organ systems must be undertaken; treatment should only be given if there are signs of organ disease.
- Sulfadiazine, pyrimethamine, and folinic acid for 6–12 months.

Prevention: Avoidance of exposure to cat litter, unwashed vegetables, and undercooked/cured meat in pregnancy.

Herpes simplex virus 1 and 2
Virus characteristics: HHV-1 and 2, DNA viruses.

Epidemiology:
- Adult seroprevalence—HSV-1 40–90%, HSV-2 10–60%.
- Frequency of genital herpes in pregnancy: 1% (most are recurrences).
- Seroconversion rate for HSV in pregnancy: 3.7%.
- Incidence of neonatal herpes infection 0.2/1000 live births.
- Both HSV 1 and 2 perinatal infections may cause severe neonatal disease.

Transmission and incubation period:
- Maternal infection may be primary or due to reactivation of HSV (viral load higher in primary).
- Genital lesions present at birth.

- Prolonged rupture of membranes.
- Use of scalp monitors.
- Symptoms may appear 4–5 days after birth—most disseminated infections becoming apparent by 11–12 days.

Clinical features:

- *Skin, eye, mouth disease:* Vesicles/crusted lesions on the skin or mucous membranes, especially where trauma occured in the first week of life—may have retinitis, and progress to CNS disease in the second week. Skin recurrences are frequent and up to 30% have long-term neurological sequelae.
- *Encephalitis:* infants usually become symptomatic in second week of life, rash is only present in up to 30%. The baby may be encephalopathic with seizures; cerebrospinal fluid (CSF) pleocytosis and raised protein are common. If untreated: has at least 50% mortality and very high morbidity.
- *Disseminated infection:* present as if with severe sepsis at around day 4–6; in 50% there is a rash. Other manifestations include: pneumonitis, liver failure, coagulopathy, encephalitis. If untreated has 100% mortality—clues are rapidly worsening hepatitis and clotting tests.

Diagnosis: HSV DNA by PCR on blood, CSF, swabs from mouth, conjunctiva, skin, or mucosal lesions.

Management: IV high-dose aciclovir is recommended treatment for disseminated neonatal herpes/herpes encephalitis and Skin, Eye and Mouth Disease. Treatment must be started immediately on suspicion, do not wait for test results. High-dose aciclovir should be given for at least 3 weeks, or longer if there are ongoing symptoms. Relapses are common and many clinicians will give long-term oral suppressive therapy to prevent recurrence for at least the first year of life.

Prevention:

- Screening of symptomatic women in pregnancy (but most have no symptoms).
- Treatment of diagnosed maternal infections with aciclovir.
- Elective caesarean section delivery if very active primary genital herpes lesions are present at term.

Chlamydia trachomatis

Pathogen characteristics: Aerobic, intracellular pathogen.

Epidemiology: 2–10% asymptomatic infection in young women. After vaginal delivery to an infected mother, 25% of infants develop conjunctivitis within 7 days. This is usually mild, but may be severe and clinically indistinguishable from gonococcal ophthalmia neonatorum.

Clinical features and sequelae: Up to 5% of infants with eye disease may develop pneumonia (after 4–12 weeks). This may present with a staccato cough in a baby who is often systemically well. Fever and hypoxia may or may not be present.

Diagnosis: PCR/culture.

Management: Treat infant with erythromycin (20% relapse rate). Arrange genitourinary screening and treatment for mother and partner.

Pregnancy interventions to prevent or treat intrauterine infections

Table 10.2 lists possible interventions to prevent or minimize damage caused by congenital infections.

Table 10.2 Interventions to prevent or treat congenital infections

Maternal screening for infection:	HBV, HCV, HIV, HTLV-1, syphilis, rubella, CMV, *Toxoplasma*
Pre-pregnancy or during pregnancy (national screening protocols differ)	
Maternal immunization	Currently rubella
	Possibly in future: VZV, CMV
Fetal monitoring:	
Invasive to detect infection	CMV, rubella, *Toxoplasma*, parvovirus B19
Non-invasive to detect viral damage	
Maternal + fetal treatment considered	*Toxoplasma*, HSV, VZV, parvovirus B19, HBV, HIV

Future research

- Improved antenatal diagnostic tests.
- Further clinical trials in the antenatal and postnatal treatment.
- Improved evidence base for screening for rarer infections.

Further reading

Health Protection Agency. Available at: 🔊 www.hpa.org.uk/ (accessed 22 March 2010).

Long SS. *Principles and Practice of Pediatric Infectious Diseases.* Edinburgh: Churchill Livingstone, 2008.

Newell ML, McIntyre J. *Congenital and Perinatal Infections: Prevention, Diagnosis and Treatment.* Cambridge: Cambridge University Press, 2000.

Yeung S, Kenny J. Infection in the foetus and neonate. *Medicine*, 2009:**37**:613–20.

Chapter 11

Conjunctivitis

📖 see also Chapters 31, 46, 57, 68, 77, 105

Introduction

Conjunctivitis is the most frequently presenting disorder of the eye. It is usually self-limiting and the risk of long-term complications is low. It involves inflammation of the conjunctiva; associated corneal involvement gives rise to keratoconjunctivitis.

Conjunctivitis may be due to bacterial or viral infection or allergic hypersensitivity (not addressed here).

Causative organisms

Bacteria are responsible for 33–78% of cases (especially in infants and toddlers).
- More likely in non-epidemic conjunctivitis.
- Most common organisms involved are *Haemophilus influenzae*, *Streptococcus pneumoniae* (especially serotypes 19F, 6A, and 14 in Europe), and *Moraxella catarrhalis*.
- Conjunctivitis-otitis syndrome occurs in 20–73% of cases of bacterial conjunctivitis (most cultures yield *H. influenzae*).
- Role of staphylococcal species in pathogenesis is controversial—they are isolated from the conjunctivae of children with conjunctivitis and asymptomatic children at equal rates.
- *Neisseria meningitidis* rarely causes conjunctivitis.
- Neonatal conjunctivitis (ophthalmia neonatorum) is usually caused by *Neisseria gonorrhoeae* (<1 week of age), or *Chlamydia trachomatis* (>1 week of age).
- Other bacteria occasionally implicated in neonatal infection include *Staphylococcus aureus* and *Staphylococcus epidermidis*, *Pseudomonas aeruginosa*, and viridans streptococci.

Viral conjunctivitis is more common in school-age children and adolescents.
- Adenoviruses are responsible for 20% of all cases of conjunctivitis.
  - Serotype 3 (and occasionally 4 or 7) causes pharyngoconjunctival fever.
  - Other serotypes (especially 8, 19, and 37) cause epidemic keratoconjunctivitis.
- HSV type 1 also causes conjunctivitis, usually in preschool children. HSV type 2 is usually responsible for neonatal infections.
- Molluscum contagiosum may be implicated in adolescents.

- Acute haemorrhagic conjunctivitis (AHC), mainly occurring as epidemics in the tropics, is caused by two picornaviruses: Coxsackie type A24 and enterovirus type 70 (also, rarely adenovirus 11).

Transmission is by direct contamination (fingers, towels etc.) with respiratory or ocular secretions. Wearing contact lenses increases the risk of getting conjunctivitis. Adenovirus is particularly contagious with an infection rate in household contacts of around 25%. The virus remains in the conjunctiva for 14 days and the faeces for 30 days. The incubation period for adenovirus is 3–29 days (mean 11 days) and 1–3 days for most bacterial infections (except for those caused by *C. trachomatis*, for which it is 5–14 days).

UK and European epidemiology

Infective conjunctivitis is common worldwide. Approximately one in eight schoolchildren has an episode of acute infective conjunctivitis each year. This means there are more than one million episodes per year in the UK, accounting for 1% of consultations in primary care. The prevalence of bacterial conjunctivitis increases in the winter and spring, and viral conjunctivitis is more common in the summer and autumn.

Enterovirus 70 thrives for longer periods in areas of high humidity, hence the reason that AHC is found mainly in the tropics (especially Asia).

The widespread use of the pneumococcal conjugate vaccine may significantly reduce *S. pneumoniae* isolates in conjunctivitis.

Clinical presentation and differential diagnosis

The symptoms and signs are similar in viral, bacterial, and allergic conjunctivitis. They include itching, burning, mucopurulent or purulent discharge, eyelid oedema, and conjunctival erythema. Itching is more common in allergic conjunctivitis. Associated pharyngitis, and/or preauricular adenopathy suggest a viral aetiology (usually adenovirus). Purulent discharge with gluey or sticky eyelids is highly suggestive of bacterial conjunctivitis (probability of 96% in one study), as is associated otitis media. Papillae on the conjunctiva and bilateral disease are also more likely in bacterial infections. However, one cannot reliably predict the aetiology on clinical examination alone.

Ocular pain and photophobia are uncommon, except in adenovirus keratoconjunctivitis. The differential diagnosis includes measles and Kawasaki disease.

Adenovirus conjunctivitis

Adenovirus conjunctivitis usually presents as one of three recognized conditions and the symptomatic phase lasts from 4 to 14 days.
- Follicular conjunctivitis—is the most common type. Follicles develop from aggregation of lymphocytes and appear as small, pale, avascular

areas, surrounded by a network of blood vessels. Typical features include:
- Preauricular adenopathy
- Hyperaemia
- Watery discharge
- Oedema of eyelids
- Rhinitis
- Pharyngitis
- Itching.

- Pharyngoconjunctival fever—transmission may be linked to poorly chlorinated pools and ponds. Typical features include:
  - Pharyngitis
  - Fever
  - Chemosis
  - Hyperaemia
  - Preauricular adenopathy
  - Occasional small petechial haemorrhages.

- Epidemic keratoconjunctivitis—this usually occurs in older children and adults. There is an early follicular response and a late papillary response. Punctate epithelial defects are seen with fluorescein and later subepithelial corneal infiltrates develop. In severe cases, conjunctival pseudomembranes and eyelid swelling develop. Typical features include:
  - Severe discomfort
  - Photophobia
  - Conjunctival oedema
  - Blurred vision.

HSV conjunctivitis

HSV conjunctivitis may be associated with a primary infection or a recurrence. Transmission occurs via direct contact with another person or autoinoculation, and 80% of cases are unilateral. There is a follicular inflammatory response and keratoconjunctivitis occurs in 50%. It is difficult to differentiate clinically from adenoviral infection. Typical features include:
- Serous discharge
- Preauricular adenopathy
- Keratitis
- Occasional lid vesicles
- Associated upper respiratory tract infection and gingivostomatitis.

Acute haemorrhagic conjunctivitis

AHC is highly contagious. Symptoms develop in <48 hours, last for 3–5 days and resolve over 10 days. Typical features include:
- Sudden onset of hyperaemic conjunctiva
- Chemosis
- Oedema of eyelids
- Excessive tears
- Photophobia
- Discomfort.

Ophthalmia neonatorum

Gonococcal conjunctivitis tends to occur 3–5 days after birth but can present later. Chlamydial conjunctivitis usually has a later onset than gonococcal conjunctivitis; the incubation period is 5–14 days.

Typical features of gonococcal conjunctivitis include:
- More severe than other causes of ophthalmia neonatorum
- Purulent conjunctivitis, which usually is bilateral
- Corneal involvement has been reported, including diffuse epithelial oedema and ulceration that may progress to perforation of the cornea and endophthalmitis
- May be systemic manifestations.

Typical features of chlamydial conjunctivitis:
- Range from mild hyperaemia with scant mucoid discharge to eyelid swelling, chemosis, and pseudomembrane formation
- May be associated with extraocular involvement, including pneumonitis.

Investigations

Routine bacterial and viral eye swabs for culture are not usually required on the grounds of time delay and cost. Viral culture may be appropriate in epidemic case clusters.

Exceptions
- Suspected HSV—viral culture, PCR, and/or antigen detection tests should be performed. Fluorescein stains required to look for associated dendritic ulcers. Appropriate viral culture medium is needed and the best samples are vesicle aspirates. Conjunctival scrapings have a lower sensitivity.
- Ophthalmia neonatorum—ensure that eye swabs are sent for microscopy and culture and that laboratory is aware that *N. gonorrhoeae* is being tested for, so that appropriate culture media are chosen. A special conjunctival swab for chlamydia culture is also required. Enzyme immunoassays, direct fluorescent antibody assays, and PCR testing are also suitable for chlamydia detection in conjunctival specimens.

Management and treatment

Excellent infection control measures are required in the clinical setting and in the community to prevent further spread:
- Thorough handwashing, glove use, instrument disinfection, and use of eye drops in individual or unit dose containers should be employed in clinics and hospitals.
- Affected children and their carers should wash their hands regularly with soap, especially after applying eye drops or ointments (use a different container for each eye). Sharing of towels, cups etc. should

be avoided. Regular disinfection of surfaces (e.g. taps, doorknobs) and changing of pillowcases are recommended.

- Exclusion from daycare or nursery is controversial and is not recommended in the UK.
- Supportive care is indicated for all types of conjunctivitis:
  - Cold compresses—improve swelling and discomfort
  - Artificial tears (especially in keratitis)—reduce discomfort and photophobia, and relieve itching and burning
  - Topical vasoconstrictors.
- Acute bacterial conjunctivitis is usually self-limiting and 65% of patients are clinically cured in 2–5 days. Most children do not require any topical or systemic antibiotics.
- However, topical antibiotic treatment of acute infective conjunctivitis (ointment or drops) shortens the clinical course, may reduce spread and discomfort, and allows child to return to normal activities earlier (may be attractive to working parents).
  - Evidence for more rapid clinical and microbiological remission is stronger if patients are treated early (within 2–5 days of presentation), as opposed to late (within 6–10 days). The number needed to treat is 6 for early clinical remission and 13 for late clinical remission.
  - Choice of antibiotic depends on cost and local resistance patterns.
  - Most active topical antibiotics are thought to be fluoroquinolones, but chloramphenicol, gentamicin, neomycin, tobramycin, erythromycin, trimethoprim-polymyxin, and fusidic acid all have reasonable activity.
  - Chloramphenicol is most commonly used in the UK and the risk of aplastic anaemia appears to be very small.
  - Systemic antibiotics may be required when there is associated otitis media.
- Generally, there is no place for corticosteroids (especially in HSV)—side effects include superinfection, glaucoma, and cataracts. Rarely topical steroids may be used (with ophthalmological supervision) if there is pseudomembrane formation and signs of severe inflammation or visual loss.
- Most cases of viral conjunctivitis are self-limiting, particularly adenovirus, and secondary bacterial infection is uncommon.
  - There is no specific anti-adenoviral agent for local infection.
  - Cidofovir may be used systemically for immunocompromised patients with disseminated adenoviral infection.
- Children with suspected ocular HSV infection should be seen by an ophthalmologist and are usually treated with a topical antiviral agent, such as aciclovir or valaciclovir. Neonates with suspected herpetic infection should be treated with systemic aciclovir. Infants with neonatal HSV keratitis should also receive a topical antiviral agent such as trifluridine, iododeoxyuridine, or vidarabine.
- Ophthalmia neonatorum—prompt treatment of gonococcal conjunctivitis is important, since this organism can penetrate an intact corneal epithelium and rapidly cause corneal ulceration. Because of the rapid progression of gonococcal conjunctivitis, patients with acute

neonatal conjunctivitis should be treated for gonococcal conjunctivitis until culture results are available using ceftriaxone as a single dose. Topical neomycin ointment should be used. Saline eye irrigation should be commenced immediately and at frequent intervals until the discharge is eliminated.
- Chlamydial conjunctivitis—infants with this are at risk of later pneumonitis. Oral erythromycin for 14 days is the current standard treatment.
- Conjunctivitis—sticky eyes, not otherwise thought to be due to gonococcus or *Chlamydia*, should be treated with topical neomycin until results of swabs are known.

Follow-up and outcome
- Acute infective conjunctivitis is usually a self-limiting condition which does not require specific follow-up.
- The risk of serious complications from untreated conjunctivitis is generally low, but this depends on the patient's immune status and the aetiology of the disease.
- The majority of bacterial cases resolve by 5 days without treatment.
- In viral disease, the symptomatic phase usually lasts for a maximum of 2 weeks, but some symptoms may persist for up to 6 weeks. The infection usually starts in one eye, but spreads easily to the other eye.
  - Pharyngoconjunctival fever usually lasts for 4 days.
  - AHC typically resolves within 5–7 days.
- Children with keratoconjunctivitis should be seen by an ophthalmologist, as severe cases may lead to conjunctival desiccation, and eventually scarring and adhesion of the palpebral and bulbar conjunctivae. Asymmetrical scarring can result in amblyopia in young children.
- Primary HSV disease is usually self-limiting, but recurrent disease may lead to corneal opacification and visual loss. These patients should be followed up by an ophthalmologist.
  - Infection in newborns tends to be more severe due to their impaired immunity, absence of conjunctival lymphoid tissue, and lack of tears. Serious systemic complications, such as encephalitis, may occur.
- Mothers whose babies are diagnosed as having either gonococcus or chlamydial infection need referral for treatment and contact tracing etc.

Future research
- With the increasing trend towards no antibiotic treatment for acute infective conjunctivitis, more data are needed on the risk of adverse events when no treatment is given and the effect on transmission rate.
- More work is needed to establish whether antibiotic use for suspected bacterial cases may be cost effective, e.g. by preventing time off work for parents.
- There is scope to try to find rapid and reliable diagnostic tools to differentiate between bacterial and viral conjunctivitis.

- Further research into antiviral therapies is required:
  - Purified, concentrated human IgG has been shown to have antiviral properties against adenoviral serotypes *in vitro* and in rabbits.
  - Zalcitabine and stavudine (nucleoside reverse transcriptase inhibitors) have demonstrated antiviral activity against adenovirus serotypes 3, 4, 8, 19, and 37 in cell culture studies.
  - Povidone-iodine 0.8% may potentially reduce contagiousness in adenoviral infections.

Further reading

Rose P. Management strategies for acute infective conjunctivitis in primary care: a systematic review. *Expert Opin Pharmacother* 2007;**8**:1903–21.

Sheikh A, Hurwitz B. Antibiotics versus placebo for acute bacterial conjunctivitis. *Cochrane Database Syst Rev* 2006;**2**:CD001211.

Teoh DL, Reynolds S. Diagnosis and management of pediatric conjunctivitis. *Pediatr Emerg Care* 2003;**19**:48–55.

Diarrhoea and vomiting

📖 see also Chapters 46, 54, 59, 60, 61, 66, 67, 69, 73, 92, 100, 104, 114, 118

Introduction

Diarrhoea and vomiting, alone or together, are extremely common presentations to healthcare in childhood. Diarrhoea is often defined as loose or watery stools at least twice as frequent as normal for that child. While acute gastroenteritis is the most common cause of diarrhoea and vomiting, other causes must be considered. Vomiting may be the presenting feature of surgical conditions such as intussusception or appendicitis, systemic illness, and non-enteric sepsis, e.g. urinary tract infection (UTI). Enteral rehydration using oral rehydration solution (ORS) remains the cornerstone of management.

There are three broad classifications of diarrhoea:
- Acute watery diarrhoea
- Acute bloody diarrhoea—also called dysentery
- Persistent diarrhoea—lasting 14 days or longer.

Epidemiology

- Acute gastroenteritis presenting with diarrhoea and/or vomiting is extremely common in childhood, and responsible for an estimated 1.5 million deaths annually in children <5 years due to dehydration.
- In the UK each year, 0.7% of children <5 years are admitted to hospital with gastroenteritis, with those between 6 and 24 months at special risk.
- Only a small proportion of cases present to healthcare, even to primary healthcare, with most treated at home.
- Gastroenteritis occurs all year round, with seasonal winter/spring peaks in temperate climates due mostly to rotavirus.
- In tropical settings, there are fewer seasonal patterns, with less predictable timing of outbreaks.
- Risk factors for developing gastroenteritis include non-breastfeeding and out-of-home childcare.

Aetiology

- An infectious agent can be identified in up to 70% of episodes of community acquired gastroenteritis. New agents continue to be identified.

- Rotavirus is the most common cause of sporadic gastroenteritis in children, followed by the caliciviruses norovirus (formerly Norwalk-like agent) and sapoviruses (formerly Sapporo-like agent). Other viral causes include astroviruses and adenovirus (types 40 and 41).
- 95% of rotavirus infections are due to the four most common serotypes. There are around 13 000 reports of rotavirus infection in the UK in children each year, virtually all in the preschool group.
- *Campylobacter*, *Salmonella*, and less commonly *Aeromonas* species are significant enteric pathogens in the UK, while in resource-poor settings *Shigella* is a major pathogen.
- In resource-poor settings bacterial pathogens assume greater importance for residents (*Campylobacter*, *Shigella*, and *Salmonella* species) and tourists (especially enterotoxigenic *Escherichia coli*).
- *Cryptosporidia* and *Giardia* are important pathogens, especially in childcare and resource-poor settings, but rarely cause severe acute disease.
- *Clostridium difficile* is a major nosocomial pathogen, as are rotavirus and norovirus.

Pathophysiology

- Most enteric pathogens are transmitted by the faecal-oral route.
- Contaminated food is a risk factor for bacterial pathogens and norovirus. Water-borne transmission is more common with bacteria and protozoa.
- Rotavirus infects mature enterocytes of jejunal and ileal villi. Cell destruction and loss of villous architecture results in a massive reduction in absorptive surface area, and exposure of the immature enterocytes at the base of the villi, increasing fluid loss. Net loss of water and salt in the faeces manifests as diarrhoea. On day 2–5 of symptoms, adjacent villi fuse to help reduce surface area of immature cells and decrease fluid loss. Between day 6 and 10 villous architecture is restored. Rotavirus enterotoxin NSP4 also contributes to the enteritis.
- Invasive bacteria (*Shigella*, *E. coli*, *Salmonella*, *Campylobacter*, *Yersinia*, *Aeromonas*) typically cause an enterocolitis, with white cells and blood more commonly present in the faeces.
- Bacterial enterocolitis can result from a number of mechanisms, including mucosal ulceration and inflammation, and toxin production affecting cellular processes.
- Enteritis-producing *Bacillus* species and *Staphylococcus aureus* have preformed toxins, while *Vibrio cholerae* and *E. coli* produce toxins following infection, including the entero-haemorrhagic *E. coli* toxin responsible for haemolytic-uraemic syndrome (HUS).

Clinical manifestations

- Acute diarrhoea and/or vomiting in early childhood may also be associated with common infections of other organ systems, including upper and lower respiratory tract infections, as well urinary tract infections.

- In childhood, it is extremely difficult to differentiate between community-acquired gastroenteritis pathogens based on clinical presentation.
- Seizures with gastroenteritis strongly indicate *Shigella* as a likely cause in *Shigella*-prevalent areas; seizures have also been described with rotavirus.
- Rotavirus gastroenteritis classically occurs following a short 1–3 day incubation period. Vomiting is common early in the illness, with hospital studies describing it in up to 97% of patients. Fever is common, with fever >39°C present in up to a third.
- Dehydration (usually isotonic) varies in frequency: it is seen in 7% of cases in community cohorts, and up to 63% admitted to hospital.
- The degree of dehydration is rated by the WHO on a scale of 3:
1. Early dehydration—no signs or symptoms, history of significant diarrhoea and vomiting
2. Moderate dehydration (4–6%):
   - Delayed central capillary refill time >2 seconds
   - Restless or irritable behaviour (tricky as almost all young children in the emergency department in the evening are restless and irritable)
   - Decreased skin elasticity
   - Sunken eyes
3. Severe dehydration (≥7%):
   - Symptoms become more severe
   - Shock, with diminished consciousness, lack of urine output, cool, moist extremities, a rapid and feeble pulse, low or undetectable blood pressure (late sign), and pale skin.

Upper respiratory tract symptoms and signs may be seen in up to 40% of cases of gastroenteritis.

Differential diagnoses

Differential diagnoses should always be considered, especially in the presence of persistent abdominal pain or isolated vomiting. They include:
- Urinary tract infection
- Appendicitis and other surgical causes of acute abdomen
- Other infections or, rarely, metabolic conditions, e.g. newly diagnosed diabetes.

Investigations

Most children with acute gastroenteritis do not require investigation.
- Serum electrolytes and glucose should be tested if there is any sign of severe dehydration, history of prolonged vomiting or diarrhoea, prior therapy with hypertonic or hypotonic fluids, or 'doughy' skin suggestive of hypernatraemia.
- Urine microscopy and culture is warranted if there are other suggestive features.

The decision to test for gastroenteritis pathogens is based on several factors, including:
   - To allow assessment of organism epidemiology

- To detect potential foodborne outbreaks that may require intervention
- For unusual presentations (such as significant bloody diarrhoea)
- To enable cohorting in hospitals to minimize nosocomial transmission
- For nosocomially acquired cases to detect hospital outbreaks.
- Faecal microscopy:
  - The presence of 5 leucocytes per high power field suggests an invasive enteritis. Fresh microscopy of faecal concentrate may reveal *Cryptosporidia*, *Giardia*, and other parasites.
- Antigen testing (latex agglutination or enzyme-linked immunosorbent assays (ELISA)) are often used to detect common viral pathogens, and sometimes protozoa.
- Culture is useful for bacterial pathogens for community-acquired gastroenteritis.
- Toxin assays for *C. difficile*-associated gastroenteritis have largely replaced culture.
- More sensitive molecular assays such as reverse-transcription PCR are especially useful for noroviruses, but as asymptomatic infection may be common with many enteric viral pathogens, the results must be interpreted carefully.

Management

- Admission is based on signs of severe dehydration, altered mental status, young age—<1 year, bloody diarrhoea, persistent vomiting or profuse diarrhoea, social factors.
- Shock should be treated with urgent IV crystalloid with 20ml/kg boluses.
- Enteral fluid replacement with ORS is the mainstay of therapy of acute gastroenteritis, either orally or via nasogastric tubes.
  - The composition of typical low osmolarity ORS includes 75 mmol/l sodium, 65 mmol/l chloride, 75 mmol/l glucose, 20 mmol/l potassium, and 10 mmol/l citrate.
  - For children <5 years who are being treated at home, around 50 ml/kg over 4–6 hours corrects moderate dehydration. Continue maintenance fluids.
  - Polymer (rice, wheat, sorghum, or maize)-based ORS has been shown to have some advantages over normal ORS and has higher osmolarity.
  - Probiotic supplementation in combination with rehydration may shorten the illness or reduce faecal output.
- Rapid enteral replacement of fluid deficit over 6 hours in most cases has been shown to be safe and allow earlier discharge.
- Calculate and add maintenance fluids to replacement.
- Measure and add ongoing losses—they may be very significant.
- After treatment of shock, IV replacement of fluid deficit occurs over 24 hours.
- Even in acute bacterial gastroenteritis, antibiotics are rarely used. Empiric antibiotics have been shown to shorten the course of traveller's diarrhoea.

- Advise parents that the usual duration of diarrhoea is up to 7 days. There needs to be in place a clear 'safety net' for the parents to return if the child is not improving.
- Bowel antispasmodic agents are contraindicated in children. Clear advice on signs of deterioration need to be given to the family, preferably in a written form.
- Post-gastroenteritis lactose and cow's milk protein intolerance is now rare in Europe. Persistent diarrhoea with failure to thrive should lead to stool testing for reducing substances and a trial of a lactose-free, cow's milk-free elemental milk for 3–6 months.

Prevention

Clean water and food precautions reduce the risk of bacterial gastroenteritis but impact little on viral acute gastroenteritis. Alcohol-based hand hygiene has been shown to decrease rotavirus transmission in school settings.

Effective and safe vaccines are available for cholera, typhoid, and rotavirus. Oral typhoid vaccine has some efficacy against *E. coli* travellers' diarrhoea. The first licensed rotavirus vaccine was withdrawn after being associated with intussusception in the following 14 days, especially when the first dose was administered after 3 months of age. The new rotavirus vaccines, the monovalent Rotarix™ (GSK) and pentavalent Rotateq™ (Merck) have not been associated with intussusception in large-scale safety and efficacy trials.

Future research

- Cost efficacy of different approaches to clinical management of gastroenteritis in ambulatory paediatric settings.
- Other novel methods of reducing admissions and IV treatment of gastroenteritis in children in Europe.
- The role of zinc supplementation.

Useful websites

World Health Organization. Gastroenteritis. Available at: ℘ www.who.int (accessed 1 February 2011).

Health Protection Agency. Available at: ℘ www.hpa.org.uk (accessed 1 February 2011).

Chapter 13

Emerging and re-emerging infections

📖 see also Chapters 14, 45, 63, 80, 116

Introduction

- Among infectious diseases, a number of infections remain a constant threat to humans. In addition are the **emerging**, **re-emerging** (or re-surging), **newly recognized**, and **deliberately emergent** infectious diseases.
- Emerging and re-emerging infections are often a consequence of complex interactions between the pathogen, host, and the environment:
  - Pathogens, particularly viruses, have a selective advantage in adapting to new ecological niches because of their high replication rates and their genetic plasticity, which allows them to acquire new biological characteristics through mutation, recombination, and reassortment.
  - Host factors include: population growth and migration; increase in international travel, trade, technology and industry; behavioural changes; ageing population; the use of broad-spectrum antibiotics and immunosuppressive drugs; breakdown of public health measures; war; poverty and social inequality; and intentional biological attacks.
  - Environmental factors (many of them induced by humans) include: climate and weather changes; agricultural development and land use; changing ecosystems; livestock farming; changing relationships between humans and animals; deforestation; reforestation; urbanization; famine; and flooding.
- **Emerging infections** refer to infections that have newly emerged in a population:
  - Around 75% of emerging infections are zoonotic and arise when humans encroach on environments where they become exposed to microbes that they would otherwise not have encountered, or when there is close and prolonged contact between humans and animals, which allows microbes the opportunity to jump the species barrier (Box 13.1).

Box 13.1 Examples of recent emerging infections

Severe acute respiratory syndrome (SARS): The first emerging infection of the new millennium began in the Guandong province of South China, which has a high population density of humans and wild and domestic animals. The aetiological agent, a previously unknown coronavirus, jumped across the species barrier from its natural reservoir, the bat, to susceptible animals such as civets and raccoons, and then to humans. The infection spread so rapidly across the world such that, in a short period of time, it was responsible for over 8000 cases and almost a thousand deaths in 30 different countries.

New variant Creutzfeldt—Jakob disease (vCJD): Transmissible spongiform encephalopathies (TSEs) are a rare group of progressive neurological conditions characterized by loss of neuronal tissue causing a typical sponge-like appearance of the brain. Unlike our common perception that all pathogens required nucleic acid to direct their replication, the aetiological agent in TSE is the prion protein, which is normally found on the surface of many cells in the body, including the brain. In TSE, the normal form of the prion protein undergoes a spatial conformation that makes it resistant to normal cellular degradation and sets up a chain reaction that induces other normal prion proteins to fold into the abnormal form. TSEs are unique in that their aetiology may be sporadic (sporadic CJD), genetic (familial CJD), iatrogenic (blood transfusions, neurosurgery), or infectious (ingestion of infected material). In the UK in the 1980s, the bovine spongiform encephalopathy (BSE) epidemic, commonly known as mad cow disease, and affecting over 200 000 cows, was most likely a result of cattle being fed the remains of other cattle with BSE. Contrary to all expectations, the disease crossed the species barrier and the first human case of 'mad cow disease', termed variant CJD (vCJD) was reported in the mid-1990s. Because of its prolonged incubation period (up to 40 years), the true burden of infection is not known. By October 2009, vCJD had killed 166 people in Britain and 44 elsewhere.

Viral haemorrhagic fevers: Haemorrhagic diseases caused by viruses such as Ebola and Marburg, which were identified in the 1960s and 1970s, are often classed as emerging infections because they appear suddenly and cause severe disease with a very high case fatality (75–90%). However, these episodes are rare, usually occur in a well-defined geographical location and, because of their rapid onset and high fatality, usually 'burn out' rapidly and return to their, as yet unidentified, natural host.

- **Re-emerging** or **resurging** infections refer to emergence of a known infection in a different form or in a different location (Box 13.2).

Box 13.2 Examples of factors that have contributed to emergence and re-emergence of specific infections

International travel: The classic example of an infection emerging in a new region is the West Nile virus which is a well-known cause of meningoencephalitis in Africa and the Middle East. In 1999, the virus appeared in New York through an unknown route, possibly via an infected bird or mosquito, and, since then, has spread throughout the USA, Canada, Mexico, the Caribbean, and Central America. Similarly, the chikungunya virus was first described in 1952 in Tanzania. In 2004, localized outbreaks on the coast of Kenya resulted in a rapid spread of the infection to the Indian Ocean islands and from there, to many parts of the world. In particular, the disease caused an outbreak of unprecedented magnitude in India, affecting over a million people.

Breakdown in public health measures: Infections that were previously well controlled may re-emerge if there is a reduction in public health measures either because of a change in service provision (including immunisation programmes) or reluctance in accepting a service.

Antibiotic pressure: The accidental discovery of the first antibiotic in 1928 was heralded as one of the triumphs of modern medicine. Extended use of broad-spectrum antibiotics, however, has resulted in the emergence of pathogens that were initially considered to be well controlled, such as multiresistant *Mycobacterium tuberculosis* and *Plasmodium falciparum* infections worldwide, MRSA, vancomycin-resistant enterococci (VRE), and certain multiresistant Gram-negative bacilli.

Immunosuppression: The development and successful use of immunosuppressive drugs for malignancies and autoimmune disorders has seen a rise in opportunistic bacterial, viral, fungal and parasitic infections, such as *Pneumocystis jiroveci* (previously known as *Pneumocystis carinii*) infections, toxoplasmosis, aspergillosis, cryptococcosis, atypical mycobacterial infections, disseminated adenovirus and cytomegalovirus infections, and histoplasmosis among many others.

Other factors: Other factors that may play a role in emerging and re-emerging infections include population growth and migration (e.g. *Plasmodium knowlesi* malaria in South-East Asia), climate and habitat changes (e.g. *Sin nombre* virus causing acute cardiopulmonary syndrome in south-west USA); migratory patterns of animals and birds (avian influenza); changes in agriculture practices (Argentine haemorrhagic fever; Korean haemorrhagic fever); and human practices such as building dams (Rift Valley Fever), among many others.

- **Newly recognized infectious diseases** refer to conditions that are now recognized to be caused by infections (Table 13.1).

Table 13.1 Examples of newly recognized infectious diseases recently associated with chronic diseases

Disease	Pathogen
Gastritis, gastric ulcers and stomach cancers	*Helicobacter pylori*
Cervical cancer	Human papillomavirus
Liver cancer	Chronic hepatitis B and hepatitis C
Bladder cancer	Schistosomiasis
Kaposi's sarcoma	HHV-8

- **Deliberately emergent pathogens** are those that are intentionally planned by humans through bioterrorism (Table 13.2).

Table 13.2 Examples of recent notable bioterrorist attacks

Year	Event
1984	The Bhagwan Shree Rajneesh religious group attempted to control a local election by infecting 11 restaurants and grocery stores with *Salmonella typhimurium* in Oregon, USA; >750 people developed severe gastroenteritis and several hundreds were hospitalized, although none died
1993	The Aum Shinrikyo religious group released anthrax spores in Tokyo, Japan. Although not a single person was infected in that attack (because anthrax spores are so difficult to aerosolize at high concentrations), the same group was also responsible for subsequent deadly attacks using sarin gas, a deadly nerve agent, in 1994 and 1995
2001	Letters deliberately laced with anthrax were sent to news media offices and the US Congress, killing five people

- These agents are usually found in nature, but may be altered to make them difficult to detect, increase their ability to cause disease, make them resistant to treatment and/or increase their ability to propagate in the environment.
- Bioterrorism is often used to create mass panic and cause disruption to society, out of proportion to the actual number of deaths or illness caused.
- Pathogens with a potential for use in bioterrorist attacks have been classified into category A (high-priority agents such as anthrax, smallpox, botulinum toxin, bubonic plaque, tularaemia, and viral haemorrhagic fevers), category B (moderate-priority agents such as brucellosis, ricin, melioidosis, and cholera), and category C (emerging pathogens that could be engineered for mass spread in the future).

Conclusions

- Human beings have been under constant threat of emerging and re-emerging infections and this is likely to continue in the foreseeable future.
- As our understanding of the factors associated with emergence and re-emergence of infectious diseases increases, it is becoming clear that an increasingly modern world will provide more opportunities for new and old pathogens to thrive.
- We must recognize that the emergence of new transmissible pathogens is a global risk and international collaboration is vital for surveillance, containment, and control of emerging infections.
- In the UK, the Health Protection Agency Emerging Infections and Zoonoses Department regularly reports on outbreaks, and incidents of new and emerging infectious diseases reported nationally and internationally (⌨ see Useful websites).

Useful websites

Centres for Disease Control and Prevention, USA: ℘ www.bt.cdc.gov (accessed 1 February 2011).

Health Protection Agency, UK: ℘ www.hpa.org.uk/HPA/Topics/InfectiousDiseases/InfectionsAZ/1234254470752 (accessed 1 February 2011).

World Health Organization: ℘ www.who.int/topics/emerging_diseases/en (accessed 1 February 2011).

Further reading

Ippolito G, Fusco FM, Di Caro A, *et al.* Facing the threat of highly infectious diseases in Europe: the need for a networking approach. *Clin Microbiol Infect* 2009;**15**:706–10.

Morens DM, Folkers GK, Fauci AS. Emerging infections: a perpetual challenge. *Lancet Infect Dis* 2008;**8**:710–19.

Zappa A, Amendola A, Romanò L, Zanetti A. Emerging and re-emerging viruses in the era of globalisation. *Blood Transfus* 2009;**7**:167–71.

Encephalitis

📖 see also Chapters 28, 29, 64, 77

Introduction

Encephalitis is a rare but devastating disease in children. It is defined by the presence of an inflammatory process of the brain in association with clinical evidence of neurological dysfunction. In children, it is most commonly caused by infection, usually viral, but may also have metabolic, toxin/drug mediated, autoimmune vasculitis, malignant, or genetic origins. Encephalitis in children may manifest as either acute encephalitis (direct invasion of the CNS) or postinfectious encephalitis (postinfectious immune mediated demyelination). The diagnosis of encephalitis is usually inferred from a combination of clinical findings and brain imaging; it is very rarely proved by histology which requires brain biopsy.

Meningoencephalitis describes the presence of clinical encephalitis with inflammatory changes in the CSF implying co-existing inflammation of the covering meninges. Table 14.1 gives the differential diagnosis of encephalitis in a child.

Table 14.1 Differential diagnosis of encephalitis

Inborn errors of metabolism	Ornithine transcarbamylase deficiency
	Glutaric acidaemia type I
	MCAD deficiency
	MELAS syndrome
	Leber optic neuropathy
	Adrenoleucodystrophy
	Urea cycle defects
	Maple syrup urine disease
CNS vasculitis	Systemic lupus erythematosus
	Polyarteritis nodosa
	Lymphogranulomatosis angiitis

(Continued)

Table 14.1 (*Contd.*)

Toxic encephalopathy	Reye's syndrome
	Acute toxic ingestion—drugs
	Lead or carbon monoxide intoxication
	Hyperpyrexic shock
	Fulminant hepatic failure
	Diabetic ketoacidosis
Other CNS conditions	Brainstem glioma
	Intracranial haemorrhage
	Intracranial thrombosis
	Pseudotumour cerebri
	Nonconvulsive status epilepticus

Pathophysiology

Infection-associated encephalitis can be caused by several mechanisms:
- Organisms can enter by the haematogenous route, resulting in diffuse encephalitis, e.g. HSV/measles/influenza/*Listeria*/Lyme disease.
- Viruses and selected bacteria can enter by neuronal tracts, resulting in focal encephalitis, e.g. temporal localization of HSV encephalitis due to retrograde spread of virus from a site of latency in the trigeminal ganglion.
- Immune-mediated encephalitis occurs where the host response to the infection causes secondary inflammatory changes in the CNS, most often within the white matter of the brain (e.g. after *Mycoplasma* or varicella zoster infection).
- Slow virus brain infections may lead to low-grade inflammatory neurotoxic damage, which can take years to evolve to clinical significance. This may occur with HIV encephalopathy or SSPE with mutant measles virus, manifesting clinically up to 8–10 years after primary infection.

Pathological findings
- Virus-induced cytolysis results in focal or generalized loss of neurons. Perivascular and parenchymal inflammation of the cortical grey matter, adjacent grey–white junction, basal ganglia, or brainstem is characteristic.
- Some viruses, including CMV and adenoviruses produce characteristic inclusions in a small number of infected cells.

- Inflammation can cause a localized vasculitis that leads to haemorrhage or necrosis, this can occur with HSV infection and in some cases with influenza. Some agents cause direct endothelial damage.
- In immunodeficient patients, the natural history is frequently chronic and pathological findings include cerebral atrophy, neuronal loss, and demyelination.
- Table 14.2 gives the more common causes of encephalitis in children.

Table 14.2 Infectious causes of encephalitis

Viruses	HSV
	CMV
	VZV
	HHV-6
	EBV
	Enteroviruses (including polio)
	Parechovirus
	Adenoviruses
	Influenza viruses
	Mumps virus
	Measles
	Rubella
	Rabies virus
	Lymphocytic choriomeningitis virus
	HIV
	Arboviruses (e.g. central European tick-borne encephalitis virus, West Nile virus, Japanese B, Dengue, Bunyaviruses; see Fig. 14.1)
Bacterial and other	GBS (neonatal)
	Mycoplasma pneumoniae
	Mycobacterium tuberculosis
	Toxoplasma gondii
	Listeria monocytogenes
	Borrelia burgdorferi

Incidence and aetiology

- Encephalitis is a rare disease with an estimated incidence of 4/100 000 in the UK.
- Incidence is highest in the first year of life (17/100 000) and declines with age.
- Manifestations of encephalitis depend on the host and the infecting organism; certain infections occur in both immunocompetent and immunocompromised hosts, but others only in the immunocompromised.
- Why only a tiny minority of individuals develop encephalitis with common infections is not well understood, but host susceptibility factors are beginning to be identified. This has been demonstrated for rare individuals who had recurrent HSV encephalitis, where an autosomal recessive deficiency in the intracellular protein UNC-93B, results in impaired cellular interferon-α/β and -γ antiviral responses, leading to recurrent HSV encephalitis.

Immunocompetent hosts

- Rates of epidemic encephalitis have fallen due to improved living conditions, vector control and vaccines. Prior to MMR vaccination, mumps was the commonest cause of meningoencephalitis in the UK. Primary varicella zoster infection can be associated with generalized encephalitis or a postinfectious encephalitis, which usually manifests as cerebellitis. In some parts of the world polio is still an important cause of encephalitis. Worldwide the flavivirus Japanese B is one of the commonest causes of encephalitis, occurring most often in Asia. See Figure 14.1 for the worldwide distribution of arboviruses which can cause encephalitis.
- Enterovirus infections are common, often in summer and autumn; symptoms may vary from none to meningitis or meningoencephalitis. Most children make a full recovery but some, especially those with parechovirus infection, may have long-term brain damage. Outbreaks of ECHO virus cause severe encephalitis in young children in the Far East.
- HSV is the leading cause of sporadic encephalitis in all ages (approximately 2 cases per million population per year) and neonatal HSV encephalitis occurs in 2–3 per 10 000 live births in the USA (less common in the UK). HSV encephalitis in older children and adults is neuronally spread and usually focused in the temporal lobes. In the neonate the infection is haematogenously spread, the viral inoculum is much greater and viral cytopathic damage seen throughout the brain substance. Relapse after HSV encephalitis can occur in up to a quarter of patients.
- Postinfectious encephalitis is the most common demyelinating condition seen in children; it may complicate common childhood infections (e.g. HHV-6 infection, VZV, adenovirus, measles, influenza, *Mycoplasma*). It usually occurs some time after the prodromal infection (1–3 weeks) and is part of the spectrum of acute disseminated encephalomyelitis. There is a clinical continuum of

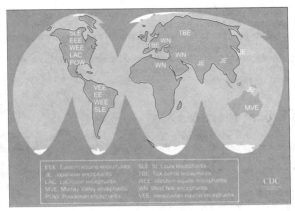

Fig. 14.1 Worldwide distribution of the major arboviruses that cause encephalitis.
(Reproduced from the Centre for Disease Control and Prevention, Atlanta USA,
🔗 www.cdc.gov/ncidod/dvbid/arbor/worldist.htm.)

such postinfectious inflammatory processes from the more diffuse
to the more specific which affect the central and peripheral nervous
systems, including: optic neuritis, transverse myelitis, acute cerebellar
ataxia, Guillain–Barré syndrome, Miller–Fisher syndrome, and
encephalomyeloradiculoneuropathy.

Immunocompromised hosts

- Congenital infections in the fetus with a poorly developed immune
  system, e.g. with members of the herpes family (CMV, VZV), rubella
  virus, syphilis, or *Toxoplasma gondii* may cause severe structural brain
  damage, and neurological symptoms present at birth.
- Infants and children with congenital immune deficiencies may present
  with encephalitis; this should always be considered in the differential
  diagnosis, e.g. infants with agammaglobulinaemia may develop chronic
  enteroviral encephalitis.
- The HIV epidemic has resulted in an increased incidence of
  neurological diseases in infected individuals. During primary HIV
  infection when there is a high level plasma viraemia, HIV crosses the
  blood–brain barrier and establishes a slow neurotoxic inflammatory
  state. In older children or adults this may eventually manifest as HIV
  dementia, with vasculitis, neuronal loss, and brain atrophy. Around
  5–10% of infants infected with HIV may present with symptomatic
  encephalopathy in the first year of life; this is associated with a very
  poor survival prognosis and often occurs with concomitant CMV
  infection. These infants often present with motor signs, microcephaly,
  and global developmental delay, and treatment may prevent further
  deterioration. Individuals with advanced HIV disease and severe

immunosuppression are also at risk of encephalitis from opportunistic infections (e.g. toxoplasmosis, VZV, CMV). They may also develop progressive multifocal leucoencephalopathy (PML) caused by polyoma virus infection (JC virus).
- Hyperpyrexic (haemorrhagic) shock with encephalopathy occurs in infants <1 year in age. Reye's syndrome is associated with antecedent viral infections including chickenpox and influenza.

Clinical features

The symptoms and severity of encephalitis depend on the age of the patient at the time of infection, the underlying aetiology, the type of virus and the part(s) of the CNS affected.
- Onset is usually acute, often preceded by a non-specific, acute febrile illness.
- In some cases onset may be subacute with altered behaviour, memory loss, personality change, etc.
- Presenting symptoms in older children are headache and malaise; infants are typically irritable and lethargic.
- Early symptoms: Fever, meningeal irritation (nausea, vomiting, neck pain and rigidity), and photophobia.
- Late symptoms: Altered level of consciousness (lethargic to confusion to coma), generalized or focal CNS abnormalities (tremor, seizures, loss of bowel or bladder control), or unprovoked emotional outbursts.
- Monitor coma using Paediatric Glasgow Coma Scale (GCS) regularly (Table 14.3).

Table 14.3 Paediatric GCS

	1	2	3	4	5	6
Eyes	Does not open eyes	Opens eyes in response to painful stimuli	Opens eyes in response to speech	Opens eyes spontaneously	N/A	N/A
Verbal	No verbal response	Inconsolable, agitated	Inconsistently inconsolable, moaning	Cries but consolable, inappropriate interactions	Smiles, orientated to sounds, follows objects, interacts	N/A
Motor	No motor response	Extension to pain (decerebrate response)	Abnormal flexion to pain for an infant (decorticate response)	Infant withdraws from pain	Infant withdraws from touch	Infant moves spontaneously or purposefully

Investigations and diagnosis

Important history for a suspected case of encephalitis

- Recent illness
- Exposure to ill contacts
- Place of residence (rural, urban)
- Animal exposure
- Tick or mosquito bite
- Recent travel or outdoor activities
- Medications (taken by patients or other family members)
- Evidence of immunocompromise in the host.

Lumbar puncture and CSF tests

- CSF abnormalities do not necessarily correlate with clinical severity.
- Measure opening pressure, red cells, white blood cells, glucose, protein. These may be normal, or the protein/white cell count may be slightly elevated. A mononuclear predominance is most common.
- Routine microscopy, rapid antigen and culture for bacteria, mycobacterium, and fungi.
- PCR is the most sensitive method to diagnose viral causes. HSV PCR may be falsely negative in the first 72 hours, and sensitivity will also be reduced after treatment with aciclovir. Bacteria specific PCRs, or the 16S ribosomal PCR may be use to try to detect bacterial infections where antibiotic treatment has already been started.
- CSF serology and PCR can be used to detect syphilis or Lyme disease.
- If SSPE is suspected then paired serum and CSF measles antibodies must be measured.
- CSF oligoclonal bands may be requested if demyelination has occurred.

Brain imaging

- MRI is the most useful imaging modality, showing brain oedema and inflammation in the cerebral cortex, grey–white matter junction, or basal ganglia. Make sure that all appropriate imaging sequences are undertaken, and with contrast where necessary. It is always best to discuss the case with a neuroradiologist.
- Repeat brain MRI is important to demonstrate evolution of the inflammatory process; very early imaging within 24–48 hours of presentation may not demonstrate significant abnormality.
- Where postinfectious encephalitis is associated with a focus of demyelination in the white matter, e.g. in basal ganglia or spinal cord. Gadolinium contrast may improve the sensitivity of MRI in detecting vasculitis.
- CT should be used to evaluate patients with encephalitis if MRI is unavailable. This is important in the acute setting to exclude other forms of CNS disease, e.g. tumour, effusion, hydrocephalus, absces, etc.

Electroencephalography (EEG)

- A useful complementary test.
- Identifies patients with non-convulsive seizure activity who are confused, obtunded, or comatose.

- In HSV, EEG may show focal unilateral or bilateral periodic discharges localized in the temporal lobes.

Blood tests and other specimens

- Standard laboratory tests and paired sera for serological tests for any suspected virus are important.
- Blood, urine, NPA/throat swabs, eye swabs (if inflamed) and stool/rectal swabs for culture of viruses and bacteria should always be collected. Skin lesions may be biopsied and blister lesions should also be swabbed for bacteria and viruses.

Brain biopsy

- Although this is the definitive test for diagnosis of encephalitis, it is very rarely done.

Management

Early treatment of encephalitis can reduce the rate of mortality and sequelae.

Supportive treatment

- This is the mainstay of management.
- Neuroprotective measures including airway protection, lower temperature, easing of the pressure on the brain and spinal cord caused by swelling of the brain with head up midline position and mannitol as necessary.
- Treat seizures, syndrome of inappropriate antidiuretic hormone secretion (SIADH), disseminated intravascular coagulation (DIC), and arrhythmias.

Antimicrobials

- Until a bacterial cause of CNS inflammation is excluded, parenteral broad-spectrum antibiotics with good CNS penetration should be given, usually ceftriaxone.
- Always think whether this could be tuberculosis.
- Appropriate high-dose aciclovir should be initiated in all patients with suspected encephalitis, pending results of diagnostic studies. However, with the exception of HSV, CMV, or VZV, the viral forms of encephalitis are usually not treatable.
- Ganciclovir may be given for CMV encephalitis.
- Antifungals may be used, especially in immunocompromised patients.
- Antiprotozoals may also be used based on diagnostic findings and suspicion.

Steroids and other immune modulator therapies (e.g. IVIG)

- Their role is controversial; many reports suggest that they may be effective at improving neurological outcome, especially in cases of post-infectious encephalomyelitis.

Vaccines

Vaccines are available for measles, mumps, rubella, VZV, rabies, Japanese encephalitis virus, tick borne encephalitis and influenza. Rarely some of these vaccines (e.g. Japanese encephalitis virus) can also cause post infectious encephalitis and should be given following appropriate expert advice.

Outcome

Severe viral encephalitis can lead to respiratory arrest, coma and death. The overall mortality rate is 3–4%. Children less than one year have fatality rates of up to 40–50% and neonates with disseminated viral infection have a very poor prognosis. There is an overall 7–10% risk of morbidity and marked neuro-developmental impairment.

Further reading

Aicardi J. *Diseases of the Nervous System in Childhood*, 3rd edn. Clinics in Developmental Medicine. Chichester: Wiley & Sons, 2009.

Casrouge A, Zhang SY, Eidenschenk C, *et al.* Herpes simplex virus encephalitis in human UNC-93B deficiency. *Science* 2006;**314**:308–12. Available at: www.hpa.org.uk (accessed 22 October 2010).

Tunkel AR, Glaser CA, Bloch KC, *et al.* The management of encephalitis: clinical practice guidelines by the infectious diseases society of America. *Clin Infect Dis* 2008;**47**:303–27.

Chapter 15

Enlarged lymph nodes

📖 see also Chapters 25, 38, 44, 56, 65, 91, 105, 106, 113

Introduction

- Lymph nodes (LNs) are highly specialized collections of immune cells that survey and handle antigen from the extracellular fluid (Fig. 15.1).
- LN size depends on the child's age, the location of the LN, and antecedent immunological events.
- Lymphoid mass steadily increases after birth until between 8 and 12 years of age, and undergoes progressive atrophy during puberty.
- In healthy children including neonates, mobile LNs, usually measuring less than 1cm in diameter, are often palpable in the cervical and axillary regions and do not usually require investigation in the absence of other signs or symptoms.
- Inguinal LNs measuring up to 1.5cm may also be normal.
- In contrast, progressively enlarging LNs and enlarged LNs associated with other systemic or local features require investigation.
- Palpable supraclavicular, epitrochlear (lateral end of humerus), and popliteal LNs should always be considered to be abnormal and investigated.
- The differential diagnosis of LN enlargement is extensive and includes viral, bacterial, mycobacterial, fungal, and protozoal infections as well as many non-infectious causes.
- The possibility of malignancy must always be considered.

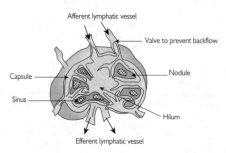

Fig. 15.1 Structure of lymph node.

Causative organisms

- The range of infectious agents causing LN enlargement are usefully considered according to the pattern of LN involvement (Fig. 15.2).
- The causative organisms and differential diagnoses to be considered according to the predominant pattern of LN involvement, are outlined in:
  - Table 15.1 (generalized)
  - Table 15.2 (cervical)
  - Table 15.3 (abdominal or mediastinal/hilar).
- The common causes of LN enlargement change with age, as outlined in Table 15.4.

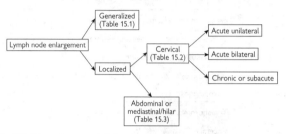

Fig. 15.2 Diagnostic approach to lymph node enlargement in children.

Table 15.1 The differential diagnosis of generalized lymphadenopathy in infants and children

Viral	EBV, CMV, and HHV-6
	Parvovirus B19
	Measles, rubella, adenovirus
	Enteroviruses, hepatitis A and hepatitis B viruses
	HIV
	Dengue fever, chikungunya virus

(Continued)

Table 15.1 (Contd.)

Bacterial	Cat scratch disease (*Bartonella henselae*, *Bartonella bacilliformis*)
	Enteric pathogens (*Salmonella typhi*, *Yersinia enterocolitica*)
	Respiratory pathogens (*Mycoplasma pneumoniae*, *Legionella pneumophila*)
	Scarlet fever (*Streptococcus pyogenes*)
	Spirochaetes—Lyme disease (*Borrelia burgdorferi*), leptospirosis (*Leptospira* sp), congenital or secondary syphilis (*Treponema pallidum*)
	Rickettsia—many including scrub typhus (*Orientia tsutsugamushi*) and ehrlichial diseases (*Ehrlichia sennetsu*)—rare
	Brucellosis (*Brucella melitensis*)—rare
	Tularaemia (*Francisella tularensis*)—rare
Mycobacteria	Tuberculosis (*Mycobacterium tuberculosis*)
Fungal	Histoplasmosis, coccidiomycosis, paracoccidiomycosis—rare
Parasitic	Toxoplasmosis
	Trypanosomiasis—rare
	Visceral leishmaniasis (Kala-azar)—rare
	Schistosomiasis and filariasis
Non-infectious causes	Malignancy (lymphomas, metastases)
	Haemophagocytic lymphohistiocytosis
	Primary immunodeficiencies (chronic granulomatous disease, Wiskott–Aldrich syndrome, Chediak–Higashi, hyper-IgE syndrome, common variable immunodeficiency)
	Rheumatological disorders (systemic onset juvenile idiopathic arthritis, systemic lupus erythematosus)
	Drug reactions (multiple, e.g. phenytoin)
	Sarcoidosis
	Chronic atopic eczema
	Miscellaneous (Table 15.5): Rosai–Dorfman disease (sinus histiocytosis with massive lymphadenopathy), Kikuchi–Fujimoto disease (histiocytic necrotizing lymphadenitis), multicentric Castleman's disease

Table 15.2 The differential diagnosis of cervical lymphadenopathy in infants and children according to the mode of initial presentation

Acute unilateral	Acute bilateral	Chronic (or subacute)
Staphylococcus aureus	EBV, CMV	Non-tuberculous mycobacterium
Streptococcus pyogenes (GAS)	HSV	
Streptococcus agalactiae (GBS)	Adenovirus	*B. henselae* (cat scratch disease)
Anaerobes (e.g. *Fusobacterium* and *Peptostreptococcus* spp.)	Enteroviruses	*T. gondii*
	HHV-6, 7, and 8 (rarely)	*M. tuberculosis*
Also: *Francisella tularensis, Pasteurella multocida, Yersinia* spp, *Streptococcus pneumoniae*, α-haemolytic streptococci, coagulase-negative staphylococci	Influenza, parainfluenza	*Actinomycetes* (*Actinomyces israelii, Nocardia* spp.)
	Measles	
	Rubella	
	Parvovirus B19	
	Mycoplasma pneumoniae	
	Corynebacterium diphtheriae	

Non-infectious cervical lymphadenopathy

Malignancy

Kawasaki disease

Periodic fever, aphthous stomatitis, pharyngitis and cervical adenitis (PFAPA)

Sarcoidosis

Miscellaneous (Table 15.5): Rosai–Dorfman disease (sinus histiocytosis with massive lymphadenopathy), Kikuchi–Fujimoto disease (histiocytic necrotizing lymphadenitis), Kimura's disease

Other neck masses

Salivary gland and thyroid masses

Head and neck malignancy

Congenital abnormalities (thyroglossal cysts, cystic hygroma, etc.)

Table 15.3 The differential diagnoses of mediastinal and abdominal lymphadenopathy in children and infants

	Mediastinal and hilar	Abdominal and retroperitoneal
Viral	Viral respiratory tract pathogens	Virus-associated gastroenteritis
	Many generalized viral infections (Table 15.1) can present predominantly with localized lymphadenopathy (e.g. EBV, HIV)	
Bacterial	Suppurative lung disease—bronchiectasis, lung abscesses M. pneumoniae	Bacterial gastroenteritis, e.g. Salmonella, Shigella, Yersinia enterocolitica
	Melioidosis	Localized abdominal infections, e.g. appendicitis
	B. henselae	
	Actinomycetes	
Mycobacterial	M. tuberculosis	Mycobacterium bovis
	Non-tuberculous mycobacterium	
Fungal	Histoplasma, Blastomyces, Coccidioides, Paracoccidioides	
	Cryptococcus	
Parasitic	Toxoplasmosis	Parasitic infections of the gastrointestinal tract, e.g. Entamoeba histolytica
Non-infectious causes	Malignancy	Crohn's disease
	Primary immunodeficiencies (e.g. chronic granulomatous disease)	Coeliac disease
	Sarcoidosis	Familial Mediterranean fever

Table 15.4 Age-specific causes of lymphadenopathy in children

Age group	Causative organism
Neonates	S. aureus
	S. agalactiae (GBS)
Infants	S. aureus
	S. pyogenes (GAS)
	Consider Kawasaki disease
1–4 years	S. aureus
	S. pyogenes (GAS)
	Non-tuberculous mycobacteria (NTM)
	Kawasaki disease
5–15 years	Anaerobic bacteria
	Toxoplasmosis
	Cat scratch disease
	Tuberculosis
	Malignancy

Table 15.5 Miscellaneous eponymous syndromes associated with lymphadenopathy

Oculoglandular syndrome of Parinaud	Unilateral chronic ulceration of the conjunctiva and ipsilateral cervical lymphadenopathy. Most commonly caused by B. henselae in childhood but associated with many other infectious agents
Rosai–Dorfman disease (sinus histiocytosis with massive lymphadenopathy)	Progressive painless bilateral symmetric or asymmetric cervical lymphadenopathy. Other LNs and extra-nodal sites may be involved. Associated with fever, anaemia, leucocytosis, raised ESR and hypergammaglobulinaemia. Occurs in first two decades of life. Diagnosed on biopsy. Generally resolves spontaneously
Kikuchi–Fujimoto disease (histiocytic necrotizing lymphadenitis)	Unilateral usually matted tender cervical lymphadenopathy associated with fever, leucopenia, and a raised ESR. Systemic features include weight loss, night sweats, malaise, and joint pains. Diagnosed on biopsy which is also required to exclude malignancy. Generally resolves spontaneously although has been associated with systemic lupus erythematosus

(Continued)

Table 15.5 (Contd.)

Kimura's disease	Unilateral chronic cervical lymph node enlargement occurring most commonly in males of Asian origin. Associated with overlying subcutaneous nodules. Benign although may be disfiguring
Castleman's disease (giant lymph node hyperplasia)	Lymphoproliferative disorder which may be localized to a single lymph node and can be treated with local excision. A disseminated form (multicentric Castleman's disease), particularly occurring in HIV-infected individuals, is strongly associated with HHV-8 infection. Patients have fever, myalgia, and weight loss associated with diffuse lymphadenopathy and hepatosplenomegaly, and a generalized inflammatory response
Gianotti–Crosti syndrome (papular acrodermatitis)	Younger children, fever, widespread lymphadenopathy, hepatomegaly, widespread papules over limbs, face, palms and soles, usually resolving in around 1 month—occurs with acute hepatitis B and other viral infections

Prevalence and epidemiology

- LNs are palpable in between 38% and 45% of otherwise healthy children and are most commonly palpable between 3 and 5 years of age.
- Most cases in children are due to infection or benign disease.
- Acute unilateral cervical lymphadenitis is caused by streptococcal or staphylococcal infection in 40–80% of cases.
- Up to 95% of cases of mycobacterial lymphadenitis are caused by non-tuberculous mycobacteria (NTM) and NTM is the commonest cause of a chronic indurated cervical abscess.
- The incidence of NTM lymphadenitis is estimated to be between 2 and 3 cases per 100 000 children up to the age of 4 years, although the distribution of NTM appears to be geographically and environmentally variable.
- Tuberculous (TB) lymphadenitis is not uncommon in UK, especially in the Asian population.
- Chronic posterior cervical lymphadenitis is the most common form of acquired toxoplasmosis and is the sole presenting symptom in 50% of cases.
- Of children requiring a LN biopsy, 50% will have benign reactive lymphadenopathy.
- The reported prevalence of malignant neoplasms in children undergoing LN biopsy varies between 4% and 13%.

Clinical presentation and differential diagnosis

- A detailed history and thorough clinical examination is critical in directing initial investigations towards the most probable and important causes.

History

- Age of the child (Table 15.4):
  - *S. aureus*, GAS, and NTM are more common in children between 1 and 4 years
  - Toxoplasmosis, cat scratch disease, and TB are more common in older children
  - Lymphadenopathy secondary to neoplasia increases in the adolescent age group.
- Rate of LN enlargement (acute, subacute, chronic).
- Site (Fig. 15.2).
- Associated local symptoms:
  - Pain (e.g. acute bacterial lymphadenitis)
  - Skin changes (e.g. erythema—acute bacterial lymphadenitis; violaceous colour—NTM).
- Associated systemic features:
  - Fever (many infectious and non-infectious causes)
  - Ear, nose and throat (e.g. scarlet fever, measles and other viruses)
  - Respiratory (e.g. TB, *Mycoplasma*, *Legionella*, fungal infections, local compression of structures associated with mediastinal LN enlargement)
  - Gastrointestinal (e.g. infectious gastroenteritis, local symptoms suggesting abdominal lymphadenopathy)
  - Musculoskeletal (e.g. arthritis—Lyme disease or rheumatological conditions; myalgia—leptospirosis)
  - Neurological—headaches, meningism (e.g. Lyme disease, leptospirosis, rickettsial disease)
  - Rash (e.g. measles and other viruses, scarlet fever, spirochaetes, Lyme disease, leptospirosis, secondary syphilis), rickettsial disease (e.g. scrub typhus), eczema, rheumatological conditions
  - Local lesions (e.g. local skin infection with inflamed draining LNs, *Bartonella*, tularaemia, scrub typhus, trypanosomiasis, leishmaniasis)
  - Conjunctivitis (e.g. measles, adenovirus, oculoglandular syndrome of Parinaud (Table 15.5), Kawasaki disease)
  - Mouth—tooth decay (anaerobes), ulcers (PFAPA or HSV)
  - Weight loss (HIV, TB, malignancy, etc.).
- Immunization status (measles, rubella, diphtheria, hepatitis A and B, Bacille Calmette Guérin (BCG)).
- Travel history:
  - TB endemic areas
  - *Brucella* (worldwide but predominant in Mediterranean, Middle East, Indian subcontinent, parts of Central and South America and Africa)
  - Tularemia (worldwide, predominantly in the northern hemisphere, particularly North America, but cases also reported in Europe)

- Melioidosis (South East Asia; also reported in Northern Australia, India and Central America)
- *Rickettsia* (many geographical distributions according to species, e.g. scrub typhus—South East Asia and Oceania)
- Fungi (e.g. *Histoplasma*—many parts of world outside Europe; *Coccidioides*—certain semi-arid parts of North America extending into Central and South America)
- Trypanosomiasis (sub-Saharan Africa, Central and South America)
- Leishmaniasis (Central and South America, Southern Europe, North and East Africa, Middle East, Indian subcontinent)
- Schistosomiasis (predominantly sub-Saharan Africa, also areas of South America, Middle East and South East Asia)
- Filariasis (worldwide tropical distribution)
- Dengue fever (worldwide tropical distribution).
- Contact with domestic and non-domestic animals—ask about unusual pets! (*Bartonella*, tularemia, *Brucella*, *Rickettsia*).
- Ingestion of unpasteurized milk (e.g. *Brucella*, *Mycobacterium bovis*).
- Tick bites (Lyme disease, *Rickettsia*, tularemia).
- Risk factors for HIV (link to high-incidence country, maternal health, risk factors for horizontal acquisition), hepatitis B (maternal health, risk factors for horizontal transmission), and TB (family and other contacts, travel and immigration).
- History suggestive of primary or secondary immunodeficiency (e.g. recurrent abscesses).

Examination

Standardized description of the LNs should include:
- Size, location
- Single or multiple
- Consistency (soft, firm, rubbery, fluctuant)
- Attachment (superficial or deep)
- Skin changes (local abrasions and overlying skin changes)
- Tenderness.

Full systemic examination guided by findings from the history but not forgetting:
- Examination of other LN groups—head and neck, supraclavicular, axillary, epitrochlear, inguinal, popliteal
- Identification of splenomegaly and hepatomegaly
- Examination for infection in tissues drained by nodes (remember the mouth, teeth and gums)
- Eyes—conjunctivitis
- Skin—viral exanthema, other rashes
- Documentation of fever and weight loss.

Clinical syndromes and associated causes

Generalized lymphadenopathy

- Defined as enlargement of more than two non-contiguous LN groups.
- Large differential diagnosis but most often associated with systemic viral illness (Table 15.1).
- HIV is an important differential diagnosis to consider as widespread generalized lymphadenopathy may be present in isolation before other symptoms and signs develop.
- Malignancy should also be considered because of the dangers of delay.
- In a newborn, generalized lymphadenopathy associated with hepatosplenomegaly is likely to indicate a congenital infection (HIV, rubella, CMV, *T. gondii*, *T. pallidum*)

Localized lymphadenopathy

Most causes of generalized lymphadenopathy may present with predominantly localized disease.

Cervical lymph node enlargement

- Cervical lymphadenopathy most commonly represents a transient reactive response to a benign local or generalized infection, but occasionally it might be a sign of a more serious disease (e.g. malignancy).
- A child presenting with cervical lymphadenopathy will generally fall into one of three categories (Table 15.2) distinguished on initial history and physical examination:
  - Acute unilateral (pyogenic) cervical lymphadenitis
  - Acute bilateral cervical lymphadenopathy
  - Chronic or subacute cervical lymphadenopathy.

Acute unilateral cervical lymphadenopathy

- A child with a warm, tender, enlarged (>2–3cm) LN, which may be fluctuant and associated with overlying erythema and a fever, is likely to have an acute pyogenic cervical lymphadenitis, although other neck masses such as cystic hygroma may also become infected.
- Cervical lymphadenitis represents over 90% of acute lymphadenitis in childhood, although lymphadenitis at other sites, such as in the axillary or inguinal regions, should usually be approached in the same way.
- *S. aureus* and *S. pyogenes* (GAS) account for up to 80% of cases (Table 15.2).
- GBS is a further important cause in the neonatal period and is likely to be associated with systemic features of sepsis.
- Oral anaerobes must also be considered in older children particularly in the presence of dental caries/periodontal disease.
- Kawasaki disease is an important differential diagnosis to consider in a child with acute cervical lymphadenopathy which is typically unilateral although may be bilateral. Early treatment with immunoglobulin decreases the probability of coronary artery aneurysm development.

Acute bilateral cervical lymphadenopathy

- A common response to acute viral pharyngitis and systemic viral infections in children and does not generally require detailed investigation.
- The LNs are usually small and multiple. They may or may not be tender, and are not associated with warmth or erythema.
- Likely infectious agents (Table 15.2) may be indicated by their associated symptoms and signs:
  - Splenomegaly/hepatomegaly (EBV/CMV)
  - Gingivostomatitis (HSV)
  - Pharyngitis/conjunctivitis (adenoviruses, measles, Kawasaki disease)
  - Rash (enteroviruses, CMV, HHV-6, rubella, measles, parvovirus, Kawasaki disease)
  - Respiratory symptoms (*Mycoplasma*).

Chronic or subacute cervical lymphadenopathy

- A clinical presentation that is inconsistent with an acute lymphadenitis or a failure to respond to antibiotic therapy should prompt a search for alternative infectious and non-infectious causes.
- Typically the LNs are painless or minimally tender and are not associated with an increase in skin temperature.
- NTM, cat scratch disease, and toxoplasmosis are the most common infectious causes (Table 15.2).
- Most children with NTM infection present with:
  - A firm, painless, discrete mass or masses
  - 'Cold' abscess formation (the mass enlarges and becomes fluctuant as disease progresses)
  - The overlying skin can develop a characteristic violet colour
  - Spontaneous drainage with sinus tract formation occurs in around 10%.
- *M. tuberculosis* may manifest with a suppurative LN identical to that of NTM—remember that supraclavicular LN in TB is secondary to a pulmonary focus.
- Suppurative adenopathy occurs in between 10% and 35% of patients with cat scratch disease in axilla, cervical, or epitrochlear nodes.
- Congenital lesions (thyroglossal duct cyst, cystic hygroma, haemangioma, etc):
  - Present at birth or identified soon after
  - Painless, diffuse, soft and compressible
  - Transilluminate, usually red or blue in colour
  - Cystic malformations may become infected.
- PFAPA may be considered in a child presenting with recurrent bilateral cervical lymphadenopathy, periodic fever, aphthous stomatitis, and pharyngitis. Not all features are required and the diagnosis is made clinically.

Abdominal and mediastinal lymphadenopathy

- Many of the causes of generalized lymphadenopathy can present with LN enlargement which is predominantly localized to the mediastinal/hilar LNs or the abdominal/mesenteric/retroperitoneal LNs. These may be identified when imaging studies are undertaken, sometimes as an incidental finding.

- In addition, local infections of the respiratory or gastrointestinal tracts may result in enlargement of the draining LNs. In this case the cause is likely to be identified from the associated symptoms and signs prompting relevant investigations (e.g. stool sample).
- An outline of some of the more specific causes is provided in Table 15.3. Consider an underlying immune system defect in children who are diagnosed with infection caused by *Actinomycetes*, *Histoplasma*, *Cryptococcus*, and *Coccidioides* or disseminated NTM disease.
- Investigations and management must be guided by a detailed history and thorough clinical examination directing the clinician towards the most probable and important causes.

Malignancy
- Malignancy (especially lymphomas in teenagers) needs to be considered in all children presenting with localized LN enlargement. Specifically:
  - The adenopathy is usually non-tender, firm and rubbery with no warmth or erythema of the overlying skin (although the possibility of secondary infection should not be forgotten).
  - The nodes can become fixed, hard, bulky and grow rapidly.
  - Supraclavicular LN enlargement is uncommon following infection and malignancy should specifically be considered in this case. Left supraclavicular node—Virchow's node, drains lymphatics from thorax, and abdomen. However, other LN groups are often involved and an absence of supraclavicular lymphadenopathy should not be considered to be reassuring.

Investigations

- Most cases of lymphadenopathy in children are benign, usually associated with viral illness and do not generally require any investigation.
- Laboratory tests, imaging and biopsy may be indicated if serious underlying disease is suspected.

A list of investigations is given below, some of which may be useful **if there is a compatible history and clinical examination**. However, the ordering of investigations indiscriminately, without reasonable clinical suspicion, is not recommended. Most children need no investigation.
- Throat/nasal swab/nasopharyngeal aspirate or blood sample for virus identification.
- Full blood count ± blood film.
- Inflammatory markers (CRP, ESR).
- Liver enzymes, LDH (malignancy) and ferritin (systemic onset juvenile idiopathic arthritis (JIA), haemophagocytic lymphohistiocytosis).
- Blood cultures.

- Serology (acute ± convalescent) including: EBV, CMV, HHV-6, HIV, measles, parvovirus, GAS, *Mycoplasma*, *Borrelia*, syphilis (VDRL), *Leptospira*, *Brucella*, *Bartonella*, histoplasmosis, and coccidiomycosis.
- Stool sample for virus, bacteria, ova, cysts, and parasites.
- Tuberculin skin (Mantoux) test ± further investigations for TB.
- Immunological tests (e.g. neutrophil function).

Imaging

Ultrasound scan

- To confirm origin of swelling (LN versus other neck masses).
- To identify abscess formation.
- To guide core-needle biopsy if needed.

Chest X-ray (lung fields plus associated hilar/mediastinal lymphadenopathy)

- A normal chest X-ray does not exclude significant hilar lymphadenopathy which may require a CT scan.

CT or MRI

- To identify other sites of lymphadenopathy.
- To identify LNs with a malignant appearance.
- To delineate the solid, viable part of the LN for biopsy.

Pathology

- Biopsy may be required for definitive diagnosis and to exclude malignancy.
- Fine needle aspiration (FNA) is a very useful quick investigation in older children, with a very low complication rate.
- Excision biopsy ensures that adequate representative tissue is obtained. This is also definitive treatment for localized NTM disease.
- Tissue should always be sent for both:
  • Histopathological examination (including microbiological stains)
  • Bacterial (including anaerobic), mycobacterial and fungal culture
  • It is extraordinary how often this still does not happen!
- Discussion with microbiology and histopathology (and the surgeon) is strongly encouraged prior to obtaining samples to ensure they are processed appropriately to maximize the chances of identifying organisms for which prolonged culture may be required (e.g. *Mycobacteria* or *Brucella*) or which have fastidious growth requirements (*F. tularensis*) and to ensure appropriate stains are carried out on the tissue to identify infectious agents. Samples may also be stored for future analysis by PCR or other techniques.

Readers are referred to the disease-specific chapters for further details regarding the specific investigations appropriate for lymphadenopathy caused by individual organisms.

Management and treatment

Generalized lymphadenopathy

- The treatment of a child presenting with generalized lymphadenopathy is largely governed by the underlying cause.
- Most cases require no treatment.

Localized lymphadenopathy

- Treatment of bilateral cervical lymphadenitis depends on the underlying cause.
- Most cases are self-limited and require no specific treatment other than observation.
- Treatment will largely be symptomatic/supportive in the child with normal immune function.
- In the majority of children with acute pyogenic lymphadenitis empirical antibiotic therapy will be warranted and should provide adequate coverage for both *S. aureus* and *S. pyogenes* pending culture and sensitivity results.
- Choice of agent:
  - Co-amoxiclav or second-generation cephalosporin (± metronidazole if anaerobes suspected)—beware rash with amoxicillin and EBV infection.
  - Clindamycin is an alternative single-agent treatment.
  - Oral flucloxacillin is not generally recommended as it is poorly tolerated, the liquid preparation tastes unpleasant and it requires administration every 6 hours.
- Route of administration:
  - In a well child with few systemic features initial oral therapy may be appropriate with close monitoring.
  - In a child who is systemically unwell, has severe cervical lymphadenitis, or is unable to tolerate oral therapy, IV antibiotics are warranted.
- Duration of therapy should be 7 days—this may be extended in the neonate and in other children depending on the associated clinical features.
- Failure to respond to initial therapy may indicate:
  - Abscess formation requiring surgical drainage
  - The presence of a less common organism requiring alternative treatment following identification by biopsy or FNA
  - The presence of a resistant organism—is community-acquired MRSA likely?
  - Failure to take or tolerate the prescribed oral medication.
- Children <1 year of age and those in whom the LN has been present for >48 hours are more likely to require surgical intervention.
- Failure of the lymphadenopathy to regress after 4–6 weeks may be an indication for a diagnostic biopsy.
- Indications for early excision biopsy:
  - LN larger than 3cm
  - Unusual location, e.g. supraclavicular area
  - Previous history of malignancy

- Associated symptoms (weight loss, night sweats, hepatosplenomegaly).
- NTM lymphadenitis is best treated with surgical excision which offers the best chance of cure for children with NTM cervicofacial lymphadenitis and is generally considered to be the gold standard.
- The current recommendation for the treatment of isolated TB lymphadenitis is 2 months of isoniazid, rifampicin, pyrazinamide, and ethambutol, followed by 4 months of isoniazid and rifampicin. This may be modified according to patterns of resistance.

Future research

- Currently, there are no strongly evidence-based clinical algorithms and protocols for referral or management of children with enlarged superficial LNs.
- Introduction of coordinated problem-based referral and management pathways is warranted.

Further reading

Anne S, Teot LA, Mandell DL. Fine needle aspiration biopsy: role in diagnosis of pediatric head and neck masses. *Int J Pediatr Otorhinolaryngol* 2008;**72**:1547–53.

Leung AK, Davies HD. Cervical lymphadenitis: etiology, diagnosis, and management. *Curr Infect Dis Rep* 2009;**11**:183–9.

Luu TM, Chevalier I, Gauthier M, Carceller AM, Bensoussan A, Tapiero B. Acute adenitis in children: clinical course and factors predictive of surgical drainage. *J Paediatr Child Health* 2005;**41**:273–7.

Menon K, Bem C, Gouldesbrough D, Strachan DR. A clinical review of 128 cases of head and neck tuberculosis presenting over 10-year period in Bradford, UK. *J Laryngol Otol* 2007;**121**:362–8.

Nield LS, Kamat D. Lymphadenopathy in children: when and how to evaluate. *Clin Pediatr (Phila)* 2004;**43**:25–33.

Timmerman MK, Morley AD, Buwalda J. Treatment of non-tuberculous mycobacterial cervicofacial lymphadenitis in children: critical appraisal of the literature. *Clin Otolaryngol* 2008;**33**:546–52.

Haemolytic-uraemic syndrome

📖 see also Chapters 66, 104, 106

Introduction

- The clinical condition of HUS is characterized by:
  - Coombs' negative microangiopathic haemolytic anaemia
  - Thrombocytopenia
  - Acute renal failure.
- It can be associated with infective diarrhoea, systemic illnesses, invasive pneumococcal infections, or use of various medications.
- A subset of HUS is associated with complement dysfunction, classified recently as 'non-classical' primary immunodeficiency.
- A very similar disease called thrombotic thrombocytopenic purpura (TTP) presents with the above triad plus fever and CNS involvement, but despite similarities in presentation the pathogenesis and treatment are different.

Classification

- The most clinically useful classification of HUS distinguishes:
  - Diarrhoea associated (D+) or typical
  - Without diarrhoea (D−) or atypical.
- In resource-poor countries, D+ HUS is usually associated with *Shigella dysenteriae* infection.
- In the Western world, diarrhoea is usually caused by enterohaemorrhagic *Escherichia coli* (EHEC), which produces a potent exotoxin responsible for target organ damage.
- In the UK, most D+ HUS is caused by *E. coli* H7 O157 strain.
- HUS can also develop during invasive pneumococcal disease (pneumonia, empyema, or meningitis).
- HUS can be associated with other conditions such as systemic lupus erythematosus, antiphospholipid syndrome, following bone marrow transplantation, as a *de novo* disease in a renal graft, and after cytotoxic drug administration.
- D− (atypical) HUS occurs when there is uncontrolled dysregulation of the complement system due to different gene mutations.

Transmission

- The pathogenic organism is usually transmitted via contaminated food and water. Undercooked beef, contaminated with faeces while processing, is a common route of spread in EHEC. Visits to an animal petting farm and poor hygiene are frequent causes of HUS. Appropriate hand, fruit, and vegetable washing, as well as adequate meat preparation and cooking are the best measures in preventing disease.

D+ HUS

Pathogenesis

- *E. coli* O157, during either sporadic or epidemic infection, secretes a potent endotoxin similar to *Shigella* toxin (SHT1):
  - The endotoxin is cytopathic to the renal (Vero) cells of a green monkey, hence termed verocytotoxin (VCT): VCT1 is almost identical to SHT1
  - Once released from the bacteria, SHT (VCT) passes through the intestinal wall into the blood stream, and is carried by peripheral polymorphic neutrophils to specific receptors on the endothelial, tubular epithelial and mesangial cells in the kidneys, brain, and pancreas, causing disease.
- SHT is made of two units, A and B:
  - The latter binds to specific glycolipid globotriaosylceramide receptor Gb3.
  - SHT1 has lower affinity than SHT2 for Gb3 and causes less severe HUS.
  - Once bound to the cell, subunit A is endocytosed and transported into cytosol, where it inhibits protein synthesis.
- Endotoxin also stimulates production of inflammatory cytokines from macrophages and monocyte-derived cells.
  - Cytokines activate polymorphonuclear cells, which enhance endothelium cell injury.
  - Platelets and fibrin bind to damaged endothelium causing microthrombi, which lead to small blood vessels occlusion.
  - This process in glomerular blood vessels results in acute renal failure.
  - In the brain, this produces CNS symptoms (seizures, coma, stroke).
  - Similarly, diabetes mellitus or cardiomyopathy can also occur if the pancreas or cardiac vessels are involved.

Clinical presentation

- Diarrhoea usually precedes HUS in the D+ form.
  - The stools are bloody in three-quarters of patients.

- However, there are cases of HUS with positive *E. coli* serology but without a history of diarrhoea. When diarrhoea is present, it is often associated with vomiting, which explains why half of the patients at admission are dehydrated and hypovolaemic.
- When oliguria/anuria is not recognized and the child is maintained on liberal volumes of hypotonic fluids, hypervolaemia, hypertension, and hyponatraemia occur.
- Anaemia and thrombocytopenia precede renal failure, resulting in pallor and jaundice, and when/if the platelet count is <20 000/ml, petechial rash or overt bleeding can be noted.
  - While red blood cell transfusion is indicated, platelet transfusion is contraindicated unless patient needs surgery or is actively bleeding.
- Acute renal failure develops suddenly in three-quarters of patients.
  - It can be anuric or oliguric, rarely polyuric.
  - If the child is not anuric, urine may be red in colour either because of haematuria or haemoglobinuria secondary to haemolysis.
  - Due to diarrhoea, many patients in acute renal failure are hypokalaemic.
  - Hypertension in the acute phase is usually volume related, but can also be renin mediated particularly in the later stage of the illness.
- CNS symptoms or signs are present in up to 20% of children.
  - They can present non-specifically with irritability, confusion or lethargy, or more dramatically with seizures and coma.
  - Patients with CNS involvement should be transferred to paediatric intensive care unit (PICU).
  - Seizures and other abnormal neurology may also reflect low serum sodium, ischaemia-hypoxia, or cerebral oedema rather than CNS vessels thrombosis.
- Diabetes mellitus has been reported in <5%.
- *E. coli* may cause severe colitis leading to toxic colitis and even intestinal perforation.
  - Rectal prolapse is common.
  - As a rule, patients infected with EHEC are not febrile because there is no bacteraemia unlike with *Shigella* infection, when children typically present with bacteraemia and shock; hence they require urgent aggressive antibiotic treatment.

Investigations

- Anaemia with fragmented erythrocytes on blood film and thrombocytopenia is typical.
- Electrolyte disturbances are in keeping with acute renal failure.
- Polymorphonuclear leucocytosis correlates with the severity of renal disease—a high number of neutrophils at the beginning of the disease is a poor prognostic marker.
- Liver enzymes can be elevated at the beginning of disease.
- LDH is elevated.
- When urine output is maintained, a dipstick test shows presence of blood and/or haemoglobin and proteinuria.

Treatment

- Supportive management is of key importance to this condition.

- • Meticulous correction and maintenance of biochemistry, fluid status and acid–base balance is essential.
- • Patients with worsening uraemia either in isolation or combined with acid–base, fluid, or biochemical disturbances that cannot be corrected require renal replacement treatment: about three-quarters of patients will need dialysis, usually peritoneal dialysis.
- It is important to maintain good nutrition.
- Blood transfusion is indicated when haemolysis is ongoing and haemoglobin concentration falls to <6g/l.
- Platelet transfusion should be avoided if possible as there is evidence it may aggravate the disease process.
- If hypertension develops, either calcium channel blockers and/or an angiotensin-converting enzyme inhibitor should be considered.
- Antimotility agents should be avoided, as by reducing gut peristalsis, there is prolonged contact of the pathogenic bacteria with the intestinal mucosa. Antibiotics for gut decontamination are not recommended.
- Vitamin E, methylprednisolone, and endotoxin-absorbing agents are not recommended.
- While plasma exchange is a key treatment in patients with TTP and some with atypical D– HUS, its use in patients with D+ HUS is not routinely recommended. Many clinicians, however, use plasma exchange in children with overt CNS disease.

Histopathology

- Histological changes in D+ HUS differ from those in D– HUS
- Three distinctive histological findings are reported in HUS patients:
  - • glomerular thrombotic microangiopathy
  - • arterial thrombotic microangiopathy
  - • cortical necrosis.
- Glomerular type is the characteristic histological picture in D+ HUS with platelets, fibrin, and erythrocyte deposits. Thrombi originate from the glomerular tuft and extending towards the afferent arteriole.
- Arterial thrombotic microangiopathy and the associated cortical necrosis are the hallmarks of D– HUS.

Prognosis of D+ HUS

- High neutrophil count (>15 000/ml) at presentation, anuria lasting >10 days, and the need for dialysis for >2 weeks are markers of poor prognosis (either isolated proteinuria, hypertension, renal failure, or their combination).
- Rectal prolapse, severity of colitis, and younger age may also be weakly associated with a poor prognosis.
- The reported early mortality rate in the order of 1.5–5% is related mainly to CNS involvement.
- Renal function fully recovers in 80%, while 5% develop severe chronic renal failure. Patients who progress to end-stage renal failure can safely receive a transplant. D+ HUS does not occur in the transplanted kidney.
- The remaining 15% are left with varying degrees of chronic kidney disease such as proteinuria, decreased glomerular filtration rate (GFR), hypertension.

- Even among patients with apparent full recovery of kidney function there are reports of late development of proteinuria, decline in GFR, or hypertension even decades later; for that reason patients with HUS, especially those with abnormal GFR, proteinuria, and hypertension a year post disease should have lifelong follow-up.
- Of children who develop diabetes mellitus, approximately a third will require long-term insulin treatment; the remaining two-thirds will recover.

HUS associated with pneumococcal infection

- Though infection related, this form is classified as D- HUS.
- Pneumococcus produces an enzyme neuraminidase, which cleaves sialic acid on glomerular endothelial cells and platelets exposing the Thomsen-Friedenreich antigen to IgM antibodies.
  - This antibody-antigen binding interaction results in endothelial damage and thrombosis with microangiopathic haemolytic anaemia and target organ damage (acute renal failure).
  - Therefore fresh frozen plasma should be avoided in these patients as it contains IgM antibodies.
- HUS related to pneumococcal infection often affects younger children, some as young as <2 years.
  - These children must be treated with antibiotics as the pneumococcal infection itself is often severe and life-threatening.
  - These patients have more severe kidney disease requiring longer dialysis.
  - They require more red cell and platelet transfusions.
- Data suggest much higher mortality in children with pneumococcal HUS (24%). The excess mortality is due to the severe pneumococcal infection rather than the renal failure.
- Renal recovery is similar to D+ HUS.
- When managing these patients, it is essential to actively manage the sepsis, septic shock, and DIC.
  - The acute renal failure in DIC is related to acute tubular necrosis whereas in HUS, renal failure is due to thrombotic microangiopathy and ischaemia.
  - In HUS, fibrinogen, prothrombin, and partial prothrombin time are either normal or slightly elevated.
  - It is important to note the direct Coombs' test is positive unlike in other forms of HUS.

D- (atypical) HUS

- D- HUS is uncommon, accounting for <10% of all HUS cases.
  - Most cases of atypical HUS are associated with dysfunction of the complement system regulatory pathway; a large body of research over the recent years has managed to characterize many of the genetic mutations responsible.

- The genetic mutations can be either dominantly or recessively inherited and include fluid phase regulatory proteins H and I, the membrane cofactor protein (MCP) or CD46 and (gain of function in) C3 protein. Recent data suggest that genetic defects result in abnormal protein structure, which allows the development of autoantibodies against elements of the pathway such as factor H, which leads to atypical HUS.
- Prognosis is much worse than in D+ disease, with half remaining on dialysis from first presentation.
- D– HUS due to these defects has a relapsing course and recurrence rate after renal transplantation is high (except in patients with CD46 mutation, which is abundantly present on glomerular cells), so that almost 90% of kidneys with recurrent disease will be lost. In cases where antibodies are present regular plasma exchange is warranted.
  - When dysfunctional protein is present, regular plasma infusions can be effective.
  - Very recently, humanized monoclonal antibody directed against C5a (eculizumab) has become available in clinical trials.

Further reading

Botto M, Kirschfink M, Macor P, Pickering MC, Wurzner R, Tedesco F. Complement in human diseases: Lessons from complement deficiencies. *Mol Immunol* 2009;**46**:2774–83.

Garg AX, Suri RS, Barrowman N, *et al.* Long-term renal prognosis of diarrhoea-associated hemolytic uremic syndrome: a systematic review, meta-analysis, and meta-regression. *JAMA* 2003;**290**:1360–70.

Pessach I, Walter J, Notarangelo LD. Recent advances in primary immunodeficiencies: identification of novel genetic defects and unanticipated phenotypes. *Pediatr Res* 2009; **65**:3R–12R.

Tarr PI, Gordon CA, Chandler WL. Shiga-toxin-producing *Escherichia coli* and haemolytic uraemic syndrome. *Lancet* 2005;**365**:1073–86.

Taylor CM, Chua C, Howie AJ, Risdon RA. Clinico-pathological findings in diarrhoea negative HUS. *Pediatr Nephrol* 2004;**19**:419–25.

Trachtman H, Cnaan A, Christen E, *et al.* Effect of an oral Shiga binding agent on diarrhoea associated HUS in children: a randomized controlled trial. *JAMA* 2003;**290**:1337–44.

Wong C, Jelacic S, Habeeb RL, Watkins SL, Tarr PI. The risk of the HUS after antibiotic treatment of *E coli* O157 infections. *N Engl J Med* 2000;**342**:1930–6.

Healthcare-associated infections

📖 see also Chapters 21, 60, 92, 105

Introduction

Healthcare-associated infections (HCAIs) are infections that are acquired as a result of healthcare interventions. Infections presenting >48 hours after admission to hospital are generally considered to be hospital acquired.

HCAIs are important for many reasons:
- They are costly
- They cause excess morbidity and mortality to patients
- They can be disruptive to running the hospital
- They can result in adverse publicity and/or legal action.

With consistent application of good infection control measures a large proportion of HCAIs are preventable. Growing recognition of this in recent years has led to many initiatives to control and prevent HCAIs.

In the UK and Europe much of the focus has been on *Clostridium difficile* and bloodstream infections with MRSA, conditions that are less common in paediatrics. However, this does not mean that HCAIs are less of a problem in paediatrics.

Epidemiology

Reasons why patients in hospital are at risk of HCAI
- Close proximity to other patients colonized or infected with important microorganisms: This risk can be compounded by movement of patients, within and between hospitals, and overcrowding.
- Underlying illnesses or chronic medical problems increasing susceptibility to infection.
- Surgery introduces risk of many types of infection.
- Other manipulations involving breach of normal host defences also increase the risk of infection, e.g. intravascular devices, mechanical ventilation, urinary catheterization, etc.
- Antibiotics used to prevent or treat infections themselves carry a risk of causing superinfections with resistant microorganisms.

HCAIs in children are less well studied than in adults. However, there are important differences:

- Infection is a more common reason for children being admitted to hospital: community-associated childhood infections such as rotavirus, norovirus, and respiratory virus infections may therefore spread in hospitals.
- Children are less likely to be immune to viral infections such as chickenpox.
- Children appear to be less susceptible to some common healthcare-associated pathogens, e.g. *C. difficile*, MRSA.
- Modes of treatment of children and adults may differ. For example, urinary catheters are used much less frequently in children.

Incidence

At any one time 8–10% of hospitalized adults have an infection that was acquired in hospital. However, these data underestimate the risk of acquiring an infection in hospital because they do not take account of length of stay or of infections that do not present until after discharge: up to 20% of patients discharged from hospital may later develop an HCAI.

The incidence of HCAI also depends on the types of patient treated: the incidence is highest in patients in intensive care (especially neonatal intensive care), recipients of solid organ and bone marrow transplantation and those with burns.

Sources of infection

HCAIs may be:

- Endogenous: infections caused by opportunist pathogens that the patient is already colonized with
- Exogenous: infections caused by microorganisms that are acquired in hospital.

Types of HCAI

HCAIs can occur at any site of the body. Many are associated with indwelling invasive devices. Rates of infection are best expressed as a proportion of how many days the device has been sited. 📖 See Chapter 8, Central venous catheters, p. 68.

Blood stream infections are the commonest cause of HCAI in children in the USA, and responsible for around a third of all reports to the National Nosocomial Infections Surveillance (NNIS) system in the USA. A study of adult patients in 273 acute hospitals in the UK and Ireland showed that four types of infection accounted for two-thirds of all HCAIs.

There are fewer comparable data for hospitalized children in the UK and Europe, but the prevalence of HCAI may be even higher than in adults, and the common types of infection will certainly differ. For all rates of nosocomial infection it is important to have clear denominator data that are comprehensive, easily collectable, and reproducible.

Table 17.1 shows the distribution of various types of HCAI.

Table 17.1 Commonest sites of HCAI in the most recent UK and Ireland prevalence survey

Infection type	Per cent of all HCAIs
Gastrointestinal tract	22.0
Urinary tract	19.7
Pneumonia	13.9
Surgical site	13.8

Infections that may be transmitted between patients and between patients and healthcare workers

- Diarrhoea
- *Staphylococcus aureus* infections (including MRSA)
- GAS infections
- Tuberculosis
- Varicella zoster
- Measles, mumps, rubella
- Influenza
- Respiratory virus infections, e.g. RSV.

Infections mainly transmitted between patients and healthcare workers

- Bloodborne viral infections
- HSV infections
- CMV infections
- Meningococcal disease.

Infections mainly transmitted between patients

- Infections caused by antibiotic-resistant bacteria
- *C. difficile* infection.

Infections that may be acquired from the hospital environment

- Legionnaires' disease
- Aspergillosis
- Infections caused by Gram-negative bacteria, e.g. *Pseudomonas*, *Acinetobacter*
- *C. difficile* infections
- Glycopeptide-resistant enterococcal infections.

Causative microorganisms

See Tables 17.2–17.6

Table 17.2 Gram-positive bacteria causing HCAIs

Species	High-risk patient groups	Types of HCAI
Staphylococcus aureus	Surgical	Surgical site infections
	Neutropenia	Bloodstream infection
	Ventilated patients	Pneumonia
	Patients with indwelling medical devices	Central venous catheter-related infections; shunt-associated meningitis; dialysis catheter-related peritonitis
	Cardiac surgery	Endocarditis
CONS	Ventilated neonates	Pneumonia
	Patients with indwelling medical devices	Central venous catheter-related infections; shunt-associated meningitis; dialysis catheter-related peritonitis
	Cardiac surgery	Endocarditis
	Neonatal intensive care	Pneumonia; bloodstream infection
Streptococcus pyogenes	Burns	Skin and soft tissue infections
	Surgical	Surgical site infections
Enterococcus spp.	Patients with multiple antibiotic exposure	Bloodstream infections
	Liver unit; gastroenterology	Intra-abdominal infections
	Patients with indwelling medical devices	Central venous catheter-related infections; catheter-associated urinary tract infections

Table 17.3 Gram-negative bacteria causing HCAIs

Species	High-risk patient groups	Types of HCAI
Enterobacteriaceae (*Escherichia coli*, *Klebsiella*, *Enterobacter*, etc.)	Neutropenia	Bloodstream infection
	Ventilated patients	Pneumonia
	Liver unit; gastroenterology; surgical	Intra-abdominal infections
	Renal	Urinary tract infection
	Neonatal intensive care	Pneumonia; bloodstream infection
Pseudomonas aeruginosa	Neutropenia	Bloodstream infection
	Ventilated patients	Pneumonia
	Burns	Skin and soft tissue infections
Acinetobacter spp.	Patients with multiple antibiotic exposures	Bloodstream infections
	Burns	Skin and soft tissue infections
	Patients with indwelling medical devices	Central venous catheter-related infections; shunt-associated meningitis
Legionella	Immunocompromised	Pneumonia

Table 17.4 Anaerobic bacteria causing HCAIs

Species	High-risk patient groups	Types of HCAI
Clostridium difficile	Recent/current antibiotic exposure; immunocompromised	Diarrhoea

Table 17.5 Fungi causing HCAIs

Species	High-risk patient groups	Types of HCAI
Candida spp.	Patients with multiple antibiotic exposures	Bloodstream infections; oesophagitis
	Patients with indwelling medical devices	Central venous catheter-related infections; catheter-associated urinary tract infection
	Neutropenia	Bloodstream infection
	Intensive care	Pneumonia; bloodstream infection
	HIV infection	Mucosal candidiasis
Aspergillus spp.	Bone marrow transplantation	Pneumonia
	Some primary immunodeficiencies (e.g. chronic granulomatous disease (CGD))	

Table 17.6 Viruses causing HCAIs

Virus	High-risk patient groups	Types of HCAI
Rotavirus	Infants	Diarrhoea
RSV	Infants	Bronchiolitis
	Immunocompromised children (all ages)	Respiratory infections
Varicella zoster	All non-immune patients	Chickenpox (risk of severe disseminated disease in neonates and immunocompromised)
CMV	Immunocompromised patients (especially post bone marrow or solid organ transplant)	Severe disseminated infection
EBV	Immunocompromised patients (especially post bone marrow or solid organ transplant)	Disseminated disease; post-transplant lymphoproliferative disorder (PTLD)
Herpes simplex	Immunocompromised patients (especially post bone marrow or solid organ transplant); neonates	Severe disseminated infection
Adenoviruses	Immunocompromised patients (especially post bone marrow or solid organ transplant)	Severe disseminated infection
Hepatitis B, hepatitis C, HIV	All	Bloodborne virus infections

Prevention

Many elements contribute to prevention of HCAI, including:
- An effective infection prevention and control service
- Hospital design
- Environmental cleanliness
- Effective decontamination of reusable medical devices
- Infection control policies and protocols
- Isolation of patients
- Hand hygiene
- Care of indwelling medical devices
- Screening and surveillance
- Prevention and management of inoculation injuries
- Appropriate antimicrobial prescribing
- Immunization.

Effective infection prevention and control service

Infection control must be embedded into clinical practice, and applied consistently by everyone. This depends on good management and organisation, underpinned by good education, training, information and communication, and an assurance framework.

Key elements
- Board-level responsibility for preventing and controlling HCAIs.
- A director of infection prevention and control who is accountable to the organization's board and responsible for its infection control team.
- An infection control team consisting of an adequate and appropriate mix of nursing and medical staff, with administrative and analytical support.
- An antimicrobial management team, typically consisting of microbiologists, clinicians and an antibiotic pharmacist.

Hospital design

Hospitals should be designed and maintained to minimize opportunities for transmission of infection. This includes provision of:
- Adequate isolation facilities
- Adequate space between beds or cots
- Appropriate air quality and ventilation in specialist areas
- Clinical areas that are uncluttered and easy to clean
- Proper separation of clean and dirty medical equipment
- A programme of ongoing maintenance.

Environmental cleanliness
- Poor environmental cleanliness is linked to the risk of HCAI.
- Cleaning schedules should be clear and well publicized, and supported by a monitoring programme.

Effective decontamination of reusable medical devices

Reusable devices must be decontaminated in accordance with manufacturers' instructions. Decontamination must be tracked throughout, together with systems to identify patients on whom devices have been used. Devices that are designated for single use or single patient use must not be used outside those restrictions.

Infection control policies and procedures

All hospitals should have and adhere to evidence-based infection control policies and procedures to ensure that clinical practice is safe for both patients and staff. Many of the other elements of good infection prevention and control described in this section will be covered by these policies.

Isolation of patients

There are two main types of isolation:
- **Source isolation** is used to prevent transmission of pathogenic microorganisms from infected patients to other patients or staff
- **Protective isolation** is used to protect susceptible individuals from potential pathogens carried by their attendants or present in the environment.

Key elements of isolation
- Patient nursed in a single room. Where the number of infected persons exceeds availability of single rooms, cohort isolation of patients with the same infection may be employed.
- Hand hygiene on entering and leaving the room.
- Wearing of appropriate personal protective equipment by all persons entering the room.
- Numbers of people entering the room minimized.

Hand hygiene

Hand hygiene is the single most important measure in preventing HCAI. The WHO has developed the 'Five Moments' strategy towards hand hygiene that identifies the moments when hand hygiene is required to effectively interrupt microbial transmission during the patient care sequence (Fig. 17.1):
1. Before patient contact
2. Before an aseptic task
3. After body fluid exposure risk
4. After patient contact
5. After contact with patient surroundings.

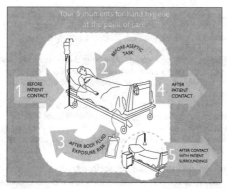

Fig. 17.1 The WHO Five moments strategy.

Source: Reproduced from H. Sax, B. Allegranzi, I. Uçkay, E. Larson, J. Boyce, D. Pittet (2007) 'My five moments for hand hygiene': a user-centred design approach to understand, train, monitor and report hand hygiene. *Journal of Hospital Infection* 2007:**67**;9–21, with permission from Elsevier.

Care of indwelling medical devices

Indwelling devices such as urinary catheters, intravascular catheters, and endotracheal tubes are a frequent source of invasive infections. Adherence to good practice during the insertion and care of these devices can significantly reduce the risk of infection.

Key elements of management of indwelling medical devices

- Indwelling devices only used where there is no suitable alternative.
- Where used, kept in place for as short a time as possible.
- Insertion always undertaken by, or supervised by, trained and competent staff.
- Manipulation after insertion always undertaken, or supervised, by trained and competent staff.
- Removal always undertaken, or supervised, by trained and competent staff.

Screening and surveillance

Screening is used to detect people who are asymptomatic carriers of a microorganism that might later cause infection in that individual and/or be transmitted to other individuals. Persons who are screen-positive can be offered appropriate management to reduce their risk.

MRSA screening: Many countries now advocate screening of patients admitted to hospital. Coupled with decolonization treatment for those found to be positive, this approach can reduce the risk of infection for the individual patient and help prevent transmission of MRSA to others. The place for universal screening of hospitalized children is unclear, because rates of colonization and infection in children are lower than in adults.

However, screening of patient groups at higher risk of invasive infection with MRSA (such as neonates, PICU admissions, patients with indwelling medical devices) may be justified. Different hospitals have different risk-based screening strategies for children.

Surveillance is the process of monitoring the rates of microorganisms or infections that may give rise to hospital outbreaks. Monitoring infection rates is increasingly regarded as an important contributor to safe and high quality healthcare. Surveillance can:

- Allow comparison of infection rates with other hospitals
- Inform planning, and allow monitoring of benefits, of infection control initiatives
- Allow early detection of increases in rates of infection, so that remedial control measures can be implemented.

Appropriate antimicrobial prescribing

Antibiotic use is directly linked to the selection and maintenance of antibiotic resistance. However, antibiotic use can also increase transmissibility and pathogenicity of multiresistant bacteria, thus contributing directly to increasing the number of HCAIs.

Increasingly, point prevalence surveys (PPSs) are performed to determine the rates, type, and indications for antibiotic use in hospitals. All hospitals, including children's hospitals, should be performing regular PPSs. In children this is more complicated as no single methodology has been validated.

Optimization of antimicrobial therapy for hospitalized patients ensures cost-effective therapy, improved patient outcomes, and reduced risks of antibiotic resistance and of HCAI.

Components of antibiotic control in hospitals

- Antibiotics prescribed only where clinical evidence of bacterial infection.
- Antibiotic formulary and prescribing guidelines that restrict use of broad-spectrum agents.
- Recommendations on duration of therapy for specific infections. For most patients:
  - IV therapy can be limited to 48 hours, and total treatment to 5–7 days
  - Surgical prophylaxis can be limited to single dose in most cases.
- Control measures including prescriber education, regular review of drug charts, audit, and restricted availability of certain antibiotics.

Immunization

Both active and passive immunization is used to control HCAIs, e.g.:

- Active immunization of non-immune staff, e.g. against hepatitis B, measles, chickenpox, influenza
- Hepatitis B immunization of high-risk patients groups
- Active and/or passive immunization against hepatitis B after inoculation injuries

- Passive immunization with VZIG for non-immune high-risk contacts of persons with chickenpox
- Passive immunization with human normal immunoglobulin for non-immune high-risk contacts of measles.

Future research

Much of the research on hospital infection control has focused on adults rather than children. There are many opportunities to investigate the prevalence, epidemiology, and prevention of healthcare-associated infections in children.

Further reading

Fraise AP. *Ayliffe's Control of Healthcare Associated Infection. A Practical Handbook*, 5th edn. Oxford: Oxford University Press, 2009.

Gould IM. Antibiotic policies to control hospital-acquired infection. *J Antimicrob Chemother* 2008;**61**:763–5.

Hambraeus A. Lowbury lecture 2005: Infection control from a global perspective. *J Hosp Infect* 2006;**64**:217–23.

Humphrey H, Newcombe RG, Enstone J, *et al.* Four country HCAI prevalence study 2006: risk factor analysis. *J Hosp Infect* 2008;**69**:249–57.

Mayhall CG, ed. *Hospital Epidemiology and Infection Control*, 3rd edn. Philadelphia: Lippincott, Williams & Wilkins, 2004.

Chapter 18

Acute hepatitis

📖 see also Chapters 17, 62, 64, 65, 75, 76, 117

Introduction

- Acute inflammation of the liver can be caused by drugs, autoimmune disease, metabolic disease, and infection, especially viruses.
- Acute hepatitis resolves by definition within 6 months. Children with persistent infection or inflammation of the liver after this time have chronic hepatitis. Acute viral hepatitis may cause subclinical disease, self-limited symptomatic disease or rarely fulminant hepatic failure.
- Acute viral hepatitis is mostly caused by the hepatitis viruses A, B, and E. Infrequent causes of viral hepatitis include adenovirus, CMV, EBV, and rarely, HSV, measles, rubella, varicella zoster, enteroviruses, HIV, parvovirus, and HHV-6.
- Most acute viral hepatitis in children is due to hepatitis A infection, which is often subclinical or very mild.

Name and nature of organisms

- Hepatitis A virus is a non-enveloped positive-stranded RNA Picornavirus.
- Hepatitis E virus is a non-enveloped, spherical, single-stranded RNA Hepevirus.

Epidemiology

Hepatitis A

- Hepatitis A occurs worldwide and is common in the Middle East, Africa, Asia, and Central and South America. Most people in these regions are infected when they are young children. Children from Europe who visit friends or relatives in these countries are particularly at risk of infection.
- The incidence of hepatitis A in developed countries has fallen greatly over the past few decades. Seroprevalence in England and Wales increases with age: 4% in those aged 1–4 years, 9% in those aged 1–9 years, 26% in those aged 25–44 years, 74% in those aged >60 years. Seroprevalence is higher amongst those of non-white ethnicity.
- Travel may be an important risk factor for hepatitis A infection with many of those of South Asian origin acquiring their infection abroad. Bloodborne transmission of hepatitis A virus can occur, but is rare.

Hepatitis E

- Hepatitis E is endemic in regions of the world where sanitation is poor, particularly in parts of Asia, Central America, and Africa.
- Sporadic cases occur in developed countries and can be associated with travel to endemic regions.
- Most children with hepatitis E infection have few symptoms. Symptomatic hepatitis E infection is more common in young adults and in pregnant women. Pregnant women have up to a 25% risk of mortality from hepatitis E and their baby may also be infected.
- There were 186 cases of hepatitis E in the UK between 1996 and 2003, 69% of which had recently travelled to endemic countries, especially the Indian subcontinent (Bangladesh). Very few of these were children.

Transmission and incubation period

Hepatitis A

- Hepatitis A virus is excreted in the bile and shed in the stools of infected persons. Transmission is by the faecal-oral route.
- Peak excretion occurs during the 2 weeks before the onset of jaundice. Patients are therefore infectious from 2 weeks before the onset of symptoms and may continue to be infectious for 1 week or more after. Children may excrete the virus for longer than adults, although a chronic carrier state does not exist.
- Foodborne outbreaks can occur due to contamination of food.
- The incubation period of hepatitis A infection is 15–45 days (average 4 weeks).
- Person-to-person spread is the most common method of transmission in developed countries. Children <6 years are particularly effective transmitters of hepatitis A infection. Transmission within households is very common and can also occur in nurseries and primary schools.

Hepatitis E

- Hepatitis E virus is transmitted by the faecal-oral route.
- Foodborne transmission also occurs.
- Direct person-to-person transmission is uncommon.
- The incubation period for hepatitis E is 40 days (range 15–60 days).

Clinical presentation and differential diagnosis

- Young children who are infected with hepatitis viruses usually remain asymptomatic. Acute hepatitis A, B, and E are all more severe in adults than in children.
- Typical symptoms of acute hepatitis are: general malaise, anorexia, nausea, vomiting, abdominal pain, arthralgia, and low grade fever.

Some children then develop jaundice, dark urine, pale stools, tender hepatomegaly, splenomegaly, or rash.
- Examination findings include an enlarged, tender liver and jaundice in more severe cases.
- Fulminant hepatic failure may occur in 1% of cases within 8 weeks of the onset of symptoms of acute hepatitis. It is defined as acute onset of liver disease in the absence of pre-existing liver disease, with the onset of hepatic encephalopathy and coagulopathy. Encephalopathy may be difficult to detect or less severe in infants and small children. Detection of coagulopathy is thus important in the absence of encephalopathy (prothrombin time (PT) >20 seconds or international normalized ratio (INR) >2.0 not corrected by parenteral vitamin K; in the presence of encephalopathy PT >15 seconds or INR >1.5).
- The mortality rate of fulminant hepatitis is very high, particularly if recognition and transfer are delayed. Deterioration can occur rapidly so all children with acute hepatitis should have a coagulation screen. Those with coagulopathy should be discussed immediately with a paediatric hepatologist.

Diagnosis

- Liver function tests (LFTs) in acute viral hepatitis show raised aminotransferase levels (from a few hundreds to >1000 U/l) and raised bilirubin. Some children have a cholestatic hepatitis with an elevated alkaline phosphatase level, instead of the typical picture of elevated aminotransferase levels.
- Severe cases of acute hepatitis may progress rapidly to acute liver failure, marked by poor hepatic synthetic function (low serum albumin, abnormal coagulation—see above).
- Cases of acute viral hepatitis are not clinically distinguishable from other types of hepatitis.
- Specific diagnosis is made by viral serology. This should include hepatitis A IgM and IgG plus hepatitis B surface antigen, and anti-hepatitis B core antigen IgM. Negative serology taken <5 days after the onset of illness may not exclude hepatitis A and a repeat sample should be obtained. Testing for other viruses (EBV, CMV, hepatitis E) should be done if hepatitis A and B serology is negative, depending on clinical features.

Management and treatment

- Many cases resolve over 4–12 weeks, provided that acute viral hepatitis does not progress to fulminant hepatic failure.
- Acute viral hepatitis may evolve into chronic hepatitis. Although patients with hepatitis A and hepatitis E do not progress to chronic hepatitis, chronic hepatitis B occurs in 90% of infants infected at birth, 20–50% of those infected aged 1–5 years, and in 6–10% of children infected when >5 years.

Treatment

- There is no specific treatment for hepatitis A or E infection. Treatment is thus supportive. Acute hepatitis B infection also resolves spontaneous in the majority of cases and is not usually an indication for antiviral therapy.
- The majority of children with acute hepatitis can be cared for at home. Hospital admission should be considered for those with persistent vomiting and is required for children with fulminant hepatitis. If children with acute hepatitis are admitted to hospital, standard universal precautions should be taken when handling blood and other body fluids.
- Children with fulminant hepatitis should be discussed urgently with a paediatric hepatologist.

Management of the child with hepatitis A

- Advise good hygiene practices (to avoid faecal-oral spread).
- Exclude from school or nursery until 7 days after the onset of jaundice.
- Identify possible source of infection.

Prevention

Hepatitis A

Primary prevention

Infection is prevented by good hygiene; especially handwashing, provision of safe drinking water, and good food hygiene. Vaccination can be used to prevent hepatitis A infection in high-risk groups. The following children are recommended to receive hepatitis A vaccination:[1]

- Anyone travelling to areas of moderate or high risk (the Indian subcontinent, the Far East, and Eastern Europe) for prolonged periods, particularly if sanitation and food hygiene is likely to be poor
- Patients with chronic liver disease or haemophilia.

Prevention of secondary cases[2]

Prevention of secondary cases should be discussed with a consultant for communicable disease control. For household contacts seen within 14 days of exposure to index case:

- Offer hepatitis A vaccine to healthy contacts aged 1–50 years
- If the healthy contact is aged <12 months:
  - Vaccinate carers to prevent tertiary infection

OR

- Offer hepatitis A vaccine to the infant if ≥2 months (unlicensed)

OR

- Exclude from childcare until 40 days after exposure.

Infants <12 months very rarely develop symptomatic hepatitis A infection. However, infants are at risk of developing subclinical infection and infecting others. If all those involved in nappy changing are vaccinated against hepatitis A this should prevent the spread of infection. If it is not feasible to vaccinate all carers, infants aged ≥2 months can be vaccinated with hepatitis A vaccine or excluded from childcare settings until 40 days after exposure to hepatitis A.

Hepatitis E

Primary prevention

- Infection is prevented by good personal hygiene (especially handwashing), use of safe drinking water/food, and proper disposal of sanitary waste.
- For travellers to highly endemic areas, the usual food hygiene precautions are recommended. These include: avoiding drinking water and/or ice of unknown purity; not eating uncooked shellfish or uncooked fruits; and not eating vegetables that are not peeled or prepared by the traveller.
- Currently, there is no vaccine for hepatitis E.

Future research

Development of a vaccine for hepatitis E.

Key references

1 Hepatitis A. In: *Immunisation against Infectious Disease*, 3rd edition. London: Department of Health, 2006. ℜ http://www.dh.gov.uk/dr_consum_dh/groups/dh_digitalassets/documents/digitalasset/dh_092124.pdf (accessed 1 February 2011).
2 Thomas L and the Hepatitis A Guidelines Group. *Guidance for the Prevention and Control of hepatitis A Infection.* Health Protection Agency. ℜ http://www.hpa.org.uk/ (accessed 1 February 2011).

Human immunodeficiency virus infection

📖 see also Chapters 4, 20, 24, 55, 61, 62, 91, 96, 113

Introduction

- The key to HIV pathogenesis is the impact of immunodeficiency through loss of T helper or CD4$^+$ cells and subsequent development of opportunistic infections. HIV also directly damages other cells causing focal organ disease. AIDS is advanced HIV disease defined by the presence of severe opportunistic infections or specific organ disease.
- The impact on morbidity and mortality in parts of the world with the greatest burden of HIV has been profound with catastrophic changes in population structures and demography.
- After years of little or no effective therapy against HIV, we have seen the advent of combination antiretroviral therapy (ART) that has remarkably altered the outlook for those with access to these drugs.
- The advent of ART and the associated benefits has meant that HIV has moved from being a fatal condition to a chronic one and the impact on children has been that of increased survival into adulthood.
- There are, however, important issues regarding adherence to therapy, stigma, and multidrug resistance that make the management of HIV more complex and different from other chronic conditions.

Causative organisms

- HIV is an enveloped RNA virus of the family *Retroviridae*.
- There are two major types—type 1 (HIV-1) and type 2 (HIV-2). HIV-1 is by far the commonest and predominates outside West Africa.
- There are also several different clades or sub-types (designated A, B, C, D, E, F, G, H, J, and K) in different geographical regions.
- As HIV is a retrovirus, its life cycle involves integration into the target cell genome as a provirus and the viral genome is copied during DNA replication to complete viral replication.
- Latent virus can persist in infected people for life.

Epidemiology

- Humans are the only known reservoir of HIV infection, although related viruses, perhaps genetic ancestors, have been identified in chimpanzees and monkeys (called simian immunodeficiency viruses).
- Established modes of HIV transmission include the following:
  - Sexual contact (vaginal, anal, or orogenital)

- Mother-to-child transmission during pregnancy, around the time of labour and delivery, and postnatally through breastfeeding
- Percutaneously through contaminated needles or other sharp instruments
- Contaminated blood products.
- The WHO estimated that in 2008 there were about 33.4 million people living with HIV/AIDS, including 2.1 million children <15 years age.
  - A total of 2.7 million people were newly infected, including 430 000 children, and there were 2 million AIDS deaths, including 280 000 children.
  - Africa represents almost two-thirds (67%) of the global total of 33 million people living with HIV/AIDS, and three-quarters (75%) of all AIDS deaths
  - Asia represents almost a fifth (15%) of the global total of people living with HIV/AIDS.
  - In Europe (Central and Western) and North America, there were an estimated 2.3 million people living with HIV/AIDS of which 1.2 million were in the USA.
  - The large majority of new infections in children occurred in Africa and Asia through mother-to-child transmission, with fewer than 500 children becoming newly infected in Europe and North America.
- The epidemiology of paediatric HIV infection reflects the pattern of infection in women because of the importance of vertical transmission.
- In resource-rich countries, injecting drug use had been a major risk factor for infection in women, but this has now been overtaken by acquisition via heterosexual sex, which is the major route of acquisition of maternal infection in resource-poor countries and worldwide.

Epidemiology of HIV infection in the UK

- In the UK and Ireland, the major risk factor for infection is vertical infection from women who acquired their infection in high-prevalence areas, particularly sub-Saharan Africa.
- A total of 1560 children in the UK were reported to the Collaborative HIV Paediatric Study (CHIPS, www.chipscohort.ac.uk) by the end of March 2009.
- The median age at first presentation of those born in the UK and Ireland has remained relatively constant at around 6 months. For children born abroad it increased from <3 years up to 1991 to >9 years in 2008. The majority of children with HIV in Europe are now teenagers.
- Children very rarely get sick, with the rate of hospital admission now around 0.1/child/year. Of the around 1000 children under care, fewer than 5 children die each year.
- Vertical transmission rates of HIV-1 infection historically varied between15% and 25% in USA and Europe and 25% and 35% in Africa. Risk factors for vertical transmission include maternal factors (primary infection, advanced clinical disease, low CD4 counts, high viral load, and presence of sexually transmitted infections (STIs)/chorioamnionitis), mode of delivery (prolonged rupture of membranes, premature delivery), and breastfeeding.
- The introduction of universal routine antenatal HIV testing and the use of combination ART in pregnancy has reduced the vertical transmission rate in Europe to generally less than 1%. A higher proportion of

women with undetectable viral loads during pregnancy are choosing to have normal vaginal deliveries, with very low rates of vertical transmission. There remain a few babies still born with HIV in Europe where the mother has either not integrated with antenatal testing and treatment, or where there have been system failures in the antenatal screening programme. Data on HIV in pregnancy and outcomes in the UK are available from the National Study of HIV in Pregnancy and Childhood (℘ www.nshpc.ucl.ac.uk).

Clinical presentation and differential diagnosis

- Updated guidance on the management of children with HIV can be obtained from the UK Children's HIV Association website (℘ www.chiva.org.uk).
- HIV infection in children and adolescents causes a broad spectrum of disease manifestations and a variable clinical course. The management of HIV is complex and should only be undertaken as part of a clinical network with a recognized paediatric HIV specialist. In the UK this will be through the Department of Health's Children's HIV National Networks).
- AIDS represents the most severe end of the clinical spectrum.
- Box 19.1 and Table 19.1 outline the Centers for Disease Control and Prevention (CDC) 1994 classification of HIV/AIDS in children based on clinical and immune categories.

Box 19.1 Revised HIV paediatric classification system—clinical categories[a]

Category N: Not symptomatic

Children who have no signs or symptoms considered to be the result of HIV infection or who have only one of the conditions listed in category A.

Category A: Mildly symptomatic

Children with two or more of the conditions listed below but none of the conditions listed in categories B and C.
- Lymphadenopathy, hepatomegaly, splenomegaly
- Dermatitis
- Parotitis
- Recurrent or persistent upper respiratory tract infection (URTI), sinusitis, or otitis media

Category B: Moderately symptomatic

Children who have symptomatic conditions other than those listed for category A or C that are attributed to HIV infection. Examples of conditions in clinical category B include but are not limited to:
- Anaemia (<8g/dl), neutropenia (<1000 /mm^3), or thrombocytopenia (<100 000/mm^3) persisting ≥30 days

Box 19.1 (Contd.)

- Bacterial meningitis, pneumonia, or sepsis (single episode)
- Candidiasis, oropharyngeal (thrush), persisting (>2 months)
- Cardiomyopathy
- CMV infection, with onset before 1 month of age
- Diarrhoea, recurrent or chronic
- Hepatitis
- HSV stomatitis, recurrent (more than two episodes within 1 year)
- HSV bronchitis, pneumonitis, or oesophagitis
- Herpes zoster (shingles) involving at least two distinct episodes or more than one dermatome
- Lymphoid interstitial pneumonia (LIP)
- Nephropathy
- Persistent fever (lasting >1 month)
- Toxoplasmosis, onset before 1 month of age
- Varicella, disseminated (complicated chickenpox)

Category C: Severely symptomatic—AIDS-defining disease

Children who have any condition listed in the 1987 surveillance case definition for acquired immunodeficiency syndrome, with the exception of LIP (which is a category B condition).

- Serious bacterial infections, multiple or recurrent
- Candidiasis, oesophageal or pulmonary (bronchi, trachea, lungs)
- Coccidioidomycosis, disseminated
- Cryptococcosis, extrapulmonary
- Cryptosporidiosis or isosporiasis with diarrhoea persisting >1 month
- CMV disease with onset of symptoms at age >1 month (at a site other than liver, spleen, or lymph nodes)
- Encephalopathy
- HSV infection causing a mucocutaneous ulcer that persists for >1 month; or bronchitis, pneumonitis, or oesophagitis for any duration
- Histoplasmosis, disseminated
- Kaposi's sarcoma
- Lymphoma
- *Mycobacterium tuberculosis*, disseminated or extrapulmonary
- *Mycobacterium*, other species or unidentified species, disseminated (at a site other than or in addition to lungs, skin, or cervical or hilar lymph nodes)
- *Mycobacterium avium* complex or *Mycobacterium kansasii*, disseminated (at site other than or in addition to lungs, skin, or cervical or hilar lymph nodes)
- *Pneumocystis jiroveci* pneumonia (PcP)
- Progressive multifocal leucoencephalopathy
- Salmonella (non-typhoid) septicaemia, recurrent
- Toxoplasmosis of the brain with onset at >1 month of age
- Wasting syndrome in the absence of a concurrent illness other than HIV infection.

[a] Modified from Centers for Disease Control and Prevention. Revised classification system for human immunodeficiency virus infection in children less than 13 years of age. *MMWR* 1994;**43**:1–10.

Table 19.1 Revised HIV paediatric classification system 1994—immune categories based of age-specific CD4$^+$ T lymphocytes and percentage[a]

Immunological category	Number/µL (%)		
	<12 months	**1–5 years**	**6–12 years**
1: No suppression	≥1500 (>25)	≥1000 (≥25)	≥500 (≥25)
2: Moderate suppression	750–1499 (15–24)	500–999 (15–24)	200–499 (15–24)
3: Severe suppression	<750 (<15)	<500 (<15)	<200 (<15)

[a] Modified from Centers for Disease Control and Prevention. Revised classification system for human immunodeficiency virus infection in children less than 13 years of age. *MMWR* 1994;**43**:1–10.

- Paediatric AIDS is defined by the appearance of a number of diseases including failure to thrive and encephalopathy.
- Opportunistic infections: PcP is the commonest reported opportunistic infection, seen most often in infants where the mother was not known to have HIV in pregnancy. It occurs most frequently at around 2–4 months of age, often when the CD4 cell count is relatively high, and has a high mortality. CMV may cause disseminated disease, especially early in life when it may accompany PcP infection. Atypical mycobacterial infection and cryptosporidiosis are seen in children with severe immunosuppression.
- Severe bacterial infections: the commonest organisms causing infection are *Streptococcus pneumoniae, Haemophilus influenzae*, and *Salmonella* species.
- Failure to thrive: poor oral intake, HIV enteropathy or secondary gastrointestinal infection are all important factors that contribute to poor growth and weight gain.
- HIV encephalopathy: developmental delay or motor signs, such as spastic diplegia, are common presentations in the early years of life. Neuroimaging studies show cortical atrophy and sometimes basal ganglia calcification.
- LIP causes widespread nodular miliary shadowing on chest radiographs: LIP is seen in 30–40% of vertically infected children and often accompanied by persistent bilateral parotid enlargement (a good clinical sign of HIV infection). In most cases it is asymptomatic and only diagnosed on radiological investigation, where it looks like miliary TB in a child who clinically looks just far too well to have miliary TB! Recurrent pneumonia may occur in some children and subsequently result in bronchiectasis and chronic lung disease.

Investigations

- In children >18 months, enzyme immunoassays are widely used for HIV antibody testing and are highly sensitive and specific. Confirmation using western blot analysis or indirect immunofluorescence antibody assays is usually done. A positive HIV antibody test result in a child ≥18 months is usually indicative of infection.
- Due to the transplacental transfer of maternal antibody, the use of antibody-based assays for diagnosis of HIV infection in infants is problematic. The median time to loss of maternal antibody is 10 months and by 18 months all infants will have lost antibody. Plasma HIV RNA PCR is therefore used to diagnose HIV infection in infants.
- Infants born to HIV-infected mothers should initially be tested by either a RNA or DNA PCR during the first 48 hours of life, with a second test at 1–2 months of age (at least 2 weeks after any neonatal PEP ART has stopped) and a third test at 2–4 months of age. An infant is considered infected if two separate samples are positive and uninfected with two or more negative results, one at >3 months of age, and provided that the mother is not breastfeeding.
- For initial assessment of a child newly diagnosed with HIV, see Table 19.2.

Table 19.2 Initial assessment of a child newly diagnosed with HIV

HIV parameters	HIV RNA PCR (viral load)
	Baseline HIV resistance test (+ maternal resistance if an infant)
	CD4 count
	HLA B5701
Haematology	Full blood count and film
	Sickle screen (if appropriate racial group)
	Ferritin
	Consider malaria film if recently arrived from endemic area
Biochemistry	Urea and electrolytes (U&E), creatinine, total protein (globulin), Ca, PO₄, albumin, liver function tests, lipids, glucose, amylase, thyroid-stimulating hormone (TSH), vitamin D
Serology	Hepatitis A IgG, HBsAg, anti-HBsAg, HCV IgG, syphilis serology, IgG for EBV, CMV, HSV, VZV and toxoplasmosis
	In children >1 year: measles, mumps, rubella IgG
	Immunization responses: *H. influenzae* type b, tetanus
	(<18 months, serology may reflect maternal antibodies, and should be repeated)

Table 19.2 (Contd.)

Viral PCRs	Plasma CMV PCR should be undertaken in infants and children with advanced disease
	Hepatitis C virus PCR should be undertaken in infants at risk of exposure and those with advanced disease
Cultures	According to symptoms/travel history: stools/urine/throat swabs/blood cultures/malaria films/gastric washings also for TB (Mantoux test), IGRA testing (where available)/sexual health screen if sexually active
Clinical investigations	Formal ophthalmological examination for infants
	Blood pressure, urinalysis, height/weight/head circumference/pubertal stage/BCG scar
Radiology	Baseline chest radiograph
	Bone age if small for age
	Infants/children with neurological signs: MRI of brain

IGRA, interferon gamma release assay.

Management

- Therapy for specific opportunistic and other infections is discussed under the individual diseases in other chapters. Management will focus on prophylaxis, prevention, and ART.

Prophylaxis against opportunistic infections

(see 🐾 www.chiva.org.uk)
- Prophylaxis with co-trimoxazole is highly effective at preventing life-threatening infections such as PcP and also reducing bacterial infections.
- Prophylaxis should be given to all HIV-infected infants from diagnosis until their first birthday. In older children, prophylaxis should be given to all those with low CD4 counts (below 200–250 cells/mm^3 or 15%).
- Prophylaxis against other infections, including CMV, atypical mycobacteria and fungal infections, has been suggested for those with very low CD4 counts.

Prevention of bacterial infection

- Immunization against *H. influenzae* and *S. pneumoniae* is recommended for all children with HIV infection.
- Prophylactic antibiotics may be beneficial in children with LIP and recurrent chest infections.

Immunization

- Children with HIV should receive all immunizations except for the BCG vaccine.

Antiretroviral therapy

Updated guidance on ART can be obtained from the Paediatric European Network for the Treatment of AIDS website (PENTA Guidelines on the use of ART, ℘ www.pentatrials.org).

When to start?
- All infants <1 year of age, irrespective of clinical or immunological status.
- All children with CDC stage B or C disease.
- Asymptomatic older children based on age-specific CD4 counts.

Table 19.3 2009 PENTA-recommended CD4 thresholds for initiating antiretroviral therapy

Marker	<12 months	1 to <3 years	3 to <5 years	≥5 years
Clinical Stage	Start all	CDC C or severe B	CDC C or severe B	CDC C or severe B
CD4% and CD4 count	Start all	<25% or <1000 cells/mm^3	<20% or <500 cells/mm^3	≤350 cells/mm^3

CDC, Centers for Disease Control and Prevention.

What to start with?
- Children should start combination ART nearly always as triple therapy, usually a dual nucleoside reverse transcriptase inhibitor (NRTI) backbone together with either a ritonavir-boosted protease inhibitor (most commonly lopinavir/ritonavir) or a non-NRTI (either nevirapine or efavirenz).
- The child's age, HLA-B*5701 status (denotes an increased susceptibility to severe allergic reactions with abacavir), previous drug exposure, resistance profile, available formulations, and likely adherence should be taken into account when constructing a first-line regimen.

Monitoring ART
- The aim of ART is to achieve an undetectable viral load (<50 copies/ml plasma) and CD4 reconstitution; viral load and CD4 counts should be monitored approximately every 3 months once established on ART.
- More frequent clinical and laboratory monitoring is required in infancy, if adherence is poor, soon after starting or changing therapy, and when giving other medications such as antituberculous therapy.

When to switch?
- The best time to switch to second- and third-line therapy remains uncertain.
- Switching treatment when there are ongoing problems with adherence may lead to loss of efficacy of further classes of ART.
- Resistance testing should be performed prior to switching regimens.

- Expert interpretation of resistance tests is required.
- In general avoid substituting single drugs in a failing regimen.

Stopping treatment and treatment interruptions
- Treatment interruptions cannot be recommended and starting ART currently means lifelong therapy.
- Treatment may be stopped due to adherence issues or drug toxicity.
- Stopping non-NRTIs requires a substitution or staggered stop to reduce the risk of developing non-NRTI resistance.

Social/psychological management
- Caring for children with HIV requires an expert multidisciplinary team, ideally involving specialist paediatric nurses, psychologists, pharmacists, and others working together to support the family.
- Testing of mothers and children can be performed by any competent professional who has adequate knowledge of the condition and implications of a positive diagnosis.
- Disclosure is complex and usually occurs in a phased approach over many years.
- Adherence requires a multidisciplinary approach.
- Adolescent issues need to tackled in close collaboration with adult services and should be part of a clearly planned transition programme into to adult services.

Prevention

- Reduction of vertical transmission: Full updated antenatal and postnatal HIV guidelines are available on the British HIV Association website (℞ www.bhiva.org):
  - Antenatal HIV testing should be universal and integrated into routine antenatal care
  - Antiretroviral therapy in pregnancy: zidovudine monotherapy commenced at 24–28 weeks gestation (mother not requiring or willing to take combination therapy) or combination therapy with ≥3 drugs starting after first trimester (if indicated for maternal health as per adult guidelines)
  - Obstetric management of pregnancy and delivery: pre-labour caesarean section (women on zidovudine monotherapy or on combination therapy but detectable viraemia) or elective vaginal delivery (women on combination therapy with no detectable viraemia)
  - Management of infants born to HIV-infected mothers: zidovudine monotherapy for 4 weeks or triple therapy as post-exposure prophylaxis (PEP) (for infants born to untreated mothers or mothers with detectable viraemia).
- Infant feeding: Exclusive formula feeding for all babies.

Future research

- Vaccine development has been very disappointing so far.
- Newer treatment strategies to minimize toxicity of long-term treatment, combined with optimal efficacy and reduced pill burden.
- Continued follow-up of vertically infected young people for long-term outcomes (growth, neurocognitive function, fertility, malignancy, and long-term drug toxicity).

Further reading

de Ruiter A, Mercey D, Anderson J, et al. British HIV association and children's HIV association guidelines for the management of HIV infection in pregnant women 2008. *HIV Med* 2008;**9**:452–502.

Welch S, Sharland M, Lyall EG, et al. PENTA 2009 guidelines for the use of antiretroviral therapy in paediatric HIV-1 infection. *HIV Med* 2009;**10**:591–613.

Immunocompromised children with infection

📖 see also Chapters 2, 3, 4, 19, 23, 24

Introduction

- The main groups of immunocompromised children at increased risk of infection are given in Table 20.1. These include primary immunodeficiencies and acquired or secondary immunodeficiencies. Alteration of the mucosal and skin barriers or normal microbial flora can also be characterized as secondary immune deficiencies, leaving the host open to infections.
- The most likely type of infection can be predicted by knowledge of the child's underlying immune deficit. Although broad-spectrum empirical treatment is usually started, an understanding of the type of immune deficit allows the clinician to optimally target investigations and therapy.

Table 20.1 Major types of immunocompromise with an increased risk of infection

Primary	Secondary
B cell defects:	Human immunodeficiency virus
X-linked agammaglobulinaemia	Malignancies
IgG subclass deficiency	
Common variable immunodeficiency	Transplantation
Selective IgA deficiency	Bone marrow—stem cell
Hyper-IgM syndrome	Solid organ
	Cancer chemotherapy
	Burns

(Continued)

Table 20.1 (Contd.)

T cell defects:	Sickle cell disease
DiGeorge syndrome	Cystic fibrosis
CD8 lymphocytopenia	Diabetes mellitus
Cytokine deficiencies	Immunosuppressive drugs
Defective T cell receptor	
Combined B and T cell defects	Asplenia
Severe combined immunodeficiency	Malnutrition
Wiskott–Aldrich syndrome	Implanted foreign body
Ataxia telangiectasia	
Hyper-IgE syndrome	
Omenn's syndrome	
Phagocyte defects:	
Leucocyte adhesion disorder	
Chediak–Higashi syndrome	
Myeloperoxidase deficiency	
Chronic granulomatous disease	
Leukopenia	
Kostmann's syndrome	
Schwachman–Diamond syndrome	
Defective opsonization—complement deficiencies	

Causative organisms

- Most common pathogens also cause infection in children with immunodeficiencies. In addition, organisms that are usually considered to be avirulent in immunocompetent hosts can be pathogenic in hosts with a limited immune system.
- Table 20.2 summarizes the most common cause of infection in immunocompromised children.

Table 20.2 Most common cause of infection in immunocompromised children

Bacteria	Viruses
Escherichia coli	Varicella zoster virus
Pseudomonas aeruginosa	Cytomegalovirus
Klebsiella spp.	Herpes simplex virus
Enterobacter spp.	Epstein–Barr virus
Haemophilus influenzae	Human herpesvirus 6
Staphylococcus aureus	Respiratory and enteric viruses
Staphylococcus coagulase-negative	Adenoviruses
Streptococcus pneumoniae	
Neisseria meningitidis	
Corynebacterium spp.	
Viridans streptococci	
Listeria monocytogenes	
Enterococcus faecalis	
Clostridium spp.	
Burkholderia cepacia	
Mycobacterium spp.	
Nocardia spp.	

Fungi	Protozoa
Candida spp.	*Toxoplasma gondii*
Aspergillus spp.	*Cryptosporidium parvum*
Cryptococcus neoformans	
Zygomycetes	
Pneumocystis jiroveci	

* Patients with defects in the B cell arm of the immune system fail to produce appropriate antibody responses, and this antibody deficiency predisposes to infections with encapsulated organisms such as *S. pneumoniae, H. influenzae,* and *N. meningitidis*. However, rotavirus, enteroviruses, and *Giardia* can also cause severe and persistent infections.
* Children with cell-mediated deficiency are susceptible to viral, fungal, and protozoan infections.

- Children with combined B cell and T cell defects may manifest a variable disease spectrum depending on the extent of the defect.
- Children with abnormalities of the phagocytic and neutrophil system have mainly bacterial and fungal infections.
- Children with defective opsonization (congenital asplenia, splenic dysfunction due to haemoglobinopathies or those who have undergone splenectomy) are at risk of serious infections from encapsulated bacteria including *S. pneumoniae*, *H. influenzae*, *N. meningitidis*, and *Salmonella*.
- If left untreated, the profound effects of HIV infection on the T cell arm leads to susceptibility to the same types of infections as with primary T cell immunodeficiencies.
- In children with cancer, the major abnormality associated with infection is neutropenia. Neutropenia is defined as an absolute neutrophil count less than 1000 cells/mm^3 and can be associated with significant risk of severe infections particularly when the absolute count is less than 500/mm^3. The most common causes of infection are Gram-positive cocci (including coagulase-negative staphylococci, *S. aureus* and *S. pneumoniae*). However, Gram-negative organisms such as *P. aeruginosa*, *E. coli*, and *Klebsiella* can cause life-threatening infection and must be considered in the empirical treatment regimen. Other Gram-negative pathogens such as *Enterobacter* and *Acinetobacter* are increasing in prevalence as well. Patients with prolonged neutropenia who have received broad antimicrobial therapy are at increased risk for opportunistic fungal infections, especially with *Candida* and *Aspergillus*.
- Children with transplants are at risk for infections caused by many of the same microbial agents that cause disease in children with primary immunodeficiencies. Differences in the type and timing of infections after transplantation exist between patients depending on the type of transplantation performed, the type and amount of immunosuppression given, and the child's previous immunity to specific pathogens.
- Intracellular pathogens, including mycobacteria are seen in children receiving anti-tumour necrosis factor (TNF) therapy.

Epidemiology

- No comprehensive data are available on the prevalence and epidemiology of infections in immunocompromised children with different disorders.
- Increasing numbers of children survive with primary immunodeficiencies or receive immunosuppressive therapy for treatment of malignancy, autoimmune disorders, or transplantation.

Clinical presentation and differential diagnosis

- In antibody deficiencies such as X-linked agammaglobulinaemia, common variable immunodeficiency and hyper-IgM syndrome, children are usually asymptomatic until 5–6 months of age, when maternal passive antibody wanes. These children then begin to develop recurrent episodes of otitis media, bronchitis, pneumonia, bacteraemia, and meningitis. On the contrary, the significance and impact of specific IgG subclass deficiencies is less well understood and their association with recurrent severe infection remains controversial. In the presence of selective IgA deficiency, some of the patients will have mild to moderate disease at sites of mucosal barriers, and recurrent sinopulmonary infection and gastrointestinal disease are the major clinical manifestations.
- In cell-mediated deficiency, clinical manifestations include chronic diarrhoea, mucocutaneous candidiasis, pneumonia, rhinitis, and otitis media.
- In combined B cell and T cell defects, complete immunodeficiency is found with severe combined immunodeficiency syndrome (SCID), whereas partial defects can be present in such states as ataxia-telangiectasia, Wiskott–Aldrich syndrome, and hyper-IgE syndrome. Children with SCID present within the first 6 months of life with recurrent severe infections caused by bacteria (both Gram-positive and Gram-negative), fungi, or viruses. Failure to thrive, chronic diarrhoea, mucocutaneous or systemic candidiasis, *P. jiroveci* pneumonitis, and CMV infection are common early in life. Children with ataxia-telangiectasia develop late-onset recurrent sinopulmonary infections from both bacteria and respiratory viruses. In Wiskott–Aldrich syndrome infections with *S. pneumoniae* or *H. influenzae* are common, as is *P. jiroveci* pneumonitis. In addition, affected boys (it is an X-linked recessive disease) have thrombocytopenia and eczema. Children with hyper-IgE syndrome have recurrent episodes of *S. aureus* abscesses of the skin, lungs, and musculoskeletal system, and they are at increased risk for fungal infections.
- In abnormalities of the phagocytic and neutrophil system, disease manifests as recurrent infections of the skin, mucous membranes, lungs, liver and bones. Children with leucocyte adhesion defects may have a history of delayed cord separation and recurrent infections of the skin, oral mucosa, and genital tract; ecthyma gangrenosum and pyoderma gangrenosum also occur. Children with chronic granulomatous disease have recurrent infections due to *S. aureus*, *Serratia marcescens*, *Burkholderia cepacia*, and *Aspergillus* spp., especially involving the lungs, liver, and bone. Primary congenital neutropenia (Kostmann's syndrome) most often presents during the first year of life with cellulitis, perirectal abscesses, or stomatitis caused by *S. aureus* or *P. aeruginosa*.
- In defective opsonization or complement deficiency, encapsulated bacteria can cause sepsis, pneumonia, meningitis, and osteomyelitis.

- In HIV infection, the severity and frequency of infections is related to CD4 cell numbers as well as percentages. 📖 See details in Chapter 19, Human immunodeficiency virus infection, p. 153.
- In malignancies, the type, duration, and intensity of anticancer therapy remain the major risk factors for infections. The degree and duration of neutropenia have long been relied on as accurate predictors of the risk of infection. However, the lack of neutrophils can lead to a loss of inflammatory response and fever may be the only manifestation of infection. Because patients with fever and neutropenia may only have subtle signs and symptoms of infection, the presence of fever warrants thorough physical examination with careful attention to the oropharynx, lungs, perineum and anus, skin, nailbeds, and areas around intravascular catheter sites.
- Infections following BMT and stem cell transplantation (SCT) can be classified as occurring during the pretransplantation period, pre-engraftment period (0–30 days after transplantation), postengraftment period (30–100 days), or late post-transplantation (>100 days). The majority of infections that occur during the pretransplantation time period are caused by aerobic gram-negative bacilli and are manifest as local infections of the skin, soft tissue, and urinary tract. In the pre-engraftment period, bacterial infections predominate. Bacteraemia is the most common documented infection and occurs in 40–50% of all BMT or SCT recipients. Gram-positive cocci, Gram-negative bacilli, yeast, and, less commonly, other fungi all cause infection during this period. *Aspergillus* has been identified in 4–20% of BMT recipients, most often after the third week of neutropenia. Viral infections also occur during this period: reactivation of herpes simplex infection in previously infected patients and nosocomial viral infections (e.g. respiratory syncytial virus, influenza, adenovirus, rotavirus) represent the most important source of infection during this time period. In the postengraftment period, opportunistic pathogens predominate: PCP, severe CMV disease (primary infection as well as reactivation), reactivation of *T. gondii* and hepatosplenic candidiasis are the most important causes of infectious diseases. In late post-transplantation, infection is unusual in the absence of chronic graft-versus-host disease (GVHD). Viral infections (primarily reactivation of VZV) are responsible for more than 40% of infections, bacterial infections (particularly of the upper and lower respiratory tract) account for approximately one-third, and fungal infections account for less than 20%.
- After solid organ transplantation, infectious complications typically develop in one of three time intervals: early (0–30 days after transplantation), intermediate (30–180 days), and late (>180 days). Early infections usually result as either a complication of the transplant surgery itself or the presence of indwelling catheters. Infections during the intermediate time period typically result as a complication of the immunosuppression, which tends to be at its greatest intensity during the first 6 months following transplantation. This is the time period of greatest risk for infections due to opportunistic pathogens such as CMV and *P. jiroveci*. Anatomical abnormalities developing as a consequence of the transplant surgery can also predispose to recurrent

infection that present in this time period. Infections developing late after transplantation typically result as a consequence of uncorrected anatomic abnormalities, chronic rejection or exposure to community-acquired pathogens. Compared to the earlier period, community-acquired infections in the late period are usually benign because levels of immunosuppression are typically maintained at significantly lower levels. However, certain pathogens, such as VZV and EBV, may be associated with severe disease even at this late time period. Primary EBV infection may lead to uncontrolled PTLD, including post-transplant lymphoma.

Investigations

- Children with recurrent and severe infections in the first 2 years of life should be considered for screening measurement of immunoglobulin levels and lymphocyte subpopulations as well as HIV status.
- Children with hyper-IgE syndrome have markedly elevated levels of IgE, marked eosinophilia, and poor cell-mediated responses to neoantigens.
- Bone marrow evaluation shows a failure of maturation of myeloid precursors in primary congenital neutropenia.
- In febrile neutropenia, a comprehensive laboratory evaluation including a complete blood cell count, serum creatinine, blood urea nitrogen, and transaminases should be obtained. Blood cultures should be obtained from each port of any central venous catheter, and a peripheral venous sample should be obtained as well. Other microbiological studies should be done if there are associated symptoms: nasal aspirate for viruses in patients with upper respiratory tract symptoms; stool for rotavirus and *C. difficile* in patients with diarrhoea; urine culture in young children or in older patients with symptoms of urgency, frequency, or dysuria; biopsy and culture of cutaneous lesions. Chest radiographs should be obtained in any individual with respiratory symptoms. Abdominal CT scan should also be considered in children with profound neutropenia and abdominal pain.
- Specific investigations in transplant recipients vary according to the type of transplantation performed, the timing from transplantation, the type and amount of immunosuppression given, and the child's previous immunity to specific pathogens.

Management and treatment

- The principles of treatment in immunocompromised children include early empirical treatment on suspicion of infection, start with broad cover and narrow when results are in, and increased use of imaging and invasive procedures to obtain specimens.
- Local protocols are often directed to the most common pathogens.
- Antimicrobial agents directed against the most likely pathogens based on the immune deficit should be used for the treatment of suspected infection. In several cases, including febrile neutropenia,

the use of empirical combinations of antibiotics able to cover Gram-positive, Gram-negative and eventually fungal infections are required. These often include an extended spectrum penicillin (e.g. piperacillin + tazobactam) combined with an aminoglycoside. IV therapy is recommended. The decision to use monotherapy versus an expanded regimen of antibiotics depends on the severity of illness of the patient, history of previous colonization with resistant organisms, and the presence of a possible catheter-related infection.

• It is critical to carefully evaluate the patient for response to therapy, development of secondary infections, or adverse effects. Patients should be reassessed daily. Those who become afebrile and are clinically well may continue on the same regimen, although consideration should be given to discontinuing vancomycin if it was included initially. Those who remain febrile with clinical progression warrant the addition of vancomycin if not included initially and where risk factors exist, as well as consideration for a change of the other antibiotics. If fever persists for more than 4–5 days, the addition of an antifungal agent is generally warranted.

• The use of antiviral agents is not recommended without specific evidence of viral disease.

• Antimicrobial prophylaxis with trimethoprim/sulfamethoxazole and itraconazole in chronic granulomatous disease, with penicillin in complement deficiency and asplenia, with trimethoprim/ sulfamethoxazole in children undergoing active treatment for malignancy and with various antimicrobials depending on the history of the patient and type of transplantation in transplant recipients may be recommended to reduce the incidence of severe infections.

• Replacement of antibody with IVIG is the mainstay of treatment for most of the primary antibody deficits. The exception to this are deficiencies of specific IgG subclasses as there is little evidence of increased susceptibility to severe infections. Where there is complete IgA deficiency and IVIG is indicated, care must be taken as these patients can develop antibody against the minute amounts of IgA found in the immunoglobulin preparations with a subsequent increased risk of anaphylaxis.

• Many of the neutropenic syndromes respond to colony-stimulating factor.

• Influenza vaccination should be strongly recommended in immunocompromised children as well as their household contacts.

• Vaccines to *H. influenzae* type b, *S. pneumoniae*, and *N. meningitidis* should be administered to all children with defective opsonization or complement deficiency as well as to all the other immunocompromised patients.

• Live attenuated vaccines are contraindicated in children with primary T cell abnormalities or with acquired immunodeficiency and severe immunosuppression.

Follow-up and outcome

- Infection is a major cause of morbidity and mortality in children with immunocompromise. Rates of infection are falling with improved treatment in some clinical areas (e.g. HIV with increased use of ART, transplantation with improved conditioning and the wider use of prophylaxis). Increasingly marrow ablative chemotherapy (e.g. for relapse oncology) is associated with higher rates of infectious complications.
- In BMT and SCT recipients, the development of infection during the pretransplantation period neither delays engraftment nor alters the success of engraftment. In pre-engraftment and post-engraftment periods, infections increase both morbidity and mortality.
- Children receiving organ transplants have frequently been hospitalized for long periods and have received many antibiotics, thus recovery of bacteria with multiple antibiotic resistance is common after all types of organ transplantation. Infections due to *Aspergillus* are less common but occur after all types of organ transplantation and are associated with high rates of morbidity and mortality. Among viral infections, primary infection due to CMV or EBV is associated with the greatest degree of morbidity and mortality. The highest risk is in a naïve host who receives an organ from a donor who was previously infected with one of these viruses.

Future research

- Future studies should focus on the comparative prevalence and epidemiology of infections in different types of immunocompromised children using the newer, less invasive diagnostic techniques. There are few updated cohort data.
- Information on the long-term outcome of infections in children with malignancy and in those who received transplantation is required.
- Paediatric trials on efficacy, safety, and pharmacokinetics of antibacterials, antifungals and antivirals, off-label for children and adolescents, but useful for severe infections in patients with immunodeficiency, remain very important.

Further reading

Kesson AM, Kakakios A. Immunocompromised children: conditions and infectious agents. *Paediatr Respir Rev* 2007;**8**:231–9.

Simon A, Schildgen O, Schuster F. Viral infections in paediatric patients receiving conventional cancer chemotherapy. *Arch Dis Child* 2008;**93**:880–9.

Thomas L, Baggen L, Chisholm J, Sharland M. Diagnosis and treatment of aspergillosis in children. *Expert Rev Anti Infect Ther* 2009;**7**:461–72.

Chapter 21

Infection control in community settings

📖 see also Chapter 17

Introduction

There are numerous settings where the prevention and control of infection in children and babies is important, and these include:

- The home
- Preschool (crèche, nurseries, and child-minders)
- Schools and after-school clubs
- Residential care (children's homes, hospices)
- Community healthcare settings, such as general practices and dentists
- Children's play areas.

Principles of infection control

Applying the principles of infection control in all childcare settings should make a major contribution to preventing infection. By removing or controlling any one of these three main links in the chain of infection, the spread of infection may be interrupted.

- Link one—Sources of infectious agents
- Link two—Pathways or vehicles of transmission
- Link three—Susceptible hosts

Link one—sources of infectious agents

These include:

- Animate sources (humans, animals, and insects) and contained in blood, faeces, urine, vomit, pus, respiratory droplets, sputum, skin rashes, and food and fluids contaminated by these body fluids
- Inanimate sources (soil, water, food).

It is possible to remove or control certain sources of infection in community childcare settings, such as:

- Preventing children with known infection, or with symptoms of possible infection such as diarrhoea, from attending during the infectious period. This is known as 'exclusion'.

- Prohibiting the introduction of potentially contaminated food and fluids into the setting, e.g.:
  - Avoiding high-risk foods, such as soft cheeses, pâtés, eggs, and raw meat
  - Purchasing only pasteurized milk and fruit juices
  - Removing soil from fresh vegetables and washing them prior to consumption.
- Guidance on the exclusion of children with infections from childcare settings is available on the HPA website (℘ www.hpa.org.uk).
- Outbreaks are defined as two or more people with the same infection or symptoms linked in terms of time, place, or common exposure, or as a greater than expected rate of infection compared with that usually expected. Outbreaks should be reported to local health authorities.

Link two—pathways or vehicles of transmission

It is not always possible, practical, or imperative to remove sources of infection from childcare settings. For example, children with minor health problems such as colds, head lice, or hand, foot, and mouth infection would not usually be excluded. Some infections are most infectious before symptoms have appeared.

For this reason, targeting vehicles of transmission or protecting susceptible hosts are important interventions.

Infection may be transmitted by the following means:
- Direct contact with an infectious individual or with other sources of infection
- Indirect contact with contaminated articles or environment
- Contact with airborne infectious respiratory secretions or aerosolized body fluids such as vomit.

The risk of transmission may be reduced by avoiding or controlling exposure to infectious agents by practising standard infection control precautions. These include:
- Hand hygiene
- Personal protective equipment (PPE)
- Environmental and equipment hygiene
- Food hygiene
- Safe disposal of waste.

Hand hygiene
- Contaminated hands are a common vehicle of transmission via direct and indirect contact.
- Simple handwashing to remove pathogens or reduce them to a safe level is usually adequate in childcare settings.
- Alcohol hand gels can be effective when used on socially clean hands, and are convenient in situations where soap and water are not readily available.

- Whichever method of hand hygiene is employed, a good technique is essential.
- Facilities should be available for hand hygiene in toilets, kitchens, baby changing rooms, and clinical rooms.
- In children's toilets, handwash basins, towel dispensers, and soap should be at an appropriate height.
- Young children should be encouraged to wash their hands, with supervision.

Handwashing technique
1. Remove hand jewellery and wristwatches, and roll up sleeves.
2. Wet hands under warm running water.
3. Apply liquid soap.
4. Rub this into all parts of the hands vigorously, without applying more water for at least 10–15 seconds.
5. Rinse hands under running water.
6. Dry thoroughly ideally using paper towels or a clean cotton towel.

Using alcohol hand gels:
1. Apply 5ml of alcohol hand gel to visibly clean hands
2. Rub product into all parts of the hands until the alcohol has evaporated—especially between the fingers, palms, and the back of the hand and wrists.

Personal protective equipment
Commonly used types of PPE include:
- Gloves
- Aprons/coveralls
- Face protection (masks and eye protection)

Gloves
- Gloves are recommended for use whenever contamination with blood and body fluids is anticipated.
- If gloves are not available, good hand hygiene should be used to remove pathogens from the hands.

Aprons
- Plastic aprons are often used in healthcare and are worn when undertaking procedures where contamination of clothing/uniform is anticipated.

Face protection
- Face masks and eye protection are used to prevent contact with, and inhalation of, airborne or aerosolized microorganisms.
- Controllable exposure by this pathway is unlikely in community childcare settings, therefore face protection should not be necessary other than in healthcare.

Environmental and equipment hygiene
Contaminated equipment, utensils, furniture, toys, and general environment can act as vehicles of spread. Accumulations of dust, dirt, and liquid residues in the environment will increase infection risks and can be

reduced by regular cleaning and drying, and ensuring fittings and fixtures are kept in good repair.

Management of the spillage of blood

- Any spillages of blood must be dealt with quickly and effectively wearing gloves (ideally disposable) and a disposable apron if available.
- In community childcare settings the waste should be contained in a plastic bag that is securely tied and discarded in the household waste. In clinical settings contaminated materials and debris is treated as clinical waste.
- Surface disinfection is usually recommended, using a chlorine-releasing agent such as bleach or sodium dichloroisocynate (NaDCC). Specific precautions should be taken to avoid exposure to these agents. If not available, detergent and water can be used.

Food hygiene

Food may pose a risk of infection if not handled correctly and food-borne outbreaks may occur. Food poisoning can cause serious illness or death, especially in young children and infants. Managers and staff must be aware of food hygiene legislation and good practice. The local environmental health department can advise on this.

Safe disposal of waste

- Local policies should be in place and staff trained in the correct procedures.

Management of sharps and inoculation injuries and bites

- Every organization should have an inoculation injury policy in place.
- Sharps include: needles, scalpel blades, stitch cutters, and cannulae used in clinical care, and sharp objects such as broken glass that is contaminated with blood.

Risk of transmission

- Risks of bloodborne viral infection are associated with **inoculation** of an **infectious dose** of **infected body fluid** into a **susceptible recipient**.
- A simple injury, which does not break the skin, or does not involve the inoculation of body fluid, is unlikely to lead to the transmission of infection.

Procedures for managing an inoculation injury include:
- Encourage bleeding (but do not suck or rub the wound)
- Rinse wounds and contaminated mucous membranes with water or emergency eye wash solution
- Cover wound with a waterproof dressing
- Seek advice from local emergency department, occupational health or GP as soon as possible.

Link three—susceptible hosts

There are many factors that increase an individual's risk of infection, and children may have all or any of these, which include:
- Extremes of age

- Underlying health conditions, such as diabetes mellitus, cancer and immunocompromised conditions such as leukaemia, and HIV and AIDS
- Medications such as steroids, cytotoxics, antibiotics
- Pregnancy
- Invasive medical devices such as indwelling urinary catheters, feeding tubes.

The key intervention aimed at removing this link in the chain is immunization:
- The childhood immunization schedule in England is described in *Immunisation Against Infectious Diseases* (known as the Green Book), which is available on the Department of Health website (ℰ www.dh.gov.uk/en/Publichealth/Immunisation/Greenbook/index.htm).
- Vulnerable children may require additional vaccinations and consult their GP should they be exposed to infectious diseases such as chickenpox.

Protection of vulnerable groups:
- In general vulnerable children and adults in the risk groups above do not need to be excluded from community childcare settings, unless unwell themselves or seriously immunocompromised. Targeting the other links in the chain will minimize infection risks.
- Pregnant women and vulnerable children should seek medical advice if they are in close contact with an infectious disease such as chickenpox, rubella, measles, or parvovirus.

Preventing zoonotic infections

- Zoonotic infections can be acquired by contact with animals, their excreta, and environment.
- They include infections caused by *Escherichia coli* O157, *Campylobacter*, and *Salmonella*, cryptosporidiosis, psittacosis, toxoplasmosis, and toxocariasis.
- There may be contact with pets in childcare settings or during visits to farms, petting zoos, and other animal centres.
- Children <5 years and pregnant women are particularly at risk of complications of infection.

Reducing infection risks during visits to farms and zoos
- Check that the farm/centre is well managed and the grounds and public areas are clean.
- Check that there are good handwashing facilities accessible for children.
- Ensure everyone washes their hands thoroughly after contact with animals and their environment, before eating or drinking, and before departure. Parents or teachers should supervise children when handwashing.
- Do not allow children to eat, drink, or put anything in their mouths when touring the farm.
- Clean footwear of any faecal matter and soil, washing hands afterwards.
- Pregnant women should avoid contact with sheep and lambs.

Also see the advice on the Health and Safety Executive website (𝄞 www.hse.gov.uk/pubns/ais23.pdf).

Further reading

Department of Health. *Immunisation Against Infectious Disease*. London: The Stationery Office, 2010.

Hawker J, Begg N, Blair I, Reintjes R, Weinberg J. *Communicable Disease Control Handbook*. Oxford: Blackwell Publishing, 2005.

Health Protection Agency Poster. *Guidance on Infection Control in Schools and Other Child Care Settings*, 2010. Available at: 𝄞 www.hpa.org.uk/web/HPAwebFile/HPAweb_C/1194947358374 (accessed 1 February 2011).

Chapter 22

Intra-abdominal infections

📖 see also Chapters 47, 48, 50, 54, 66, 69, 74

Introduction

This chapter focuses on community-acquired intra-abdominal infections in childhood. Suggested empirical antibiotic regimens should be viewed in the context of local microbial resistance patterns and modified accordingly, as there is considerable regional variation in the prevalence of resistant organisms implicated in intra-abdominal infections, particularly *Enterococcus faecalis* (e.g. VRE), *Staphylococcus aureus* (e.g. MRSA) and *Pseudomonas aeruginosa*.

Liver abscess

Introduction

Liver abscess is rare in children, and predominately affects immunocompromised hosts. Hepatoportoenterostomy (Kasai procedure) and liver transplantation are further predisposing factors. Liver abscess can result from bacterial spread from a variety of sources:

- Contiguous spread from an adjacent structure (e.g. cholangitis, cholecystitis, pancreatitis)
- Penetrating hepatic trauma
- The portal vein (from an intestinal focus, umbilical catheters)
- The systemic circulation.

In approximately half of cases no definitive cause can be established (cryptogenic liver abscess). An underlying primary immunodeficiency (e.g. chronic granulomatous disease) should be considered.

Causative organisms

- Bacterial: Frequently Gram-negative organisms, including *Escherichia coli*, *Enterococcus*, *Klebsiella*, *Pseudomonas*, *Proteus*, and *Bacteroides* species.[1] *S. aureus* is a common causative agent in children.[2,3] *Streptococcus milleri* group organisms are also relatively common.
- Fungal: Mainly *Candida albicans* (typically multiple small foci—hepatosplenic candidosis). Almost exclusively in immunocompromised hosts (e.g. primary immunodeficiency and neutropenic patients) and premature neonates.
- Parasitic: *Entamoeba histolytica* (amoebic liver abscess; rare in Europe).

Epidemiology

- There are no definitive published data on the incidence, specifically in children.
- A population-based study in Denmark reported an overall annual incidence of 11/1 000 000, highlighting the rarity of this entity in the European setting.[1]
- Liver abscesses are considerably more common in resource-poor countries.

Clinical presentation

- The symptoms associated with liver abscess are often non-specific (e.g. anorexia, malaise) and the infectious focus may therefore not be apparent (consider hepatic abscess in fever without focus).
- Most patients are febrile, but some have only low-grade pyrexia.
- Approximately half of the cases report pain or tenderness in the right upper abdominal quadrant; there may also be radiation of pain to the right shoulder.
- Hepatomegaly is rarely present.
- Jaundice and other features indicating hepatic disease are relatively uncommon.

Differential diagnosis

- Solitary liver cyst
- Polycystic disease of the kidneys and liver
- Choledochal cyst
- Hepatic haematoma (following trauma), haemangioma
- Hydatid disease (*Echinococcus granulosus* and *Echinococcus multilocularis*).

Investigations

- Hepatic and biliary parameters (AST, ALT, bilirubin, alkaline phosphatase (ALP), γ-glutamyl transferase (γ-GT)) may be only mildly elevated or even within normal range.
- Inflammatory parameters (WBC, CRP, ESR) are usually elevated.
- Blood cultures generally fail to isolate the causative organism.
- Consider stool microscopy and serology for *E. histolytica* in patients with a history of travel to an endemic area.
- Abdominal ultrasound is the preferred radiological investigation for initial screening, and is also useful for monitoring progress.
- Abdominal CT provides the most detailed information.

Management and treatment

- Pyogenic liver abscesses require drainage. This can generally be achieved via ultrasound- or CT-guided percutaneous drainage. In multiple or multiloculated abscesses surgical drainage can be necessary.
- The purulent material obtained during the intervention should be sent for Gram-staining and culture.
- The initial empirical parenteral antibiotic treatment should provide adequate cover for *S. aureus* and Gram-negative organisms (including *Pseudomonas*), as well as anaerobes. The treatment should be

rationalised once the causative organism and the susceptibilities are known.

- Amoebic liver abscesses require treatment with metronidazole, followed by a course of diloxanide furoate. Whether drainage is indicated in these patients remains controversial, since the majority respond to medical therapy alone.

Follow-up and outcome

- Progress should be assessed by monitoring inflammatory parameters and by performing serial ultrasound scans.
- Prolonged antibiotic therapy over several weeks is required in most cases.
- Immunodeficiency should be considered and investigated.
- Pyogenic liver abscess is a potentially life-threatening condition. In 1989, a literature review estimated the overall majority to be 15%.[2] However, a more recent publication of 15 patients over a 10-year period from the UK reported no fatalities.[3]

Cholangitis

Introduction

Cholangitis is the collective term for inflammation of the biliary system. Bile is generally sterile; infectious cholangitis is usually the result of bacterial colonization (bacterobilia). In adults cholangitis typically occurs in association with cholelithiasis,[4] but this pathogenesis is rare in children. In the paediatric age group predisposing factors include: congenital bile duct abnormalities (e.g. Caroli's syndrome and choledochal cysts), hepatoportoenterostomy (Kasai procedure) and liver transplantation. Cholangitis is also more common in children with primary or acquired immunodeficiency.[5]

Causative organisms

- Bacterial: Gram-negative, enteric organisms are responsible for the majority of episodes. E. coli, Klebsiella, Enterococcus, Enterobacter, Pseudomonas, Proteus, and Bacteroides species are the most commonly implicated pathogens.[6]
- Viral: Viruses play a minor role. However, cholangitis due to cytomegalovirus, and hepatitis B and C viruses has been reported.
- Fungal: Fungal cholangitis is rare, and predominately occurs in immunocompromised patients (mainly C. albicans).
- Parasitic: Ascaris lumbricoides, Fasciola hepatica and Opisthorchis species can cause cholangitis, but are rare in the European setting. In immunocompromised patients (e.g. HIV infection and transplant recipients) Cryptosporidium parvum and Isospora belli have been reported.

Epidemiology

- Cholangitis is rare in children. There are no definitive incidence data.
- However, cholangitis is a common complication after Kasai procedure, and typically occurs within the first 3 months post surgery.

Clinical presentation

- The classical presentation is known as Charcot's triad: fever, jaundice, and right upper quadrant abdominal pain.
- In some patients the pain is exacerbated by food intake.
- Other possible features include: malaise, anorexia, pruritus, and acholic (pale) stools.
- Particularly in immunocompromised individuals, symptoms can be mild or absent.

Differential diagnosis

- Hepatitis
- Pyogenic liver abscess
- Cholelithiasis and cholecystitis
- Primary sclerosing cholangitis (associated with inflammatory bowel disease)
- Drug-induced cholestasis (e.g. antibiotics: cephalosporins, erythromycin, sulfonamides; anticonvulsants: phenobarbital).

Investigations

- Biliary tract enzymes (ALP, γ-GT) and serum conjugated bilirubin are generally elevated. AST and ALT are also frequently elevated. Inflammatory parameters (WBC, CRP, ESR) are usually elevated.
- Blood cultures are positive in approximately 10–25% of patients.
- Abdominal ultrasound scans are useful for identifying biliary obstruction (e.g. cholelithiasis), and can help to identify underlying anatomical abnormalities.
- IV cholangiography, helical CT scans, magnetic resonance cholangiopancreatography (MRCP), endoscopic retrograde cholangiopancreatography (ERCP), and hepatobiliary scintigraphy (hepatobiliary iminodiacetic acid (HIDA) scans) can be useful in selected cases.

Management and treatment

- The patient should be kept nil by mouth and started on IV fluids. Provide adequate pain relief, manage hypovolaemia/shock.
- Broad-spectrum, IV antibiotics providing adequate cover for Gram-negative bacteria (including *Pseudomonas*) and anaerobe organisms should be started empirically, e.g. (i) a combination of a third generation cephalosporin and an aminoglycoside or (ii) a combination of piptazobactam (piperacillin-tazobactam) and an aminoglycoside.[4,6] Addition of metronidazole provides additional cover for anaerobic bacteria.
- In cases with biliary obstruction intervention via ERCP or surgery is indicated, although the optimal timing still remains debated.

Follow-up and outcome

- The mortality associated with acute cholangitis remains considerable (up to 10%), despite improvements in antimicrobial treatment and intensive care support.

Cholecystitis

Introduction

Cholecystitis can be classified as calculous or acalculous, depending on the presence or absence of cholelithiasis. The vast majority of adult cases are calculous, but in childhood up to half of the cases are acalculous. Risk factors for calculous cholecystitis include: haemolytic disease (sickle cell disease, thalassaemia, hereditary spherocytosis), biliary dyskinesia, distal ileal resection and short gut syndrome (loss of bile salts), pregnancy, prolonged fasting, and total parenteral nutrition.[7,8] Risk factors for acalculous disease are: critical illness, trauma, burns, sepsis, Henoch–Schönlein purpura, systemic lupus erythematosus, and Kawasaki disease.

Causative organisms

- The range and frequency of bacterial organisms in the pathogenesis of cholecystitis are similar to those reported for cholangitis.
- Acalculous cholecystitis has been described in association with systemic bacterial infections (e.g. typhoid fever, brucellosis, streptococcal infections, *S. aureus*).
- Cholecystitis caused by viral infections (e.g. CMV, EBV) has been described, but appears to be rare.
- In immunocompromised patients fungal cholecystitis (*Candida* and *Aspergillus* species) has also been reported.

Epidemiology

- Cholecystitis is rare in children.[7] The incidence increases with age (in the paediatric age group highest in adolescents).

Clinical presentation

- Typically pain in the right upper abdominal quadrant or epigastric region is reported. The pain may be constant or colicky in nature. There is often tenderness and guarding on palpation of the liver edge/ the gallbladder (Murphy's sign). Food intake may exacerbate the pain.
- Anorexia, nausea, and vomiting. Jaundice can also be present.

Differential diagnosis

- Gastric and duodenal ulcers
- Pyogenic liver abscess
- Cholangitis, hepatitis, pancreatitis.

Investigations

- Laboratory investigations may reveal leucocytosis, elevated biliary parameters (ALP, γ-GT, bilirubin) and elevated hepatic enzymes (AST, ALT).
- Abdominal ultrasound findings include thickening and increased echogenicity of the gallbladder wall; with or without cholelithiasis.
- HIDA scans are useful for identifying biliary dyskinesia.

Management and treatment

- The management is largely identical to that for cholangitis.

- Cases with suspected biliary obstruction or calculous cholecystitis should be discussed with the surgical team (decompression and/or cholecystectomy may be necessary).[9]

Follow-up and outcome

- The most common complication of cholecystitis is perforation of the gallbladder, which can result in pericholecystic abscess formation or peritonitis.
- Cholelithiasis may be complicated by pancreatitis.

Pancreatitis

Introduction

The pancreas has endocrine (insulin) and exocrine functions (digestive enzymes). Most of the digestive enzymes (trypsin, chymotrypsin, elastase and carboxypeptidases) are secreted into the pancreatic duct as inactive proenzymes, which are converted to active enzymes upon reaching the intestinal lumen. Activation of these enzymes within the pancreas results in inflammation and autodigestion.[10] In contrast, lipase and amylase do not induce tissue damage.

Pancreatic inflammatory disease can be classified as acute or chronic. The spectrum of acute pancreatitis ranges from oedematous pancreatitis, which is generally mild and self-limiting, to severe necrotizing pancreatitis, a potentially life-threatening condition. Mild disease only requires supportive treatment. Children with severe disease should be managed by a multidisciplinary team in a high-dependency or intensive care unit.[11]

Aetiology and causative organisms

In children, a considerable proportion of pancreatitis is caused by microbial infections. In adults, cholelithiasis and alcohol abuse are the most common causes. In approximately 10–20% of the cases no aetiology can be established (idiopathic pancreatitis).

Infectious causes

- Bacterial: Organisms causing intestinal infections, including *Campylobacter jejuni*, *Yersinia enterocolitica*, *Yersinia pseudotuberculosis* and *Salmonella* species. Other bacterial organisms: *Mycoplasma pneumoniae*, *Legionella pneumophila* (Legionnaires' disease), *Mycobacterium tuberculosis*, *Mycobacterium avium* complex, and *Leptospira* species.
- Viral: mumps virus, coxsackie viruses (most commonly coxsackie B4), echoviruses, CMV, EBV, hepatitis viruses (HAV, HBV, HEV), adenoviruses, measles virus, HIV.
- Protozoal: *Cryptosporidium parvum* and *Toxoplasma gondii* (rare, mainly immunocompromised patients); malaria (rare).
- Helminthic: *A. lumbricoides* (via migration into the common bile duct or pancreatic duct) and liver flukes (*F. hepatica*, *Clonorchis sinensis*, *Opisthorchis viverrini*).

Non-infectious causes
- Trauma: Blunt abdominal trauma, abdominal surgery, ERCP.
- Anatomical abnormalities: Obstruction of the common bile duct, pancreatic duct or ampulla of Vater; annular pancreas; pancreas divisum (controversial); choledochal cyst.
- Endocrine: Hypercalcaemia (e.g. hyperparathyroidism).
- Medication: Among others, antibiotics (erythromycin, metronidazole, nitrofurantoin, rifampicin, sulfonamides, tetracyclines), antivirals (didanosine), anticonvulsants (carbamazepine, valproate), diuretics (thiazides, furosemide), immunosuppressive and chemotherapeutic agents (azathioprine, cytarabine, ciclosporin A, glucocorticoids, mercaptopurine) and non-steroidal anti-inflammatory drugs.
- Vasculitis: Kawasaki disease, systemic lupus erythematosus.
- Other: cystic fibrosis, α_1-antitrypsin deficiency, hereditary pancreatitis, hyperlipidaemias, lymphoma, Crohn's disease, renal failure, Reye's syndrome.

Epidemiology
- Pancreatitis is uncommon in childhood.
- The overall incidence (adults and children combined) in the UK has been estimated to range from 150 to 420 cases per million population.[11]

Clinical presentation
- The majority of children with pancreatitis present with abdominal pain and tenderness. However, unlike in adults, who often report pain in the epigastric region or right upper abdominal quadrant, localization of pain is often less typical in children (e.g. periumbilical or diffuse abdominal pain). In about a third of the cases radiation of pain is reported (e.g. back and lower abdomen). The pain is typically described as sharp in nature and often moderate to severe.
- Children frequently adopt an antalgic position with flexion of the hips and knees, while sitting upright or lying on the side.
- Nausea and vomiting are common features.
- Pyrexia is not universally present.
- Physical examination may reveal epigastric tenderness and guarding on palpation, rebound tenderness, abdominal distension and ascites. Bowel sounds may be decreased or absent.
- Cullen's sign and the Grey Turner's sign (ecchymosis in the periumbilical area or flanks, respectively) are rarely present and indicative of severe disease (haemorrhagic pancreatitis).
- Potential complications include pancreatic abscess, pancreatic pseudocyst, hypotension, shock and multiorgan dysfunction.

Differential diagnosis
- Gastric and duodenal ulcers
- Cholelithiasis, cholecystitis, hepatitis
- Ileus/intestinal obstruction, appendicitis
- Nephrolithiasis
- Myocardial infarction, porphyria, Addisonian crisis.

Investigations

- Serum amylase and lipase concentrations are elevated (note: amylase can also be elevated in other conditions, including parotitis, sialadenitis and alcohol intoxication; both enzymes can be elevated in renal failure). In pancreatitis amylase concentrations rise and decline faster than lipase. Therefore, lipase may be within the normal range in early presentation. Inflammatory parameters (WBC, CRP, ESR) are often elevated.
- Hepatic parameters (ALT, AST, γ-GT, ALP, bilirubin) may be within the normal range or elevated. Other possible laboratory findings include hypocalcaemia, hyperglycaemia, elevated LDH, hypoalbuminaemia and abnormal clotting profile.
- Additional investigations may aid in identifying the underlying cause, and should be considered on the background of history and examination (e.g. serology, stool microscopy and culture).
- Abdominal ultrasound helps in confirming the diagnosis and identifying the underlying cause (e.g. cholelithiasis), as well as complications, such as abscess and pseudocyst formation.
- Abdominal CT or MRI scans are not routinely indicated. However, abdominal CT has been recommended in the following circumstances: persisting organ failure, signs of sepsis, or deterioration of clinical status 6–10 days after admission.[11]
- ERCP should be considered in cases where obstruction is suspected to be causative (ampulla of Vater, common bile duct, pancreatic duct).

Management and treatment

- Adequate fluid management is crucial. Hypovolaemia and shock should be treated with crystalloids or colloids.
- Provide adequate analgesia and consider antiemetics.
- Traditionally patients have been kept nil by mouth during the initial stage of the illness. Recent data in adults suggest that early enteral feeding is likely to be safe in mild pancreatitis.
- The role of prophylactic antibiotics to prevent suppurative complications remains controversial.[11,12] Many experts recommend starting antibiotics in cases with severe pancreatic necrosis.
- Additional management depends on the underlying aetiology (e.g. discontinuation of medication in drug-induced cases; treatment of causative microorganisms).
- Approximately 4% of acute pancreatitis cases develop a pancreatic abscess, which requires antibiotic therapy and generally surgical or radiological drainage (📖 see also Intra-abdominal abscess, p. 190).

Follow-up and outcome

- In 80–90% of cases pancreatitis is a benign, self-limiting disease that resolves within 1 week.
- In contrast, the mortality associated with pancreatic abscess and haemorrhagic pancreatitis remains considerable.
- In cases with recurrent pancreatitis further investigations to elucidate the underlying cause should be arranged.

Future research
- Further studies are required to better define high-risk patients who benefit from prophylactic antibiotic cover.
- Further research is needed to establish whether early enteral feeding is a safe option in children with mild pancreatitis.

Appendicitis

Introduction
- The diagnosis of appendicitis is generally based on the history and characteristic clinical findings, although laboratory and radiological investigations can be useful in supporting the presumptive diagnosis.
- Timely management is critical in order to prevent perforation and secondary suppurative complications.

Aetiology and causative organisms
- Appendicitis is thought to primarily be the result of obstruction of the appendiceal lumen (e.g. caused by inspissated faeces or faecaliths, enlarged lymphatic tissue or helminths) resulting in distension, oedema, and ultimately ischaemia of the appendix. Ischaemia facilitates translocation of intraluminal bacteria and may result in perforation with release of faecal contents into the peritoneal cavity. Both processes can result in intra-abdominal abscess formation or peritonitis.
- A large variety of organisms have been isolated from the appendiceal lumen in patients with appendicitis; however, in most instances their role in the pathogenesis remains unclear. The spectrum includes, among others, parasites (e.g. *A. lumbricoides*, *Enterobius vermicularis*, *Taenia solium* and *Taenia saginata*, *Cryptosporidium parvum*), bacteria (e.g. *E. coli*, *S. milleri* group, *Shigella*, *Salmonella*, *Campylobacter*, *Yersinia*, *Bacteroides* and *Fusobacterium* species), and viruses (e.g. coxsackie viruses, adenoviruses).

Epidemiology
- Appendicitis is the commonest cause of acute abdomen in Europe.
- The individual lifetime risk for developing appendicitis has been estimated to be approximately 5–10%.
- Appendicitis occurs across all age groups, although it is uncommon in children <5 years, and very rare in infants.
- The peak incidence is in the second decade of life.
- There are some data indicating that the incidence of acute appendicitis in the UK has declined over the past decades.

Clinical presentation
- Abdominal pain is almost universally present. The pain may initially be periumbilical, with later shift into more typical location in the right lower abdominal quadrant/the right iliac fossa. The pain can be constant or colicky in nature and is usually not severe.
- In young children who are unable to report symptoms, fever, irritability, restlessness and anorexia can be the only presenting features.

- Most patients adopt an antalgic position with flexion of the right hip. Movement (e.g. walking, jumping, coughing) exacerbates the pain.
- Vomiting typically occurs only after the onset of pain. Both constipation and diarrhoea (usually mild) can occur. Dysuria is only infrequently reported.
- Low-grade pyrexia is present in more than two-thirds of the cases. High-grade pyrexia (>39°C) is uncommon, and more commonly associated with perforation. Importantly, absence of pyrexia does not rule out appendicitis.
- Palpation typically reveals right iliac fossa tenderness and guarding. In older children the point of maximum tenderness is frequently at McBurney's point (at the junction between the lower and middle thirds of an imaginary line between the right anterior superior iliac spine and the umbilicus). Rebound tenderness is commonly present; Rovsing's sign and the psoas sign (pain on flexion of the right leg against resistance) may also be positive.
- Tenderness may be absent in cases with atypical location of the appendix (e.g. retrocaecal and pelvic appendix).
- Bowel sounds are often reduced. Complete absence frequently indicates perforation.

Differential diagnosis

- Intestinal: Gastroenteritis, mesenteric lymphadenitis, infectious colitis (e.g. *Yersinia* and *Campylobacter* species), ileus/intestinal obstruction, intussusception, volvulus, Meckel's diverticulitis, necrotizing enterocolitis, Crohn's disease, constipation.
- Renal: Nephrolithiasis, pyelonephritis, cystitis.
- Genital tract: Testicular torsion, ovarian torsion, ovarian cyst, salpingitis, pelvic inflammatory disease, ectopic pregnancy.
- Other: lower lobe pneumonia, spontaneous bacterial peritonitis, psoas abscess, sickle cell crisis, Henoch–Schönlein purpura, diabetic ketoacidosis, porphyria.

Investigations

- Laboratory tests are not particularly useful, but may support the presumptive diagnosis of appendicitis.
- Inflammatory parameters (WBC, CRP, ESR) are often elevated. However, unremarkable results do not rule out appendicitis.
- Urine analysis may reveal presence of red and/or white blood cells (beware erroneous diagnosis of urinary tract infection).
- The routine use of abdominal ultrasound remains debated. However, selective abdominal ultrasound can provide useful information in cases where the diagnosis is uncertain. The sensitivity of this technique ranges from 87–95% in suspected appendicitis.[13]

Management and treatment

- Patients with suspected appendicitis should be kept nil by mouth.
- Appendectomy remains the standard treatment for appendicitis. Removal of the appendix can be performed either via laparoscopic or open surgery, depending on locally available facilities.[14]

- All patients with appendicitis should be commenced on antibiotic therapy.[15] Empirical regimens that have been proposed include:[15]
  - Piptazobactam (piperacillin-tazobactam) or timentin (ticarcillin-clavulanate) or co-amoxiclav
  - Ceftriaxone, cefotaxime, or ceftazidime in combination with metronidazole
  - Gentamicin or tobramycin in combination with metronidazole or clindamycin and with or without ampicillin.
- There are some data in adults suggesting that selected cases with uncomplicated appendicitis can be successfully managed with antibiotic therapy alone (i.e. without surgery).[16] However, the currently available evidence to support this strategy is still limited.
- Patients with perforation and/or diffuse peritonitis should be managed as a surgical emergency.

Follow-up and outcome

- Perforation complicates the course of appendicitis in 5–20% of cases.
- The case fatality rate in the UK is currently significantly below 1%.

Future research

- Further research is needed to better define patient groups that can be safely managed without surgical appendectomy.

Peritonitis

Introduction

Peritonitis is defined as inflammation of the peritoneum, a serosal membrane that lines the abdominal cavity and the intra-abdominal organs. The inflammation can be caused by irritants (e.g. gastric and pancreatic secretions, bile, blood or urine) or infectious agents. Peritonitis can be classified as primary (or spontaneous) or secondary.[17–19] Primary peritonitis is thought to predominately result from bacterial spread via the haematogenous route (i.e. bacteraemia). Secondary peritonitis results from intra-abdominal disease processes, which lead to organ perforation or abscess formation. Peritonitis can also be the result of infections associated with intra-abdominal devices, such as peritoneal dialysis catheters and ventriculoperitoneal shunts.

Causative organisms

- Primary peritonitis: Commonly Gram-positive bacterial organisms—*Streptococcus pneumoniae*, *Streptococcus pyogenes*, *S. aureus*. Gram-negative bacteria, including *E. coli* and *Klebsiella pneumoniae*, are also common causative agents.
- Secondary peritonitis: Predominately organisms that are part of the gastrointestinal flora—*E. coli*, *Klebsiella*, *Enterococcus*, *Enterobacter*, *Pseudomonas* and *Proteus* species. Anaerobic bacteria, such as *Bacteroides* and *Peptostreptococcus* species, are also common

isolates. Infections due to gastrointestinal perforation are generally polymicrobial.

- Peritoneal dialysis: A broad range of organisms has been reported. Most commonly implicated are *Staphylococcus epidermidis*, *S. aureus*, streptococci and *Enterobacteriaceae*. *P. aeruginosa* accounts for 5–10% of the cases. Fungal peritonitis, most commonly due to *C. albicans*, can also occur in this setting. Mycobacterial peritonitis has also been reported in this patient group.
- Ventriculoperitoneal shunt: Most commonly *S. epidermidis* and *S. aureus*.
- Mycobacterial peritonitis: rare in the European setting (*M. tuberculosis*, *M. bovis*, and atypical mycobacteria).

Epidemiology

- Although there are no definitive incidence data for primary peritonitis in children, it is very rare.
- Primary peritonitis mainly affects children with pre-existing illnesses associated with ascites, e.g. liver disease and nephrotic syndrome.
- Necrotizing enterocolitis is the most common underlying aetiology of secondary peritonitis in neonates, while appendicitis is the predominating underlying cause in older children.

Clinical presentation

- Typically diffuse abdominal pain, which is moderate to severe in nature and exacerbated by movement.
- Non-specific signs and symptoms such as fever, anorexia, nausea and vomiting are frequently present.
- Examination may reveal abdominal distension, reduced or absent bowel sounds, diffuse tenderness and guarding on palpation, as well as rebound tenderness.
- Intra-abdominal fluid loss can lead to hypovolaemia and shock.

Differential diagnosis

- Gastroenteritis; food poisoning
- Mesenteric lymphadenitis
- Hepatitis; cholecystitis; cholelithiasis; cholangitis
- Pancreatitis; ileus/intestinal obstruction
- Pyelonephritis; nephrolithiasis
- Diabetic ketoacidosis
- Sickle cell crisis
- Familial Mediterranean fever
- Extrauterine pregnancy; ovarian and testicular torsion.

Investigations

- Inflammatory parameters (WBC, CRP, ESR) are often elevated.
- Depending on the underlying aetiology plain abdominal X-rays may reveal free intra-abdominal air or evidence of intestinal obstruction.
- Abdominal ultrasound and CT scans help in establishing the underlying cause.

- Analysis of intra-abdominal fluid can be useful in several ways:
  - Discoloration may indicate the underlying cause (e.g. bilious or faecal matter)
  - In peritonitis the leucocyte count in peritoneal fluid is generally >300 WBC/mm^3 (neutrophils typically predominate); in dialysate fluid >100 WBC/mm^3 is considered as indicative of peritonitis
  - Gram-staining and culture aid in identifying the causative microorganism.

Management and treatment

- The patient should be kept nil by mouth and started on IV fluids.
- Primary peritonitis is managed conservatively, unless uncertainty about the diagnosis warrants laparoscopy or laparotomy.
- In secondary peritonitis treat the underlying aetiology.
- Empirical antibiotic treatment should be started promptly. The choice of empirical antibiotic agents depends on: the type of peritonitis (primary versus secondary), and the underlying aetiology. For possible regimens in patients with intestinal perforation 🕮 see Appendicitis, p. 186. In patients with device-associated infections specialist advice should be sought.

Follow-up and outcome

- The potential complications of acute peritonitis include shock and multiorgan failure. The prognosis depends on the pre-existing morbidity, the underlying aetiology and the complications associated with surgical intervention.

Intra-abdominal abscess

Introduction

Intra-abdominal abscesses can be divided into intraperitoneal, visceral (liver (discussed above), splenic and pancreatic abscesses) and retroperitoneal abscesses. In the paediatric age group intraperitoneal abscesses, which usually result either from extension of a localised infectious focus (e.g. appendicitis) or loculation of diffuse peritonitis, are the most common.

Causative organisms

- Intraperitoneal abscess: Frequently polymicrobial; most commonly bacteria that are part of the gastrointestinal flora (🕮 p. 188).
- Splenic abscess: The majority are monomicrobial; common causative agents include staphylococci, streptococci, and *Enterobacteriaceae* (including *Salmonella* species).[20] *Candida* species have mainly been described in immunocompromised patients (typically multifocal—hepatosplenic candidiasis is a recognised complication of severe neutropenia). Splenic abscesses caused by mycobacteria, mainly in immunocompromised individuals, have also been reported. Cat scratch disease (*Bartonella henselae*) can cause microabscesses in the spleen and liver.

Epidemiology

- Intra-abdominal abscesses are rare in children. Appendicitis is the most common underlying cause.
- Predisposing factors for splenic abscess include: haemoglobinopathies, endocarditis, trauma, malignancy, and immunocompromise.
- Predisposing factors for pancreatic abscess include: cholelithiasis, pancreatitis, and trauma.

Clinical presentation

- Intraperitoneal abscess: Pyrexia is common. Symptoms and signs depend on the site of the abscess.
- Splenic abscess: Typically pyrexia, generalized or left upper quadrant abdominal pain and splenomegaly. Patients may also report left-sided chest or shoulder pain. Pleural effusion may also be present.

Investigations

- Inflammatory parameters (WBC, CRP, ESR) are elevated.
- Blood cultures should be obtained in all patients (positive in approximately half of the cases with splenic abscess).
- Abdominal ultrasound and CT scans are the initial radiological investigations of choice in patients with suspected intra-abdominal abscess.
- Purulent material obtained during drainage should be sent for Gram-staining and culture.

Management and treatment

- Supportive treatment, empirical antimicrobial therapy and drainage of the abscess form the basis of management. Antimicrobial therapy should be adjusted once culture results and susceptibilities become available.
- Drainage of the abscess can be performed via interventional radiology (ultrasound- or CT-guided) or surgically, depending on the site and extent of the infectious focus.
- Splenectomy can become necessary in patients with splenic abscess.

Follow-up and outcome

- Potential complications include disseminated infection (sepsis), peritoneal adhesions and intestinal obstruction.
- The prognosis depends on the underlying aetiology and the type and site of the abscess.

Key references

1 Hansen PS, Schønheyder HC. Pyogenic hepatic abscess. A 10-year population-based retrospective study. APMIS 1998;**106**:396–402.

2 Pineiro-Carrero VM, Andres JM. Morbidity and mortality in children with pyogenic liver abscess. Am J Dis Child 1989;**143**:1424–7.

3 Muorah M, Hinds R, Verma A, et al. Liver abscesses in children: a single center experience in the developed world. J Pediatr Gastroenterol Nutr 2006;**42**:201–6.

4 Lee JG. Diagnosis and management of acute cholangitis. Nat Rev Gastroenterol Hepatol 2009;**6**:533–41.

5 Rodrigues F, Davies EG, Harrison P, et al. Liver disease in children with primary immunodeficiencies. *J Pediatr* 2004;**145**:333–9.

6 Westphal JF, Brogard JM. Biliary tract infections: a guide to drug treatment. *Drugs* 1999;**57**:81–91.

7 Rescorla FJ. Cholelithiasis, cholecystitis, and common bile duct stones. *Curr Opin Pediatr* 1997;**9**:276–82.

8 Reif S, Sloven DG, Lebenthal E. Gallstones in children. Characterization by age, etiology, and outcome. *Am J Dis Child* 1991;**145**:105–8.

9 Heaton ND, Davenport M, Howard ER. Intraluminal biliary obstruction. *Arch Dis Child* 1991;**66**:1395–8.

10 Frossard JL, Steer ML, Pastor CM. Acute pancreatitis. *Lancet* 2008;**371**:143–52.

11 Working Party of the British Society of Gastroenterology, Association of Surgeons of Great Britain and Ireland, Pancreatic Society of Great Britain and Ireland, Association of Upper GI Surgeons of Great Britain and Ireland. UK guidelines for the management of acute pancreatitis. *Gut* 2005;**54** (Suppl 3):iii1–9.

12 Villatoro E, Bassi C, Larvin M. Antibiotic therapy for prophylaxis against infection of pancreatic necrosis in acute pancreatitis. *Cochrane Database Syst Rev* 2010;**5**:CD002941.

13 Rosendahl K, Aukland SM, Fosse K. Imaging strategies in children with suspected appendicitis. *Eur Radiol* 2004;**14** (Suppl 4):L138–45.

14 Sauerland S, Lefering R, Neugebauer EA. Laparoscopic versus open surgery for suspected appendicitis. *Cochrane Database Syst Rev* 2004;**4**:CD001546.

15 Solomkin JS, Mazuski JE, Bradley JS, Rodvold KA, Goldstein EJ, Baron EJ, et al. Diagnosis and management of complicated intra-abdominal infection in adults and children: guidelines by the Surgical Infection Society and the Infectious Diseases Society of America. *Clin Infect Dis* 2010;**50**:133–64.

16 Varadhan KK, Humes DJ, Neal KR, Lobo DN. Antibiotic therapy versus appendectomy for acute appendicitis: a meta-analysis. *World J Surg* 2010;**34**:199–209.

17 Mazuski JE, Solomkin JS. Intra-abdominal infections. *Surg Clin North Am* 2009;**89**:421–37.

18 Johnson CC, Baldessarre J, Levison ME. Peritonitis: update on pathophysiology, clinical manifestations, and management. *Clin Infect Dis* 1997;**24**:1035–45.

19 McClean KL, Sheehan GJ, Harding GK. Intraabdominal infection: a review. *Clin Infect Dis* 1994;**19**:100–16.

20 Keidl CM, Chusid MJ. Splenic abscesses in childhood. *Pediatr Infect Dis J* 1989;**8**:368–73.

Invasive fungal infection

📖 see also Chapters 2, 20, 51, 55, 96

Introduction

The incidence of IFI in children is rising. This is because of the increasing number of children undergoing intensive chemotherapy or haematopoietic stem cell transplantation (HSCT) for the treatment of malignancy, increasing use of monoclonal antibodies for the prevention and treatment of GVHD, and the wider use of novel immunosuppressive therapies for children with rheumatological and autoimmune conditions.

Historically, *Aspergillus fumigatus* and *Candida albicans* have been the most common pathogens isolated, but over the past few decades there has been an emergence of new fungal infections, with increasing rates of non-albicans *Candida*, non-fumigatus *Aspergillus*, zygomycetes and non-*Aspergillus* filamentous moulds. The last decade has seen the development of a number of novel therapies and new rapid diagnostic tests. Unfortunately, despite this, the mortality and morbidity from IFI remains high.

Epidemiology

Candida

- This remains the most common pathogen responsible for IFI, although rates have reduced in comparison to invasive mould infections. This is because of the increasing use of prophylactic fluconazole, which has activity against *Candida* but not *Aspergillus*.
- Main portal of entry is from the gut, especially if mucosal integrity is disrupted by cytotoxic drugs in the face of neutropenia. Skin transmission is possible, especially with a CVC *in situ*.
- Can cause single organ infection or disseminated infection, especially to the lungs, liver, kidney, and brain.
- Rates in neonates > children > adults
  - Neonatal rates are approximately 150 per 100 000 admissions.
- *Candida albicans* remains the most common species isolated—*Candida albicans* (50%), *Candida parapsilosis* (20%), *Candida tropicalis* (10%); *Candida glabrata*, and *Candida krusei* remain infrequent.
  - Increasing rates of *C. parapsilosis* have been reported in the neonatal and paediatric populations, especially with CVC use.
  - Increasing use of fluconazole has resulted in higher rates of *C. glabrata* and *C. krusei*, which have increased resistance to amphotericin B.

Aspergillus

- *Aspergillus* is found in air, soil, water and grows on decaying vegetation. Local building works, contaminated ventilation and water sources have all been responsible for invasive aspergillosis in immunocompromised children.

- Invasive pulmonary disease is most common and follows the inhalation of conidia (spores). Angioinvasion of germinating hyphae leads to invasive disease. Sinusitis and gastrointestinal aspergillosis occur less frequently. Disseminated disease, especially CNS infection, can occur.
- *Aspergillus fumigatus* remains the most common species isolated, with *Aspergillus flavus, Aspergillus terreus, Aspergillus nidulans,* and *Aspergillus nigrans* less frequent. *A. nidulans* preferentially infects patients with CGD, with a predisposition to bone infection and lack of angioinvasion.
- Rates of invasive aspergillosis are similar in adults and children. Rates of mould infection are increasing, because of the increasing use of fluconazole prophylaxis and the use of anti-TNFα drugs such as infliximab. TNFα is a key molecule in the initial innate immune response to *Aspergillus*.

Other fungi

Cryptococcus

- Infection is most commonly caused by *Cryptococcus neoformans*, which lives in soil and organic matter containing high concentrations of bird excreta.
- *C. neoformans* is neurotropic, leading to CNS infection.
- Risk factors for invasive infection include lymphoma, AIDS, and steroid use.
- The 10-year prevalence in children with HIV used to be 1%, but it has reduced to virtually zero since the introduction of highly active antiretroviral treatment.
- There has been an increasing incidence of non-neoformans *Cryptococcus* strains in the past few decades, especially *Cryptococcus laurentii* and *Cryptococcus albidus*.

Zygomycetes

- Include *Rhizopus, Mucor, Rhizomucor, Absidia,* and *Cunninghamella*.
- Transmission is mainly airborne and requires impaired phagocytic function or disruption of mucosal surfaces to cause disease. Common sites of infection include sinuses, pulmonary, cutaneous and gastrointestinal.
- Zygomycetes have a predilection for invasion of blood vessels, causing thrombosis and infarction.
- Neonatal infection is associated with increased rates of dissemination and higher mortality.
- Tend to be resistant to most azoles and echinocandins.

Fusarium

- A filamentous mould similar to *Aspergillus*.
- Presents with fungaemia and disseminated skin and soft tissue lesions.
- Often resistant to amphotericin B and the echinocandins.

Saccharomyces cerevisiae (Baker's yeast)

- Invasive disease has been associated with its use as a probiotic in immunocompromised patients.

Risk factors for IFI include:

- Host factors such as immunodeficiency and neutropenia, rather than virulence factors associated with the individual fungus, contribute most significantly to the development of IFI.
- Neutropenia is the most significant risk factor for IFI, especially significant neutropenia for prolonged periods. Moderate neutropenia of $0.1–0.5 \times 10^9$ /l for <1 week carries considerably less risk (Table 23.1).
- Invasive candidiasis tends to occur after 1–2 weeks of neutropenia, whereas invasive aspergillosis tends to occur after recurrent and prolonged periods of neutropenia.
- The overall mortality of invasive candidiasis in children may be up to 10–20%. Prior colonization almost invariably precedes invasive candidiasis. This risk increases if more than one site is colonized or if colonization is heavy. Neonates have the highest rate of infection, although it remains rare. The highest rates are seen in extremely low birthweight (ELBW) infants.
- The overall mortality of invasive aspergillosis in children may be as high as 50%.

Table 23.1 Risk factors for the development of invasive candidiasis and invasive aspergillosis

Invasive candidiasis	Invasive aspergillosis
Immunosuppression Prolonged/severe neutropenia	Haematological malignancy (acute myeloid leukaemia (AML)/allogeneic HSCT > acute lymphocytic leukaemia (ALL) > lymphoma)
Colonisation ≥2 sites	Prolonged/severe neutropenia
Mucosal disruption and gastrointestinal colonization	Use of TNFA blocking drugs
Portal of entry, i.e. central venous catheters	HSCT
Total parenteral nutrition (TPN) Broad-spectrum antibiotic use Neonatal risk factors: • Extreme prematurity and ELBW • Use of H_2 blockers • High glucose levels • Lack of enteral feeding	For HSCT recipients: • Peripheral blood stem cell transplant > BMT • T cell depleted/CD34+ selected > whole marrow • GVHD (grade III/IV > grade I/II)

Risk stratification

Risk stratification allows patients to be identified as low, intermediate, or high risk for developing IFI. A model for risk stratification,[1] which has been summarized in Box 23.1, has been validated only in an adult cohort. Explicitly categorizing patients on the basis of risk may lend weight to the results of diagnostic tests and may allow therapeutic interventions to be targeted most accurately. To date, no such model has been developed for paediatric patients.

Box 23.1 Stratified risk of invasive fungal infection, based on adult data[a]

- Low risk
  - Autologous HSCT
  - Childhood acute lymphocytic leukaemia
  - Lymphoma
- Intermediate risk
  - Neutropenia $0.1–0.5 \times 10^9/l$ for 1–5 weeks' duration
  - Colonized ≥2 sites
  - Allogeneic matched sibling donor HSCT
  - Acute myeloid leukaemia
  - TBI (by causing severe mucositis/gastrointestinal damage)
  - CVL *in situ*
  - Recent bacteraemia
- High risk
  - Neutrophils $<0.1 \times 10^9/l$ for >3 weeks or $<0.5 \times 10^9/l$ for >5 weeks duration
  - Unrelated or mismatched HSCT especially T cell depleted peripheral blood SCT
  - GVHD (grade III/IV)
  - Corticosteroids >2 mg/kg for >2 weeks
  - Chemotherapy with fludarabine or high-dose cytosine arabinoside

[a]Adapted from Prentice *et al.*[1]

Preventative strategies

Despite the identification of high-risk patients and the early initiation of treatment, IFI carries a high risk of mortality and morbidity. Up to 70% of premature infants with blood or CNS fungal infection either die or have neurodevelopmental sequelae. For this reason, preventative strategies are required to reduce the risk of IFI:

- Avoidance where possible of prolonged broad spectrum antibiotics use in neonates
- Enhancing enteric colonization with early feeding of neonates
- Prophylactic use of antifungal drugs

- Use of granulocyte colony-stimulating factor (G-CSF) during the period of neutropenia in high-risk patients. However, small retrospective studies have raised concerns about a possible association between the use of G-CSF in allogeneic BMT patients, and the subsequent development of GVHD. Therefore the use of G-CSF should be limited to patients receiving autologous HSCT and considered in children receiving allogeneic peripheral blood stem cell transplants[2]
- Granulocyte infusions may be considered in neutropenic patients with invasive aspergillosis, until neutrophil recovery occurs.

Prophylactic use of antifungal drugs

- Prophylactic antifungal drugs have been shown to reduce the risk of IFI when used in high risk patients during periods of greatest risk. These periods include severe myelosuppression, during cytotoxic therapy induced mucosal damage and augmented immunosuppression such as during the treatment of GVHD.
- Paediatric data support the use of prophylactic fluconazole and amphotericin B in targeted populations. More recent adult data suggest that itraconazole maybe superior in reducing IFI compared to fluconazole. However, unpredictable bioavailability and drug interactions may limit its use.
- The use of prophylactic drugs is not indicated for all neutropenic patients and clinical trials have shown no reduction in overall mortality apart from in the highest risk patients.
- 6 weeks of fluconazole in ELBW infants has been shown to reduce the rate of IFI by up to 75%. The risk–benefit analysis of routine use of fluconazole prophylaxis is complex and depends on local factors, including rates of TPN usage, surgery, antibiotic policies and current rates of IFI. Many neonatal units have a targeted policy of fluconazole prophylaxis based on the risk factors of VLBW, abdominal surgery, prolonged TPN and broad-spectrum antibiotics.
- Adult data support the use of posaconazole as primary prophylaxis in patients at high risk of developing invasive aspergillosis, showing superiority to both fluconazole and itraconazole.[3]

The diagnostic process

Active surveillance and diagnostic programmes can reduce the mortality from IFI significantly. This was seen in Dijon, France, when the strengthening of diagnostic facilities and improved management resulted in the mortality rates of invasive aspergillosis falling from 60% to 12% over a 6-year period.[4]

Microbiology/histopathology

- Microscopy and culture, along with histopathology, has traditionally been the gold standard for diagnosing IFI. Testing can be performed on blood, bronchoalveolar lavage (BAL) fluid, fluid from sterile sites and tissue specimens.

- Microscopy has a higher yield than culture alone, especially in BAL samples. Fluorescent staining can improve the sensitivity, allowing septate and non-septate moulds to be distinguished and appropriate therapy to be initiated in a timely manner.
- All fungi obtained from sterile sites including blood, peritoneal dialysis fluid and CVC tips should be identified to species level by referring them to a specialist laboratory.
- There is uncertainty about the usefulness of identifying *Candida* obtained from BAL fluid to a species level, although the recognition of *Cryptococcus neoformans* is important.
- In the absence of an alternative diagnosis, abnormal CSF should be tested for cryptococcal antigen and cultured for fungi.
- All histology samples for suspected IFI should be stained with a fungal stain such as silver stain concurrently with conventional haematoxylin and eosin stain.
- However, all these tests are limited by the difficulty in obtaining adequate specimens, their prolonged time of culturing and their relatively low sensitivities. The sensitivity of microscopy and culture of BAL fluid for *Aspergillus* is only approximately 30%.

Imaging

- In adults, the use of serial high-resolution CT (HRCT) of the chest has allowed invasive aspergillosis to be diagnosed earlier. Characteristic radiological features include the halo sign (an area of ground glass opacity around a nodule) and air crescents (due to lung tissue destruction). When *Aspergillus* is isolated in BAL fluid or respiratory secretions, HRCT changes allow respiratory tract colonization to be distinguished from invasive disease.
- Unfortunately, these characteristic radiological features are found far less commonly in children. Non-specific changes may represent invasive aspergillosis in a child, which means that HRCT has a lower specificity for diagnosing invasive pulmonary aspergillosis in children than in adults. The radiation risk of serial CT scans must also be considered in children. The commonest CT sign is persistent focal abnormalities. CT changes are often much more remarkable than chest radiograph appearances in invasive aspergillosis.
- Ultrasound scanning can be used to identify hepatosplenic and renal fungal lesions. The sensitivity can be increased by using a linear probe.
- MRI can be used to identify other potential sites involved, and to guide biopsies and surgical intervention.
- The role of positron emission tomography (PET) has not been fully established in the paediatric population, but may be useful to identify sites of infection.

More recently, the detection of fungal wall products has enabled invasive fungal infection to be diagnosed more rapidly than using clinical and radiological suspicion alone.

Galactomannan

- The galactomannan ELISA test allows the detection of *Aspergillus* galactomannan. The test has predominantly been validated in serum, but studies support its use for BAL and CSF fluid. Two or more positive results from consecutive serum samples are required to make a diagnosis (or one from BAL/CSF fluids).
- Paediatric studies suggest a sensitivity of 70% and specificity of 90%, when an optical density index cut-off of 0.5 is used.
- False positive results may occur with B-lactam antibiotics, especially piperacillin-tazobactam and amoxicillin-clavulanate, because of cross-reactivity. Cross-reactivity also occurs with bifidobacteria present in infantile gut microflora and food groups such as rice and pasta, which may translocate across damaged gut mucosa.
- False-negative results may occur when antifungal drugs are being concurrently used. In addition, lower fungal burdens in non-neutropenic patients may result in false negative results.

Mannan

- The mannan ELISA detects mannan, a Candidal surface protein. Studies support its use in serum and CSF.
- However, the results of mannan detection in serum have been variable, with sensitivities ranging from 0–100% and specificities from 88–100%.

β-D glucan

- This assay detects (1,3)-β-D glucan, which is present in most opportunistic fungi. It has a sensitivity of 70% and specificity of about 90% in diagnosing IFI but cannot distinguish yeast and mould infections.
- Unfortunately, baseline levels in uninfected children are not yet clearly established, limiting its role in paediatrics at present.

Fungal DNA

- The use of PCR technology to diagnose IFI still remains unvalidated but will potentially enable routine screening of high-risk patients. *Candida* and *Aspergillus* PCR assays exist but are currently not standardized between laboratories and at present remain within the realms of research.

Managing the child with possible fungal infection

Empirical treatment

- The late diagnosis and delayed initiation of antifungal treatment is associated with increased mortality and morbidity. Empirical treatment of neutropenic patients remaining febrile despite broad-spectrum antibiotics is based on studies dating back to the early 1980s, which showed that giving amphotericin B to such patients reduced their rates of IFI and overall mortality.

- No individual antifungal drug has shown a superior survival benefit, although voriconazole is perhaps superior in preventing breakthrough infections and can be considered for high-risk patients such as allogeneic HSCT recipients.

Pre-emptive therapy

- Prolonged fever in a high risk patient can be caused by inadequately controlled non-fungal infection, malignancy, drugs, GVHD, engraftment post HSCT or neutrophil recovery post chemotherapy. As a result, 40–50% of high risk patients receive empirical antifungal treatment, whilst the incidence of IFI is approximately 20%.
- Adult data suggest that a pre-emptive approach, using the novel diagnostic tests outlined above, can be safely used to identify patients who require treatment, whilst avoiding unnecessary treatment in the majority of neutropenic patients with prolonged fever.[5]
- The safety of this approach relies on rapid access to these tests, and so far such an approach has not been validated in a paediatric population.

Invasive candidiasis

- This may present with acute disseminated candidiasis, hepatosplenic candidiasis, cutaneous neonatal candidiasis, or organ-specific disease such as urinary, pulmonary, osteomyelitis, peritoneal, endocarditis, meningitis, and endophthalmitis.
- First-line drug treatment includes L-amB, fluconazole, caspofungin, and micafungin. These recommendations are derived from adult data because no adequately powered paediatric comparative trials have been performed.
- Adjunctive measures include giving G-CSF if neutropenic, stopping/reducing immunosuppression if possible and consider CVL removal (see below).
- Second-line treatment includes voriconazole.
- The choice of drug used depends on drug interactions, organ impairment, whether any prophylaxis agents were used (if an azole was used as prophylaxis, use a polyene or echinocandins for treatment), the strain isolated (if *C. krusei* or *C. glabrata*, consider using an echinocandin), and the local epidemiology of circulating stains.
- The duration of treatment depends on the clinical presentation, clearance of *Candida*, resolution of clinical symptoms and whether immunosuppression has been discontinued (see Table 23.2). Funduscopy prior to the end of treatment is mandatory to rule out endophthalmitis. Candidaemia of ≥5 days in neonates is associated with increased risk of ophthalmic, renal and cardiac dissemination.
- Persisting Candidaemia in the face of treatment may indicate resistance, an infected CVC or significant immunosuppression. Consider changing treatment to a different class drug, attempt to isolate the organism to species level and perform drug susceptibility testing, reduce immunosuppression if possible, and consider CVC removal.

Table 23.2 Management of invasive candidiasis

Acute disseminated candidiasis	Continue treatment for 14 days after blood cultures become negative and symptoms have resolved. Consider switching to oral fluconazole after initial IV therapy
Chronic disseminated candidiasis (hepatosplenic *Candida*)	A prolonged treatment course is required. Consider initial treatment with 2–3 weeks of L-amB followed by oral fluconazole until resolution of symptoms and calcification of lesions. Premature discontinuation may result in relapse, especially in immunocompromised children
Candida osteomyelitis	Antifungal therapy and surgical debridement is often required. Consider 2–3 weeks IV therapy followed by up to 6 months of oral fluconazole
Candida endocarditis	If surgical replacement of the infected valve is performed, treatment should be continued for at least 6 weeks. If valve replacement is not performed, a considerably longer treatment course is required because of a high risk of relapse—consider lifelong fluconazole
Candida meningitis	Treat with L-amB and flucytosine combination therapy, to improve CNS penetration. Remove any prosthetic material such as ventriculoperitoneal shunts. Continue treatment for at least 4 weeks after normalization of CSF and resolution of all symptoms

CVC removal
- Data supporting CVC removal during IC are conflicting.[6] No high-quality RCTs have been performed, but some prospective cohort studies show no benefit. In view of the complications associated with catheter removal (especially tunnelled lines), the likely gastrointestinal origin in the majority of cases (especially during severe mucositis and neutropenia) and the difficulties faced maintaining adequate vascular assess in this population of patients, a pragmatic approach may be considered.
- Antifungal therapy given through the CVC can be continued unless the patient is haemodynamically unstable, has persisting candidaemia despite 72 hours treatment or remains symptomatic. In addition, the presence of endocarditis or thrombophlebitis would expedite line removal.

Invasive aspergillosis
- This may present as invasive pulmonary aspergillosis, chronic necrotizing pulmonary aspergillosis or organ-specific disease such as tracheobronchial, sinonasal infection, carditis, septic arthritis, endophthalmitis, peritonitis, gastrointestinal, hepatic, or renal infection.
- First-line drug treatment for invasive aspergillosis is voriconazole or L-amB. Direct comparison suggest that voriconazole is superior (see Chapter 3, p. 20), but the choice of drug depends on organ

impairment, drug interactions, and whether prophylactic/pre-emptive therapy was used. In a setting of high rates of zygomycosis infection, voriconazole may be a less useful drug for pre-emptive treatment.

- Adjunctive measures include giving G-CSF if neutropenic and stopping/ reducing immunosuppression if possible. Granulocyte infusions may also be considered to stabilize invasive aspergillosis until neutrophil recovery.
- Second-line treatment recommendations are limited by a lack of data in patients who appear refractory to first line treatment for invasive aspergillosis or experience break-through infection despite mould-active azole prophylaxis. In such situations, voriconazole levels should be checked, IV drug therapy should be used and changing/adding a drug from a different class should be considered. Suggested drugs include caspofungin, itraconazole and posaconazole.
- The duration of treatment remains unclear but depends upon the clinical, microbiological and radiological response. Oral treatment can be considered once the clinical situation is stable. For patients who remain chronically immunocompromised, treatment should be continued through the period of immunosuppression. If invasive aspergillosis has been successfully treated, secondary prophylaxis should be considered if subsequent immunosuppression is required.
- Surgical intervention should be considered for operable cerebral/ lung lesions, especially lung lesions with proximity to the great vessels or pericardium, sinus infections, skin and soft tissue infections, bony lesions, and endocarditis.
- Other filamentous fungi such as *Fusarium* and *Scedosporium* can present with a similar clinical and radiological picture. Therefore, a definitive microbiological diagnosis should be established whenever possible.

Combination therapy

The rationale behind the use of combination therapy with drugs from different classes is to achieve increased antifungal therapy through synergy, increase the spectrum of antifungal activity, especially when initiated pre-emptively or empirically, and to reduce the emergence of resistance. Unfortunately, the evidence supporting the use of combination treatment is limited to retrospective case series. Therefore, until high-quality paediatric data are available, the use of combination treatment should be limited to children with progressive or overwhelming infection. Trials of combination therapy in children are under way.

Key references

1 Prentice HG, Kibbler CC, Prentice AG. Towards a targeted, risk-based, antifungal strategy in neutropenic patients. *Br J Haematol* 2000;**110**:273–84.
2 Trivedi M, Martinez S, Corringham S, Medley K, Ball ED. Optimal use of G-CSF administration after hematopoietic SCT. *Bone Marrow Transplant* 2009;**43**:895–908.
3 Cornely OA, Maertens J, Winston DJ, et al. Posaconazole vs. fluconazole or itraconazole prophylaxis in patients with neutropenia. *N Engl J Med* 2007;**356**:348–59.
4 Caillot D, Casasnovas O, Bernard A, et al. Improved management of invasive pulmonary aspergillosis in neutropenic patients using early thoracic computed tomographic scan and surgery. *J Clin Oncol* 1997;**15**:139–47.

5 Maertens J, Theunissen K, Verhoef G, *et al.* Galactomannan and computed tomography-based preemptive antifungal therapy in neutropenic patients at high risk for invasive fungal infection: a prospective feasibility study. *Clin Infect Dis* 2005;**41**:1242–50.
6 Nucci M, Anaissie E. Should vascular catheters be removed from all patients with candidemia? An evidence-based review. *Clin Infect Dis* 2002;**34**:591–9.

Further reading

Bow EJ. Considerations in the approach to invasive fungal infection in patients with haematological malignancies. *Br J Haematol* 2008;**140**:133–52.

Pappas PG, Rex JH, Sobel JD, *et al.* Guidelines for treatment of candidiasis. *Clin Infect Dis* 2004;**38**:161–89.

Walsh TJ, Anaissie EJ, Denning DW, *et al.* Treatment of aspergillosis: clinical practice guidelines of the Infectious Diseases Society of America. *Clin Infect Dis* 2008;**46**:327–60.

Chapter 24

Investigating the child with possible immunodeficiency

📖 see also Chapters 19, 20, 26

Introduction

An increased susceptibility to infections is the hallmark of primary immunodeficiency disorders. This abnormal handling of infection may be characterised by:

- Unusual microbial causes of infection not generally seen in healthy individuals—e.g. opportunistic organisms such as *Pneumocystis jiroveci*
- Atypical features in a common infection—e.g. severe haemorrhagic chicken pox
- Excessive frequency of infections—e.g. recurrent lower respiratory tract infections.

Other non-infective clues to the presence of immunodeficiency may include:

- Family history
- Lymphoid hypertrophy
- Rashes
- Enteropathy
- Autoimmune phenomena
- Miscellaneous—e.g. delayed umbilical cord separation.

Types of immunodeficiency

Immunodeficiency disorders may affect the adaptive or innate immune systems. The adaptive system can be divided into disorders affecting both T cell mediated immunity and antibody production or just antibody mediated immunity. A large number of specific disorders are now recognized (📖 see Further reading, p. 213, Notarangelo *et al.*). Tables 24.1–24.4 list the categories and the most important disorders.

Table 24.1 Major combined (T cell and antibody) deficiency disorders

Disorder	Molecular type and inheritance	Specific features
SCID	Many different forms	Opportunistic, bacterial and fungal infections
	Main causes (by lymphocyte pattern) are:	
	B+ NK– common γ chain (X-L) or JAK3 (AR)	ADA—sensorineural hearing loss in some cases
	B+ NK+ – IL-7rα (AR)	
	B– NK– ADA deficiency (AR)	
	B– NK+ – RAGI or II; Artemis (all AR)	
Atypical (attenuated) SCID	Potentially any SCID form with 'leaky' mutation or second 'reversion' mutation	As SCID but presents later; autoimmune features (especially intestinal and pancytopenias)
	PNP deficiency (AR)	PNP—upper motor neuron symptoms/signs
	MHC2 deficiency (AR)	
	Syndromic e.g. cartilage hair hypoplasia (AR)	
	Undefined (in molecular terms)	
SCID with Omenn syndrome	Potentially any SCID form or complete DiGeorge's	Erythroderma, lymphadenopathy, hepatosplenomegaly, enteropathy
	Most commonly RAG defects	
DiGeorge syndrome (DGS)	Most associated with 22 q.11 deletion. Also CHARGE syndrome. Spectrum from none to complete T cell deficiency	Other clinical features of DGS variably present including dysmorphism, hypoparathyroidism, cardiac abnormalities
	Complete DGS occurs in <1% cases of 22 q.11 deletion	
Hyper IgM syndrome with combined immunodeficiency	Mostly caused by defect in CD40 Ligand (X-L). Rarely, CD40 defect (AR)	Bacterial and opportunistic infections; cryptosporidiosis

(Continued)

Table 24.1 (Contd.)

Disorder	Molecular type and inheritance	Specific features
X-linked lymphoproliferative disease, XLP	Type I mutations in SH2D1A coding for protein, SAP (X-L) Type 2 mutations in X-linked inhibitor of gene for apoptosis (XIAP) (X-L)	Presentations include: • Fulminant infectious mononucleosis (with HLH) • Hypogammaglobulinaemia • Aplastic anaemia • Lymphoma
Wiskott–Aldrich syndrome	Defect in Wiskott–Aldrich protein; X-L	Bacterial and occasionally opportunistic infections, thrombocytopenia, eczema, autoimmunity
Ataxia-telangiectasia	Defect in the ataxia-telangiectasia mutated, ATM gene; AR	Bacterial infections; ataxia, ocular dyspraxia, telangiectasia (late sign); malignancy

ADA, adenosine deaminase; AR, autosomal recessive; HLH, haemophagocytic lymphohistiocytosis; IL, interleukin; JAK, Janus kinase; MHC2, major histocompatibility complex 2; NK, natural killer (cell); PNP, purine nucleoside phosphorylase; RAG, recombination activating gene; SAP, slam associated protein; SCID, severe combined immunodeficiency; X-L, X-linked.

Table 24.2 Major antibody deficiency disorders

Disorder	Molecular type and inheritance	Specific features
X-linked agammaglobulinaemia	Defect in Bruton tyrosine kinase (btk) X-linked	Bacterial infections especially capsulated; giardiasis; enteroviral infections
Common variable immunodeficiency	Identifiable genetic defect in around 10% of cases, AR	Bacterial infections, autoimmunity, inflammatory disease
Hyper IgM syndromes which are pure humoral immunodeficiencies	Various subtypes. Most common is associated with activation induced cytidine deaminase (AID) defect (AR)	Similar to agamma-globulinaemia plus lymphadenopathy and autoimmunity
Minor antibody deficiency syndromes	IgA deficiency; IgG subclass deficiency Specific polysaccharide antibody deficiency	Sinopulmonary infections; invasive pneumococcal disease; coeliac disease (with IgA deficiency)

AR, autosomal recessive; X-L, X-linked

Table 24.3 Major neutrophil disorders

Disorder	Molecular type and inheritance	Specific features
Congenital neutropenia	AD form due to mutations in neutrophil elastase gene AR—HAX-1, glucose 6 phosphatase deficiency + probable others	Bacterial/fungal infections; gingivitis; lymphadenitis
Cyclical neutropenia	AD due to mutations in neutrophil elastase gene	Cyclical malaise, mouth ulcers, fevers
Chronic granulomatous disease, CGD	Defect of photo-oxidase enzyme cluster; 67% due to glycoprotein (gp) 91 (X-L) 33% gp67,47 or 21 (AR)	Bacterial/fungal pneumonias; deep-seated abscesses; non-infective granulomas especially in intestinal and urinary tract
Leucocyte adhesion deficiency	Defect in integrin molecule leucocyte function antigen 1; AR	Delayed umbilical cord separation (>3 weeks); invasive bacterial/fungal infections

AD, autosomal dominant; AR, autosomal recessive; X-L, X-linked

Table 24.4 Disorders of the innate immune system

Disorder	Molecular type and inheritance	Specific features
Hyper IgE syndrome	70% have heterozygous defect in STAT3; AD + other genes (30%)	Pneumonias (often with pneumatocoele) dermatitis, 'cold' abscesses, bony fractures, delayed loss of primary dentition
IRAK4 deficiency	Defect in IRAK 4 defective signalling through multiple toll-like receptors; AR	Bacterial infection especially pneumococcal and staphylococcal. Impaired inflammatory response
X-linked ectodermal dysplasia with immunodeficiency	Defect in nuclear factor essential modulator	Broad range of infections especially mycobacterial, pneumococcal; skin and nail abnormalities
Defects of interferon γ/ IL-12 signalling	Defect in interferon γ/IL-12 receptors; AR	Disseminated BCG or atypical mycobacterial, invasive salmonella infections

(Continued)

Table 24.4 (Contd.)

Mannan binding lectin (MBL) deficiency	Polymorphisms in structural and/or promoter region of gene resulting in low levels	General increased infection susceptibility—mainly to bacteria including meningococcus
Alternate pathway complement deficiencies	Properdin (X-linked)	Bacterial (especially *Neisseria*) infections
	Other factors (AR)	Bacterial infections, autoimmunity
Classical pathway complement deficiencies	Early components (C1–5)	Autoimmunity, bacterial infections
	Late components (C6–9)	*Neisseria* infections

AD, autosomal dominant; AR, autosomal recessive; STAT, signal transducers and activators of transcription; X-L, X-linked.

When to suspect primary immunodeficiency

Primary immunodeficiencies are rare and consequently the diagnosis is often delayed. This can have major consequences for the child. As a rule the more severe disorders present in infancy.
- Table 24.5 lists some of the more common clinical presentations and the most likely diagnoses to consider.
- Table 24.6 covers some common clinical presentations for which immunodeficiency is unlikely to be the cause.

Table 24.5 Common presenting features of primary immunodeficiency

Clinical feature	Diagnoses to consider
Interstitial pneumonitis (usually presenting in infancy) caused by *P. jiroveci* or viruses	Combined immunodeficiencies especially SCID, XHIM, MHC2 deficiency. Complete DGS
Chronic diarrhoea, either persistent enteric viral infection(s) or immune-mediated gut inflammation	Combined immunodeficiencies, IPEX syndrome (immune dysregulation polyendocrinopathy, enteritis, X-L)
Persistent superficial candidiasis	Combined immunodeficiencies, neutrophil disorders
Invasive bacterial disease: staphylococcal or Gram negative bacillary (including bacteraemia; two or more episodes)	Neutrophil disorders, antibody deficiencies, combined immunodeficiencies (especially with Omenn syndrome)
Invasive capsulated bacterial disease (including bacteraemia; two or more episodes)	Combined immunodeficiencies, antibody deficiencies

Table 24.5 (*Contd.*)

Clinical feature	Diagnoses to consider
Two or more episodes of pneumonia	Antibody deficiency (minor or major); combined immunodeficiency; innate immunodeficiencies; neutrophil disorder (especially if staphylococcal or fungal)
Four or more episodes of otitis media sinusitis or lower respiratory infections in a year	Antibody deficiency (minor or major); combined immunodeficiency; innate immunodeficiencies
Invasive fungal disease (not *Candida* associated with indwelling catheters)	Neutrophil disorders (especially CGD if *Aspergillus* infection present); combined immunodeficiencies
Disseminated atypical mycobacterial infection or invasive non-typhoidal *Salmonella* infection (in infant over 6 months of age)	Defects of interferon γ/IL-12 signalling; combined immunodeficiency; defect in nuclear factor essential modulator
Failure to thrive in infancy (with infection susceptibility)	Combined immunodeficiencies, antibody deficiencies
Severe generalized erythroderma (with or without lymphadenopathy, hepatosplenomegaly)	SCID or complete DGS with Omenn syndrome or GVHD—maternal engraftment or transfusion acquired
Maculopapular rashes (with infection susceptibility)	SCID with GVHD
Eczema and thrombocytopenia	Wiskott–Aldrich syndrome
Granulomatous rash (confirmed on biopsy)	CVID, A-T
Other congenital abnormalities, e.g. dysmorphism, cardiac, hypoparathyroidism, colobomata, choanal atresia, microcephaly, short limbs	DGS with 22 q.11 deletion or CHARGE syndrome; SCID with other abnormalities, e.g. microcephaly may be found in SCID associated with radiosensitivity defects; cartilage hair hypoplasia
Chest and ear infections with unsteady gait	Ataxia-telangiectasia (AT)
Multiple autoimmunity phenomena: multi-lineage cytopenias; polyendocrinopathy; atypical systemic lupus erythematosus	Autoimmune lymphoproliferative syndrome; combined immunodeficiencies; CVID
	Rarer causes: Autoimmune polyendocrinopathy, candidiasis, ectodermal dystrophy (APECED); IPEX syndrome in boys; complement factor deficiencies
Lymphadenopathy and splenomegaly (otherwise unexplained)	ALPS; combined immunodeficiencies; autosomal recessive hyper IgM (AID defect)

(*Continued*)

Table 24.5 (Contd.)

Clinical feature	Diagnoses to consider
HLH	XLP (type 1 or 2); perforin deficiency, defects of cytotoxic granule release, e.g. Munc4 deficiency; defects of granule release associated with pigment abnormalities—Chediak-Higashi syndrome, Griscelli's syndrome

CVID, common variable immunodeficiency; XLP, X-linked lymphoproliferative disease.

Table 24.6 Common scenarios not usually associated with primary immunodeficiency

Clinical scenario	Comments
Recurrent upper respiratory 'viral' infections without bacterial complications	Most likely related to social/schooling circumstances
Recurrent septic spots/boils in absence of other infections	Exclude diabetes mellitus; most likely represents colonization with a troublesome strain of *Staphylococcus aureus*
Recurrent tonsillitis	Consider chronic streptococcal infection; periodic fever syndrome such as PFAPA
Recurrent central line sepsis in absence of other infections	Consider treating for *S. aureus* colonization; possible MBL deficiency
Recurrent regular fevers	Periodic fever syndrome such as PFAPA, possible cyclical neutropenia
Idiopathic thrombocytopenia without other autoimmunity, infections or lymphadenopathy/splenomegaly	Most are idiopathic; consider X-linked thrombocytopenia (variant of Wiskott-Aldrich without immunodeficiency); in boys—look for small platelet volume

MBL, mannan binding lectin.

Laboratory investigations

Laboratory testing is geared towards the broad type of immunodeficiency suspected. In most cases, testing first involves a phase of confirming the presence of a real deficiency and then progresses to more specific tests to try to establish a precise diagnosis. In some instances very specific clinical features may allow focused investigation for individual conditions, for example Wiskott-Aldrich syndrome or ataxia-telangiectasia.

Discussion with the laboratory and/or a clinical immunologist prior to testing will usually help focus investigations and maximize the information gained. The interpretation of immunological assessments can be affected by:
- Age of the child
- Gestation at birth (if an infant)
- Recent administration of blood products
- Recent/current use of immunosuppressive agents including corticosteroids.

Investigation of a child with suspected immunodeficiency but no specific features of a specific genetic disorder normally follows the following pattern (Table 24.7):
- Fist line—broad screening tests for immunodeficiency—always remember HIV!
- Second line:
  - More detailed immunological tests
  - Protein-based tests to look at expression (+ sometimes function) of a particular gene product
  - Other non-immunological tests for specific disorders.
- Third line—genetic analysis:
  - Genetic tests to identify mutations in specific genes.

Table 24.7 Tests for immunodeficiency

Type of immunodeficiency suspected	First line	Second line
Combined immunodeficiency	Blood count, immunoglobulins, IgE, lymphocyte subsets, mitogen (phytohaemagglutinin (PHA)) response	Naïve/memory T cells; other lymphoid markers (class I and II MHC, CD25, CD40L; T cell receptor families and spectratypes; TRECs; antigen specific (*Candida*, tetanus) proliferative responses
		Functional molecular assays, e.g. phosphorylation of intermediates to test kinase activity
		Specific protein assays by FACS or western blot (e.g. WASP)
		ADA and PNP enzyme levels
		FISH test for 22q.11 deletion radiation sensitivity testing (skin fibroblast culture)
		α-fetoprotein (screen for A-T)
Antibody deficiency	Blood count; immunoglobulins; antibody levels (tetanus, Pneumococcus); lymphocyte subsets	B cell markers; antibody levels post vaccination; IgG subclasses; isohaemagglutinins
		Specific protein assays e.g. Btk (for X-linked agammaglobulinaemia)

(Continued)

Table 24.7 (Contd.)

Type of immunodeficiency suspected	First line	Second line
Neutrophil disorders	Blood count; nitroblue tetrazolium (NBT) test; Expression of LFA-1 CD11/18	Sequential blood counts (cyclical neutropenia); bone marrow; flow cytometric assessment of oxidative burst; neutrophil activation (CD62L shedding); assays of migration, phagocytosis, bacterial killing
		Specific protein assays, e.g. gp91 (for X-linked CGD)
Complement disorders	MBL levels; C3 and C4; total haemolytic complement (THC or CH100); alternative pathway assay (AP50)	Individual complement component assays
HLH	Perforin assay by Granule release assay (CD107 expression); SAP and XIAP protein (for type I and II XLP)	Protein expression for other proteins involved in granule release
ALPS	FACS assay for double negative (CD4 and CD8) T cells	Apoptosis assays; Fas expression

FACS, fluorescence activated cell sorting; FISH, fluorescence in situ hybridization; gp, glycoprotein; MHC, major histocompatibility complex; TREC, T cell recombination excisim circles; WASP, Wishott Aldrich syndrome protein.

Genetic and prenatal diagnosis

Storage of DNA from a child dying of an unusual infection (either EDTA blood or skin fibroblast culture) is important as it may enable a posthumous genetic diagnosis to be made with subsequent genetic counselling.

Families should be counselled about the risk of recurrence of serious immunodeficiencies in the family. Prenatal testing is available for some serious disorders:

- Chorionic villous sampling at 12 weeks if mutation(s) identified
- Amniocentesis at 14–16 weeks—for ADA- and PNP-deficient SCID
- Fetal blood sampling 19–20 weeks—for complete SCID with absent T cells

Where families choose not to have these procedures, cord blood should be collected for testing when the infant is born and appropriate prophylactic measures initiated—see 📖 Management while investigating for suspected immunodeficiency, p. 213.

It is also important also to save cord blood as a potential source of stem cells for possible future affected babies in the family.

Management while investigating for suspected immunodeficiency

New pathologies may occur while tests are being undertaken. If a diagnosis of primary immunodeficiency is strongly suspected, consider:

- SCID:
  - Commence PCP prophylaxis with co-trimoxazole
- All blood products to be CMV negative and irradiated
- Stop breastfeeding until mother's CMV status established (if negative can restart)
  - No live vaccines to be given.
- Suspected antibody deficiency (not yet commenced on immunoglobulin therapy):
  - Commence prophylactic antibiotics to cover capsulated bacterial pathogens e.g. azithromycin
  - Avoid live oral polio vaccine.
- Suspected complement factor deficiency:
  - Commence penicillin prophylaxis against meningococcal disease.

Further reading

Cant AJ, Cale C, Gennery A, Davies EG. Immunodeficiency. In: McIntosh N, Helms P, Smyth RC, Logan S, eds. *Forfar & Arneil's Textbook of Paediatrics.* 7th edn. Edinburgh: Churchill Livingstone, 2008:1139–72.

Griffith LM, Cowan MJ, Notarangelo LD, et al. Workshop summary. Improving cellular therapy for primary immune deficiency diseases: recognition, diagnosis and management. *J Allergy Clin Immunol* 2009;**124**:1152–60.

Notarangelo LD, Fischer A, Geha RS, et al. International union of immunological societies expert committee on primary immunodeficiencies. *J Allergy Clin Immunol* 2009;**124**:1161–78.

Chapter 25

Kawasaki disease

📖 see also Chapters 32, 33, 46, 106

Introduction

Kawasaki disease is a self-limiting vasculitic syndrome that predominantly affects medium and small-sized arteries. It is the second commonest vasculitic illness of childhood (the commonest being Henoch–Schönlein purpura) and is the leading cause of childhood acquired heart disease in developed countries.

Pathogenesis

- Pronounced seasonality and clustering of Kawasaki disease cases have led to the hunt for infectious agents as a cause. However, so far no single agent has been identified.
- The aetiology of Kawasaki disease remains unknown but it is currently felt that one or more widely distributed infectious agents evoke an abnormal immunological response in genetically susceptible individuals, leading to the characteristic clinical presentation of the disease.

Epidemiology

- Kawasaki disease has a worldwide distribution with a male preponderance, an ethnic bias towards oriental children, some seasonality, and occasional epidemics.
- The reported incidence of Kawasaki disease is rising worldwide, including the UK. The current reported incidence in the UK is 8.1/100 000 children <5 years old. This may reflect a truly rising incidence or increased clinician awareness.

Clinical presentation

- The principal clinical features of Kawasaki disease are:
  - Fever persisting for ≥5 days
  - Peripheral extremity changes (reddening of the palms and soles, indurative oedema and subsequent desquamation)
  - Polymorphous exanthema
  - Bilateral conjunctival injection/congestion

- Lips and oral cavity changes (reddening/cracking of lips, strawberry tongue, oral and pharyngeal injection)
- Acute non-purulent cervical lymphadenopathy.
- For the diagnosis of Kawasaki disease to be formally established five of the above six clinical features should be present.
- Children with fewer than five of the six principal features can be diagnosed with Kawasaki disease when coronary aneurysm or dilatation is recognized by two-dimensional echocardiography or coronary angiography.
- The cardiovascular features are the most important manifestations of the condition with widespread vasculitis affecting predominantly medium size muscular arteries, especially the coronary arteries. Coronary artery involvement occurs in 15–25% of untreated cases. Additional cardiac features include pericardial effusion, electrocardiographic abnormalities, pericarditis, myocarditis, valvular incompetence, cardiac failure, and myocardial infarction.
- Irritability is an important sign, which is virtually universally present although not included in the diagnostic criteria.
- Another clinical sign that maybe relatively specific to Kawasaki disease is the development of erythema and induration at sites of BCG inoculations. The mechanism of this sign is thought to be cross-reactivity of T cells in Kawasaki disease patients between specific epitopes of mycobacterial and human heat shock proteins.
- An important point is that the principal symptoms and signs may present sequentially such that the full set of criteria may not be present at any one time. Awareness of other non-principal signs (such as BCG scar reactivation) may improve the diagnostic pick-up rate of Kawasaki disease.
- Other clinical features include: arthritis, aseptic meningitis, pneumonitis, uveitis, gastroenteritis, meatitis and dysuria, and otitis.
- Infants may have few classic signs of Kawasaki disease and can present with persistent fever, signs of inflammation, and irritability—a difficult diagnosis to make. Infants also respond less well to IVIG.
- Relatively uncommon abnormalities include hydrops of the gallbladder, gastrointestinal ischaemia, jaundice, petechial rash, febrile convulsions, and encephalopathy or ataxia, macrophage activation syndrome, and SIADH.

Differential diagnosis

Conditions that can cause similar symptoms to Kawasaki disease and must be considered in the differential diagnosis include:
- Scarlet fever
- Rheumatic fever
- Streptococcal or staphylococcal toxic shock syndrome
- Staphylococcal scalded skin syndrome
- Systemic-onset JIA
- Infantile polyarteritis nodosa
- Systemic lupus erythematosus

- Infections with adenovirus, enterovirus. EBV, CMV, parvovirus, influenza virus
- *Mycoplasma pneumoniae* infection
- Measles
- Leptospirosis
- Rickettsial infection
- Adverse drug reaction
- Mercury toxicity (acrodynia).

Investigations

In cases of suspected Kawasaki disease the following investigations should be considered:

- Full blood count (FBC) and blood film
- ESR
- CRP
- Blood cultures
- Antistreptolysin O titre (ASOT) and anti-DNase B
- Nose and throat swab—bacterial and viral, and stool sample for culture (superantigen toxin typing if *Staphylococcus aureus* and/or β-haemolytic streptococci detected). Measles is best tested for with a saliva swab
- Renal and liver function tests
- Coagulation screen
- Autoantibody profile (ANA, extractable nuclear antigen (ENA), rheumatoid factor, antineutrophilic cytoplasmic antibody (ANCA))
- Serology (IgG and IgM) for *M. pneumoniae*, enterovirus, adenovirus, measles, parvovirus, EBV, CMV
- Urine M, C, and S
- Dip test of urine for blood and protein
- Consider serology for Rickettsiae and leptospirosis if history is suggestive
- Consider chest X-ray
- ECG
- Two-dimensional echocardiography to identify coronary artery involvement acutely and monitoring changes long term
- Coronary arteriography has an important role for delineating detailed anatomical injury, particularly for children with giant coronary artery aneurysms (greater than 8mm), where stenoses adjacent to the inlet/outlet of the aneurysms are a concern. Note that the procedure may need to be delayed until at least 6 months after disease onset since there could be a risk of myocardial infarction if performed in children with ongoing severe coronary artery inflammation.

Management and treatment

The treatment of Kawasaki disease comprises:

- IVIG at a dose of 2g/kg as a single infusion over 12 hours (consider splitting the dose over 2–4 days in infants with cardiac failure).

- IVIG should be started early, preferably within the first 7–10 days of the illness. However, clinicians should not hesitate to give IVIG to patients who present after 10 days if there are signs of persisting inflammation.
- Aspirin 30–50mg/kg/day in four divided doses. The dose of aspirin can be reduced to 2–5mg/kg/day when the fever settles and the child improves (disease defervescence). Aspirin at anti-platelet doses is continued for a minimum of 6 weeks.
- If the symptoms persist within 48 hours or disease recrudescence within 2 weeks a second dose of IVIG at 2g/kg over 12 hours should be considered.
- However, IVIG resistance occurs in up to 10–20% of cases.
- When a patient fails to respond to a second dose of IVIG, consider IV pulsed methylprednisolone at 15–30mg/kg daily for 3 days to be followed by oral prednisolone 2mg/kg/day once daily, weaning over 6 weeks. Some clinicians are increasingly using corticosteroids after disease recrudescence following one dose of IVIG based on the results of a recent study. This remains an area of controversy, but seems rational since this is associated in most cases with rapid resolution of inflammation.
- In refractory cases infliximab, a human chimeric anti-TNFα monoclonal antibody, given IV at a single dose of 6mg/kg has been reported to be effective, and is increasingly used for IVIG-resistant cases. Considering that rapid and effective interruption of inflammation is a primary target of Kawasaki disease therapy, anti-TNFα blockade may be a logical step following one failed dose of IVIG, particularly in very active disease with evidence of early coronary artery dilatation.
- Echocardiography should be repeated at 2 weeks and 6 weeks from initiation of treatment (refer to paediatric cardiology).
- If the repeat echocardiogram shows no coronary artery aneurysms (CAA) at 6 weeks, aspirin can be discontinued and lifelong follow-up at least every 2 years should be considered.
- In cases of confirmed CAA <8mm with no stenoses present, aspirin should be continued until aneurysms resolve.
- If CAA >8mm and/or stenoses is present, aspirin at a dose of 2–5mg/kg/day should be continued, probably lifelong. The combination of aspirin and warfarin therapy in patients with giant aneurysms has been shown to decrease the risk of myocardial infarction.
- In patients who develop CAA, echocardiography and ECG should be repeated at 6-monthly intervals and an exercise stress test considered.
- Other specific interventions such as PET, addition of calcium channel blocker therapy, and coronary angioplasty should be organized at the discretion of the paediatric cardiologist.

Fig. 25.1 summarizes the guidelines for management of Kawasaki disease.

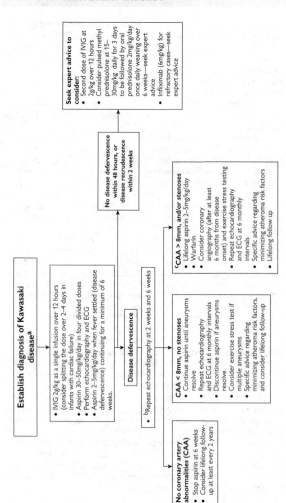

Fig. 25.1 Guideline for the management of Kawasaki's disease.

[a]Treatment can be commenced before full 5 days of fever if sepsis excluded; treatment should also be given if the presentation is >10 days from fever onset.

[b]Refer to paediatric cardiologist.

[c]Other specific interventions such as PET, addition of calcium channel blocker therapy, and coronary angioplasty at discretion of paediatric cardiologist.

Outcome

- Treatment with IVIG and aspirin reduces CAA from 25% for untreated cases to 4–9%.
- IVIG resistance occurs in up to 10–20%, and is associated with higher risk of CAA.
- The overall outlook of children with Kawasaki disease is good, with the acute mortality rate due to myocardial infarction having been reduced to <1%, in part due to the alertness of clinicians to the diagnosis and prompt treatment.
- Nonetheless the disease may contribute to the burden of adult cardiovascular disease and cause premature atherosclerosis, an area of active ongoing research.

Future research

- Further advance our understanding of the environmental triggers and host responses resulting in Kawasaki disease.
- Genetic studies of Kawasaki disease so far suggest a polygenic contribution, and ongoing international collaborative studies will hopefully provide a greater understanding of the genetic factors contributing to the pathogenesis (e.g. inositol 1, 4, 5-trisphosphate 3-kinase C (ITPKC), MBL among others).
- Peripheral blood biomarkers of vascular injury to allow reliable non-invasive monitoring of disease activity and guide therapeutic decisions.
- Optimize current treatment protocols for IVIG-resistant Kawasaki disease.
- Investigate the longer-term adult cardiovascular morbidity in children with Kawasaki disease with and without CAA.

Further reading

Biezeveld MH, Kuipers IM, Geissler J, et al. Association of mannose-binding lectin genotype with cardiovascular abnormalities in Kawasaki disease. Lancet 2003;**361**:1268–70.

Brogan PA, Bose A, Burgner D, et al. Kawasaki disease: an evidence based approach to diagnosis, treatment, and proposals for future research. Arch Dis Child 2002;**86**:286–90.

Burns JC, Mason WH, Hauger SB, et al. Infliximab treatment for refractory Kawasaki syndrome. J Pediatr 2005;**146**:662–7.

Inoue Y, Okada Y, Shinohara M, et al. A multicenter prospective randomized trial of corticosteroids in primary therapy for Kawasaki disease: clinical course and coronary artery outcome. J Pediatr 2006;**149**:336–41.

Newburger JW, Sleeper LA, McCrindle BW, et al. Randomized trial of pulsed corticosteroid therapy for primary treatment of Kawasaki disease. N Engl J Med 2007;**356**:663–75.

Newburger JW, Takahashi M, Gerber MA, et al. Diagnosis, treatment, and long-term management of Kawasaki disease: a statement for health professionals from the Committee on Rheumatic Fever, Endocarditis, and Kawasaki Disease, Council on Cardiovascular Disease in the Young, American Heart Association. Pediatrics 2004;**114**:1708–33.

Onouchi Y, Gunji T, Burns JC, et al. ITPKC functional polymorphism associated with Kawasaki disease susceptibility and formation of coronary artery aneurysms. Nat Genet 2008;**40**:35–42.

Sugahara Y, Ishii M, Muta H, Iemura M, Matsuishi T, Kato H. Warfarin therapy for giant aneurysm prevents myocardial infarction in Kawasaki disease. Pediatr Cardiol 2008;**29**:398–401.

Chapter 26

Laboratory diagnosis of infection

Introduction

The purpose of laboratory diagnosis of infection is to assist the clinician in determining whether or not a patient has a significant infection. Even when all stages of laboratory testing are conducted optimally, few if any tests are 100% accurate. Test accuracy depends partly on the inherent properties of the test itself, but it is also influenced by variables such as sample volume and quality. This is often a problem in paediatrics. It is important that the requester understands the limitations of the tests that he or she orders, so that only appropriate tests are requested, good quality samples reach the laboratory, and that the results are interpreted appropriately.

Test accuracy (Fig. 26.1) is ascertained by a comparison of measurements obtained with that test with those obtained by a reference standard. A reference (or 'gold') standard is a measure that confirms or refutes the presence or absence of the condition being tested for beyond reasonable doubt.

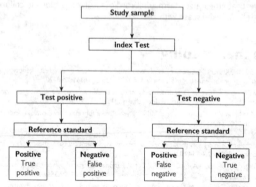

Fig. 26.1 Test accuracy.

Test accuracy can be expressed as sensitivity, specificity, and positive predictive value (PPV) and negative predictive value (NPV).
• Sensitivity is a measure of the ability of a test to identify as positive those individuals who have the condition being tested for.
• Specificity is a measure of the ability of the test to correctly identify those patients who do not have the condition.
• PPV is the probability that an individual with a positive test result has the condition.
• NPV is the probability that an individual with a negative result does not have the condition.

Calculation of test accuracy (Table 26.1)

Table 26.1 Equations for measures of test accuracy

	Condition present	**Condition not present**
Positive test	True positive (a)	False positive (b)
Negative test	False negative (c)	True negative (d)

Sensitivity = a/(a+c)

Specificity = d/(b+d)

Positive predictive value = a/(a+b)

Negative predictive value = d/(c+d)

• Sensitivity and specificity are constant measures of a test's performance.
• PPV and NPV are influenced by the prevalence of the condition in the population being tested. This is important, because when testing a population with a low disease prevalence, even a test with high specificity may only have a low PPV.

A test that is 100% sensitive and 99% specific when used on a population with a condition prevalence of only 1%, half of all positive results will be false positives, giving a PPV of only 50%. For example, a positive rapid screen for respiratory virus infection in the summer (when prevalence is low) would be more likely to be a false positive, whereas a positive rapid screen during the winter is almost certainly a true positive.

Stages in laboratory testing

Proper use of laboratory tests to diagnose and manage patients requires consideration of all stages of the testing process, from test requesting to results interpretation.

Key steps
1. Requesting of appropriate tests.
2. Collection of appropriate and good-quality samples at the appropriate time.
3. Appropriate storage and delivery of samples to the laboratory.

4. Reliable laboratory testing using techniques with an acceptable degree of accuracy.
5. Accurate and timely reporting, with appropriate interpretation of the results.

Requesting of appropriate tests

Any laboratory test requested must have a measurable benefit.

- Tests should only be requested where there is a reasonable likelihood of the patient having the disease, or where it is important to exclude a disease.
- Over-investigating patients is wasteful of time and resources.
- Indiscriminate use of tests for rare infections may lead to over diagnosis, and the wrong treatment because the PPV of the test in such a population may be low (📖 see Calculation of test accuracy, p. 221). Some children with a condition causing a current marked inflammatory activation may have false-positive anamnestic secondary immunological response leading to false acute positive serology to actual past infections.
- Tests should only be requested where the results will be available within a clinically useful timeframe. All tests should be requested with legible information on a request form. The more detail that is provided, e.g. travel history, immunocompromise, clinical signs, the more helpful the microbiological testing will be. If you want to discuss the child— ring the lab!

Examples of tests that are not usually necessary:

- Urine culture in children aged ≥3 years with uncomplicated UTI (empirical treatment is appropriate in most such circumstances)
- Urine culture in children aged ≥3 years who have leucocyte esterase and are nitrite negative on dipstick testing (they are unlikely to have a UTI)
- Skin swabs from children with uncomplicated impetigo
- Nasopharyngeal swabs for bacterial culture (usually detects only commensal flora)
- Blood cultures from well children with low-grade fever.

Sample collection

Samples of blood for serological or molecular biological investigations require no special measures, other than to ensure that sufficient sample is obtained to allow the tests requested to be undertaken.

For most other sample types, care must be taken to ensure the best possible chance of detecting pathogenic microorganisms, and without contaminating the sample with non-pathogenic microorganisms.

- Samples should be collected from sites where the infection is likely to be present.
- Samples should be timed optimally.
  - In tests that detect the organism this will be during the acute phase of the illness when microbial numbers are likely to be highest.
  - Samples for bacterial culture should ideally be taken before commencing antibiotics.

- Analyses for parasites should be undertaken at the time of day when the parasite load is likely to be highest.
- For serological assays, time must be given for the patient to mount an immune response.
- An adequate quantity of material for complete examination must be obtained. Small sample volumes may compromise sensitivity: it may be preferable to collect a second sample, rather than undertake multiple investigations on a single sample.
- Correct sampling technique must also be followed to give the best possible chance of detecting microorganisms of interest, whilst avoiding contamination.
  - When sampling dry sites moisten the swab first with sterile water or saline.
  - Take care to minimize contact with adjacent anatomical areas during swabbing.
  - Careful collection of samples such as blood cultures and urines to avoid contamination—use closed sample collection techniques, e.g. not dripping blood from a needle!

Specimen handling and transport to the laboratory

Safety is imperative:
- Samples should be contained within leak-proof containers and then sealed in a specimen transport envelope.
- Samples being transported outside the hospital require additional packaging.
- High-risk samples must be clearly identified as biohazards.

Samples must be delivered to the laboratory promptly to avoid deterioration. This is specially important for tests that depend on the presence of viable microorganisms, to avoid:
- Loss of viability of the microorganisms of interest
- Overgrowth of non-pathogenic microorganisms in the sample.

Samples that cannot be delivered immediately to the laboratory must be stored appropriately (usually in a refrigerator). Use of transport media can also help to maintain sample quality.

Laboratory processing

It is important that testing is undertaken in an appropriately accredited laboratory that participates in internal and external quality assurance. Although most microbiology testing is undertaken in the laboratory, there are some tests that can be undertaken at the point of care. Such testing must be overseen by the laboratory, to provide assurance of quality and safety. There are three broad categories of laboratory tests used to assist in the diagnosis of infection:
- Tests that involve direct detection of pathogenic microorganisms or their components in clinical samples, e.g. microscopy, culture, antigen detection and molecular biology
- Tests that demonstrate a specific immune response to a specific pathogen: usually antibody detection
- Tests that provide non-specific evidence of an infective (or inflammatory) process.

Laboratory diagnostic techniques

Microscopy

Microscopy may be used to give a rapid preliminary or definitive assessment of the cause of infection. It is most useful for examination of specimens that are normally sterile (where the presence of any microorganisms is abnormal), where pathogenic microorganisms have distinctive morphology, or where a stain that is specific to the target microorganisms is used. There are various different microscopic techniques, including:

- Light microscopy of unstained or stained preparations
- Fluorescence microscopy
- Electron microscopy

Light microscopy

Examination of unstained preparations (wet mounts) can detect specific types of microorganism, especially parasites, as well as different types of cells that may be important in evaluating infection, e.g. white and red blood cells, bacteria, squamous epithelial cells.

Many stains can be used to detect microorganisms in clinical material. The most important is the Gram stain. By observing the morphological appearance and Gram-staining reaction of bacteria (Table 26.2), their likely identity can be narrowed down to help provisionally identify the cause of infection and select appropriate antibiotic therapy. The Gram stain is quick and easy to perform:

1. Crystal violet, followed by iodine (which acts as a mordant), is applied to the heat-fixed slide and binds to the bacterial cell wall.
2. Acetone is then added as a decolourizer, followed by safranin as a counterstain. Gram-positive bacteria, which have a much thicker cell wall, retain the crystal violet stain and appear violet.
3. Gram-negative bacteria are decolourized by acetone and take up safranin to appear pink.

Table 26.2 Morphological and Gram-stain reactions of medically important bacteria

	Gram positive	Gram negative
Cocci	Streptococcus	Neisseria
	Staphylococcus	
	Enterococcus	
Bacilli	Listeria	Escherichia coli
	Corynebacterium	Klebsiella
	Bacillus	Enterobacter
	Clostridium	Salmonella
		Pseudomonas
		Haemophilus

The Ziehl–Neelsen (ZN) stain is another important stain in medical microbiology. Heat is used to drive stain (fuchsin) into the waxy cell wall of mycobacteria, which then resists decolorization with acid and alcohol (hence mycobacteria are described as alcohol and acid-fast bacteria). However, both the staining technique itself and the examination of stained preparations are relatively labour-intensive, and the ZN stain has been largely superseded as a screening test by the auramine stain (📖 see Fluorescence microscopy).

Fluorescence microscopy

Here, a fluorescent dye or fluorescent-labelled antibody targeting specific microorganisms is applied to a smear of the sample on a slide. The fluorescent reagent binds to the corresponding microorganisms in the clinical material and can be detected by fluorescent microscopy. Common examples of fluorescence tests are:

- Auramine stain for mycobacteria uses a fluorescent dye with an affinity for the waxy cell wall
- Fluorescent-labelled antirespiratory virus antibodies used to examine NPAs.

Electron microscopy (EM)

Viruses are too small to be visible using light microscopy. EM is still occasionally used to examine for viruses, especially in faeces.

Table 26.3 summarizes the value of microscopy in the investigation of infections.

Table 26.3 Advantages and disadvantages of microscopy for diagnosis of infectious diseases

Advantages	Disadvantages
Rapid	Poor sensitivity: microorganisms have to be present in large numbers to be detectable
Additional information, e.g. pus cells, may be obtainable	Gives limited information on the identity of the organisms seen
Inexpensive	May not be able to distinguish between pathogenic and non-pathogenic microorganisms

Culture

Culture is the mainstay of laboratory diagnosis of bacterial and fungal infections. Culture readily detects a wide range of different pathogens, and provides important additional phenotypic information, including a full range of antimicrobial susceptibilities, that is not readily obtainable with any other diagnostic technique.

Samples are inoculated onto culture media and then incubated (Fig. 26.2). Solid culture media are most widely used: most conventional bacteria will grow within 1–2 days. Addition of an initial enrichment culture in broth can enhance the detection rate of microorganisms present in small numbers. Mycobacteria are much slower growing than conventional bacteria and may take several weeks to grow.

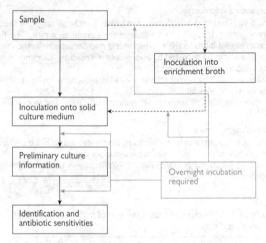

Fig. 26.2 Outline of bacterial and fungal culture.

Once a microorganism has grown, further tests (usually requiring further incubation) are required to determine its identity and antimicrobial susceptibilities.

Different microorganisms also require different cultural conditions. There are many different culture media, some of which are designed to detect particular pathogens. It is therefore important that requests for culture include sufficient clinical information for the laboratory to determine the most important culture methods.

Table 26.4 summarizes the value of culture in the investigation of infections.

Table 26.4 Advantages and disadvantages of culture for diagnosis of infectious diseases

Advantages	Disadvantages
Versatile—a large number of microorganisms can be readily detected and a wide range of additional phenotypic information is readily available	Variable sensitivity
Excellent specificity (usually regarded as the gold standard test)	Dependent on the target microorganisms remaining viable
Relatively inexpensive	May be difficult to distinguish between pathogenic and non-pathogenic microorganisms
	Takes at least 1 day (and usually longer) to obtain a definitive result

Nucleic acid amplification techniques

These are techniques such as the PCR, which use primers to anneal to target-specific sequences of the microbial genome, followed by enzymatic amplification of the target sequence, and detection of the amplification product. The range of pathogens detectable using these techniques is growing, but other than for a few pathogens they have still to establish themselves as diagnostic techniques. They are slowly replacing viral cell culture.

Table 26.5 summarizes the value of nucleic acid amplification techniques in the investigation of infections.

Table 26.5 Advantages and disadvantages of nucleic acid amplification techniques for diagnosis of infectious diseases

Advantages	Disadvantages
Potentially rapid results turnaround time (especially with modern real-time assays)	Very expensive
Potentially highly sensitive and specific	Requires expensive hardware
Not dependent on viable organisms	Limited number of organisms can be detected
	Provides limited or no additional information about the microorganisms tested

Immunological techniques

Most of these techniques detect either microbial antigens in clinical material or, more commonly, antibodies produced in response to infection. There are many different techniques, and the commonest is enzyme immunoassay (Fig. 26.3). Antibody assays can detect total antibody or specific immunoglobulin classes, usually IgG (a marker of infection at some time) and IgM (produced in response to acute infection).

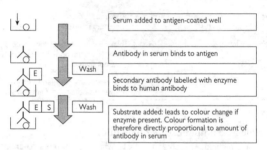

Fig. 26.3 Basic steps in enzyme immunoassay for detection of antimicrobial antibodies in serum.

A recent advance in immunological testing is the enzyme-linked immunosorbent spots (ELISPOT) test. This test detects antibody-producing T cells specific for *Mycobacterium tuberculosis* antigens.

Table 26.6 summarizes the value of immunological techniques in the investigation of infections.

Table 26.6 Advantages and disadvantages of immunological techniques for diagnosis of infectious diseases

Advantages	Disadvantages
Inexpensive	Variable accuracy
Technically straightforward	Antibody may not be present (e.g. too early in infection; if patient immunocompromised or had large proportion of blood volume replaced)
Rapid results turnaround time	Limited number of infections can be diagnosed
Not dependent on viable organisms	Provides limited or no additional information about the microorganisms tested

Tests that provide non-specific evidence of infection

Various biochemical tests may be helpful in the initial evaluation and monitoring of the patient with suspected infection.

- CRP is the most widely used acute phase reactant. However, concentrations change relatively slowly and are age-dependent.
- Pro-calcitonin (PCT) may be a better marker of sepsis. Concentrations change faster that CRP, but the sensitivity and specificity are still relatively low for prediction of infection.

Interpretation of results

Any laboratory test result must be interpreted in the context of the patient's clinical condition and the accuracy of the test. Additional interpretation is required of microbiological culture results. Relatively few microorganisms are unequivocal pathogens and the likely significance of positive cultures must be interpreted in the light of the clinical picture. Factors to consider are:

- Whether the microorganism is isolated in abundance
- Whether it is isolated in pure culture
- Whether it is isolated from deep tissues or sites that are normally sterile
- Whether it is isolated on more than one occasion
- Whether it is a microorganism that is a normal commensal
- Whether there is clinical or laboratory evidence of local inflammation
- Whether the presence of the microorganism fits with clinical picture.

Future research

- Accuracy and cost-effectiveness of newer diagnostic techniques, such as nucleic acid amplification techniques.
- Increasingly multiplex PCR techniques are being used on clinical specimens, with the potential of detecting up to 20 different pathogens. The importance of dual or triple infections and the differentiation between colonization and invasive disease requires considerable further study.
- Development and evaluation of rapid diagnostic tests for infectious diseases.

Further reading

Engelkirk PG, Duben Engel-Kirk JL. *Laboratory Diagnosis of Infectious Diseases: Essentials of Diagnostic Microbiology*. Baltimore: Wolters Kluwer Health, 2008.
Jensen HB, Baltimore RS, eds. *Pediatric Infectious Diseases*. 2nd edn. Philadelphia: WB Saunders, 2002.

Chapter 27

Lower respiratory tract infection

📖 see also Chapters 46, 58, 69, 70, 80, 81, 86, 90, 94, 95, 96, 99, 105, 106, 113

Epidemiology

- The respiratory tract is the commonest site of childhood infections and acute respiratory infections make up 50% of all illness in children aged <5 years.
- Most involve only the upper respiratory tract but about 5% will involve the larynx and lower respiratory tract.
- Lower respiratory tract infection (LRTI) is commonest in the first year of life.
- During the first decade, LRTIs occur more commonly in boys.
- Hospitalization rates vary considerably but it is estimated that 1 in 20 will be hospitalized due to respiratory infection in the first 4 years of life.
- LRTIs show marked and unexplained seasonal variation, being commonest in the coldest months. This is particularly striking for the annual winter–spring epidemics of bronchiolitis and pneumonia due to RSV in infants.

Pathogenesis

- LRTIs develop by two routes; direct respiratory droplet transmission or indirect spread from the blood stream.
- Most organisms (respiratory viruses, *Mycoplasma pneumoniae*, *Bordetella pertussis*, and *Chlamydia trachomatis*) produce infection by initial involvement of airway epithelium with progression into parenchyma. The infection typically starts in the upper respiratory tract and then spreads to the lower.
- Bacteria and certain viruses—EBV, CMV, and VZV spread from the blood stream into the parenchyma and airways.
- The development and localization of disease in the lower respiratory tract depends on a complex interaction between the organism, the host, and environmental factors (Table 27.1).
- While respiratory viral infections can involve more than one part of the respiratory tract, inflammation usually predominates at a single site.
- Certain organisms have affinities for particular parts of the respiratory tract, e.g. RSV for peripheral airways, for reasons that are not well understood.

Table 27.1 Risk factors for lower respiratory tract infections in children

Host factors	Environmental factors
Age	Passive and active smoking
Sex	Exposure to infection via:
Low birth weight	• Siblings
	• Domestic overcrowding
Neonatal lung injury	• Daycare
Congenital malformation	
Bottle-feeding	Low socioeconomic status
Obesity	Air pollution

Organisms

- The spectrum of organisms that cause LRTIs is wide (Table 27.2) and varies with age.
- In the newborn, pneumonia is usually due to organisms acquired from the mother's genital tract before or during delivery, e.g. GBS, Gram-negative bacteria, *Listeria monocytogenes*, *C. trachomatis*, *Mycoplasma hominis*, and *Ureaplasma urealyticum*, CMV and HSV.
- After the first month of life, the vast majority of respiratory infections are due to viruses (RSV, parainfluenza, influenza, human metapneumovirus, coronavirus, bocavirus, adenovirus, rhinovirus), *C. pneumoniae*, *M. pneumoniae*, and *Streptococcus pneumoniae*. *Mycoplasma* infection rarely occurs <3 months of age and is most frequent in schoolchildren.
- *S. pneumoniae* is the most common bacterial cause of childhood pneumonia. Other causes of bacterial pneumonia, e.g. *Staphylococcus aureus*, are uncommon in normal children.
- Bacterial superinfection during respiratory viral or mycoplasmal infections is rare in normal children. There are some well-recognized associations between viruses and secondary bacterial infection, (e.g. influenza and staphylococcal pneumonia) which if they occur, are often serious, e.g. with measles and adenovirus.
- Usually the specific aetiology of a LRTI cannot be determined. Developments in medical microbial diagnostic technology such as nucleic acid technology and PCR, are increasing the proportion of respiratory infections that can be identified definitively. It may be difficult to tell if an organism detected from an URT specimen is being carried or is the cause of the LRTI. PCR is now detecting dual or triple infections, increasing the complexity of the diagnosis.

Table 27.2 Relative frequency of organisms causing community-acquired pneumonia in otherwise healthy children

Most frequent	Occasional	Rare
Neonates (<1 month)		
GBS	*Haemophilus influenzae*	*Mycobacterium* spp.
Escherichia coli	S. pneumoniae	*Chlamydia* spp.
Respiratory viruses	GAS	*Listeria monocytogenes*
Enteroviruses	S. aureus	VZV
		CMV
		HSV
Young infants (1–3 months)		
Febrile		
Respiratory viruses	GBS	VZV
Enteroviruses	GAS	CMV
S. pneumoniae	H. influenzae	Mycobacteria
	B. pertussis	Gram-negative enteric
	CMV	bacilli
	U. urealyticum	
Afebrile		
Chlamydia	CMV	
Mycobacteria	U. urealyticum	
Infants and young children (3 months–5 years)		
S. pneumoniae	B. pertussis	*Moraxella catarrhalis*
Respiratory viruses	S. aureus	
	GAS	
	H. influenzae	
	Mycoplasma spp.	
	Mycobacteria	
Older children (>5 years) and adolescents		
M. pneumoniae	C. pneumoniae	S. aureus
S. pneumoniae	Mycobacteria	
Respiratory viruses		

Clinical presentation

- The clinical features of LRTIs can include cough with tachypnoea, chest indrawing, wheeze, and stridor. There are well-defined clinical syndromes (Table 27.3) and these clinical patterns are helpful in narrowing the range of likely infectious agents.
- In infants, clinical features of pneumonia are often non-specific and include fever (>38.5°C), refusal to feed and vomiting.
- The absence of tachypnoea makes pneumonia very unlikely.
- The respiratory rate is best measured by observing the chest wall over 1 minute.
- Cut-offs for diagnosing tachypnoea are: >60/min in infants <2 months; >50/min for 2–12 months old; and >40/min for >12 months.
- Bronchial breathing and reduced breath sounds are specific but insensitive indicators of pneumonia, particularly in infants where auscultation is relatively unreliable.

Table 27.3 LRTI syndromes (infection at or below the larynx) and their clinical features

Syndrome	Presenting symptoms and signs
Croup	Hoarseness, cough, inspiratory stridor with laryngeal obstruction
Tracheobronchitis	Cough and ronchi; no laryngeal obstruction or wheezing
Bronchiolitis	Expiratory wheezing with or without tachypnoea, air trapping and indrawing, end expiratory crepitations
Pneumonia	Crackles or evidence of pulmonary consolidation on physical examination or chest X-ray. Bronchial breathing

Severity assessment

- For children with pneumonia, the severity can range from mild to life threatening (Table 27.4).

Indications for admission to hospital

- Hypoxaemia is the key indication for hospital admission.

Indicators for admission to hospital in infants
- Oxygen saturation (SaO$_2$) <92%, cyanosis
- Respiratory rate >70 beats/min
- Difficulty in breathing
- Intermittent apnoea, grunting
- Not feeding
- Family not able to provide appropriate observation or supervision.

Indicators for admission to hospital in older children
- SaO_2 <92%, cyanosis
- Respiratory rate >50 breaths/min
- Difficulty in breathing
- Grunting
- Signs of dehydration
- Family not able to provide appropriate observation or supervision.

Indications for transfer to intensive care unit

Transfer to intensive care should be considered if the following features are present:
- The patient is failing to maintain an SaO_2 of >92% in fraction of inspired oxygen (FiO_2) of >60%
- The patient is shocked
- There is a rising respiratory rate and rising pulse rate with clinical evidence of severe respiratory distress and exhaustion, with or without a raised arterial carbon dioxide tension ($PaCO_2$)
- There is recurrent apnoea or slow irregular breathing.

Table 27.4 Severity assessment

Syndrome	Mild	Severe
Infants	Temperature <38.5°C	Temperature >38.5°C
	RR <60 breaths/min	RR >60 breaths/min
	Mild recession	Moderate to severe recession
	Taking full feeds	Nasal flaring
		Cyanosis
		Intermittent apnoea
		Grunting respiration
		Not feeding
Older children	Temperature <38.5°C	Temperature >38.5°C
	RR <50 breaths/min	RR >50 breaths/min
	Mild breathlessness	Severe difficulty in breathing
	No vomiting	Nasal flaring
		Cyanosis
		Grunting respiration
		Signs of dehydration

RR, respiratory rate.

Diagnosis

- The gold standard for microbial diagnosis of pneumonia is a needle aspiration obtained from the lower respiratory tract or BAL.
- In clinical practice, chest radiographs provide a pragmatic alternative. They are indicated in children with fever and clinical signs of respiratory distress.
- In children with immunodeficiency or cardiorespiratory disease, the signs of LRTI may be less obvious and a high index of suspicion is required.
- Chest X-ray changes in pneumonia do not distinguish between bacterial and non-bacterial causes.
- Chest X-ray findings may also be absent in early bacterial pneumonia. Lobar or segmental consolidation is characteristic of bacterial pneumonia but bronchopneumonia and interstitial infiltrates can occur in bacterial pneumonia, as can alveolar infiltrates in viral pneumonia. An exception is a large pleural effusion where a bacterial origin is most likely. Tuberculosis should be considered if hilar lymphadenopathy and pleural effusions are seen.
- Nasopharyngeal aspirates provide excellent material for microbial diagnosis for organisms entering via the respiratory tracts, particularly viruses.
- Rapid, sensitive and specific immunofluorescence tests are available for many respiratory viruses, most notably RSV, parainfluenza and influenza virus.
- Newer molecular testing using PCR offers greater sensitivity and is increasingly replacing immunofluorescence and serology.
- There may be polymorphonuclear leucocytosis. C-reactive protein is often raised in bacterial infections.
- Cold agglutinins frequently occur in *M. pneumoniae* infections; especially with more severe pulmonary involvement.
- Culture of nasopharyngeal swabs is an unreliable alternative because colonisation with *S. pneumoniae* and *H. influenzae* occurs, particularly in preschool children.
- Rapid, bacterial antigen detection tests are increasingly used in clinical practice.
- In severely ill or immunocompromised child, more invasive procedures such as bronchoscopy with bronchoalveolar lavage or lung biopsy may be essential to guide therapy.

Special problems

Immunocompromised children

- The lung is the common site of serious infection in immunocompromised children.
- They are prone to infection, particularly when the absolute neutrophil count falls to <500/mm^3.

- The risk increases with both the severity and duration of neutropenia. Neutropenia for longer than 2 weeks is associated with a high incidence of nosocomial bacterial and/or fungal infections.
- Prompt, accurate diagnosis of LRTI is crucial but often difficult in ill, immunocompromised children because of lack of specificity of the clinical signs and the wide range of organisms encountered.
- Bronchoalveolar lavage provides a safe and accurate method of diagnosis and may provide a specific diagnosis in 50–70% of cases.

Treatment

- Respiratory viruses, *C. pneumoniae*, and *M. pneumoniae* cause most of the cases of LRTIs. Symptomatic *Mycoplasma* infections are uncommon in children <5 years of age.
- Treatment of RSV infection is mainly supportive. Ribavirin should only be considered in children with severe immunodeficiency.
- Antibiotics should be prescribed in pneumonia because of the difficulty of differentiating bacterial from viral infections particularly in very young or very sick children. The child's age and likely pathogen can help to determine the initial choice of antibiotic. Antibiotics are not required in infants with classical RSV bronchiolitis.
- Because of the emergence of resistant strains such as penicillin-resistant pneumococci, it is important that this choice is informed by knowledge of local microbial sensitivities.
- Less severe cases of pneumonia can be managed at home.
- Antibiotics administered orally are safe and effective for children presenting with pneumonia.
- For children <5 years of age, oral amoxicillin is the first choice antibiotic because it is effective against the majority of causative bacterial organisms. A standard course of 5 days is likely to be adequate in most cases.
- Macrolide antibiotics can be used as first choice antibiotic for those >5 years of age, when *M. pneumoniae* is more prevalent. Macrolides should be used if either *Mycoplasma* or *Chlamydia* pneumonia is suspected irrespective of the child's age.
- In severe cases requiring hospitalization, IV antibiotics should be used if the child is unable to absorb/tolerate oral antibiotics or has severe respiratory distress and clinical findings. Oral treatment should be considered as soon as there is clear clinical improvement.
- IV antibiotics used in Europe for severe pneumonia include penicillin/amoxicillin, co-amoxiclav, cefuroxime, and cefotaxime/ceftriaxone. Consider staphylococcal pneumonia in an ill child with lung abscesses and/or an empyema. Lung abscesses can also be caused acutely by Gram-negative bacteria (*Pseudomonas* and *Klebsiella*) or anaerobes if following an aspiration.
- Pleural (parapneumonic) effusions can be caused by a transudate (pleural:serum protein ratio <0.5) due to non-infectious causes (heart failure/cirrhosis/hypoproteinaemia, etc.) or an exudate (pleural:serum protein ratio >0.5) due to infective or other causes (malignancy/chylothorax/surgical/auto-immune disease/intra-abdominal pathology).

The commonest acute infectious causes of a pleural effusion are pneumococcus, *S. aureus*, *H. influenzae* type b, and GAS infection. Always consider TB, especially in a non-toxic older child.

Supportive care and hospitalization

- Most children with LRTIs are managed in the community. Supportive care and antibiotics, where indicated, will be all that is required.
- About 10% will be admitted to hospital. In young children especially, this is usually needed because of respiratory distress, severe systemic features or difficulty feeding. In these more serious cases a number of specific points should be considered as follows.

Maintain an adequate airway and ensure oxygenation

- Hypoxaemia is common. Excessive handling aggravates this and should be avoided.
- The development of non-invasive monitoring has allowed oxygen saturation to be monitored routinely. Low flow oxygen administered via nasal cannulae or head box will often be sufficient to maintain the oxygen saturation in the normal range (above 92%).
- About 1–2% of infants with severe bronchiolitis will develop respiratory failure and need mechanical ventilation.

Maintain hydration and nutrition

- Children with severe LRTIs often have difficulty with feeding. Nasogastric feeding or IV fluids may be necessary to maintain nutrition and avoid dehydration.
- Children with pneumonia and bronchiolitis can develop excessive antidiuretic hormone secretion so mild fluid restriction is usually advisable.

Clear nasal secretions and encourage sputum clearance

- Gentle clearance of nasal secretions may increase comfort and aid feeding in infants.
- There is no evidence that chest physiotherapy is helpful in children with bronchiolitis or pneumonia but it may have an important role in children with impaired sputum clearance.

Treat/drain pleural effusion

- Pleural effusion with pneumonia is most commonly caused by pneumococcal disease. In a toxic ill child consider staphylococcal pneumonia and add an antistaphylococcal agent, e.g. flucloxacillin.
- Three stages of empyema have been defined.
  - Stage 1: 'exudative'—fluid within the pleural space but no loculations present.
  - Stage 2: 'fibropurulent'—the fluid becomes loculated due to the presence of fibrin.
  - Stage 3: 'organizational'—there are multiple loculations and a thickened pleural layer.
  - Empyema has not been clearly defined, but denotes a complex para-pneumonic effusion. Always think: *could this be TB?*

- When present, it may be useful to aspirate fluid for diagnostic purposes. Therapeutic aspiration may only be necessary if breathing is compromised or if the clinical response to antibiotics is poor.
- Pre-drainage localization of the fluid and selection of the optimal drainage spot using ultrasound scan is useful. Adequate sedation and analgesia are necessary for safe and painless drainage, especially in infants and young children.
- The optimal management remains controversial, with both aggressive and conservative approaches being taken across Europe. Options include conservative management with IV antibiotics only, insertion of a percutaneous chest drain (with or without a fibrinolytic) and video-assisted thoracoscopy (VATS) or decortication in very severe disease. There have been no good large randomized controlled trials comparing length of stay, cost benefit, and long-term outcome. Empyema rates are falling in Europe following the introduction of the conjugate pneumococcal vaccine.
- Installation of urokinase has been shown to reduce length of hospital stay and is used sometimes for complicated parapneumonic effusions and empyema.
- Surgery should be considered in the presence of persisting clinical and radiological signs and symptoms. The type of surgery depends in part on the expertise available locally and the severity and stage of the empyema.
- Outcome of effusions is usually very good in children, irrespective of the treatment modality as long as a good course of appropriate antibiotics is given.

Follow-up

- For children with pneumonia, careful clinical follow-up to check that the child is better and that signs have resolved is all that is necessary in uncomplicated cases.
- Further chest X-rays do not appear necessary if the clinical resolution is occurring.
- In any child with an unusual, persistent or recurrent pneumonia an underlying disorder such as immune deficiency, cystic fibrosis, or a congenital lung disorder should be excluded.

Outcome

- In developed countries, most LRTIs will resolve satisfactorily with appropriate treatment. However, LRTIs remain an important cause of childhood death.
- Pneumonia kills more children worldwide than any other childhood illness.
- A few LRTIs, particularly with specific serotypes of adenovirus (e.g. 7) can cause lasting damage to the lung—*bronchiolitis obliterans*.
- A year after recovery from pneumonia it has been found that children still have residual lung scan defects.
- Children with past respiratory illnesses show evidence of airways obstruction and lung function deficit in later childhood and young

adults with a history of LRTI in the first 2 years of life have an increased incidence of chronic cough.
- It is not yet clear whether low lung function predisposes to or is a consequence of LRTI.

Prevention

- The prevention and improved therapy of LRTIs in early infancy may be vital for later pulmonary health.
- Social and environmental determinants of LRTIs should be avoided. Breastfeeding and the high uptake of childhood immunizations should be encouraged.
- Influenza and pneumococcal vaccination for at risk groups should be arranged.
- Hospital admissions due to pneumonia and empyema have fallen significantly in the UK since the introduction of the conjugate pneumococcal vaccine PCV-7. PCV-13 may reduce disease still further.
- Immunoprophylaxis such as with high-titre RSV immunoglobulin or monoclonal antibodies may have a role in preventing lower respiratory tract infection in high-risk infants and children in the absence of an appropriate vaccine.
- One simple measure that would have a substantial impact would be a reduction in parental smoking. Parents of children admitted with a LRTI should be advised to stop smoking.

Further reading

British Thoracic Society. Guidelines for the management of community acquired pneumonia in childhood. *Thorax* 2002;**57** Suppl 1:1–24.

Lynch JP, Zhanel GG. Streptococcus pneumoniae: epidemiology, risk factors, and strategies for prevention. *Semin Respir Crit Care Med* 2009;**30**:189–209.

Osterhaus AD. New respiratory viruses of humans. *Pediatr Infect Dis J* 2008;**27** Suppl 10:S71–4.

Rudan I, Boschi-Pinto C, Biloglav Z, Mulholland K, Campbell H. Epidemiology and etiology of childhood pneumonia. *Bull World Health Organ* 2008;**86**:408–16.

Chapter 28

Mastoiditis, quinsy, and brain abscess

📖 see also Chapters 29, 44, 48, 105, 106

Mastoiditis

- Mastoiditis is a complication of acute otitis media (AOM). The incidence is around 1 per 10 000 child-years. In AOM there is inflammation of the respiratory epithelial cells lining the air cells of the mastoid. In acute mastoiditis the bony septa between the air cells break down and pus spreads either through the eustachian tube or by perforating the tympanic membrane.
- The abscess can extend laterally producing a subperiosteal abscess leading to a fluctuant swelling behind the ear or over the mastoid process. Medial spread into the petrous bone and into the cortex leads to the suppurative complications of an intracranial abscess or venous sinus thrombosis.
- There have been only a few recent studies on the microbiology of mastoiditis. The normal pathogens that cause AOM also cause mastoiditis, especially Streptococcus pneumoniae, GAS, MSSA, and rarely anaerobes.
- The diagnosis is made clinically with fever, pain, and the ear pinna being pushed forward. CT can show destruction of the air cells and bony erosion. CT with contrast or MRI may be needed to diagnose venous sinus thrombosis.
- Treatment is usually medical if there are no complications and mastoiditis often responds to IV antibiotics, for example, co-amoxiclav or ceftriaxone. Bony erosion needs to be treated as for osteomyelitis and venous sinus thrombosis may require anticoagulation. A simple mastoidectomy usually with a drainage tube insertion is performed for children who do not respond to medical treatment or have signs of subperiosteal abscess formation. Most children have no long-term consequences unless there are intracranial suppurative complications— see below.
- The role of antibiotics in preventing mastoiditis after AOM is complex. Children often present with mastoiditis as their first clinical sign of AOM. A recent large study noted that prescribing antibiotics for AOM does reduce the risk of subsequent mastoiditis, but the number of cases of AOM that would need to be given antibiotics to prevent one case of mastoiditis was around 5000.

Peritonsillar abscess—quinsy

- Quinsy is an infection of the space between the tonsillar capsule and the fauces. Rarely, it follows acute tonsillitis or glandular fever. It is more common in adolescents and young men, especially if they smoke.
- The commonest organisms isolated are GAS and MSSA or rarely anaerobes. Lemierre's disease can present with a quinsy-like picture.
- Clinically the teenager presents with worsening pain in the throat, a hoarse voice and difficulty in eating then drinking. They can appear septic or reasonably well. The classic triad includes an inability to open the mouth fully, swelling of the tonsil, and deviation of the uvula. Extremely rarely upper airway obstruction can occur.
- Treatment is by surgical drainage of the abscess. IV antibiotics include co-amoxiclav or clindamycin. The outcome is usually very good. The role of antibiotics in the treatment of pharyngitis to prevent quinsy is very limited. Current evidence suggests that quinsy is very rare in children and many thousands of children with tonsillitis would require treatment with antibiotics to prevent one case of quinsy.

Brain abscess

This is a focal infection within the brain tissue that develops into a purulent collection with a fibrous capsule, commonly associated with surrounding cerebral oedema.

Causes

- **Contiguous spread** (sinusitis, otitis media, mastoiditis, dental and orbital infections, or meningitis): abscesses mostly solitary and superficial.
- May lead to a subdural empyema which can spread rapidly across the subdural space and cause cerebral thrombophlebitis.
- **Haematogenous spread** (skin and soft tissue infections, pulmonary infections, osteomyelitis, endocarditis, other causes of bacteraemia): abscesses mostly multiple and deep seated.
- Following **penetrating head injury or a neurosurgical procedure**.
- In 15–30% the source of infection remains obscure (**cryptogenic abscess**).

Epidemiology

Rare in childhood with a reported incidence of 4/1 000 000, usually between 4 and 7 years. Prevalence is higher in at-risk populations, such as patients with congenital heart disease and neonates, and in the context of immunosuppression, such as in transplant recipients, patients on chemotherapy or steroids, and patients with HIV infection.

Risk factors (Table 28.1)

Table 28.1 Sources of underlying risk identified for brain abscesses

Sinusitis	6–8%
Otitis media, mastoiditis	6–34%
Cyanotic congenital heart disease	30–50%
Pulmonary infections (bronchiectasis, foreign bodies, aspiration)	0.7–10%
Congenital and acquired immune deficiencies	12%
Penetrating head injury	4–13%
Complication of neurosurgical procedure	8–10%
Endocarditis	9–10%
Septicaemia	23%

Microbiology

Brain abscesses may arise from infection with bacterial, fungal, or proto-zooic pathogens (Table 28.2).

Table 28.2 Bacteria most commonly cultured from brain abscesses

Anaerobic and aerobic streptococci (*Streptococcus pyogenes*, Viridans group streptococci)	60–79%
Anaerobic Gram-negative bacilli	20–40%
Enterobacteriaceae	20–30%
S. aureus	10–15%
Mixed flora	13–30%

Mechanism of spread and host characteristics define the likely spectrum of causative pathogens and empirical antibiotic management:

- **Continuous spread:** *Streptococcus* spp. (*S. pyogenes*, *S. milleri*), *Haemophilus*, *Pseudomonas aeruginosa*, *Bacteroides*, *Peptostreptococcus*, *Fusobacteria*, *Proteus mirabilis*, other anaerobes
- **Haematogenous spread:** Streptococci, *S. aureus*, *Staphylococcus epidermidis*, *Bacteroides*, *Pseudomonas*, *Klebsiella*
- **Lower respiratory tract infection, bronchiectasis:** Streptococci, *S. aureus*, *Pseudomonas*, *Bacteroides*
- **Cyanotic congenital heart disease (CCHD):** Streptococci including viridans group streptococci, *Haemophilus*, *Peptostreptococcus*

- **Post head trauma or postoperatively:** *Staphylococcus* or *Streptococcus* species, *Clostridium*, *Enterobacter*
- **Immunocompromised host:** any of the above as well as fungi (*Candida*, *Aspergillus*, *Histoplasma*, *Cryptococcus*), *Toxoplasma*, *Nocardia*, *Klebsiella*, Mycobacteria, *Actinomyces*.

Clinical presentation

A high level of suspicion is needed since signs and symptoms of a cerebral abscess are not pathognomonic. The **classic triad of fever, headache, and neurological deficit** only presents in 15–30% of cases.

- Fever (30–85%)
- Headache (35–70%)
- Vomiting (60–80%)
- Neurological deficit (14–50%) depending on location of the lesion:
  - Motor weakness, visual field defects, ataxia (5–15%)
  - Cranial nerve palsies (10–20%)
  - Hemiparesis (20–30%)
- Altered level of consciousness (30–40%)
- Seizures: generalized tonic-clonic (GTC) and/or focal, 16–50%
- Meningism (25–35%)
- Signs of raised intracranial pressure (ICP), bulging fontanelle, increasing head circumference, papilloedema.

Investigation

History and clinical findings combined with a high level of suspicion are key to diagnosis of a cerebral abscess. Inflammatory markers will be raised in most cases.

Microbiological

- Blood cultures should be obtained prior to starting antibiotics.
- Material obtained from the lesion during neurosurgical intervention must be sent for microbiological investigations.
- Lumbar puncture commonly yields non-specific CSF findings. However, it is potentially dangerous in case of an associated mass effect, and therefore not routinely indicated in the management of confirmed cerebral abscess. It may be considered in cases where raised ICP can be ruled out and there is a strong suspicion of associated meningitis, ventriculitis, or rupture of the abscess into the ventricular system.

Imaging

- CT scan with contrast classically shows a ring-enhancing lesion reflecting the purulent collection surrounded by a well-vascularized, and therefore strongly enhancing, capsule. Changes on CT lag behind clinical signs. Early CT changes can show either a focal area of oedema or a hypodense area only. A normal CT does not exclude an abscess.
- MRI with contrast is more sensitive than a CT especially in detecting the early stages of an abscess and for diagnosis of brainstem or cerebellar (i.e. posterior fossa) lesions.
- Other (cranial ultrasound, radiolabelled leucocyte scan, etc.).

Management

Treatment of brain abscesses usually involves a combination of neurosurgical and medical approaches:

1. Address life-threatening complications

Such as septicaemia or raised intracranial pressure and stabilize the patient.

2. Neurosurgical

Most abscesses will require surgical intervention to reduce raised ICP and avoid ventriculitis, confirm the diagnosis, obtain a microbiological specimen and guide antimicrobial therapy:

- Stereotactic aspiration via burr hole
- Excision via craniotomy
- Neuroendoscopy.

Medical management under serial imaging follow-up alone might be considered in selected patients if the following applies:

- The patient is neurologically intact
- There is no raised ICP
- The pathogen is known with reasonable certainty, e.g. from sinus washouts or ear swab
- The abscess has a diameter of 2.5cm or less
- Surgical intervention is not feasible owing to location of the lesion, multiple abscess formations, an unstable patient or presence of a coagulopathy
- Duration of illness <2 weeks.

New operative and imaging techniques now make surgical intervention possible for patients who may until very recently have been considered only for conservative treatment and close liaison with a specialist neurosurgical centre for expert advice should be sought.

3. Antimicrobial

When choosing the antibiotic the presumed source of infection, suspected organism, and CNS penetration of the chosen agent need to be taken into consideration.

Empirical treatment: Broad-spectrum antibiotics until culture results available:

- Third-generation cephalosporin (such as ceftriaxone or cefotaxime) IV

Plus

- Metronidazole IV

Plus sometimes one of the following as necessary:

- Vancomycin IV—if *Staphylococcus epidermidis*/*S. aureus*/MRSA suspected, in cases associated with penetrating head injury, endocarditis, ventriculoperitoneal shunts, associated meningitis
- Ceftazidime if *Pseudomonas* suspected
- Antifungals if immunosuppressed
- Amikacin or gentamicin if neonate.

Specific treatment: Adjust antibiotic treatment to culture results once available.

Duration of treatment: Usually 4–6 weeks antibiotics is given after surgical management, and 6–8 weeks if treated conservatively, adjusted to the individual patient. The optimal time to change the patient from intravenous to oral antibiotics in children is not known, but may be guided by a fall in inflammatory markers in the context of clinical improvement.

4. Steroids

The use of steroids is controversial. Current practice discourages use of steroids unless there is a clinically significant mass effect or an impending risk of herniation.

5. Anticonvulsants

- Given the high prevalence of seizures associated with brain abscesses, patients should be started on anticonvulsants (valproic acid or carbamazepine) and continue treatment for at least 3 months to 1 year (some advise 2 years) when a trial can be made to stop medication, provided the EEG findings are normal at this point.
- It is important to be aware that in most cases, the onset of seizures will occur only after a latency period of several months (mean time of onset 3 years), and less than 50% of seizures manifest within the first 12 months.

6. Treatment of the original focus of infection

Outcome

Close follow-up including serial imaging during and following treatment is vital in order to monitor the efficacy of treatment; 3–25% of aspirated and up to 6% of excised abscesses reoccur, highlighting the importance of close clinical and radiological follow-up, generally for 12 months.

Morbidity

Brain abscesses are associated with significant morbidity and about 30% of surviving children are left with neurological deficits. Poor prognostic factors with regard to neurological outcome are:

- Low GCS scores at presentation
- Higher number/large/deep-seated abscesses present
- Larger size of the lesion
- Intraventricular rupture
- Associated meningitis
- Young age (<1 year).

Most common neurological sequelae:

- Long-term seizure disorder (10–72%)
- Persisting motor weakness/limb paresis or other focal neurological deficit
- Delayed obstructive hydrocephalus
- Impaired cognitive function or subsequent developmental and psychomotor delay, especially in infants and toddlers—close developmental long-term follow-up is imperative.

Mortality

Cerebral abscess in children is associated with a significant mortality of 6–14%, higher in cases with low GCS at presentation, patients with multiple abscesses, and those with significant comorbidities, especially the immunocompromised.

Further reading

Ciurea AV, Stoica F, Vasilescu G, Nuteanu L. Neurosurgical management of brain abscess in children. *Child Nerv Syst* 1999;**15**:309–17.

Infection in Neurosurgery Working Party of the British Society for Antimicrobial Chemotherapy. The rational use of antibiotics in the treatment of brain abscess. *Br J Neurosurg* 2000;**14**:525–30.

Lu C-H, Chang W-N, Lui C-C. Strategies for the management of brain abscess. *J Clin Neurosci* 2006;**16**:979–85.

Lumbiganon P, Chaikipinyo A. Antibiotics for brain abscesses in people with cyanotic congenital heart disease (Review). *Cochrane Database of Syst Rev* 2007;**3**:CD004469.

Saez-Llorens X. Brain abscess in children. *Sem Pediatr Infect Dis* 2003;**14**:108–14.

Meningitis

📖 see also Chapters 14, 28, 69, 70, 87, 106, 113

Introduction

- Meningitis is inflammation of the meninges, although the arachnoid and pia mater are also usually inflamed, i.e. leptomeningitis.
- Most cases are culture negative, i.e. aseptic meningitis, and are usually caused by viruses.
- Meningitis due to encapsulated bacteria has become less frequent since the introduction of highly effective conjugate vaccines against *Neisseria meningitidis*, *Streptococcus pneumoniae*, and *Haemophilus influenzae* type b in the past two decades.
- **The priority is prompt diagnosis and treatment of bacterial pathogens.**

Causative organisms

Bacterial meningitis

The predominant bacteria responsible vary depending on age:
- **Neonates (<1 month)**: GBS (45% of bacterial cases), *Escherichia coli* (20%), other Gram-negative organisms (10%), *S. pneumoniae* (6%), *Listeria monocytogenes* (5%)
- **1–3 months**: Organisms from either group
- **>3 months**: *N. meningitidis*, *S. pneumoniae*, *H. influenzae* type b (Hib).

Aseptic meningitis

- Characterized by CSF pleocytosis and raised protein, with absence of microorganisms on Gram stain and routine culture.
- Viruses are the commonest cause, most frequently enteroviruses. Other viral causes include mumps, HSV, CMV, EBV, VZV, adenoviruses, HIV, measles, rubella, influenza, parainfluenza, and rotavirus.
- Other infectious causes include:
  - Partially treated bacterial meningitis
  - Non-pyogenic bacteria, e.g. Mycobacteria, *Leptospira*, *Treponema pallidum*, *Borrelia*, *Nocardia*, *Bartonella*, and *Brucella*
  - Atypical organisms, e.g. *Chlamydia*, *Rickettsia*, and *Mycoplasma*
  - Fungi, e.g. *Candida*, *Cryptococcus*, *Histoplasma*, and *Coccidioides*
  - Protozoa and helminths, e.g. roundworms, tapeworms, flukes, amoebae, and *Toxoplasma*.

Epidemiology

Bacterial meningitis (📖 **also see Chapters 70, 87, 106**)

Neisseria meningitidis

- Peak incidence of disease occurs in children aged 6 months – 2 years, with a second smaller peak at 15–19 years.
- The incidence of meningococcal disease across Europe is 2–89 per 100 000 per year in children <1 year and 1–27 per 100 000 per year in 1–4 year olds, with high rates in the UK and Ireland; 60–90% have meningitis, with or without septicaemia.
- The majority of disease in Europe is caused by serogroup B and C organisms. The serogroup C conjugate vaccine (introduced in the UK in 1999 and subsequently across Europe) resulted in a 10-fold drop in the incidence of serogroup C disease. Serogroup B organisms now cause 85–90% of cases in the UK.
- Serogroup Y accounts for a substantial proportion of cases in North America. An ACYW–135 conjugate vaccine has been introduced in the USA for adolescents.
- Epidemics in Africa are usually associated with serogroup A, and more recently serogroups W-135 and X.

Streptococcus pneumoniae

- The peak incidence of disease is in children <2 years.
- In Europe the incidence of pneumococcal meningitis was 1–8 cases per 100 000 per year in children <5 years prior to widespread use of the 7–valent pneumococcal conjugate vaccine (PCV7).
- PCV7 contains polysaccharides from serotypes 4, 6B, 9V, 14, 18C, 19F, and 23F and was introduced into the routine UK immunization schedule in September 2006.
- Five years after introduction of PCV7 into the USA, in children <2 years:
  - The incidence of pneumococcal meningitis decreased by 64% overall, from 10 per 100 000 per year to 3.7 per 100 000 per year
  - There was a decrease in PCV7-serotype meningitis of 93%
  - The incidence of PCV7-serotype meningitis was 0.6 per 100 000 per year and of non PCV7-serotype meningitis was 2.9 per 100 000 per year
  - The most common serotypes were 14 and 23F prior to widespread use of PCV7, and 19A and 22F afterwards.
- Two years after introduction of PCV7 for vaccination of 'high risk' children in France there was a 39% reduction in the incidence of pneumococcal meningitis in all children <2 years.
- New conjugate vaccines containing 10 and 13 polysaccharides have now been licensed in Europe.

Haemophilus influenzae type b

- Most Hib disease occurs in children <5 years.
- Before use of Hib conjugate vaccines the incidence of invasive Hib disease in Europe was 12–54 per 100 000 per year in children <5 years; approximately 60% had meningitis.

- Most European countries implemented routine Hib conjugate vaccination between 1992 and 1996, leading to >90% reduction of disease in all countries.
- From 1999 there was a resurgence in the number of cases in the UK, predominantly in children aged 1–4 years. In 2003, a further catch-up campaign occurred and a routine booster dose was introduced into the immunization schedule in 2006, resulting in a decrease in disease.

Neonatal bacterial meningitis
- The incidence of bacterial meningitis has been 0.2–1 per 1000 live births in developed countries since the 1980s.
- Up to 30% of neonates with sepsis have associated bacterial meningitis.

Aseptic meningitis
- Approximately 95% of children presenting with meningitis in the highly immunized populations of developed countries will have aseptic meningitis.
- The epidemiological pattern depends on the causative pathogen, which is only identified in approximately 10% of cases because diagnostic investigation is often incomplete.
- Approximately 85% of cases are due to enteroviruses, which are more common in summer and autumn in temperate climates.
- In the largest published study, in Finland, the annual incidence of viral meningitis was 219 per 100 000 in infants <1 year and 27.8 per 100 000 in all children <14 years.
- The incidence of viral meningitis in neonates is approximately 0.05 per 1000 livebirths.
- Most TB cases in the UK occur in non-UK born children (37 per 100 000 per year vs 2.5 per 100 000 per year), especially those born in Africa and those of south Asian ethnic origin, and rates of disease are increasing in these groups.
- TB meningitis has been reported in up to 6% of children with TB disease, and is most common in those <6 years. It usually occurs 2–6 months after the initial infection and is associated with miliary TB in 50% of cases.
- Fungal meningitis is usually associated with immunocompromised hosts and neonates.

Predisposing factors
- Young age
- Male gender
- Malnutrition or chronic illness
- Recent head trauma, neurosurgery or presence of a ventriculo-peritoneal shunt
- Local anatomical defects
- Close contact with:
  - A colonized carrier (*N. meningitidis*, *S. pneumoniae*, Hib)
  - An individual with disease (*N. meningitidis*, Hib, TB, viruses, rarely *S. pneumoniae*)

- An individual with a sputum-positive smear (TB)
- Certain animals (e.g. reptiles—*Salmonella*, domestic animals—*Listeria*).
- Consumption of unpasteurized dairy products in pregnancy (*Listeria*)
- Swimming in water contaminated by urine from infected animals (*Leptospira*)
- Recent tick bite (*Borrelia*, *Rickettsia*)
- Lack of immunization (mumps, Hib, *S. pneumoniae*, *N. meningitidis*)
- Immunosuppression:
  - Deficiencies in terminal complement components (*N. meningitidis*)
  - Hyposplenism, e.g. post-splenectomy, congenital asplenia (*S. pneumoniae*, *H. influenzae*)
  - Immunosuppressive drugs (fungi, TB)
  - Hypogammaglobulinaemia (enteroviruses)
  - HIV infection (*S. pneumoniae*, CMV, HSV, VZV, fungi, TB, *Toxoplasma*)
  - Defects in cell-mediated immunity (fungi, TB, CMV, HSV, VZV).
- Sickle cell disease (*S. pneumoniae*, Hib, *Salmonella*)
- Malignant neoplasia
- Risk factors for TB include:
  - Travel to an area with a high incidence of TB
  - Belonging to an ethnic minority originating from areas with a high incidence of TB.
- Risk factors for neonatal fungal infection include:
  - Prematurity (gestational age <32 weeks)
  - Very low birth weight (<1500 g)
  - Prolonged intubation or indwelling vascular devices
  - Parenteral nutrition and delayed enteral feeding
  - Treatment with broad spectrum antibiotics, corticosteroids or H_2-receptor blockers.

Clinical presentation

- **The classical manifestations present in older children are rarely present in infants and young children.**
- Usually begins with fever, nausea and vomiting, photophobia, and severe headache. Occasionally the first sign is a seizure, which can also occur later. Irritability, delirium, and altered level of consciousness develop as CNS inflammation progresses.
- The most specific signs are neck stiffness, associated with Kernig's and Brudzinski's signs. These are often absent in children.
  - Kernig's sign—inability to fully extend knee while hip is flexed due to contraction of hamstring muscles and pain
  - Brudzinski's sign—automatic flexion of the hips and knees after passive neck flexion.
- Focal neurological abnormalities may occur. In the absence of seizures they indicate cortical necrosis, occlusive vasculitis or cortical venous thrombosis.
- In infants and young children symptoms are non-specific, and include fever or hypothermia, poor feeding, vomiting, lethargy, irritability,

jaundice, respiratory distress or apnoea, and seizures. A bulging fontanelle may be present.

- Additional manifestations tend to be associated with specific organisms:
  - Petechiae and purpura (*N. meningitidis*, possibly Hib or *S. pneumoniae*)—the rash may be blanching
  - Leg pain, cold extremities, abnormal skin colour, and shock (*N. meningitidis*)
  - Joint involvement (*N. meningitidis*, Hib)
  - A chronically draining ear or history of head trauma (*S. pneumoniae*)
  - Pleurodynia, herpangina, or unexplained rashes (enteroviruses)
  - Chronic symptoms (TB, fungi).
- Bacterial and viral meningitis cannot be reliably distinguished on clinical features alone, however:
  - Children with bacterial meningitis are more likely to have specific features and many have neck stiffness or an altered conscious level
  - Children with viral meningitis are less likely to have shock, an altered conscious level or seizures.
- TB meningitis can be staged on the basis of clinical features:
  - Stage 1—no reduced conscious level or focal neurological signs
  - Stage 2—reduced conscious level and/or focal neurological signs
  - Stage 3—coma.

Differential diagnosis

- Other CNS infection—encephalitis, intra-cranial abscess (cerebral, subdural or epidural)
- Generalized sepsis from another focus
- Leukaemia and solid CNS tumours
- Connective tissue disorders, e.g. systemic lupus erythematosus, Behçet's disease
- Kawasaki disease
- Sarcoidosis
- Drugs and toxins, including intravenous immunoglobulin and heavy metals.

Investigations

Lumbar puncture

- **CSF should ideally be obtained prior to commencing treatment, but initiation of antimicrobial therapy should not be delayed if an immediate lumber puncture (LP) cannot be performed.**
- CSF analysis by microscopy, Gram stain, culture, and PCR is the definitive method of diagnosis. Biochemistry for protein and glucose (with a plasma glucose taken at the same time) should also be performed (Table 29.1).
- Any child in whom meningitis is suspected and any drowsy or ill infant should have an LP, in the absence of any contra-indications (Box 29.1).

- CSF should be examined as soon as possible because white blood cells (WBCs) start to degrade after approximately 90 minutes.
- Initial Gram staining of CSF reveals an organism in 68–80% of bacterial meningitis cases.
- It is rare for CSF microscopy to be normal and a pathogen identified later, although this occurs most often in meningococcal meningitis (up to 8%) and in neonates.
- Consider alternative diagnoses in a seriously unwell child with normal CSF variables.
- CSF cultures are negative 2 hours after parenteral antibiotics are given in meningococcal meningitis, after 6 hours in pneumococcal meningitis, and after 8 hours in neonatal GBS meningitis.
- CSF cellular and biochemical changes remain up to 44–68 hours after the start of treatment.
- If TB meningitis is suspected CSF staining for acid-fast bacilli and appropriate culture should be done.
- *Cryptococcus* can be diagnosed by India ink staining of CSF.

Table 29.1 CSF WBC count, and protein and glucose values in normal children and changes that occur with meningitis

	Macroscopic appearance	CSF WBC count (per mm^3)[a]	CSF Protein (mg/dl)	CSF glucose (% of plasma glucose)
Normal CSF				
Neonate	Clear and colourless	0–20[b]	20–170	>60
>1 month		0–5[c]	0–40	60–70
Children with meningitis				
Bacterial meningitis	Turbid or purulent	↑↑↑[d]	↑↑↑	↓↓
Viral meningitis	Usually clear	↑	N/↑	↓/N
TB meningitis	Yellow or cloudy	↑↑[e]	↑↑↑	↓
Fungal meningitis	Usually clear	↑[e]	↑↑	↓

[a]In the case of a traumatic LP, one WBC per 500 red blood cells can be subtracted from the total CSF WBC count.
[b]WBCs in neonatal CSF is predominantly lymphocytes, although neutrophils may be present.
[c]Outside the neonatal period all CSF WBCs should be lymphocytes and the presence of any neutrophils is abnormal.
[d]CSF WBCs in bacterial meningitis are usually mostly neutrophils, although lymphocytes can be predominant in early disease; CSF WBCs in viral meningitis are usually mostly lymphocytes, although neutrophils can be predominant.
[e]In tuberculous or fungal meningitis, the majority of CSF WBCs are lymphocytes.

Box 29.1 Contraindications to LP

- Signs of raised intracranial pressure:
  - Reduced level of consciousness (GCS <9)
  - Relative bradycardia and hypertension
  - Unequal, dilated or poorly responsive pupils
  - Absent doll's eyes movements
  - Abnormal tone or posture
  - Respiratory abnormalities
  - Papilloedema*
  - Evidence of raised ICP on CT
- Abnormal focal neurological signs
- Following a prolonged convulsive seizure *or* within 30 minutes of a short convulsive seizure *or* following any tonic seizure[b]
- Cardiorespiratory instability
- Abnormal clotting studies (if available) or concurrent administration of anticoagulant therapy
- Severe thrombocytopenia (platelet count <100 × 10⁹/l)
- Extensive or extending purpura
- Localized infection at the site of LP

[a]Papilloedema is an uncommon finding in acute meningitis and its presence should prompt consideration of venous sinus occlusion, subdural empyema, or brain abscess.
[b]Prolonged: >30 minutes; short: ≤30 minutes.

If contraindications are present, LP should be delayed and performed when contraindications are no longer applicable.

Cranial CT and MRI

- **A scan should not delay the use of antimicrobial therapy.**
- **A normal CT scan does not mean it is safe to do an LP**. This decision should be based on clinical assessment. However, if a scan shows evidence of raised intracranial pressure an LP should not be performed.
- The main indication for cranial imaging is when the diagnosis is uncertain or to detect other possible intracranial pathology.
- If a CT scan is to be done, it should be undertaken urgently after stabilisation of the child.
- While CT is widely available and very useful for rapid assessment of hydrocephalus, mass lesions, haemorrhage or cerebral oedema, MRI will detect more subtle findings, particularly of vascular infarction.
- Non-contrast CT or MRI can be normal in early cases of meningitis.
- CT in cerebral oedema may show slit-like lateral ventricles, areas of low attenuation, and absence of basilar and suprachiasmatic cisterns.
- Signs of TB meningitis include obstructive hydrocephalus, basilar enhancement, and parenchymal granulomas.
- Cryptococcal meningitis usually has non-specific abnormalities on CT. There may be signs of raised intracranial pressure, hydrocephalus, or focal lesions, especially in the basal ganglia.
- Neonatal *Candida* meningitis may result in cerebral micro- or macro-abscesses.

Other investigations

- All children with suspected meningitis should have:
  - Blood culture (positive in 80–90% of antibiotic-naïve children)
  - Blood for PCR (see below)
  - FBC, CRP, clotting, U&Es, glucose.
- Bacterial meningitis is likely in those with abnormal CSF parameters who have a significantly raised WBC count and/or CRP. If bacterial meningitis is suspected clinically and an LP has not been performed, children should be managed as such regardless of blood results.
- A normal CRP and WBC count do not rule out bacterial meningitis.
- If TB meningitis is suspected, tests should include a chest X-ray, tuberculin skin test (TST) ± an interferon-γ release assay (IGRA) (📖 see Chapter 113, p. 753).

Molecular techniques

- PCR for *N. meningitidis*, *S. pneumoniae*, and Hib using CSF or for *N. meningitidis* using blood can be obtained in the UK from the meningococcal reference laboratory in Manchester.
- For *N. meningitidis*, PCR from blood has a sensitivity of 87% and specificity of 100%.
- For *S. pneumoniae*, PCR is sensitive and specific on CSF, but false positive results may be obtained from blood due to the high nasopharyngeal carriage rate in young children.
- Rapid antigen latex agglutination tests on CSF or blood (which can be used to detect *N. meningitidis*, *S. pneumoniae*, *H. influenzae*, *E. coli*, or GBS) can be done locally and rapidly, but the lack of sensitivity has limited their clinical use.
- CSF can be sent for PCR for possible viral aetiologies, including HSV, EBV, VZV, and enteroviruses.
- If TB meningitis is suspected, prolonged culture is required and CSF should be analysed by specific PCR if acid-fast bacilli are seen on microscopy.

Clinical decision rules

- Meningitis in developed countries is predominantly aseptic, so clinical decision rules have been developed since the introduction of the Hib conjugate vaccine to distinguish bacterial from aseptic meningitis, to reduce antibiotic and corticosteroid use and hospitalization.
- The 'Bacterial Meningitis Score' is the only rule which has been sufficiently validated in a large number of children, and classifies patients with CSF pleocytosis (WBC count >10 per mm^3) as very low risk of bacterial meningitis if they fulfil the following criteria:
  - Negative CSF Gram stain
  - CSF neutrophil count <1000 per mm^3
  - CSF protein <80 mg/dl
  - Blood neutrophil count <10 × 10^9/l
  - No seizure prior to presentation.

- In a Hib-immunized population, this score had a negative predictive value of 100% (95% CI 97% to 100%) prior to routine use of PCV7, and 99.9% (95% CI 99.6% to 100%) when validated after introduction of the vaccine.
- In a very large study only 1.3% of children with a CSF WBC count <300 per mm^3 had bacterial meningitis, increasing to 10% and 28% for those with a CSF WBC count >500 per mm^3 and >1000 per mm^3, respectively.
- Early studies probably underestimated the prevalence of bacterial meningitis in children with CSF pleocytosis because they excluded 23% of eligible children, including those with critical illness, purpura, immunosuppression, and previous antibiotic administration.
- No data are available from countries where the meningococcal serogroup C conjugate vaccine is routinely used.
- Clinical decision rules need further validation before they can be routinely implemented to determine treatment of children with suspected meningitis.

Management

- **Any child with suspected meningitis should be transferred to a hospital immediately**.
- **All children should be assessed for dehydration, shock, and raised intracranial pressure**.
- Many children, particularly those with meningococcal meningitis, will have coexisting septicaemia and shock. Standard resuscitation guidelines should be followed with the expectation that prompt and adequate fluid resuscitation may be required.

Antimicrobial therapy (Table 29.2)

- For suspected meningococcal disease (presence of a purpuric or petechial rash), antibiotic therapy with parenteral benzylpenicillin is often given before admission to hospital and is recommended in the UK. There is no reliable evidence to support or refute this practice and the priority of transfer to hospital should remain.
- **In hospital, antibiotic therapy for suspected acute bacterial meningitis must be started immediately, before the results of CSF culture and antibiotic sensitivity are available**.
  - All ages: initiate antibiotics if CSF WBC count is abnormal (Table 29.1)
  - Neonates: bacterial meningitis should still be considered if other clinical features are present, irrespective of CSF WBC count.
- Intravenous antibiotics are required to achieve adequate serum and CSF levels.
- Choice of empirical agent(s) should consider current local data regarding circulating pathogens and their antibiotic resistance patterns. Specific therapy may need to be adjusted once a pathogen is cultured and antibiotic susceptibility results are available.
- The possibility of TB meningitis should be considered in all cases.

Empirical therapy for children aged >3 months
- Monotherapy with a third-generation cephalosporin, e.g. ceftriaxone or cefotaxime (ceftriaxone preferred as once-daily dosing).
  - Broad spectrum of activity against Gram-positive and Gram-negative organisms, highly resistant to β-lactamase, and penetrate the blood–brain barrier.
  - Neonatal deaths have been reported due to an interaction between ceftriaxone and calcium-containing products, so ceftriaxone should not be administered simultaneously with calcium containing infusions. In this situation cefotaxime should be used.
- Overall 20–45% of *S. pneumoniae* strains worldwide are resistance to penicillin. In regions where there is a high prevalence of resistance, or in children with recent prolonged or multiple exposure to antibiotics, or those who have recently travelled to an area with a high rate of pneumococcal resistance, adding vancomycin should be considered.

Specific therapy for children aged >3 months
- Specific therapy with ceftriaxone is recommended for convenience and cost-effectiveness of once daily dosing. The duration of antibiotic therapy depends upon the infecting organism: 7 days for *N. meningitidis*, 10 days for *H. influenzae*, 14 days for *S. pneumoniae*.
- Treat unconfirmed, uncomplicated but clinically suspected bacterial meningitis with ceftriaxone for at least 10 days depending on clinical features and course.

Empirical therapy for children aged <3 months
- Amoxicillin/ampicillin (to cover *Listeria*) plus cefotaxime.
- Ceftriaxone may be used as an alternative to cefotaxime, but should be avoided in infants who are jaundiced, hypoalbuminaemic, acidotic or born prematurely as it may exacerbate hyperbilirubinaemia. Ceftriaxone should not be administered at the same time as calcium-containing infusions.
- Vancomycin should be added for indications as above.
- Consider meropenem instead of cefotaxime in settings with high rates of community-acquired extended spectrum β-lactamase producing Gram-negative organisms.
- Add aciclovir if there is a possibility of HSV infection.

Specific therapy for children <3 months
- There are no controlled clinical trials to guide duration of therapy.
- GBS: Cefotaxime should be continued for at least 14 days after initiation, but should be extended to at least 3 weeks in complicated cases.
- Gram-negative organisms: Cefotaxime should be given for 21 days, but this may be modified based on local resistance patterns and sensitivities of the specific organism.
- *L. monocytogenes*: Therapy is recommended for 21 days with amoxicillin, adding gentamicin for at least the first 7 days.

- Unconfirmed but clinically suspected: Administer amoxicillin/ampicillin plus cefotaxime for at least 14 days. If the course is complicated consider extending treatment duration of treatment and consultation with an expert in paediatric infectious diseases.
- Repeat LP should be performed in neonates after 48–72 hours only if there is worsening or no improvement of clinical condition and/or laboratory parameters.

Specific therapy for aseptic meningitis

- TB meningitis: Current UK guidelines recommend treatment with rifampicin, isoniazid, pyrazinamide plus a fourth drug (e.g. ethambutol) for the first 2 months, followed by rifampicin and isoniazid alone for a further 10 months.
- Fungal meningitis: Infection of HIV-affected children with *Cryptococcus* or *Histoplasma* involves treatment with amphotericin B, fluconazole, and flucytosine. Amphotericin B and fluconazole are the agents of choice for neonatal *Candida* meningitis.

Table 29.2 Empirical and specific therapy for bacterial meningitis

Age group	Empirical therapy	Specific therapy
>3 months	Ceftriaxone or cefotaxime ± vancomycin	Ceftriaxone: • 7 days for *N. meningitidis* • 10 days for Hib • 14 days for *S. pneumoniae* • ≥10 days for unconfirmed organism
<3 months	Amoxicillin/ampicillin + cefotaxime (or ceftriaxone or meropenem) ± vancomycin Consider aciclovir	GBS: ≥14 days cefotaxime Gram-negative organisms: 21 days cefotaxime *Listeria*: 21 days amoxicillin/ampicillin with gentamicin for first 7 days No confirmed bacterial diagnosis: ≥14 days amoxicillin/ampicillin plus cefotaxime

Corticosteroid therapy

- The use of corticosteroid therapy in bacterial meningitis remains controversial, principally because of the lack of data relevant to the post-conjugate vaccine era. There are no studies examining the use of steroids in aseptic meningitis and guidelines emphasize the need to target steroid use to children who are most likely to have bacterial meningitis.
- **Children >3 months should receive corticosteroids if they have**:
  - Bacteria on CSF Gram stain
  - *Or* a CSF WBC count >1000 per mm^3
  - *Or* CSF pleocytosis and CSF protein >100 mg/dl (consider the possibility of TB meningitis if the protein is very raised).
- Corticosteroids should ideally be administered before or with the first antibiotic dose, but they may be beneficial up to 12 hours later.
- Corticosteroids reduce meningeal inflammation and modulate cytokine secretion to reduce pro-inflammatory responses.
- In clinical trials corticosteroids reduced the rate of severe hearing loss in bacterial meningitis from 11.0% to 6.6%. The majority of children in these trials had meningitis due to Hib and a CSF WBC count >1000 per mm^3, but there was also a trend for better outcome in non-*Haemophilus* meningitis. In adults, steroids appeared to reduce mortality in addition to the improved hearing outcomes.
- Most studies used a 4-day course of 0.1–0.15 mg/kg/dose four times daily of dexamethasone.
- The safety of corticosteroids in aseptic or neonatal meningitis has not been adequately addressed.
- For children in resource-poor countries, the use of corticosteroids is not recommended as there is no evidence of benefit.
- Children with TB meningitis should receive corticosteroids for 2–3 weeks, followed by gradual withdrawal.

Ongoing fluid management

- **Fluid therapy should be guided by clinical assessment of hydration status, signs of raised intracranial pressure, and shock combined with regular electrolyte measurements.**
- Both over- and under-hydration are associated with adverse outcomes.
- Over 50% of children have hyponatraemia at presentation attributed to increased concentrations of antidiuretic hormone (ADH), and this is a marker of severe disease. There are differing opinions as to whether hyponatraemia is due to dehydration or SIADH.
- Enteral fluids or feeds should be used where appropriate, and isotonic fluid when intravenous therapy is required.
- After correction of dehydration, full maintenance fluid should be given to prevent hypoglycaemia and maintain electrolyte balance.
- In settings with high mortality and where children present late, full maintenance fluid therapy was associated with reduced spasticity, seizures, and chronic severe neurological sequelae. Where children present early and mortality rates are lower there is insufficient evidence, so fluid restriction should not be employed routinely.

- If there is evidence of raised intracranial pressure or circulatory failure, initiate emergency management for these conditions and discuss ongoing fluid management with a paediatric intensivist.

Other supportive treatment
- A possible need for management in a PICU setting should be considered.
- Adequate oxygenation.
- Treatment and prevention of hypoglycaemia.
- Anticonvulsant treatment for seizures.
- Reduction of raised intracranial pressure (treat if clinically evident or signs on CT scan):
  - 30° bed head elevation;
  - Maintenance of normal pCO_2 through mechanical ventilation;
  - Treatment with mannitol and furosemide.
- Children with severe sepsis will require circulatory support with inotropes.

Prevention of secondary cases

- Chemoprophylaxis against meningococcal disease with rifampicin, ciprofloxacin, or ceftriaxone should be given as soon as possible and ideally within 24 hours of diagnosis to:
  - Household members who have had prolonged close contact with the index case
  - Those who have had transient close contact with the index case if they have been directly exposed to large particles or respiratory droplets/secretions (e.g. healthcare workers).
- Chemoprophylaxis against Hib disease is only indicated if the index case is <10 years old or there is a vulnerable individual (immunosuppressed, asplenic or <10 years of age) in the household. In such cases rifampicin should be given to:
  - The index case
  - All household contacts if there is a vulnerable individual in the household.
- Following Hib disease, Hib immunization should be given to:
  - The index case if <10 years of age *and* incompletely immunized or convalescent antibody levels <1µg/ml or hyposplenic
  - All incompletely immunized children <10 years of age in the same household.
- Household contacts of a child with TB meningitis should be screened using a TST ± an IGRA, with further assessment as indicated. Other close contacts should also be assessed for any child with smear-positive TB.
- Following contact with smear-positive TB:
  - All children <2 years should receive isoniazid while screening tests are being performed;
  - Children of any age should receive BCG if the Mantoux test is <6 mm.
- Maternal intrapartum antibiotics for cases at high-risk of neonatal GBS reduce early-onset GBS disease (first week of life) but have no effect on late-onset disease.

Outcomes

Outcome depends on multiple factors, including age, time and clinical stability prior to treatment, organism, and host inflammatory response.

Bacterial meningitis
- Early complications:
  - Seizures
  - SIADH.
- Later complications of acute disease:
  - Subdural effusions in one-third, often asymptomatic with spontaneous resolution. They may manifest with enlargement of head circumference, vomiting, seizures, bulging fontanelle, focal neurological signs or persistent fever
  - Focal neurological abnormalities
  - Hydrocephalus, more often in younger infants
  - Brain abscesses, especially in newborns infected with *Citrobacter diversus* or *Proteus*.
- Long-term complications (occur in 10–30% overall):
  - **Sensorineural hearing loss—all should have hearing screening after discharge**
  - Epilepsy
  - Motor and cognitive impairment
  - Blindness and optic atrophy
  - Learning and behavioural problems.
- In the developed world, case fatality rates are <10% overall and <5% for meningitis due to *N. meningitidis* or Hib.
- For neonatal bacterial meningitis, mortality is approximately 5–10% overall. Disability at 5 years is 50% for GBS and *E. coli*, and 78% following infection with other Gram-negative organisms.

Aseptic meningitis
- Full recovery is usual in uncomplicated viral meningitis, although neuro-psychological sequelae can occur, including fatigue, irritability, reduced concentration, and muscle pain, weakness or spasm. Some infants have an increased risk of delayed language development.
- HSV in neonates can result in severe neurological sequelae.
- TB meningitis has almost 100% survival in stage 1 disease, but only 80% in stage 3 disease, with significant long-term disability in survivors. Sequelae include hydrocephalus, blindness, deafness, motor and cognitive impairment, intracranial calcification, and diabetes insipidus.
- Invasive neonatal candidiasis has a mortality rate of around 30%.

Future research

- Development of vaccines against serogroup B *N. meningitidis*.
- Prevention of neonatal GBS and *E. coli* infection through maternal vaccination or use of specific antibody preparations.
- More sensitive tests, such as amplification of 16S rRNA gene by PCR, for diagnosis in antibiotic pretreated patients.

- Assessment of new antimicrobial agents against resistant pneumococcal strains.
- Benefit of corticosteroids in the era of widespread coverage of Hib, pneumococcal and meningococcal serogroup C vaccine coverage, and in neonates.
- Further evidence regarding the risk or benefit from fluid restriction.

Further reading

Maconochie I, Baumer H, Stewart ME. Fluid therapy for acute bacterial meningitis. *Cochrane Database Syst Rev* 2008;**1**:CD004786.

National Collaborating Centre for Chronic Conditions. *Tuberculosis. Clinical Diagnosis and Management of Tuberculosis, and Measures for its Prevention and Control.* London: Royal College of Physicians, 2006.

National Collaborating Centre for Women's and Children's Health. *Bacterial Meningitis and Meningococcal Septicaemia in Children: The Management of Bacterial Meningitis and Meningococcal Septicaemia in Children and Young People Younger than 16 years in Primary and Secondary Care.* London: RCOG Press, 2010.

van de Beek D, de Gans J, McIntyre P, Prasad K. Corticosteroids for acute bacterial meningitis. *Cochrane Database Syst Rev* 2007;**1**:CD004405.

Chapter 30

Neonatal infection

📖 see also Chapters 10, 64, 68, 69, 75, 76, 77, 83, 99, 101, 105, 106, 107

Introduction

- Infections are a frequent and important cause of morbidity and mortality in the neonatal period.
- As many as 1–2% of fetuses are infected *in utero*, and up to 10% of infants have infections in the first month of life.
- The timing of exposure, inoculum size, immune status, and virulence of the aetiologic agent influence manifestations of disease in a fetus or newborn infant.
- A wide variety of agents infect the newborn, including bacteria, viruses, fungi, protozoa, and mycoplasmas.
- With advances in neonatal intensive care, increasingly immature, very low birth rate (VLBW) newborns are surviving and remain in the hospital for a longer time, an environment that puts them at ongoing risk for infections.

Causative organisms

- Infections acquired in utero can be viruses (rubella virus, CMV, parvovirus B19, HBV, HIV, VZV), bacteria (*Listeria monocytogenes*, *Treponema pallidum*, *Mycobacterium tuberculosis*) or protozoa (*Toxoplasma gondii*).
- Intrapartum infections are often due to bacteria (GBS, enteric organisms (*Escherichia coli*, *Serratia* spp., *Enterobacter* spp., *Citrobacter* spp. *Pseudomonas* spp., *Salmonella* spp.), gonococci and *Chlamydia trachomatis*) and in a minority of cases viruses (HIV, HSV, HBV).
- Postpartum infections are mainly due to CONS, *Staphylococcus aureus*, *Streptococcus pneumoniae* and Gram-negative bacilli (*E. coli*, *Klebsiella pneumoniae*, *Salmonella*, *Enterobacter*, *Citrobacter*, *Pseudomonas aeruginosa*, *Serratia*), enterococci, and GBS. Viruses play a minor role, even though CMV, RSV, influenza viruses, parainfluenza viruses, adenovirus, and rotavirus can cause outbreaks of nosocomial infection. Fungi (mainly *Candida*) are responsible for an increasing number of systemic infections in children admitted to neonatal intensive care units (NICU).

Epidemiology

- Neonatal infections can be divided by age at onset of symptoms in the neonatal period (early-onset if in the first 48–72 hours of life, late-onset if after 48–72 hours of life).
- Intrapartum infections cause mainly early-onset infections, i.e. infections that are symptomatic in the first week of life.
- Several factors influence the incidence of neonatal infections including prematurity, low birth weight, maternal age, maternal immunization status and the presence of maternal infections, such as chorioamnionitis. Also the prevalence of organisms in the community, socioeconomic status, race, sexual practices, conduct of labour, and environmental conditions in the nursery and at home, can influence the incidence. Finally, invasive procedures, presence of indwelling vascular catheters, ventricular shunts, and endotracheal tubes, alterations in the skin and mucous membrane barriers may favour infections.
- Previous use of antibiotics increase the likelihood of infections caused by more resistant bacteria.
- In industrialized countries, CMV infection is the most frequent congenital viral infection with a rate of around 0.5/1000 livebirths. Congenital rubella is very rare where the vaccine is systematically used. The same is true for hepatitis B. In resource-poor countries, perinatal HIV infection is a major concern.
- In industrialized countries, the incidence of neonatal sepsis is between 1 and 4/1000 livebirths and that of meningitis between 0.2 and 0.4/1000 livebirths. In premature infants, especially if admitted to the NICU, these values can be 10-fold higher. These incidences are significantly increased in resource-poor countries.
- Neonates may be infected at different times via three different routes: *in utero* (transplacental), intrapartum (ascending), and post partum (nosocomial or community).
- Transplacental infections are the result of a clinical or subclinical maternal infection.
- Perinatal infections are acquired just before or during delivery, with vertical transmission from mother to neonate.
- Postnatal infections are transmitted by direct contact from various human sources, such as the mother, family contacts, and hospital personnel; from breast milk (HIV, CMV); or from inanimate sources, such as contaminated equipment.

Clinical presentation and differential diagnosis

- Clinical signs and symptoms do not help make a specific aetiological diagnosis, but rather raise suspicion of infection. The initial signs of sepsis are often non-specific. It is very important to re-evaluate infants over time to determine whether the symptoms have progressed.

- Infection acquired *in utero* may result in spontaneous abortion, stillbirth, congenital malformations, intrauterine growth retardation, premature birth, acute disease in the neonatal period, or asymptomatic persistent infection with neurological sequelae later in life.
- First trimester infection may alter embryogenesis, with resulting congenital malformations.
- Late gestational infections may lead to a delay in clinical manifestations until some time after birth (e.g. syphilis).
- Presenting signs and symptoms of infection in the neonate are:
  - General—fever or temperature instability; change in activity/feeding
  - Gastrointestinal—abdominal distension, vomiting, diarrhoea or hepatomegaly
  - Respiratory—apnoea, dyspnoea, tachypnoea, retraction, flaring, grunting or cyanosis
  - Renal—oliguria
  - Cardiovascular—pallor, mottled, cold, clammy skin, tachycardia, hypotension, bradycardia
  - Central nervous system—irritability, lethargy, tremors, seizures, hyporeflexia, hypotonia, irregular respirations, full fontanelle or high-pitched cry
  - Haematological—jaundice, splenomegaly, pallor, petechiae, purpura or bleeding.
- Specific clinical findings and presentations:
  - *Fever*: Only 50% of infected neonates have a fever (axillary temperature >37.8°C) and the presence of fever is not always due to infection (e.g. may be due to dehydration, overheating). A single temperature elevation is infrequently associated with infection; fever sustained over 1 hour is more likely to be due to infection. In premature infants, look for hypothermia or temperature instability rather than fever.
  - *Rash*: Cutaneous manifestations of infection include impetigo, cellulitis, mastitis, omphalitis, and subcutaneous abscesses. Ecthyma gangrenosum is highly suggestive of pseudomonal infection. A vesicular rash is characteristic of HSV infection. Dermal erythropoiesis (purple papulonodular lesions referred to as 'blueberry muffin', see 🕮 p. 79) can be associated with CMV, rubella, or parvovirus infection, as well as congenital neoplastic disease and Rh haemolytic disease.
  - *Omphalitis*: Infection of the umbilical cord is usually caused by bacteria that colonize the maternal genital tract or the environment. Early manifestations include erythema or serous or purulent discharge; cellulitis can be progressive and other complications include necrotizing fasciitis and spread of infection via the umbilical or portal vessels to cause sepsis.
  - *Pneumonia*: Early signs and symptoms are frequently non-specific (such as poor feeding, irritability, lethargy, cyanosis, temperature instability). Classic signs on physical examination are very difficult to appreciate in a neonate. Tachypnoea, retractions, nasal flaring may be observed. As the degree of respiratory compromise increases,

progressive respiratory failure may develop. GBS, a common bacterial cause of pneumonia, can lead to fulminant infection, whereas atypical bacteria (e.g. *Chlamydia*) are associated with an indolent course.

• *Sepsis*: Despite its multisystem involvement, sepsis can initially manifest with signs affecting only one organ system (e.g. tachypnoea with recession). Late manifestations include signs of respiratory failure as a result of acute respiratory distress syndrome, pulmonary hypertension, cardiac failure, shock, renal failure, hepatocellular disease with hyperbilirubinaemia and elevated enzymes, cerebral oedema or thrombosis, adrenal haemorrhage and/or insufficiency, bone marrow dysfunction (neutropenia, thrombocytopenia, anaemia), and DIC.

• *Meningitis*: Signs of meningitis in babies, especially premature babies, may be very difficult to detect. Characteristic features found in infants may not occur and non-specific signs of illness are common (see Sepsis above).

Investigations

Evaluation of a neonate with suspected infection or sepsis should include the following:

• Detailed history to identify specific risk factors:
  • Maternal infections during gestation or at delivery (type and duration of antimicrobial therapy, urinary tract infection, chorioamnionitis, sexually transmitted infections)
  • History of GBS infections during prior pregnancies
  • Maternal colonization with GBS (screening may be universal or for selected high-risk groups depending on national policy)
  • History of previous sexually transmitted infections (gonorrhoea, syphilis, chlamydia, herpes)
  • Gestational age/birthweight
  • Multiple birth
  • Duration of membrane rupture
  • Complicated delivery
  • Fetal tachycardia
  • Age at onset (in utero, birth—early or late)
  • Medical interventions (scalp electrodes, vascular access, endotracheal intubation, parenteral nutrition, surgery).
• Identification of underlying conditions that can favour sepsis:
  • Congenital malformations (e.g. neural tube malformations)
  • Respiratory tract disease
  • Necrotizing enterocolitis.
• Detailed physical examination:
  • Abnormal vital signs (in relationship to age)
  • Other important observations include feeding, stools, urine output
  • General appearance, neurological status, movement of extremities
  • All organ systems should be examined, including skin and skeletal systems.

- Laboratory studies—signs of sepsis include evidence of:
  - Infection (culture from normally sterile sites, such as blood, cerebrospinal fluid, urine; demonstration of an organism in tissue or fluid; antigen detection in urine and cerebrospinal fluid; maternal or neonatal serology for syphilis, toxoplasmosis, CMV, rubella, HIV, HBV)
  - Inflammation (leucocytosis, increased immature/total neutrophil count ratio, acute phase reactants such as C-reactive protein and procalcitonin, pleocytosis in cerebrospinal fluid or synovial or pleural fluid, fibrin split products for DIC; histological, e.g. placenta)
  - Multiorgan system involvement (pH and pCO_2 for metabolic acidosis; PO_2 and PCO_2 for pulmonary function; blood urea nitrogen and creatinine for renal function; bilirubin, ALT, AST, ammonia, prothrombin time (PT), partial thromboplastin time (PTT) for hepatic function; neutropenia, anaemia, thrombocytopenia for bone marrow function).

Treatment

- Treatment is determined by the pattern of disease and the organisms that are common for the age of the infant and the local flora of the nursery.
- Once bacterial infection is suspected and appropriate cultures have been obtained, intravenous antibiotic therapy must be instituted immediately.
- Narrow-spectrum antibiotics should always be used wherever possible to reduce the pressure on antimicrobial resistance. Broad-spectrum cephalosporins should be avoided if possible on neonatal units.
- Initial empirical treatment of early-onset bacterial infections is based on penicillin or ampicillin and an aminoglycoside, usually gentamicin.
- Initial empirical treatment of late-onset bacterial infections is based on ampicillin or flucloxacillin and an aminoglycoside, usually gentamicin, but the combination chosen should be based on knowledge of local antibiotic resistance patterns.
- Flucloxacillin may be substituted with vancomycin if methicillin-resistant staphylococci are known to be endemic. Otherwise, in order to avoid the emergence of vancomycin resistance, vancomycin should be limited to severely ill neonates with an indwelling intravascular catheter and therapy should be discontinued after 2–3 days in the case of negative blood cultures.
- Piperacillin, ticarcillin, carbenicillin, or ceftazidime and an aminoglycoside should be administered when necrotic skin lesions suggest the presence of *Pseudomonas aeruginosa*.
- Empiric antifungal therapy should be considered in VLBW infants who have had previous antibiotic therapy, have mucosal colonization with *Candida albicans*, and who are at high risk for invasive disease (especially gastrointestinal disease, e.g. necrotizing enterocolitis).

- A third-generation cephalosporin together with ampicillin or penicillin ± an aminoglycoside, should be initiated for presumed bacterial meningitis.
- Once the pathogen has been identified and the antibiotic sensitivities determined, the most appropriate narrow spectrum drug(s) should be selected.
- The rational use of antibiotics in neonates involves using narrow-spectrum drugs when possible, treating infection and not colonization, and limiting the duration of therapy.
- Therapy for most bloodstream infections should be administered for 7–10 days or for at least 5 days after the clinical response. In the case of meningitis, 14–21 days of therapy are recommended.
- Cultures taken 24–48 hours after initiation of therapy should yield negative results. If the culture results remain positive, a change in antibiotics and/or removal of an existing catheter may be indicated.
- HSV requires specific antiviral treatment with aciclovir for 21 days.
- Supportive therapy includes correction of hypovolaemia, hyponatraemia, hypocalcaemia, and hypoglycaemia.
- Fluids should be limited if inappropriate secretion of diuretic hormone is diagnosed.
- Inotropic agents, fluid resuscitation, and mechanical ventilation can be useful to manage shock, hypoxia, and metabolic acidosis.
- Adequate oxygenation of tissue should be maintained, eventually with mechanical support.
- Refractory hypoxia may require extracorporeal membrane oxygenation.
- Hyperbilirubinaemia should be monitored and treated aggressively with phototherapy and/or exchange transfusion (the risk of kernicterus increases in sepsis or meningitis).
- DIC is usually treated by management of the primary infection. However, if bleeding occurs, fresh frozen plasma, platelet transfusion, or whole blood should be considered.
- The use of G-CSF or granulocyte macrophage colony-stimulating factor (GM-CSF) abolishes sepsis-induced neutropenia, but the effect of these cytokines on sepsis-related mortality is unclear.
- The use of IVIG has been shown to decrease mortality in patients with sepsis. A single dose of 500–750 mg/kg as adjunctive therapy is recommended by many experts. However, the overall benefit is currently uncertain and is awaiting further clinical trial data.

Follow-up and outcome

- Infections acquired *in utero* may cause late sequelae, even if the infant is asymptomatic at birth. These adverse outcomes include sensorineural hearing loss, visual disturbances (including blindness), seizures, and neurodevelopmental abnormalities.
- Complications of bacteraemic infections include endocarditis, septic emboli, abscess formation, septic joints with residual disability, and osteomyelitis, and bone destruction. Recurrent bacteraemia is rare.

- Candidaemia may lead to vasculitis, endocarditis, endophthalmitis, and abscesses in the kidneys, liver, lungs, and brain. Sequelae of sepsis may result from septic shock, DIC, or organ failure.
- Reported mortality rates in neonatal sepsis varies from 2% to 35% and depends on the definition of sepsis as well as the proportion of VLBW babies in the study population. The sepsis case fatality rate is highest for Gram-negative and fungal infections.
- The case fatality rate for neonatal bacterial meningitis is between 10% and 35%. Many of these cases have associated sepsis. Risk factors for death or for moderate or severe disability include duration of seizures for >72 hours, coma, necessity for the use of inotropic agents, and leucopenia. Immediate complications of meningitis include ventriculitis, cerebritis, and brain abscess. Late complications of meningitis occur in 40–50% of survivors and include hearing loss, abnormal behaviour, developmental delay, cerebral palsy, focal motor disability, seizure disorders, and hydrocephalus. A number of these sequelae may also be encountered in infants with sepsis but without meningitis as a result of cerebritis or septic shock.

Prevention

- Several intrauterine infections are preventable by means of immunization (including hepatitis B, polio, rubella, tetanus, varicella).
- Early onset GBS infections can be prevented by the administration of antibiotics during labour. Either a risk-based or swab-based screening strategy may be used to identify mothers at highest risk.
- Toxoplasmosis is preventable with appropriate diet and avoidance of exposure to cat faeces.
- Congenital syphilis is preventable by timely diagnosis and appropriate early treatment of infected pregnant women.
- Neonatal infection with *C. trachomatis* can be prevented by identification and treatment of infected pregnant women.
- Mother-to-child transmission of HIV is significantly reduced by maternal antiretroviral therapy during pregnancy, labour, and delivery and treatment of the infant at birth.
- Attention to hygiene in the nursery and in the NICU (including handwashing, avoidance of overcrowding, special isolation precautions, meticulous neonatal skin care, decreasing the number of venepunctures and heelsticks, minimizing the risk of catheter contamination, reducing the duration of catheter and mechanical ventilation days, promoting oral feeding, reducing the duration of parenteral nutrition and providing education and feedback to nursery personnel) is the basis for a reduction of nosocomial infection.
- Monitoring of the circulation of pathogens in the nursery and in the NICU is essential.
- Prophylactic use of IVIG is associated with a small reduction in neonatal infections but has no effect on mortality.

Future research

- More studies are required to define key interventions for reducing the incidence and improving the outcome of neonatal sepsis and meningitis.
- Further research on off-label anti-infective drugs for neonates are urgently warranted for the treatment of complicated neonatal infections.
- Development of rational European guidelines for neonatal units are required for optimizing treatment while minimizing overuse of broad-spectrum agents.

Further reading

Burke C. Perinatal sepsis. *J Perinat Neonatal Nurs* 2009;**23**:42–51.

Fernando AM, Heath PT, Menson EN. Antimicrobial policies in the neonatal units of the United Kingdom and Republic of Ireland. *J Antimicrob Chemother* 2008;**61**:743–5.

Galiza EP, Heath PT. Improving the outcome of neonatal meningitis. *Curr Opin Infect Dis* 2009;**22**:229–34.

Chapter 31

Ocular infections

see also Chapters 11, 38, 44, 46, 48, 57, 58, 62, 68, 77, 105, 111

Introduction

Ocular and intraocular infections in children require a rapid review and diagnosis because they are potentially sight-threatening. Prognosis depends on extent and site of infection (Fig. 31.1). In most cases a prompt review by an ophthalmologist is required. This chapter discusses keratitis, endophthalmitis, uveitis, retinitis, and orbital infections.

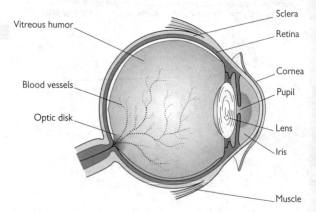

Fig. 31.1 The various anatomical sites in the eye where infections may occur.

Keratitis

- *Definition*—inflammation of the cornea.
- Potentially affects vision, therefore requires urgent ophthalmology review, particularly if associated with corneal ulceration.
- Unlike conjunctivitis, it is characterized by variable loss of vision at presentation.
- Photophobia and reflex blepharospasm make examination difficult particularly in younger children.
- Corneal scrapings may be used to identify causative organism.

Causative organisms

1. Bacterial

- **Most common**.
- Usually caused by direct inoculation, i.e. trauma, contact lens use.
- Dry eyes predispose to bacterial infection.
- Endophthalmitis/corneal perforation results if treatment is delayed.

Neonates

- *Neisseria gonorrhoeae*

Child

- *Staphylococcus aureus*
- *Streptococcus pneumoniae*
- *Pseudomonas aeruginosa*—usually associated with contact lens use
- *Klebsiella pneumoniae*—less commonly *Bacillus cereus*, atypical *Mycobacterium*
- *Chlamydia trachomatis*—extremely common in developing countries and can follow follicular conjunctivitis

Presentation

- Extremely painful.
- Hyperaemia.
- Chemosis, conjunctival injection, focal haziness, corneal opacification.
- Associated purulent conjunctivitis.
- Corneal ulcers.
- Hypopyon—pus in the anterior chamber of the eye, usually collects at the bottom of the chamber and may be seen as a fluid level.

Investigations

- Corneal scrapings, for culture and microscopy after topical anaesthesia under sterile technique.
- May be helpful to culture material from conjunctiva, eyelids, contact lenses.
- Giemsa, Gram, and silver staining required from scrapings.

Differential diagnosis

- Foreign body
- Corneal abrasions

Treatment

- Small ulcers—topical antimicrobials, usually chloramphenicol, fusidic acid, or gentamicin depending on organism suspected.
- Frequency depends on severity of infection; usually begin with drops 2 hourly and tailored accordingly.
- Topical ciprofloxacin or gentamicin, or polymyxin B if *P. aeruginosa* infection is suspected.

2. Viral

- HSV types 1/2—either herpetic conjunctivitis or perinatally acquired. Use of topical steroid drops can exacerbate infection, which can then involve deeper stromal structures and lead to blindness. Acute disease is usually self-limited. Recurrences are common and can lead to a wider area of injury that is thought to be immunologically mediated.

- VZV—with disseminated disease particularly in immunocompromised patients.
- Adenovirus—highly contagious, particularly subgroup D types 8, 19, and 37 which cause epidemic keratoconjunctivitis.
- Molluscum contagiosum, measles, and EBV are rarer causes.

Presentation
- HSV and VZV:
  - Decreased corneal sensation
  - Characteristic dendritic ulcers on fluorescein stain
  - Stromal disease may progress to necrotizing inflammation
  - VZV may cause a nummular keratitis—with fine granular infiltrates in the anterior corneal stroma.
- Adenovirus:
  - Begins unilaterally, pink hyperaemia
  - Clear watery discharge and photophobia
  - Diffuse punctuate keratitis on fluorescein staining
  - Spread to other eye common
  - Acute keratitis lasts 2–3 weeks, followed by subepithelial infiltrates
  - Associated with preauricular lymphadenopathy.

Investigations
- Corneal scrapings should be collected into viral transport media by sterile technique.
- Should have same day inoculation for cell culture.
- PCR is useful for rapid diagnosis for, e.g. HSV, VZV.

Treatment
- HSV:
  - Topical aciclovir five times daily. Continue for at least 3 days post healing, usually for 10–14 days
  - Oral aciclovir or valaciclovir for 7–14 days has adequate corneal penetration and may be preferable in paediatric patients. Oral agents may be used for up to 12 months to prevent recurrence at prophylactic doses.
- VZV:
  - Topical antimicrobials to prevent secondary infection
  - Systemic aciclovir in severe disease or immunocompromise for 7–14 days or until lesions have healed
  - In severe keratitis topical corticosteroids may be used in conjunction with above.
- Adenovirus:
  - Artificial tears ± cycloplegics.

3. Fungal
- Rare risks include underlying immunocompromise, corneal trauma.
- *Candida* most common, filamentous fungi, e.g. *Fusarium*, *Aspergillus* less so in children.

Presentation and differential
- Slowly enlarging corneal ulcers with feathery margins.
- Central corneal opacification.
- Candida associated with yellowish white microabscesses.

Investigations
- Corneal scrapings for extended culture.
- Silver staining or calcoflour white staining may be required for microscopy.

Treatment
- Topical fluconazole 1% intravenous solution, miconazole 10mg/ml or amphotericin B (0.15–1%).
- May be used in conjunction with systemic therapy if severe.

Endophthalmitis

- *Definition*—infection of intraocular fluid and/or intraocular structures
- Emergency therefore requires prompt recognition.
- Requires urgent review by ophthalmology.
- Most commonly caused by penetrating trauma or associated systemic infection.
- Culture/smear of aqueous, vitreous fluids, and conjunctiva required to identify organism.

Causative organisms

Trauma/postoperative infection
Acute (within 48–72 hours)
- Coagulase-negative staphylococci
- *S. aureus*
- Streptococci
- *Pseudomonas*
- *B. cereus*—characterized by abrupt onset of symptoms 12–24 hours after eye injury, and a ring corneal infiltrate. Most eyes lose all vision even with prompt treatment
- *Candida*, usually *Candida parapsilosis*
- *Aspergillus*, rarely *Fusarium* species
Delayed
- Coagulase-negative staphylococci
- *Propionibacterium acnes*
- *Candida*
- *Aspergillus*

Endogenous (haematogenous)
- Streptococcus, most commonly *S. pneumoniae*
- Staphylococcus
- *Candida*, most commonly *C. albicans* as more virulent
- *N. meningitidis*
- *B. cereus*
- Enteric Gram-negative bacilli

Presentation
Depends on infecting organism, bacterial load, virulence and host defence mechanisms:

- Eye pain, redness, lid swelling
- Decreased visual acuity
- Photophobia
- Conjunctival oedema
- Blepharospasm
- Hypopyon
- Fundoscopy shows:
  - Chorioretinitis
  - Vasculitis
  - Retinal haemorrhage and vitreous cellular reactions resembling cottonwool balls are characteristic of *Candida*.

Differential diagnosis

- Post-traumatic inflammatory response.
- Drug reactions most notably with rifabutin, cidofovir.
- Tumours, e.g. retinoblastoma, lymphoma.

Investigations

- Culture of aqueous, vitreous, and conjunctiva must be obtained under general anaesthesia.
- Extended cultures may be required.
- Gram, Giemsa, and silver staining for microscopy.
- Endogenous endophthalmitis requires systemic review and culture of urine, blood and CSF.

Treatment

Trauma or postoperative infection

- Vitrectomy then intravitreal, regular periocular, and topical antibiotics.
- Although systemic antibiotic penetration into the vitrea is poor, it will require consideration.
- If no or poor response within 3 days, a repeat vitrectomy may be required.
- Organism present on smears should guide initial therapy—often broad-spectrum antibiotics commenced initially.
- Intravitreal agents are used after diagnostic tap.

Bacterial

- Intravitreal ceftazidime and vancomycin at separate locations with separate syringes.
- Vancomycin with either amikacin, gentamicin, or tobramycin. Aminoglycosides may cause retinal damage.

Fungal

- Choice of the antifungals depends on organism suspected, commence with amphotericin B.
- Prognosis better if treated early.
- May require repeat intravitreal injection.

Corticosteroids may be used in addition to above, using antifungals both the intravitreal and oral routes as fibrovascular proliferation and possible retinal detachment may complicate infection.

Endogenous infection

- Systemic antimicrobial therapy will be required depending on systemic disease and organism isolated.
- The prognosis is better if systemic antifungals are commenced early if fungal disease is suspected.
- Intravitreal antimicrobials/antifungals will be required in addition if optic nerve/macula involvement or severe vitritis is present.

Complications

- Corneal oedema and glaucoma
- Retinal detachment
- Panophthalmitis
- Orbital abscess
- Cavernous sinus thrombosis

Uveitis, retinitis, and optic neuritis

Definition—Inflammation of the internal structures of the eye.

Uveitis

- This is the inflammation of iris (anterior), ciliary body, and choroid (posterior).
- Acute inflammation—usually lasts 2–6 weeks with chronic inflammation being more insidious.
- More commonly caused by autoimmune disease, than infection.
- Organisms associated:
  - HSV as part of disseminated HSV infection, more common in neonates
  - VZV
  - Rubella
  - Human immunodeficiency virus
  - *Mycobacterium tuberculosis*, often associated with HIV infection
  - *Borrelia burgdorferi*
  - *Toxoplasma gondii*
  - *Bartonella henselae*
  - *Treponema pallidum*
  - *Histoplasma*—rarely found in children.

Presentation

- Insidious irritation in one or both eyes.
- Dilatation of vessels at corneal-conjunctival junction known as limbal flush.
- Blurred vision.
- Photophobia.
- May present with cataracts/vitreous haze.
- Slit-lamp examination shows haziness and precipitates.
- Miliary tubercles or tuberculoma found in ocular tuberculosis.

Differential diagnosis

- Traumatic iritis
- Juvenile rheumatoid arthritis
- Behçet's syndrome

- Ankylosing spondylitis
- Sarcoidosis

Diagnosis
- Careful history including travel, pets, contacts, immune status, medication, diet, family history of autoimmune disease.
- Tests include: chest radiograph, FBC, ESR, CRP, ANA, rheumatoid factor, angiotensin-converting enzyme (ACE), HLA-B27, serology (for HSV, rubella, HIV, rubella, *Toxoplasma*, *Bartonella*, *Borrelia*), TB ELISPOT and Mantoux, PCR of ocular fluid for HSV, *Toxoplasma*.

Treatment
- Ophthalmology review.
- Treat systemic disease.
- Topical corticosteroids in anterior uveitis, prednisolone 1% 2 hourly tapered according to response.
- Intermediate uveitis treated with periocular methylprednisolone injections.
- Chronic uveitis may be treated with methotrexate or ciclosporin under expert review.

Complications
- Cataracts
- Deposition of cellular debris on iris
- Raised intraocular pressure
- Decreased visual acuity

Retinitis
- Defined as inflammation of the retina or choroid or both.
- May be unilateral or bilateral and may be a manifestation of systemic disease.
- When the macula is involved blindness may result.

Organisms
- HSV, VZV, CMV—all are acquired perinatally (or later in life) depending on immune status. Infect epithelial cells and cause neurotropism. Usually presents as haemorrhagic retinitis, with yellow patches, or a blanched retina with areas of haemorrhage (Fig. 31.2).
- Rubella—congenital infection.
- *T. gondii*—infection is usually congenital or due to congenital reactivation. Presents as a retinochoroiditis, with focal necrosis and additional anterior chamber inflammation. Chorioretinal pigment clumping causes deposition around peripheral zone of inflammation. Often associated with central nervous system calcification.
- *B. henselae*—indirect ophthalmoscopy typically shows a macular star or stellate retinopathy.
- *Toxocara canis*—pica or exposure to dog excrement resulting in ocular larva migrans. Inflammation occurs after larval death with eosinophilic and mononuclear cell infiltration. Indirect ophthalmoscopy shows a granulomatous mass associated with vitritis.
- *T. pallidum*—presents with both an interstitial keratitis and retinitis.
- HIV—retinopathy typically associated with haemorrhagic vasculitis.

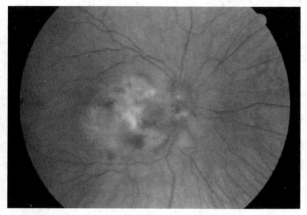

Fig. 31.2 Cytomegalovirus retinitis showing granular retinitis with perivascular sheathing.

(Reproduced from National Eye Institute, National Institutes of Health)

Presentation—may be indolent or fulminant
- Decreased visual acuity
- Photophobia
- Diminished red reflex
- Ocular floaters
- Photopsia
- Ophthalmoscopy shows patchy areas of white or haemorrhage on the retina with vitreous haze

Differential diagnosis
- Retinal haemorrhage post trauma
- Systemic lupus erythematosus (SLE)
- HIV retinopathy
- Aicardi's syndrome
- Retinoblastoma

Investigations
- CXR, FBC, ESR, CRP, ANA, rheumatoid factor, ACE, HLA-B27, serology (for HSV, rubella, HIV, VDRL, *Toxocara*, *Toxoplasma*, *Bartonella*, *Borrelia*), PCR of ocular fluid for HSV, *Toxoplasma*.

Treatment
- HSV/VZV:
  - Intravenous aciclovir for 5–10 days which reduces risk of infection in second eye by 50%
  - Followed by oral aciclovir or valaciclovir for 4–6 weeks.
- CMV:
  - Ganciclovir or foscarnet or cidofovir intravenously as induction therapy for 2–3 weeks

- Followed by long-term maintenance therapy for months. Ganciclovir can be implanted as a sustained release system to last 4–6 months.
- Rubella—supportive treatment.
- Syphilis—treat as tertiary syphilis, benzylpenicillin every 4–6 hours for 14 days.
- Toxoplasmosis
  - Congenital toxoplasmosis should be treated with pyrimethamine twice daily for 2 days, then once daily for 6 months, then three times a week for 6 months and sulfadiazine (twice daily for 12 months), with leucovirin (three times a week) for a year. Corticosteroids may be added under expert advice.
  - Older children are generally not treated unless immuno-compromised or the lesions are close to the optic nerve or macula.
- *Toxacara*:
  - Usually not treated unless associated with visceral larva migrans, which requires ivermectin, albendazole, or tiabendazole.

Orbital infections

Preseptal cellulitis

- Preseptal cellulitis differs from orbital cellulitis in that it is confined to the soft tissues that are anterior to the orbital septum.
- Common infection of the eyelid and periorbital soft tissues are characterized by acute eyelid erythema and oedema.
- Results from local spread of adjacent upper respiratory tract infection, external ocular infection, or following trauma to the eyelids.
- Approximately 80% of preseptal infection occurs in children <10 years of age, most <5 years. Patients with preseptal cellulitis tend to be younger than patients with orbital cellulitis.

Causative organisms
Bacterial
- *S. pneumoniae*, *S. aureus*, *H. influenzae* type b, more commonly in prevaccination era
- Anaerobes

Presentation
- Pain.
- Conjunctivitis.
- Periorbital erythema and oedema (sometimes so severe that patients cannot voluntarily open the eye).
- Sinus tenderness, rhinorrhea, adenopathy, and other hallmarks of upper respiratory tract infection may be present.

Differential diagnosis
- Nephrotic syndrome
- Allergic reaction
- Conjunctivitis
- Contact dermatitis

Investigations
- CRP and WCC are usually elevated, blood culture is usually negative.
- Samples of conjunctival discharge, eyelid lesions, and lacrimal sac material should be sent for culture.

Treatment
- Mild preseptal cellulitis—oral co-amoxiclav or a first-generation cephalosporin. Flucloxacillin or clindamycin if S. aureus suspected.
- In more severe preseptal cellulitis or if the child fails to respond within 48–72 hours, consider intravenous antibiotics. Usually IV co-amoxiclav or cefuroxime for 24–48 hours followed by oral antibiotics.
- Clinical improvement should be seen within 24–48 hours. If the patient worsens, then consider an underlying orbital process or resistant organisms.

Complications
- Orbital cellulitis.
- Spread along tissue planes to cause subperiosteal abscess, orbital abscess, or cavernous sinus thrombosis.
- Intracranial infection, high-risk features include age >7 years, subperiosteal abscess, headache and fever persisting despite intravenous antibiotics.
- Patients who are immunocompromised have a higher likelihood of developing fungal infections and orbital extension.

Orbital cellulitis
- Infection of the soft tissues of the orbit posterior to the orbital septum.
- Involve ophthalmology and ENT early.
- Median age of children hospitalized with orbital cellulitis is 7–12 years.
- Caused by extension of an infection from the periorbital structures, most commonly from the paranasal sinuses, direct inoculation of the orbit from trauma or haematogenous spread from bacteraemia.

Causative organisms
Bacteria
- *Streptococcus* species
- *S. aureus*
- *H. influenzae* type b, more commonly in prevaccination era
- *Pseudomonas*
- *Klebsiella*
- *Enterococcus*

Polymicrobial infections with aerobic and anaerobic bacteria are more common in patients aged ≥16 years.

Fungal
- *Mucor* and *Aspergillus* most common, usually associated with immunocompromise.

Presentation
- Conjunctival chemosis.
- Lid oedema.
- Rhinorrhoea, purulent nasal discharge may be present.

- Orbital pain and tenderness are present early.
- Vision may be normal early, but it may become difficult to evaluate in very ill children with marked oedema.
- Dark red discoloration of the eyelids, chemosis, hyperaemia of the conjunctiva.
- Proptosis and ophthalmoplegia develop as infection progresses.
- Late signs are increased orbital pressure, reduced corneal sensation.

Differential diagnosis
- Thyroid exophthalmos
- Idiopathic inflammation—sarcoidosis orbital myositis, orbital pseudotumour, Wegener's granulomatosis
- Neoplasm with inflammation—lymphoma, histiocytosis X, leukaemia, retinoblastoma, rhabdomyosarcoma.

Investigations
- FBC—leucocytosis common, blood cultures prior to the administration of any antibiotics, although they are unlikely to reveal the responsible organism. Swab purulent material from the nose for Gram stain, and culture on both aerobic and anaerobic media.
- Needle aspiration of the orbit is contraindicated.
- Lumbar puncture if any signs of meningism.
- CT with contrast or MRI (MRI better if cavernous sinus thrombosis suspected).
- If ethmoidectomy performed, culture and stain aspirate, request extended aerobic and anaerobic culture.
- Continuing deterioration on antibiotic therapy suggests abscess formation and repeat imaging will be required.

Treatment
- Urgent iv antibiotics—e.g. ceftriaxone IV and metronidazole, or high dose co-amoxiclav. Clindamycin may be added.
- Ophthalmology and ENT review.
- Sinus surgery may be required.
- Consider orbital surgery, in every case of subperiosteal or intraorbital abscess, particularly if; decrease in vision occurs, an afferent pupillary defect develops, proptosis progresses despite appropriate antibiotic therapy or the size of the abscess does not reduce on CT scan within 48–72 hours after appropriate antibiotics have been administered.
- In cases of fungal infection, surgical debridement of the orbit is indicated together with high-dose antifungal treatment, usually amphotericin B or Ambisome IV.
- Neurosurgical involvement if cerebral abscess on imaging.

Complications
- Subperiorbital or orbital abscess
- Permanent vision loss from corneal damage
- Meningitis
- Cavernous sinus thrombosis
- Intracranial, epidural, or subdural abscess formation

Table 31.1 presents a comparison of the two types of cellulitis.

Table 31.1 Preseptal versus orbital cellulitis

	Preseptal	Orbital
Proptosis	Absent	Present
Ocular motility	Normal	Painful and restricted
Visual acuity	Normal	Reduced in severe cases
Colour vision	Normal	Reduced in severe cases
Relative afferent papillary defect	Normal	Present in severe cases

Reproduced from Denniston A, Murray P (2006). *Oxford Handbook of Ophthalmology*, with permission from Oxford University Press.

Further reading

Brook I. Microbiology and antimicrobial treatment of orbital and intracranial complications of sinusitis in children and their management. *Int J Pediatr Otorhinolaryngol* 2009;**73**;1183–6.

Fan JC, Niederer RL, von Lany H, Polkinghorne PJ. Infectious endophthalmitis: clinical features, management and visual outcomes. *Clin Experiment Ophthalmol* 2008;**36**:631–6.

Rodriguez-Adrián LJ, King RT, Tamayo-Derat LG, Miller JW, Garcia CA, Rex JH. Retinal lesions as clues to disseminated bacterial and candidal infections: frequency, natural history, and etiology. *Med (Balt)* 2003;**82**:187–202.

Thordsen JE, Harris L, Hubbard GB 3rd. Pediatric endophthalmitis. A 10-year consecutive series. *Retina* 2008;**28** Suppl:S3–7.

Chapter 32

Periodic fever syndromes

📖 see also Chapter 33

Definition

- Periodic fever syndromes are also known as 'autoinflammatory diseases'.
- The term refers to a group of conditions characterized by hereditary recurrent or periodic episodes of systemic inflammation.
- Usually present as fever associated sometimes with rash, serositis, lymphadenopathy or arthritis.

Types of periodic fever syndromes

- Familial Mediterranean fever (FMF)
- Tumour necrosis factor (TNF) receptor-associated periodic fever syndrome (TRAPS)
- Hyper IgD syndrome (HIDS)
- Cryopyrin-associated periodic fever syndromes (CAPS)
- Periodic fever, aphthous stomatitis, pharyngitis, and adenitis syndrome (PFAPA).

Familial Mediterranean fever

Epidemiology

- Most common periodic fever syndrome.
- Usually seen in people from eastern Mediterranean regions (Sephardic Jews, Armenians, Turks, and North African populations).
- Usually autosomal recessive—carrier frequency of 1 in 4 in some populations.
- Almost 80% of cases have onset in childhood or adolescence.

Clinical features

- Fever with painful serositis (peritonitis, pleuritis, arthritis—large joint, rarely pericarditis).
- Peritonitis can mimic acute abdomen—more usually painful all over.
- Erysipelas like rash on lower part of legs.
- Headache, arthritis, and chest pain also seen in some children.
- Elevated inflammatory markers, CRP, WCC.
- High risk of amyloid in untreated patients.

- Attacks are often short lived, but can last for 1–3 days—no fixed pattern of attacks—can be menstruation related.

Diagnosis
- Mainly clinical—needs to be thought of—often long delay before diagnosis.
- DNA analysis for known genotypes (mutations in *MEFV* gene, which codes for pyrin) can be very helpful.
- Most laboratories offer only limited genotype analysis.

Treatment
- Colchicine very effective as a prophylactic agent to reduce frequency and severity of attacks.
- Acute attacks need supportive therapy—anti-inflammatories.
- IL-1 inhibitors (e.g. anakinra, a recombinant IL-1 receptor antagonist) are effective in colchicine-resistant patients.

TNF receptor-associated periodic fever syndrome

TRAPS was previously known as 'Familial Hibernian fever'.

Epidemiology
- Autosomal dominant.
- Mainly affects people of Northern European extraction but seen in all ethnic groups.

Clinical features
- Usual onset during childhood or adolescence.
- Variable clinical picture.
- Episodes can last for 1–3 weeks.
- Episodes characterized by fever associated with myalgia, arthralgia, abdominal pain, or chest pain.
- Skin lesions include erythematous rash with oedema or on occasions serpiginous plaques.
- Conjunctivitis and periorbital oedema are also seen in some children.
- Amyloidosis is seen in 25% of patients with TRAPS.

Diagnosis
- Mutation analysis reveals mutation in the gene for TNF receptor superfamily 1A (TNFRS F1A) in affected children.
- Not all known mutations may be screened in labs.

Treatment
- Fever episodes do respond to steroids.
- Some patients have response to anti-TNF drugs such as etanercept.
- Growing evidence than IL-1 inhibitors (anakinra) may be effective in this condition.

Hyper IgD syndrome

Epidemiology

- Autosomal recessive disease.
- Initially described in Dutch and north European populations.
- Reported in all ethnic groups.
- Disease onset early in life, almost always present in paediatric age group.

Clinical features

- Recurrent episodes of fever every 4–6 weeks.
- Last for 3–7 days.
- Fever may be associated with lymphadenopathy, abdominal pain, diarrhoea and vomiting, mucocutaneous lesions, and arthritis.
- Headaches are also seen in some patients.
- Can resolve in adult life in some patients.

Diagnosis

- High serum IgD seen usually but not always.
- High IgA seen in 80% of cases.
- High inflammatory markers.
- Mevalonic acid in urine during attacks
- Mutations in mevalonic kinase (*MVK*) gene can be identified in most patients.

Treatment

- Fever attacks may respond well to steroids.
- Non-steroidal anti-inflammatory drugs (e.g. naproxen) and statin therapy have been reported to be of benefit in some patients.
- Recent reports show a good response to anti-TNF agents (etanercept) and IL-1 inhibitors (e.g. anakinra, a recombinant IL-1 receptor antagonist).

Cryopyrin-associated periodic fever syndromes

Epidemiology

- Includes Muckle Wells syndrome (MWS), familial cold urticaria syndrome (FCAS) and CINCA/NOMID syndrome (chronic infantile neurological, cutaneous and articular syndrome/neonatal onset multisystem inflammatory disorder).
- Autosomal dominantly inherited conditions with varying severity.
- Most reported patients of European ancestry but seen in all ethnic groups.

Clinical features

Familial cold urticaria syndrome

- Intermittent episodes of urticarial rash associated with exposure to cold.
- Fever and arthralgia also seen.
- Other symptoms include nausea, drowsiness, and sweating post episode.

Muckle Wells syndrome

- Recurrent episodes of urticarial lesions.
- Associated with fever, malaise, limb pain.
- Development of sensorineural hearing loss in early childhood.
- Risk of amyloidosis in uncontrolled disease.

CINCA syndrome

- Also known as NOMID (neonatal onset multisystem inflammatory disorder).
- Most severe of CAPS syndromes.
- Presents in neonatal period.
- Characterised by urticarial rash, typical facies with frontal bossing, saddle nose, and mid-face hypoplasia.
- Bony overgrowth of patella.
- Chronic polyarthritis.
- Aseptic meningitis, severe uveitis, chronic papilloedema, sensorineural hearing loss also seen.

Diagnosis

- Raised acute phase reactants.
- Mutations in *NLRP3/CIAS1* gene.
- Several mutations identified.

Treatment

- All CAPS patients respond dramatically to IL-1 inhibitor (anakinra).
- Therapy results in marked improvement in children.
- Newer long acting IL-1 inhibitors are currently being trialled.

Periodic fever, aphthous stomatitis, pharyngitis, and adenitis syndrome

PFAPA is also known as Marshall's syndrome.

Clinical features

- Onset <5 years of age.
- Episodes of sudden onset high fever every 2–6 weeks lasting for 2–6 days.
- Aphthous ulcers are the key symptom.
- Febrile episodes associated with pharyngitis and cervical adenitis.
- Headache, abdominal pain, and arthralgia may also be present.

Diagnosis
- Negative for mutations of other periodic fever syndromes.
- Diagnostic criteria not very helpful.

Treatment
- Controversial—improves as child gets older anyway.
- Fever attacks respond to 1–3 day course of steroids.
- Some reports of resolution of attacks with tonsillectomy.

Future research

The optimal management of most of these conditions is poorly evidence based, with very few randomized trials to support treatment advice.

Further reading

Gattorno M, Federici S, Pelagatti MA, *et al.* Diagnosis and management of autoinflammatory diseases in childhood. *J Clin Immunol* 2008;**28** Suppl 1:S73–83.

Lachmann HJ, Hawkins PN. Developments in the scientific and clinical understanding of autoinflammatory disorders. *Arthritis Res Ther* 2009;**11**:212.

Yao Q, Furst DE. Autoinflammatory diseases: an update of clinical and genetic aspects. *Rheumatology (Oxf)* 2008;**47**:946–51.

Pyrexia of unknown origin

📖 see also Chapters 32, 34

Introduction

- In 1961, Petersdorf and Beeson defined pyrexia of unknown origin (PUO) as fever higher than 38.3°C (101°F) on several occasions, persisting without diagnosis for at least 3 weeks, with at least 1 week of investigation in hospital.
- True PUO (or FUO, fever of unknown origin) is a not a common paediatric problem. In most children presenting with fever, the child recovers before a definitive diagnosis has been made and a viral infection is assumed to be the cause. Children with a real, persistent fever may have a serious underlying disease.
- The three commonest causes are malignancy, an autoimmune condition or an unusual infection (e.g. TB, HIV, or *Salmonella*) where a delayed diagnosis can be very important to the child and the family. In addition, children presenting with PUO may need prolonged hospital admission and multiple investigations, which have cost and resource implications.

Definition

- With the development of newer diagnostic tests and increasing cost of hospitalization, the PUO definition has been changed. The classic definition of fever for 3 weeks has been replaced by a: *fever on three outpatient visits or 3 days in the hospital without elucidation of a cause* or *fever where no cause is found after 1 week of 'intelligent and invasive' ambulatory investigations.*[1] In addition, there are three other categories added to this new definition: nosocomial PUO, neutropenic PUO, and HIV-associated PUO.[1]
- Table 33.1 outlines the different definitions of PUO with possible causes.

Differential diagnosis

There is a wide differential diagnosis for cases presenting with PUO. The broad categories include infection, autoimmune/rheumatological conditions, malignancy, inflammatory bowel disease, and a miscellaneous group. The disorders listed in Table 33.2 are those which may be encountered in Europe and North America. A simple mnemonic to remember these

Table 33.1 Definitions of PUO with possible causes

	Definition	Causes
Classic PUO Revised PUO	Temperature >38.3°C Duration >3 weeks 1 week of inpatient evaluation Evaluation of at least 3 days in hospital/3 outpatient visits/1 week logical and intensive testing	Infection, Rheumatological conditions, malignancy, Others
Nosocomial PUO	Temperature >38.3°C Patient hospitalized >48 hours, negative blood cultures, no fever incubating on admission	HCAI, including *C. difficile*, drug-induced, catheter related, pulmonary embolism
Neutropenic PUO	Temperature >38.3°C, negative blood cultures, neutrophil count <1 × 10⁹, evaluation of at least 3 days	Febrile neutropenia, other opportunistic bacterial infection, CVC infection, fungal or viral infection
HIV-associated PUO	In known HIV patients: Temperature >38.3°C, negative blood cultures, duration >4 weeks outpatient OR >3 days inpatient	CMV, mycobacterial (atypical and typical), PcP, malignancies, depends on CD4 count

broad groups on the ward round is 'If you don't know what this can be, think of TB, SLE and malignancy'.

- A very thorough travel history is important to both include and exclude specific infections.
- Ask about common and unusual pets—snakes, parrots, pigeons all may be important. Ask about hobbies—a water sport raises the possibility of leptospirosis, forest walking of Lyme disease.
- A family history of autoimmune disease, immunodeficiency, or recurrent/unusual infections should be taken.
- A detailed drug history is required, as drug allergy may present with a fever and no rash.

Table 33.2 Disorders that may be encountered in Europe and North America

Bacterial	Tuberculosis, Brucellosis, cat scratch disease, *Salmonella typhi* infection, *Campylobacter* infection, *Spirochaete* infection, rheumatic fever
	Localized or occult bacterial infection, abscess, sinusitis, osteomyelitis, pyelonephritis, arthritis, endocarditis, meningitis
Viral	EBV, CMV, HIV infection, hepatitis, enterovirus
Atypical	*Mycoplasma*, *Chlamydia*, *Rickettsia*

Table 33.2 (*Contd.*)

Parasitic	Malaria, toxoplasmosis, giardiasis, toxocariasis, trypanosomiasis
Fungal	*Histoplasma*
Autoimmune diseases	SLE, polyarteritis nodosa, systemic-onset JIA, vasculitis, sarcoidosis, post-infectious inflammatory syndromes
Neoplastic	Leukaemia, lymphoma, solid tumors (Wilm's tumour, neuroblastoma), histiocytosis
Miscellaneous	Endocrine diseases (thyroiditis); Kawasaki disease; Kikuchi Fujimoto syndrome; drug fever; inflammatory bowel disease; head injury; periodic fever, factitious fever

Management

A good clinical history and a thorough clinical examination repeated every day remains the mainstay in the diagnosis of PUO. Frequently new signs arise that were not present on admission, including the evanescent rash of JIA, which only comes in the evening when the consultant has gone home, or the slowly enlarging lymph nodes in lymphoma.

Investigations should be directed by clues from the history and examination. A stepwise approach to investigations should be taken and a period of inpatient observation is very useful, as some conditions evolve over time. There is an art to the investigation of PUO, minimizing unnecessary investigations, while obtaining the correct diagnosis as quickly as possible. The child, the family, and often the doctor find the uncertainty difficult to deal with.

Table 33.3 summarizes some of the common presenting symptoms and likely diagnoses.

Table 33.3 Common presenting symptoms and likely diagnoses

History	Likely diagnosis	Investigations
Fever—type, duration, pattern	Quotidian fever—systemic-onset JIA	Raised inflammatory markers
	Tertian/quartan (rare)—malaria	Malarial film
	Recurrent fever—periodic fever, brucellosis	Genetic studies, IgD
	Nocturnal fever—tuberculosis, lymphoma	Mantoux test, QuantiFERON, tissue biopsy, bone marrow
Travel abroad	Asia, sub-Saharan Africa—malaria, typhoid	📖 See Chapter 27
	North America—Rocky mountain fever, Lyme's disease	
	East Asia—filariasis, dengue	

(*Continued*)

Table 33.3 (Contd.)

History	Likely diagnosis	Investigations
Exposure to wild/domestic animals	Toxoplasmosis, leptospirosis Lyme's disease	Specific serology test
Rash	JIA	
Lymphadenopathy	Infections, autoimmune diseases, malignancies	Serology, autoimmune test, biopsy, bone marrow
Abdominal pain, gastrointestinal symptoms	Inflammatory bowel disease Intra-abdominal collection Gastrointestinal infection	Barium studies, endoscopy and biopsy, ultrasound
Uveitis	Sarcoidosis, JIA, SLE, Kawasaki disease	Angiotensin-converting enzyme level, inflammatory markers, autoimmune screen
Chorioretinitis	CMV, toxoplasmosis, syphilis	Virus isolation, PCRs, specific serology
Weight loss	TB, malignancies, inflammatory bowel disease	Tests for TB, bone marrow, endoscopy

Investigations

Investigations should be directed by the history. It is not a good idea to send hundreds of tests for every possible diagnosis. Table 33.4 gives guidance regarding initial investigations that may be considered. Further investigations are directed towards the clinical picture and organ involvement if any. Blind imaging studies such as bone scans and whole body MRI or bone marrow aspiration are rarely helpful.

Table 33.4 Investigations for evaluating children presenting with PUO

Baseline investigations should include	Other investigations that may be included if the history is suggestive
Haematology – FBC, blood film, ESR, malaria films (if travelled)	Mantoux test, QuantiFERON® gamma
Chemistry—CRP, LFTs, U&Es, bone profile	Thyroid function tests, ferritin, triglycerides, genetic studies—haemophagocytic lymphohistiocytosis, periodic fever
Microbiology—blood cultures × 3, urine, stool culture, CSF, throat swab	Autoimmune tests – autoantibodies, ANA, dsDNA, immunoglobulin, complements, lymphocyte subsets
Serology—ASOT, Mycoplasma, EBV, Lyme serology	
Viral isolation /PCR—EBV, CMV, adenovirus	
Radiology—chest radiograph, ultrasound abdomen	Radiology—ECHO, CT, MRI, Barium studies, endoscopy, bone scan, white cell scan, angiogram
	Histology—Bone marrow, lymph node, liver, skin biopsy

Outcome

In studies no cause has been found for PUO in between 5% and 35% cases. Consideration should also be given to the possibility of factitious illness and periodic fever syndromes. Table 33.5 shows the final diagnosis of PUO in different paediatric studies conducted in the past 10 years.

Table 33.5 Summary of final diagnoses of PUO

First author, country	No of patients	Infection (%) (commonest causes)	Autoimmune/ rheumatology (%)	No cause found (%)
Pasic, Belgrade[2]	185	37.8 (EBV, Leishmania)	12.9	29.1
Bakashvili, Russia[3]	52	61 (respiratory, UTI)	3.8	13.4
Chouchane, Tunisia[4]	67	56.7 (Leishmania, hydatid)	20.9	19.4
Cogulu, Turkey[5]	80	58.7 (respiratory, UTI)	13.2	19.4
Chantada, Argentina[6]	113	36.2 (respiratory, TB)	13.2	19.4

Future research

A key area of research is the development of the most cost-effective and time efficient algorithms in the management of PUO.

Key references

1 Durack DT, Street AC. Fever of unknown origin——re-examined and redefined. *Curr Clin Top Infect Dis* 1991;**11**:35–51.
2 Pasic S, Minic A, Druric P, et al. Fever of unknown origin in 185 paediatric patients: a single-centre experience. *Acta Paediatr* 2006;**95**:463–6.
3 Bakashvili LZ, Makhviladze MA, Pakava EK, et al. Fever of unknown origin in children and adolescents in Georgia: a case review of 52 patients. *Georgian Med News* 2006;**135**:66–9.
4 Chouchane S, Chouchane CH, Ben Meriem CH, et al. Prolonged fever in children. Retrospective study of 67 cases. *Arch Pediatr* 2004;**11**:1319–25.4.
5 Cogulu O, Koturoglu G, Kurogol Z, et al. Evaluation of 80 children with prolonged fever. *Pediatrics International* 2003;**45**:564–569.
6 Chantada G, Casak S, Plata JD, et al. Children with fever of unknown origin in Argentina: analysis of 113 cases. *Pediatr Infect Dis J* 1994;**13**(4):260–3.

Chapter 34

Rash: making a diagnosis

📖 see also Chapters 10, 42, 57, 64, 71, 77, 78, 79, 84, 86, 87, 88, 90, 93, 101, 102, 105, 106, 115

Introduction

- Skin rashes or exanthems are among the most common clinical presentations in childhood. They are associated with diseases ranging from benign self-limiting illnesses caused by viruses to severe life-threatening bacterial infections.
- Enanthems are eruptions on mucous membranes—inside the body.

Causative organisms

Rashes in childhood are most commonly caused by viruses, but may also be bacterial or non-infectious in origin (Table 34.1).

Table 34.1 Aetiology of different types of rash in children

Type of rash	Viral	Bacterial	Other infections	Other
Maculo-papular	Measles	Staphylococcal and streptococcal toxic shock	Toxoplasmosis	Kawasaki disease
	Rubella		*Rickettsia*	Pityriasis rosea
	EBV, CMV	Scarlet fever	*Mycoplasma*	Juvenile chronic arthritis
	Erythema infectiosum (parvovirus B19)	*Borrelia*	Psittacosis	
		Typhoid		Drug reaction
	Roseola infantum (HHV-6 and 7)	Brucellosis		Eczema
		Arcanobacterium haemolyticum		SLE
	Enterovirus			Dermatitis
	Adenovirus			
	Dengue			

Table 34.1 (Contd.)

Type of rash	Viral	Bacterial	Other infections	Other
Petechial/ purpuric	Enterovirus	Meningococcus	*Rickettsia*	Henoch–Schönlein purpura
	EBV	Pneumococcus	Malaria	
	Papular purpuric gloves and socks syndrome	Leptospirosis	Leishmaniasis	Haemolytic uraemic syndrome
		Bacterial endocarditis		
	Viral haemorrhagic fevers			Idiopathic thrombocytopenic purpura
	Congenital CMV/rubella			Leukaemia
				Neuroblastoma
Vesicular/ bullous	Varicella	Staphylococcal scalded skin	*Mycoplasma*	Stevens–Johnson syndrome
	HSV			
	Enterovirus, especially Coxsackie	Staphylococcal and streptococcal impetigo		
Scaly			Fungal, e.g. tinea	Eczema
				Psoriasis
				Pityriasis rosea

Epidemiology

- In recent studies with modern molecular diagnostic techniques, the proportion of rashes that have a cause found approaches 50%.
- In the UK and Europe the most commonly identified causes of a maculopapular rash are:[1]
  - Parvovirus B19 (17%)
  - GAS (15%)
  - HHV-6 (6%)
  - Enterovirus (5%)
  - Adenovirus (4%).
- The incidence of varicella is around 25/10 000 in Europe.
- Although measles and rubella account for fewer than 1% of cases in these highly immunized populations, the number of cases is increasing in the UK and several other European countries.
- According to the Health Protection Agency, the number of laboratory-confirmed cases of measles in the UK in 2007 was 990, which increased by almost 40% to 1370 in 2008.
- Studies undertaken outside Europe feature dengue fever and measles as common causes of rash and these should therefore be considered when a child presenting with a rash has recently travelled abroad.

Clinical presentation and differential diagnosis

- Most of the organisms associated with rashes discussed in this chapter are detailed in other specific chapters, so the emphasis here is the clinical distinction between different causes of rash.
- Diagnosis is particularly important in:
  - Severe infection
  - The immunocompromised host
  - When there is contact with a pregnant woman.
- The causes of rash in childhood are frequently difficult to differentiate from each other. However, the incidence of many infections peaks in specific age groups and the aetiology can be narrowed down by careful history and examination.

History

Prodromal symptoms

- Most infectious rashes in childhood are associated with systemic symptoms such as fever, and these symptoms may precede the onset of rash (Table 34.2).
- The differential diagnosis of prodromal symptoms such as fever, conjunctivitis, and lymphadenopathy includes Kawasaki disease and adenoviral infection, both of which also manifest with a rash.

Table 34.2 Prodromal symptoms associated with common exanthems

Infection	Duration	Symptoms
Measles	3–4 days	Fever, coryza, conjunctivitis, cough
Rubella	1–5 days	Fever, lymphadenopathy, conjunctivitis (rare in children)
Varicella	1–2 days	Fever, cough, coryza, sore throat (less in children)
Erythema infectiosum	2–3 days	Mild fever, malaise (less in children)
Roseola infantum	3 days	High fever which defervesces when rash appears
Scarlet fever	1–2 days	Fever, sore throat, headache, abdominal pain

Evolution of the rash

- Some rashes appear as generalized rashes over the entire body at onset, while others change in nature or distribution.
- The rash of chicken pox starts as macules and papules and then develops into vesicles that eventually crust over. Lesions at different stages exist at the same time.

- The rash of rubella starts with a facial rash that spreads to the remainder of the body.
- The rash of erythema infectiosum starts as an erythematous rash on the cheeks that may also progress to include a lacy rash of the trunk and limbs.
- The rash of roseola infantum starts on the neck and trunk and then spreads to the face and limbs.
- The rash of Rocky Mountain Spotted Fever starts on the hands and feet and spreads up the limbs to the trunk (remember—climb UP the mountain).
- The rash of Lyme disease classically begins with a circular red annular lesion expanding outward from the site of the tick bite, which develops into a bulls eye lesion (erythema chronicum migrans). After several days macular lesions may develop at other sites on the body, distant from the original bite.
- Several rashes desquamate with time, including scarlet fever, Kawasaki disease, syphilis, and various toxin-mediated infections.

Associated symptoms

- Respiratory symptoms may be associated with roseola infantum and more severely with pneumonitis in measles, chicken pox, and psittacosis.
- Gastrointestinal symptoms may be a feature of measles, roseola infantum, toxic shock syndrome, typhoid, and leptospirosis.
- Hepatitis may occur in roseola infantum, Gianotti–Crosti syndrome, and leptospirosis.
- There may be coexisting meningitis in meningococcal sepsis, enteroviral infection and leptospirosis, or rarely an encephalitic picture with measles, rubella, chicken pox, erythema infectiosum, and roseola infantum.
- Joint symptoms may be associated with rubella, erythema infectiosum, psittacosis, and brucellosis, and at a late stage in Lyme disease.

Exposure to infections

- Contact with other people with similar symptoms is important as some diseases are highly infectious, for example chicken pox and erythema infectiosum.
- Exposure to insects that might transmit infections is relevant, for example in Lyme disease (deer ticks) and dengue fever (mosquitos).
- Contact with animals that might transmit infections is relevant, for example in leptospirosis (rats), toxoplasmosis (puppies and kittens) and psittacosis (birds).

Foreign travel

- With increasing worldwide travel, imported infections are an important cause of rashes.
- Typhoid fever is a common infection in febrile children who have returned from travelling, which may present with rose spots on the abdomen in older children.
- Dengue fever is the most commonly identified cause of maculopapular rash in endemic areas. Dengue haemorrhagic fever can also present with a haemorrhagic rash.

- Malaria is a common infection and a rare cause of purpuric rash.
- Countries other than tropical countries are also the source of infections, for example Rocky Mountain Spotted fever and West Nile virus in the USA, and leishmaniasis in southern Europe.

Time of year
- Many infections are seasonal, so awareness of prevailing microorganisms is important.
- Enterovirus infections (echovirus, Coxsackie virus, and enterovirus) occur predominantly in the summer and autumn months.
- Erythema infectiosum tends to occur in late winter and early spring.
- Tropical infections also have seasons of increased incidence, for example dengue fever and malaria (including associations with school holiday periods).

Immunization history—a mild rash may be seen around 6–10 days post MMR vaccination.

Drug history
- A widespread rash after the administration of amoxicillin for sore throat suggests EBV as the aetiology.
- Drugs may cause rash, even without a concomitant infection, and may be due to allergy or side effect. Drugs with rash as a well-recognized side effect include anti-epileptics, antibiotics, and antimalarials.
- Sun exposure may exacerbate rashes caused by drugs.
- Drugs may cause different types of rash, e.g. maculopapular, urticarial, erythema multiforme and severely, Stevens–Johnson syndrome.

Examination

Nature of the rash
- The key to diagnosis is the nature of the rash—maculopapular, petechial/purpuric, vesicular/bullous or scaly (Table 34.1).
- Some organisms cause several different types of rash, e.g. enteroviruses which can cause maculopapular, petechial, and vesicular rashes.
- In chicken pox, different stages of the rash can occur at the same time—maculopapular, vesicular, and crusted. Historically this differentiated it from smallpox where all the vesicles had similar morphology.
- Some rashes have a classic morphology, e.g. the rash of toxic shock syndrome which is described as looking like sunburn, the bullseye lesions in Lyme disease, the sandpaper rash of scarlet fever, and the salmon pink macules in juvenile chronic arthritis.

Rash distribution
- The distribution of the rash also differentiates between pathogens. It may change with time, so history of its evolution is important.
- The main classifications regarding distribution are local versus generalized (Table 34.3), and centripetal versus centrifugal.

Table 34.3 Distribution of childhood rashes

Localized rashes		Generalized rashes
Infection	Rash site	Infection
Erythema infectiosum	Cheeks	Measles
Hand foot and mouth disease	Hands, feet, perioral, buccal cavity	Enterovirus infection other than hand foot and mouth
Shingles	One or two dermatomes	Rubella
Herpes simplex	Mouth, genitals, fingers	Roseola infantum
Gianotti–Crosti syndrome	Extensor surface of the extremities, face, buttocks	Chicken pox
Unilateral laterothoracic exanthem	Axilla, flank	Adenovirus
Papular purpuric gloves and socks syndrome	Hands, feet	EBV (especially with amoxicillin)
Lyme disease	Site of tick bite	Acute HIV infection
Typhoid fever	Abdomen	Scarlet fever
Psittacosis	Face	Meningococcal septicaemia
Early Rocky Mountain Spotted fever	Palms, soles	Toxic shock syndrome
Bacterial endocarditis	Ends of fingers and toes	Leptospirosis
Pityriasis rosea	Trunk, often a single lesion	Kawasaki disease
Fungal infections	Scalp or skin but often a single or few lesions	Juvenile chronic arthritis
SLE	Face	Leukaemia
Henoch–Schönlein purpura	Legs and buttocks	Drug reaction

- Centripetal rashes predominate or start on the extremities, and include hand foot and mouth disease, syphilis, Rocky Mountain spotted fever, dengue fever, and historically smallpox, which was one of the ways to differentiate it from chicken pox.
- Centrifugal rashes predominate or start on the trunk, and include measles, rubella, chicken pox and scarlet fever.

Oral enanthems
- Several skin rashes have associated oral lesions (enanthems) that can easily be missed if the buccal cavity is not specifically examined (Table 34.4).

Table 34.4 Oral enanthems associated with common exanthems

Infection	Symptoms
Measles	Koplik's spots—white spots on the buccal mucosa
Rubella	Forscheimer's spots—red papules on the hard palate
Varicella	Vesicles which may ulcerate
Erythema infectiosum	Red macules on palate and buccal mucosa, erythematous tongue
Roseola infantum	Nagayama's spots—erythematous papules on the soft palate
Scarlet fever	Red exudative tonsils, strawberry tongue, palatal petechiae
EBV	Red enlarged tonsils, palatal petechiae
Coxsackie herpangina	Erythematous lesions on hard palate that become vesicular

Other clinical findings

- Conjunctivitis may occur in measles, rubella, adenovirus infection, scarlet fever, and Kawasaki disease.
- Mucosal changes may be a feature of scarlet fever, Kawasaki disease, toxic shock syndrome, and drug reactions including Stevens–Johnson syndrome.
- Lymphadenopathy may occur in rubella, EBV, scarlet fever and Kawasaki disease.
- Hepatomegaly and/or splenomegaly may be found in EBV infection, rubella, acute HIV infection, leukaemia, juvenile chronic arthritis.
- Genital lesions may be found in herpes simplex infection, Kawasaki disease and Stevens–Johnson syndrome.

Immunocompromised individuals

Rashes associated with benign self-limiting illnesses in immunocompetent children may have a much more severe course in the immunocompromised host. See specific chapters for more details, but examples are:

- Measles—may be *no* rash with measles in the immunocompromised child
- Varicella—multidermatomal zoster may be a sign of immunocompromise
- Erythema infectiosum
- Roseola infantum.

Pregnant women

Several infections with rashes have severe consequences for the fetus if transmitted to a non-immune pregnant woman, and may also present with a rash in the neonatal period. See specific chapters for more details, but examples are:

- Rubella
- Toxoplasmosis
- CMV
- Syphilis
- HSV
- Varicella
- Erythema infectiosum.

Specific rashes not covered elsewhere

Gianotti–Crosti syndrome (papular acrodermatitis of childhood)

- The commonest cause is EBV, and other infectious agents implicated include hepatitis B, enteroviruses, respiratory viruses, parvovirus B19 and CMV.
- There are a few reports of Gianott–Crosti syndrome following immunizations.
- It is generally a self-limiting condition usually lasting 10–14 days and predominantly affecting pre-school children. The exanthem is an erythematous papular or vesicular rash affecting the extensor surface of the extremities, face, and buttocks which may be pruritic. The rash is often asymmetrical and lesions may coalesce to form plaques.
- It is associated with fever and/or lymphadenopathy in about a third of individuals.
- Occasionally acute hepatitis develops, particularly when the causative organism is hepatitis B, EBV, or CMV, and very rarely this may become chronic.
- Treatment is symptomatic.

Unilateral laterothoracic exanthem (asymmetrical periflexural exanthem of childhood)

- No single causative organism has been identified although parvovirus B19 and EBV have been associated.
- It usually occurs in winter and early spring.
- It is most common in children aged 1–5 years, and rare in adults.
- There is usually a prodrome of low grade fever and mild respiratory and gastrointestinal symptoms.
- The rash begins unilaterally on the trunk, most frequently in the axilla and may be accompanied by an enlarged axillary lymph node. It is a morbilliform papular or eczematous rash that may spread bilaterally but retains a unilateral predominance. It is self-limiting and usually resolves in about 4 weeks without complication.

Papular purpuric gloves and socks syndrome

- This exanthem is most commonly caused by parvovirus B19. HHV-6 and 7, CMV, and measles virus have also been implicated in the aetiology.

- Erythema, oedema, and pruritus of the hands and feet in a glove and sock distribution are associated with mild fever. The erythema progresses to petechiae and purpura on the palms and soles, which may be painful.
- Treatment is symptomatic with antihistamines, and the rash usually resolves in 1–2 weeks without sequelae.

Pityriasis rosea

- This is an exanthem of unknown origin, although a viral cause is suggested by seasonal and geographical clustering.
- It predominantly affects older children and young adults.
- A sore throat may precede the exanthem, and constitutional symptoms such as headache and low grade fever may accompany the rash.
- The rash is characterized by pink or red scaly oval lesions, often with a single herald patch on the back before others develop, predominantly on the trunk. It may be pruritic, and treatment with antihistamines provides symptomatic relief.
- The rash usually resolves within several weeks without treatment. Ultraviolet light has been used anecdotally to shorten the course in pityriasis, but comparative studies in a few patients have not shown good evidence for its use.

Rickettsial rashes

- Classical rickettsial infection is Rocky Mountain spotted fever, caused by the bacterium *Rickettsia rickettsii*.
- The infection is transmitted by ixodid ticks, which can be associated with both deer and domestic dogs. It occurs across most of eastern and central USA as far as the Rocky Mountains, as well as Canada, Central and South America.
- Rocky Mountain spotted fever has a prodromal phase of fever, headache, myalgia, and nausea lasting several days.
- The rash frequently starts as a maculopapular rash on the palms and soles that spreads up the limbs to the trunk, and progresses to a petechial rash.
- Treatment is with doxycycline for up to 10 days.
- Without antibiotic treatment mortality is up to 30%.
- Mediterranean spotted fever—or Boutonneuse fever due to *Rickettsia connori* occurs in southern Europe, and may present with a fever, maculo-papular rash, and an eschar (black necrotic tissue).

Investigations

Investigation of rash in childhood should initially be tailored towards likely causes, and may include the following:
- Culture—of blood, respiratory specimens, CSF, and stool for bacteria and viruses
- Serology—IgM, paired IgG
- PCR—most viral exanthems can be diagnosed by PCR of blood or CSF, including the herpes viruses, measles, rubella, parvovirus B19, adenovirus, and enterovirus
- Antigen tests—poor sensitivity so less frequently used, although urine pneumococcal antigen test may be useful in children >5 years
- Specific tests:
  - Salivary IgA for measles
  - Immunofluorescence of vesicle fluid for varicella or herpes
  - Immunofluorescence of nasopharyngeal aspirate for adenovirus.

In most studies of childhood rashes no cause is identified in about half of patients.

Management and treatment

Management of the different causes of rash is dealt with in specific chapters.
- As most causes of rash are benign and self-limiting, treatment is usually supportive:
  - Fluids—where needed
  - Antipyretics—may provide symptomatic relief
  - Antihistamines—for itchy rashes, for example chicken pox.

Follow-up and outcome

The outcome of different causes of rash is dealt with in specific chapters.
- Many of these rashes are highly infectious and contact tracing may be necessary if there is contact with an immunocompromised person or pregnant woman.
- It is useful to know the incubation and infectivity periods for common childhood rashes (Table 34.5).

Table 34.5 Incubation and infectivity periods for acute viral exanthems

Exanthem	Incubation (days)	Duration of infectivity
Measles	8–12	2 days before prodrome to 5 days after rash appears
Rubella	14–21	7 days before rash to 5 days after rash appears; in congenital infection viral shedding can persist for months
Varicella	10–21	2 days before rash to 5 days after rash appears
Erythema infectiosum	4–14	Prior to the onset of the rash
Papular-purpuric gloves and socks syndrome	10	During shedding of virus which can persist until after the rash disappears after 7–14 days
Roseola infantum	9	During shedding of virus which can persist
Hand foot and mouth	4–7	During shedding of the virus which can persist in the stool for several weeks

Future research

There is a need to update the commonest presentation and clinical diagnosis of rashes in childhood and the role of multiplex PCR in rapid diagnosis.

Key reference

1 Ramsay M, Reacher M, O'Flynn C, *et al.* Causes of morbilliform rash in a highly immunised English population. *Arch Dis Child* 2002;**87**:202–6.

Refugees and internationally adopted children

📖 see also Chapters 19, 42, 75, 76, 107, 113

Introduction

Child migration is an important international problem. The pattern of migration varies from country to country and year to year and so appropriate facilities will vary.

Children may arrive in Europe from abroad for short-term stays on holiday or visiting relatives. These children will not usually come in contact with health services unless they become acutely unwell. This circumstance is covered in other chapters. On the other hand, there are children who come here intending to stay long term. Some already have European citizenship and data on how many children this may be are not readily available. There are also those who are seeking asylum or are being adopted ('inter-country adoption'). It is these two groups who are the subjects of this chapter.

Epidemiology

In 2007, 3525 unaccompanied asylum seeking children aged ≤17 years applied for asylum in the UK.

- 32% (1135) were from Afghanistan, 26% (900) from sub-Saharan Africa (mainly Somalia and Eritrea), 21% (735) from the Middle East and North Africa, 9% (315) from China, 8% (295) from the Indian subcontinent, and 2% (80) from Europe (mainly Eastern Europe).
- A further 3825 children were dependents of asylum seekers. These children tended to be younger (46% <5 years old and only 9% 15–17) and the distribution of countries of origin was different—39% (1500) were from sub-Saharan Africa, 22% (825) from the Indian subcontinent, 15% (570) from Middle East and North Africa, 6% (240) from Europe, and 3% (125) from China.
- In 2008, the Department for Children Families and Schools received 2232 applications for inter-country adoption: 41% (920) from China, 11% (252) from Russia, 9% (202) from India, 8% (170) from Guatemala, 6% (123) from USA, and 5% (116) from Thailand.
- In addition, there are an unknown number of undocumented children.

All these groups of children are scattered throughout the country, in private homes, foster care, detention centres, etc. In 2009, the House of Commons Home Affairs Committee was told that 'Nearly 1000 children a year are detained in UK Border Authority's immigration detention centres. On average, children spend over a fortnight in detention. Detention for up to 61 days is not uncommon. On 30 June 2009, 10 of the 35 children in detention had been held for between 29 days and 61 days.'

The majority of these children come from countries where the healthcare systems are very different, as is the spectrum of endemic infectious illnesses. Many of the children will not have received the basic preventative health measures in their country of origin and may be harbouring unrecognised infectious diseases.

In terms of healthcare related to infectious diseases there are three issues:
- Screening for current infection
- Prevention of future infection
- Protection of carers and household members.

Arrangements should be made for all children to sign on with a general practitioner. Children for adoption should have an inter-country adoption form (ICAF), or something similar, completed. Unfortunately documentation relating to potential adoptees from abroad may be inaccurate or even fraudulent. Unless the source is known and can be trusted, it may be best to ignore the information and not let it influence management in relation to infection and immunization.

Screening for current infection

Many of the countries from which the children arrive have relatively high prevalence of infectious diseases; however, there are few data on infectious diseases in child immigrants in UK. Most originates from USA.

In a US study of children adopted from China in the early/mid 1990s:
- 9/242 (4%) were positive for hepatitis B surface antigen
- None of those tested were HIV positive
- 21/184 (11%) had parasites in their stools—*Giardia* in 13; *Ascaris* in 5; *Dientamoeba* in 1; and 1 child had both *Giardia* and *Ascaris*
- Of stool cultures from 86 children, four were positive for *Salmonella*, two for *Campylobacter*, two for both *Salmonella* and *Campylobacter*, and one for *Clostridium difficile*
- 6/164 (4%) had a positive Mantoux test, but none had symptoms and all had normal chest X-rays.

Although exact proportions vary, this is a common pattern.

There are some data suggesting that children with latent TB have an increased risk of developing clinical disease on moving to temperate climates. It is therefore important to determine whether the child has latent TB and treat accordingly.

The British Association for Adoption and Fostering (BAAF) has made recommendations in 'Health Screening of Children Adopted from Abroad'.[1] These could equally well be applied to refugees, except that where refugees are accompanied by parents/relatives, more information may be available allowing one to reduce the number of investigations. Table 35.1 is based on BAAF recommendations. It only applies to asymptomatic children. The recommendations are very similar to those of the American Academy of Pediatrics (AAP), except that AAP recommends screening all adoptees for hepatitis B, hepatitis C, and HIV. As it is often difficult to assess risk in these circumstances, it is probably better to screen, unless there is good reason not to.

Table 35.1 Screening for infection in international adoptees or asylum seekers

Condition	Investigation	When to do	Comments
Tuberculosis (if >3 months old)	Mantoux test	On arrival—if negative and malnourished, repeat in 6 months	A positive result may be difficult to interpret, if BCG has been given previously
Hepatitis B	Hepatits B surface antigen	On arrival and routinely after 3 months[a] for all children with an increased risk of horizontal or vertical transmission or from endemic areas	If present, indicates ongoing infection, which may be acute or chronic. If persists for 6 months, is likely to indicate chronic carriage
			Susceptible household contacts should be immunized[b]
	Hepatitis B core antibody		If present, indicates past or present infection, depending on the presence of hepatitis B surface antigen
	Hepatitis B surface antibody		If present, may be due to past infection or immunization. In the latter case hepatitis B core antibody is absent
Hepatitis C	Hepatitis C antibody	On arrival and routinely after 3 months[a] for all children with an increased risk of horizontal or vertical transmission or from endemic areas	If present, indicates past or present infection. Further investigation is required

(Continued)

Table 35.1 (Contd.)

Condition	Investigation	When to do	Comments
HIV	HIV 1 and 2	On arrival and routinely after 3 months[a] for all children with an increased risk of horizontal or vertical transmission or from endemic areas	If the child is <18 months, a positive result may be due to transmission of maternal antibodies rather than infection.
Syphilis	VDRL	On arrival	
Gastrointestinal infections and infestations	Stool for ova, parasites and cysts Stool culture if symptomatic	On arrival	Children may carry parasites without any obvious symptoms and signs. Any parasites found, should be appropriately treated

[a]Seroconversion may occur after arrival in the UK and therefore these tests should be repeated after an interval of 3 months.

[b]Transmission has been recorded within households even in the absence of obvious risk factors.

Prevention of future infection

- A full immunization history should be taken and any records consulted.
- Where immunizations that are part of the local schedule have been omitted, they should be given in line with the standard protocol.
- When there is doubt as to whether a vaccine has been given, it should be assumed not to have been given and the schedule completed accordingly.
- If BCG vaccine has not been given, depending on the country of origin of the child, it may need to be given after a Mantoux test has been administered.
- If the child is to travel back to the country of origin, the appropriate immunizations should be given. Other advice, e.g. about antimalarial medication and other precautions, should be given.

Protection of carers and household members

- All routine immunizations, including routine boosters, should be up to date. Measles, mumps, and rubella have been transmitted to adopters in USA, by children incubating infection on arrival in the country.
- If adopting or caring for a child who is at high risk of hepatitis B, all household contacts should be immunized, unless the child is reliably known not to be hepatitis B surface antigen positive.

The above recommendations relate only to infection. All children moving into a country from abroad need a much broader assessment. This should include a full medical history, including checking which screening tests have been done.

Future research

There is very little literature on the rates of infections and health outcomes of children migrating to Europe.

Key reference

1 British Association for Adoption and Fostering. Practice note 46: *Health Screening of Children Adopted from Abroad*, 2004. Available to purchase at: ✆ www.baaf.org.uk (accessed 1 February 2011).

Further reading

Miller LC. International adoption: infectious diseases issues. *Clin Infect Dis* 2005;**40**:286–93.

Chapter 36

Sepsis syndrome

📖 see also Chapters 39, 70, 83, 87, 105, 106

Introduction

- Infections remain a major cause of childhood mortality and morbidity in the UK. Although most infections are of viral origin and self-limiting, a minority are bacterial, some of these leading to sepsis syndrome. Adverse outcomes are often mediated *via* septic shock. Most children who develop septic shock present first with fever, although some, especially in the first weeks of life, may become hypothermic.
- Differentiating between self-limiting illnesses and potentially life-threatening bacterial infections is an increasing diagnostic challenge: rapid evolution of the clinical picture further complicates the problems of assessment and diagnosis, especially in younger children.
- Parents and clinicians perceive a need to improve recognition of the causes of fever in order to offer early treatment to those with evolving sepsis.
- Some children with fever have symptoms and signs suggesting a serious infection, such as the non-blanching rash of meningococcal septicaemia, so facilitating early treatment. Many children have a fever without apparent source.

Terminology and definitions

Sepsis in children is defined as *systemic inflammatory response syndrome* (SIRS) in the presence of, or as a result of, suspected or proven *infection*.

   SIRS is defined as the presence of at least two of four criteria, one of which must be abnormal temperature or leucocyte count (see Box 36.1 and Table 36.1).

   Infection is defined as a suspected or proven infection caused by any pathogen *or* a clinical syndrome associated with a high probability of infection (see Box 36.1). Evidence of infection includes positive findings on clinical exam, imaging, or laboratory tests (e.g. WBCs in a normally sterile body fluid, perforated viscus, chest radiograph consistent with pneumonia, petechial or purpuric rash, or purpura fulminans).

   Severe sepsis is defined as sepsis plus one of the following: cardiovascular organ dysfunction *or* acute respiratory distress syndrome, *or* two or more other organ dysfunctions (see Box 36.2).

   Septic shock is defined as sepsis and cardiovascular organ dysfunction (see Box 36.2).

Table 36.1: Age-specific vital signs and laboratory variables (lower values for heart rate, leucocyte count, and systolic blood pressure are for the 5th and upper values for heart rate, respiration rate, or leucocyte count for the 95th percentile) (after Goldstein B, et al, 2005)

Age Group	Heart rate (beats/min) Tachycardia Bradycardia		Respiratory rate (breaths/min)	Leucocyte count (leucocytes x10³/mm³)	Systolic blood Pressure (mm Hg)
0 days to 1 wk	> 180	< 100	> 50	> 34	< 65
1 wk to 1 mo	> 180	< 100	> 40	> 19.5 or < 5	< 75
1 mo to 1 yr	> 180	< 90	> 34	> 17.5 or < 5	< 100
2–5 yrs	> 140	NA	> 22	> 15.5 or < 6	< 94
6–12 yrs	> 130	NA	> 18	> 13.5 or < 4.5	< 105
13 to > 18 yrs	> 110	NA	> 14	> 11 or < 4.5	< 117

NA, not applicable.

Box 36.1 Definitions of systemic inflammatory response syndrome

SIRS

The presence of at least two of the following four criteria, one of which must be abnormal temperature or leucocyte count:

- Core temperature of >38.5°C or <36°C
- Tachycardia, defined as a mean heart rate >2SD above normal for age in the absence of external stimulus, chronic drugs, or painful stimuli; or otherwise unexplained persistent elevation over a 0.5–4-hour time period; or for children <1 year old: bradycardia, defined as a mean heart rate <10th percentile for age in the absence of external vagal stimulus, β-blocker drugs, or congenital heart disease; or otherwise unexplained persistent depression over a 0.5-hour time period
- Mean respiratory rate >2SD above normal for age or mechanical ventilation for an acute process not related to underlying neuromuscular disease or the receipt of general anaesthesia
- Leucocyte count elevated or depressed for age (not secondary to chemotherapy-induced leukopenia) or >10% immature neutrophils

Causative organisms

Organisms responsible for sepsis syndrome in infants and children include *Neisseria meningitidis* (most common), *Escherichia coli*, *Klebsiella* spp., *Salmonellae*, *Haemophilus influenzae* type b, and other Gram–negative bacteria. *Streptococcus pneumoniae* and *Staphylococcus aureus* are the most frequent Gram–positive pathogens. Group B Streptococci, *E. coli*, and *Listeria monocytogenes* are the most common bacterial causes of sepsis syndrome <3 months of age. Occasional cases are caused by viruses.

Immunosuppressed patients may develop septicaemia due to unusual and opportunistic organisms, though Gram–negative bacteria cause most mortality. Surgical patients usually develop sepsis due to enteric organisms.

Epidemiology

Up to 1% of children aged 0–5 years have a serious bacterial illness, such as meningitis, septicaemia, urinary tract infection, or pneumonia each year. The incidence of sepsis in this age group is around 10–20 per 100 000.

Epidemiology has been radically altered by immunization programmes. In the UK immunization against *H. influenzae* type b (1992), serogroup C *N. meningitidis* (1999), and *S. pneumoniae* (2006) all resulted in a dramatic drop in incidence of sepsis caused by these organisms. Serogroup B *N. meningitidis* awaits an effective vaccine.

Pathophysiology of sepsis

- Rapid bacterial multiplication produces bacterial toxins in the bloodstream. Sepsis is the clinical expression of the host's response to constituents of the cell wall of Gram-negative bacteria (endotoxins) or to the exotoxins of Gram-positive organisms. Infection results in activation of macrophages that produce the lymphokines γ interferon and GM-CSF, TNF, and ILs, especially IL-1 and IL-6. These substances normally benefit the host by mediating protective inflammatory responses, but in severe infection, an exaggerated, harmful response occurs and high levels of TNF and IL-1 lead to serious damage.
- Other inflammatory mediators such as prostaglandin E_2 (PGE_2) released by neutrophils, nitric acid released by macrophages and platelet activating factor, lead to endothelial cell damage which results in leakage of plasma from the circulation.
- Myocardial depression is mediated by IL-6. Resulting hypovolaemia may lead to cardiovascular dysfunction, acute respiratory distress, and other organ dysfunction.
- Meanwhile, abnormal activation of clotting can lead to DIC. The convergence of these pathways precipitates multiple organ failure and death.

Clinical presentation and differential diagnosis

Early diagnosis of sepsis syndrome depends on thorough assessment of the ill child. In the seriously ill child history and examination proceed simultaneously. Diagnostic clues, such as a spreading non-blanching rash, may be the reason for presentation.

- Immediately life-threatening features, including compromise of airway, breathing, or circulation, and decreased level of consciousness or confusion (often difficult to assess in a young child) should be sought.
- Full clinical assessment includes observations of temperature (ideally peripheral and central), pulse rate, capillary refill, respiration rate and pattern, blood pressure, skin turgor and status of mucous membranes, mental status, conscious level, and urine output. Body weight and height should be measured or estimated. Recent travel abroad should be elicited.
- Early features of sepsis typically include fever and tachycardia. Respiratory rate may be normal or mildly raised with an irregular breathing pattern. Urine output may be mildly reduced, reflecting mild dehydration. Limb pain and cold hands and feet are early signs of sepsis. Later features may include hypothermia, a marked tachycardia, sustained tachypnoea and respiratory irregularity, depressed conscious level, and a clinically appreciable reduction in urine output.
- SIRS requires deviation from age-specific vital signs (see Table 36.1). Impaired perfusion may be recognized by cold peripheries, poor capillary refill, tachycardia, tachypnoea and oliguria. A prolonged capillary refill time of 3 seconds or more in a room–warm limb suggests reduced skin perfusion and, in a tachycardic, feverish child, may indicate serious illness, particularly septic shock (see NICE guidance on fever2). Hypotension is not essential to the diagnosis of septic shock in children (Box 36.2). Blood pressure is often maintained surprisingly well especially in young children, who develop a marked tachycardia and impaired microcirculation in limbs and organs from hypovolaemia before suddenly hypotension appears. Skin core–temperature gradient (toe and rectal thermistor probes) of >3°C is a sensitive marker for severe shock, although rectal temperature measurement is not recommended in the NICE guidance. Blood pressure should be measured if heart rate or capillary refill time is abnormal in a feverish child.
- Dehydration can be assessed by considering capillary refill time, skin turgor, respiratory pattern, pulse strength, and temperature of extremities. Measurement of oxygen saturation is an essential adjunct to clinical examination. Hypoxaemia or poor cerebral perfusion results in restlessness, irritability or 'bad behaviour'.
- The source of fever and symptoms and signs associated with specific diseases should be sought. Meningococcal septicaemia presents with fever, malaise, and a non-blanching rash, (especially skin lesions >2 mm in diameter (purpura) or spreading), or capillary refill time ≥3 seconds. Meningitis should be considered if a child is feverish with decreased level of consciousness, convulsions, and/or bulging fontanelle.

Box 36.2 Organ dysfunction criteria

Cardiovascular

Despite administration of isotonic intravenous fluid bolus ≥40ml/kg in 1 hour

- Decrease in blood pressure (hypotension) <5th centile for age or systolic BP >2SD below normal for age[a]

OR

- Need for vasoactive drug to maintain BP in normal range (dopamine >5mcg/kg/min or dobutamine, adrenaline, or noradrenaline at any dose)

OR

- Two of the following
  - Unexplained metabolic acidosis: base deficit >5.0mmol/l
  - Increased arterial lactate >2 times upper limit of normal
  - Oliguria: urine output <0.5ml/kg/h
  - Prolonged capillary refill: >5s
  - Core to peripheral temperature gap >3°C

Respiratory[b]

- PaO_2/FiO_2 <300 in absence of cyanotic heart disease or pre-existing lung disease

OR

- $PaCO_2$ >65mmHg or >20mmHg over baseline $PaCO_2$

OR

- Proven need[c] or >50% FiO_2 to maintain saturation >92%

OR

- Need for non-elective invasive or non-invasive mechanical ventilation[d]

Neurological

- GCS score <11

OR

- Acute change in mental status with a decrease in GCS score ≥3 points from abnormal baseline

Haematological

- Platelet count <80 × 10^9/l or a decline of 50% in platelet count from highest value recorded over the past 3 days (for chronic haematology/oncology patients)

OR

- International normalized ratio >2

Renal

- Serum creatinine ≥2 times upper limit of normal for age or twofold increase in baseline creatinine

---

Box 36.2 (Contd.)

Hepatic

- Total bilirubin ≥40mg/l (not applicable for newborn)

OR

- ALT two times upper limit of normal for age

[a]See Box 36.1.

[b]Acute respiratory distress syndrome must include a PaO_2/FiO_2 ratio ≤200mmHg, bilateral infiltrates, acute onset, and no evidence of left heart failure. Acute lung injury is defined identically except the PaO_2/FiO_2 ratio must be ≤300mmHg.

[c]Proven need assumes oxygen requirement was tested by decreasing flow with subsequent increase in flow if required.

[d]In postoperative patients, this requirement can be met if the patient has developed an acute inflammatory or infectious process in the lungs which prevents extubation.

(After Goldstein et al.[1])

If diagnosis is not immediately apparent, look for predictors of serious illness.[2] Predictors of serious illness and septic shock, include:
- Infants <3 months with fever ≥38°C
- Infants 3–6 months with fever ≥39°C
- Bile-stained vomiting
- Unrousable
- Respiratory rate ≥60 breaths/min or grunting
- Weak, high-pitched, or continuous cry
- Pale/mottled/blue/ashen skin, especially centrally
- Severely reduced skin turgor
- Moderate/severe chest recession
- Children appearing ill to another healthcare professional.

Predictors for intermediate risk of serious illness include:
- Waking only with prolonged stimulation
- Decreased activity
- Poor feeding in infants
- Not responding normally to social cues/no smile
- Dry mucous membranes.

Infants <3 months age can have serious bacterial infection without any clinical features. They may benefit from observation for 4–6 hours, and reassessment with investigation results.

Investigations

Children with features of septic shock and a clinically evident underlying cause should have appropriate investigations taken (see Chapters 8, 17, 20, 22, 27, 29, 38, 40, 43).

If a child has fever without an apparent source but ≥1 feature predicting serious illness, tests should include:
- FBC
- Blood culture
- CRP
- Urine dipstick, microscopy, and culture.

Investigations may follow clinical assessment, including:
- Chest X-ray
- Plasma U&Es
- Blood gas
- Stool culture if diarrhoea is present.

LP should be considered at all ages, but is contraindicated with clinical evidence of septic shock, to avoid deterioration during the procedure.

In sepsis clinical deterioration progresses and rapidly accelerates. Haemoglobin may fall rapidly. The WCC may show leucocytosis >15 × 10^9 /l (or, more seriously, leucopenia <5 × 10^9 /l). Blood lactate may be elevated but blood glucose is often low. Potassium and calcium may be low and need correcting. Clinical and laboratory evidence of DIC, ARDS, acute renal failure, hepato-biliary dysfunction, and CNS dysfunction may presage multi-organ failure.

Management and treatment

Successful management requires rapid response and continuing care following diagnosis. SIRS is initiated by organisms, but sustained by an inflammatory cascade determined by genetic predisposition and inflammatory pathways, often sensitized by recent minor viral infection. Killing organisms with antibiotics takes hours, but the inflammatory cascade may self-perpetuate well beyond that time.

Management of sepsis syndrome requires;
- Urgent antibiotics to cover the likely causative organisms
- Parenteral fluid therapy (resuscitation, continuing replacement and maintenance); early drainage of purulent foci
- Vasoactive (usually inotropic) support
- Oxygen and paediatric intensive care measures.

Frequent monitoring is required, with reassessment of vital signs, signs of shock, and detection of new problems.

Immediate management

- Management recommendations are supported by consensus guidelines, but sparse evidence (e.g. ☐ see 'Early Management of Meningococcal Disease in Children', ◈ www.meningitis.org/health-professionals). Paediatric life-support guidelines should be broadly followed.
- The most experienced clinician available should stay with the child. Call for extra help, including senior nursing staff and alert the anaesthetic staff that a child with severe sepsis may require ventilatory support.

- Blood cultures should precede, but not delay, antibiotics. Causative organisms can be isolated within 24 hours. PCR can detect bacterial DNA up to 72 hours after killing by antibiotics.
- Parenteral antibiotics should be given at the earliest opportunity (ideally within half an hour after appropriate cultures have been obtained), especially if a child presents with shock, is unrousable, or showing signs of meningococcal disease, or in a child with fever and reduced levels of consciousness (meningitis might be responsible). Antibiotics should not be delayed pending the results of investigations.
- Children with suspected meningococcal disease or community acquired infection should be given a third-generation cephalosporin. Antibiotic regimens may need variation in healthcare associated infections and in surgical or immunocompromised patients, to cover them from negative sepsis. Local or tertiary centre protocols may cover certain groups (e.g. oncology patients with febrile neutropenia). In infants <3 months of age an antibiotic active against *L. monocytogenes* should be given as well (e.g. ampicillin or amoxicillin).
- Children with impaired peripheral perfusion or septic shock should receive 0.9% sodium chloride 20ml/kg over 10–30 minutes, repeated if response is poor, and then receive further boluses as necessary (see also Fluid and electrolyte balance). Albumin 4.5% can be used instead of 0.9% sodium chloride for further boluses, but must be obtained from the blood transfusion service.
- The child should be nursed in a high-dependency care area in the emergency department or paediatric ward (high-dependency unit (HDU)), where intensive care can commence if needed. Facilities for intermittent positive pressure ventilation and cardiopulmonary resuscitation should be available. Children with impaired mental state and reduced perfusion may need attention to the airway.
- Children with fever who are shocked, unrousable or showing signs of meningococcal disease should be urgently reviewed by an experienced paediatrician (i.e. senior middle grade or consultant) to consider discussion with a PICU about management and possible admission.

Fluid and electrolyte balance

- Fluid balance is calculated as: volume restoration, maintenance fluids, and replacement of ongoing losses. Intravenous (intraosseous if necessary) access for aggressive fluid resuscitation is essential. If large resuscitation volumes are needed, crystalloid at half-maintenance should be given. Ongoing fluid losses (e.g. nasogastric aspirates) should be replaced volume/volume with intravenous 0.9% saline hourly.
- Regular electrolyte and blood glucose measurements should be made. Potassium balance may need attention. If blood glucose is low, dextrose 10% infusion at 0.5 ml/kg/h should be commenced, with higher concentrations if a poor response.

Further management of septic shock

- Preventing septic shock with marked tachycardia from progressing to hypotension and cardiovascular collapse may require saline or colloid administration (initial volumes of 40–60ml/kg) until central venous pressure (CVP) is +12 to +15cm H_2O, which will reduce the core–peripheral temperature difference and improve capillary refill.

- Fluid administration should not be slowed or discontinued too early. Children with Gram–negative septic shock may ultimately require several times their own circulating volume (that is, several times 80ml/kg) of resuscitation fluid to replace capillary leakage.

Cardiovascular support

- With adequate volume replacement (normal CVP and blood pressure) persisting signs of impaired peripheral perfusion (raised pulse rate, prolonged capillary refill time) suggests that either myocardial failure due to endotoxinaemia or peripheral vasoconstriction may be present. Myocardial function can be assessed echocardiographically, measuring end–diastolic volume.
- Inotrope introduction should follow local tertiary PICU protocols, which differ across the UK and Europe. Dopamine, an inotrope with vasodilator action, is usually first–line supportive treatment when there is impaired perfusion unresponsive to volume replacement. If hypotension persists despite adequate CVP, dopamine can be increased up to a maximum of 20mcg/kg/min. In dopamine-refractory shock, adrenaline or noradrenaline may be used instead of dobutamine. Vasodilators (which include nitroglycerin, glyceryl trinitrate patch, and nitroprusside) reduce after load on the heart and improve perfusion, but a role in management of septic shock has not been established in double–blind placebo-controlled trials in children.
- The successful endpoint of resuscitation of septic shock should be the return of normal heart rate, capillary refill (i.e. <2 seconds), pulse rate, warm extremities, urine output >1ml/kg/h and normal mental state. CVP should return to +8 to +12 cmH_2O. Blood tests should show decreased lactate and improved base deficit.

Disseminated intravascular coagulation

- Septic shock causes DIC, with deranged clotting studies, thrombocytopenia, and raised fibrin degradation products. A combination of small vessel thrombosis and DIC is called *purpura fulminans* and may lead to extensive tissue necrosis or limb ischaemia. Management is supportive during correction of the underlying cause. If clotting studies are severely deranged, fresh frozen plasma or cryoprecipitate should be given. Platelet infusions (which last 6–8 hours) may be required for patients with severe thrombocytopenia and active bleeding (e.g. from puncture sites).
- Low–dose heparin for impending peripheral gangrene and severe coagulation derangement is controversial and should be discussed with PICU staff. Results of trials of specific treatments for DIC are awaited.

HDU care

Children have low functional residual capacity. They may require early intubation and ventilation, which reduces work of breathing and myocardial workload. Children with emergent septic shock should be electively intubated and ventilated, i.e. before deterioration occurs and emergency intubation is required for airway compromise or abnormalities of breathing rate or pattern. Early use of intermittent positive pressure ventilation can avert severe deterioration, which occurs during a period of unexpected decompensation, and reduces the risk of pulmonary oedema. Midazolam sedation is often used during ventilation: it is also anticonvulsant. Intravenous opiate infusions such as morphine or alfentanil convey sedative and analgesic effects.

Admission to PICU

Patients who do not respond to immediate treatment or are very ill at presentation require admission to a PICU. A senior paediatrician should contact a paediatric intensivist for early discussion. The interchange may provide relevant management advice and facilitate early transfer.

Ventilatory support is not a prerequisite for PICU admission requests, though most patients will be ventilated for transfer. Other reasons include the diagnosis, deterioration, degree of shock, treatment given, and respiratory pattern.

Transfer to PICU will be needed when children: require >40 ml/kg of intravenous fluids; need ≥1 inotrope; develop a raised respiratory rate or irregular breathing pattern (indicating emergent pulmonary oedema); and show persisting acidosis or have a significantly depressed conscious level.

Continued resuscitation and stabilization

Active management must be continued while awaiting the transfer team. Senior members of medical and nursing staff should remain with the transfer team during optimal stabilization prior to departure from the HDU.

The child should be accompanied by paediatric, anaesthetic, and nursing staff experienced in transfer care of the critically ill paediatric patient. Fluid resuscitation and inotropes should be continued. Final outcome depends on maintenance or improvement of condition during transfer.

Areas of controversy

Adrenal insufficiency in severe sepsis in children is associated with a poor prognosis. Low-dose corticosteroids to replace potential adrenal insufficiency in septic shock, are controversial. Children who have clear risk factors for adrenal insufficiency (previous steroid therapy, chronic illness or pituitary or adrenal abnormalities) should receive steroids; otherwise, hydrocortisone therapy should be used in catecholamine resistance, suspected or proven adrenal insufficiency, or when recommended by intensivists.

Plasmapheresis, haemofiltration and blood exchange have been used in PICU to reduce the concentrations of circulating endotoxin and cytokines. There is no double-blind trial evidence of their success.

There is no evidence that modulators of the inflammatory response are efficacious or safe (e.g. monoclonal antibodies against endotoxins and cytokines, nitric oxide synthase inhibitors and other agents such as activated recombinant protein C). Consensus guidelines advise against their use.

Supportive care

Postpubertal children with severe sepsis should also receive:
- Prophylaxis against deep vein thrombosis
- H_2 blocker prophylaxis against stress ulcers
- Renal replacement therapy if required with continuous veno-venous haemofiltration, (maybe clinically useful in children with anuria/severe oliguria and fluid overload)
- Correction of hypo- or hyperglycaemia
- Sedation and analgesia as required
- Blood products and (polyclonal) immunoglobulin preparations as necessary.

ECMO should be reserved for refractory paediatric septic shock and/or respiratory failure unresponsive to conventional therapies.

Follow-up and outcome

Children with sepsis syndrome should be examined at discharge for possible sequelae and followed up to detect late-onset sequelae. This is especially the case for infants who may not manifest minor neurodevelopmental sequelae or learning difficulties until school years. Children who have had septicaemia or meningitis should have audiological testing.

Children who have been immunized against *H. influenzae* type b, *Meningococcus* type C, and *S. pneumoniae* may need immunological investigations if infected with these organisms.

Future research

Diagnostic research should be aimed at differentiating emerging sepsis from non-life-threatening infections in childhood populations. Studies are needed to improve the prediction of the early signs of serious bacterial infection, which include:
- Confirm normal ranges for heart rate and respiratory rate at various body temperatures; positive predictive value of vital signs, non-specific features (such as limb pain and cold hands and feet), and blood investigations (for example, procalcitonin and CRP), alone or in combination
- Clinical scoring systems.

Research into prevention and management of sepsis with anti-infective, anti-inflammatory, or anti-sepsis drugs (often agents antagonistic to endo-toxins, the cytokines or inflammatory mediators) are required. Novel non-mortality endpoints, such as organ failure-free days or ventilator-free days, have been proposed for paediatric clinical trials given the relatively low incidence of mortality in paediatric sepsis. Biomarkers such as procalcitonin, D-dimer, IL-6, and IL-8 may also be used as primary endpoints. Longer-term outcomes such as overall level of functioning at 3- or 6-month follow-up may also be useful endpoints.

A study of replacement corticosteroids in paediatric septic shock is required.

Further reading

Annane D, Bellissant E, Cavaillon JM. Septic shock. *Lancet* 2005;**365**:63–78.

Dellinger RP, Levy MM, Carlet JM, *et al.* Surviving Sepsis Campaign: international guidelines for management of severe sepsis and septic shock: 2008. *Intensive Care Med* 2008;**34**:783–5.

Goldstein B, Giroir B, Randolph A, Members of the International Consensus Conference on Pediatric Sepsis. International pediatric sepsis consensus conference: Definitions for sepsis and organ dysfunction in pediatrics. *Pediatr Crit Care Med* 2005;**6**:2–8.

National Collaborating Centre for Women's and Children's Health. Feverish Illness in Children: Assessment and Initial Management in Children Younger than 5 years. London: National Institute for Health and Clinical Excellence, 2007. Available at: ✍ www.nice.org.uk/CG47 (accessed 1 February 2011).

National Institute for Health and Clinical Excellence (NICE). *Bacterial Meningitis and Meningococcal Septicaemia: Management in Children and Young People Under 16 years in Primary and Secondary Care.* London: National Collaborating Centre for Women's and Children's Health, October 2009 (consultation document).

Scottish Intercollegiate Guidelines Network (SIGN). *Management of Invasive Meningococcal Disease in Children and Young People: A National Clinical Guideline.* Edinburgh: SIGN, 2008.

Chapter 37

Sexually transmitted infections

📖 see also Chapters 19, 43, 58, 68, 70, 75, 76, 79, 88, 107

Introduction

- Sexually transmitted infections (STIs) in young people (<25 years) are causing a public health crisis.
- The use of barriers such as male condoms, and vaginal and anal dams, reduce the likelihood of transmission but cannot always protect against infections caused by skin-to-skin contact, such as warts.
- Multiple sexual partners increase the risks of acquisition.
- Adolescent girls are more susceptible to infection, possibly due to cervical ectopy and a relatively immature immune system.
- Findings of STIs in prepubertal children raise concerns about possible sexual abuse, but some, in young children, may have been acquired from the mother during pregnancy, delivery, or breastfeeding.
- It should be remembered that the wide variety of receptive and insertive sexual activity practised requires investigation of multiple sites.
- When postpubertal girls attend services for contraception (particularly if condoms have not been used) or are pregnant, it is appropriate to offer testing for sexual infections.

Causative organisms

Viruses

- Herpes simplex virus (HSV) types 1 and 2
- Hepatitis B
- Hepatitis C
- HIV
- Molluscum contagiosum virus
- Human papillomavirus (HPV), usually types 6 and 11

Bacteria

- *Chlamydia trachomatis*
- CT serovars 1, 2, and 3 causing lymphogranuloma venereum (LGV)
- *Neisseria gonorrhoea*
- (Bacterial vaginosis may be associated with the presence of STIs)

Spirochaetes
- *Treponema pallidum* (syphilis)

Protozoa
- *Trichomonas vaginalis*

UK prevalence

- There is often coexistence of more than one STI.
- Teenagers are the main group with a reported rise in STIs (Table 37.1).

Table 37.1 Numbers of new diagnoses in 2007 (and percentage increase from 1998) in sexually transmitted infections by age

	Males under 16	Males 16–19	Males all ages	Females <16	Females 16–19	Females all ages
C. trachomatis	406 (269)	10 002 (289)	60 798 (189)	3154 (162)	22 037 (141)	61 188 (121)
N. gonorrhoeae	80 (8)	1742 (66)	12 933 (45)	412 (31)	2120 (37)	5777 (35)
Warts	208 (4)	5311 (65)	47 239 (29)	1526 (54)	12 856 (34)	42 599 (26)
HSV	20 (−9)	718 (126)	10 031 (50)	462 (110)	3249 (63)	16 031 (52)
Syphilis (primary and secondary)	4 (0)	52 (940)	2,395 (2,561)	8 (0)	46 (143)	285 (482)

Derived from multiple sources at the Health Protection Agency.

- Part of the increased diagnoses made at genitourinary clinics may be due to reduced perceived stigma in accessing services for check-ups when asymptomatic, or for investigation of symptoms.
- The English National Chlamydia Screening Programme aims to test 35% of young people aged 15–24 in 2009–10, and in 2007 had an overall 10% positive rate averaged across different settings, with higher figures in genitourinary attendees and at abortion services.
- Figures for HIV infection in people <16 years has approximately halved, whereas those diagnosed at ages 16–18 have not changed markedly in the past 5 years.

European prevalence

It is more difficult to assess the true prevalence or percentage changes across Europe, as people access STI care in a greater variety of settings. Only some STIs in some countries require mandatory reporting, and so direct comparisons are not possible.

Clinical presentation

Mother-to-child transmission may result in presentation at birth or early childhood. The possible modes of transmission are summarized in Table 37.2.

Table 37.2 Possible modes of transmission to the infant

Infection	Mode of transmission		
	Transplacental	During labour	Via breast milk
HIV	+	+	+
Hepatitis B and C	+	+	
Syphilis	+	+	
HSV, gonorrhoea, trichomonas, warts, and chlamydia		+	

- Presentation in infants includes no symptoms, conjunctivitis, lung infections, encephalitis, rashes, failure to thrive, laryngeal warts, and hepatosplenomegaly

Prepubertal children:
- None
- Discharge
- Itching
- Dysuria, frequency or enuresis.

By definition, sexual intercourse with a prepubertal child is sexual abuse and may present with symptoms other than those due to infection, e.g. pain with defecation, soiling or withholding, and emotional problems, e.g. school refusal.

Paediatricians with concerns about possible sexual abuse should take into account whether mother-to-child transmission has been possible, and the time after which external infection is more likely, as indicated in Table 37.3. Unfortunately the evidence base is lacking, and maternal infection does not exclude subsequent acquisition by the child due to abuse. Table 37.3 is therefore only a very rough guide.

Table 37.3 Indicative likelihood of a sexually transmitted infection being acquired by vertical transmission

	Possible delay in detection/presentation if acquired via mother-to-child transmission	Index of suspicion of acquisition through sexual abuse if outside these time periods
Warts	Several months	+
Chlamydia	Up to 3 years	+++
Gonorrhoea	Up to 1 year	+++
Herpes simplex	2 weeks, possibly longer	++
Trichomonas	4 weeks	+++
HIV	Weeks to years	(Maternal testing and look back if antenatal tests done)
Syphilis	Weeks to years	(Maternal testing and look back if antenatal tests done)
Hepatitis B	Weeks to months	(Maternal testing and look back if antenatal tests done)

Sexually active teenagers:
- None (chlamydia is asymptomatic in 70% girls and 50% boys)
- Vaginal, penile or anal discharge
- Vulval itching or discomfort
- Dysuria
- Intermenstrual or post coital bleeding in girls
- Testicular pain
- Prostatitis
- Pelvic pain during intercourse
- Genital ulcers
- Genital warty lesions
- Throat infections where receptive or insertive oral sex has occurred
- Skin rashes
- Inguinal lymphadenopathy
- Tenesmus in LGV
- Later sequelae such as iritis, arthritis, ectopic pregnancy, infertility, chronic pelvic pain, cancer of cervix, oropharynx, or rectum.

Differential diagnosis

- Non-sexually transmitted infections—*Candida*, bacterial vaginosis, Group A Streptococcal (GAS) disease causing perineal erythema and bleeding in younger children.
- Physiological vaginal discharge.
- Retained tampon or self-inserted foreign body in younger children.

- Skin conditions such as lichen planus, lichen sclerosus, psoriasis, eczema, blistering conditions.
- Unscheduled, heavy, painful or prolonged vaginal bleeding related to side effects of hormonal or intrauterine contraception.

Investigations

- Swabs taken from the cervix or low vagina for nucleic acid amplification tests for chlamydia and gonorrhoea. Blind introital or low vaginal swabs, where possible, for prepubertal girls. Cervical culture where possible for antibiotic sensitivity if positive for gonorrhoea.
- First pass urines more than 1.5 hours since last voiding for chlamydia and gonorrhoea in boys and girls.
- Rectal nucleic acid amplification test for LGV.
- Viral culture for herpes from blister fluid.
- Dark ground microscopy of scrapings from the base of (usually painless) ulcers and serology for syphilis.
- Serology for HIV antibody and p24 antigen, from 6 weeks post exposure.
- Serology for hepatitis B surface antigen.
- Examination under anaesthesia may be required to look for foreign bodies in young children when other causes of symptoms have been excluded.
- Paediatricians have opportunities to consider early detection of STIs when young women present with urinary symptoms with culture-negative mid-stream urine samples, and when there are concerns about possible pregnancy.

Management and treatment

- Management will depend on the age of the child or young person, and whether safeguarding children assessment and referral are required.
- Where sexual abuse is considered, specialist examination with samples taken to preserve a forensic chain of evidence will be required.
- For young people who are having sex consensually, knowledge of the legal age of consent in different countries in the UK plus assessment of Gillick competence, using the Fraser rules to consent to treatment, must guide clinicians.
- Clinicians should be alert to the possibility of coercion, providing sex for money and trafficking.
- Partner notification is a vital public health intervention to break the chain of infection, and this is most often facilitated by health advisers in genitourinary clinics.
- Treatment must be followed by abstention from all sexual activity until all current partners have completed own treatment. Unsurprisingly this is not always followed, so re-infection occurs. Adherence to medication may be a particular concern in young people, and directly observed treatment as a single dose may be best for chlamydia.

- Antibiotics may reduce the effectiveness of combined hormonal contraceptive methods, while taking it and for the following 7 days. Liver enzyme-inducing antibiotics such as rifampicin and rifabutin, and some antiretroviral drugs lower the efficacy of oestrogens and progestogens, affecting combined hormonal methods, subdermal implants, emergency hormonal and progestogen-only oral contraception. Up-to-date evidence about which drugs cause this effect is available on ℞ www.hiv-druginteractions.org.
- Consider the need for emergency contraception if there has been recent unprotected vaginal intercourse.
- Postexposure prophylaxis for sexual exposure to HIV may be advisable in high-risk situations—see the British HIV Association website (℞ www.bhiva.org).
- Hepatitis B immunoglobulin followed by an accelerated course of immunization may also be indicated in acute situations.

Follow-up and outcome

- Health advisers contact patients to ensure compliance with treatment and advice not to restart having sex until completion of treatment for all partners. Retreatment of all partners may be required if not compliant.
- Test of cure required following treatment for gonorrhoea.
- Test of cure for chlamydia only required if young person is pregnant or has been treated with less effective medication such as erythromycin.
- Review of clinical response to treatment for warts and continuation or change of treatment if required.

Prevention

- Health promotion to help the young person consider if they feel ready to start or continue having sex and strategies to avoid peer pressure.
- Teach correct use of condoms and encourage their use with all new partners, or where the faithfulness of the current partner is in doubt (safest to always doubt).
- Interventions to reduce other related risk-taking behaviour, such as alcohol and recreational drugs.
- In England, the National Chlamydia Screening Programme aims to decrease incidence in the community by case finding on an annual basis or where there has been a partner change, and partner notification. The highest uptake for screening is currently in the white ethnic population, but the highest positivity rate is in the black Caribbean and other black groups. Scotland does not have universal screening, but targets areas of greatest prevalence.
- HPV vaccine is currently offered to girls to prevent cervical cancer.
- Hepatitis B vaccination should be offered to all young men who have sex with men, people who themselves share drug injecting equipment or whose sexual partner does so, and people who sell sex.

Future research

- Feasibility of adopting HPV vaccination for young men to prevent oro-genital warts.
- Strategies to encourage more people from ethnic communities to come forward for chlamydia screening.

Further reading

British Association for Sexual Health and HIV. *UK National Guideline on the Management of Suspected Sexually Transmitted Infections and Related Conditions in Children and Young People.* London: BASHH, 2009. Available at: ℜ www.bashh.org (accessed 1 February 2011).

General Medical Council. *0–18 Guidance For All Doctors.* 2007. Available at: ℜ www.gmc-uk.org/ (accessed 9 February 2011).

Health Protection Agency. *Sexually Transmitted Infections and Young People in the United Kingdom.* London: HPA, 2008. Available at: ℜ www.hpa.org.uk (accessed 1 February 2011).

National Chlamydia Screening Programme. ℜ www.chlamydiascreening.nhs.uk/ps/default.html.

National Institute for Health and Clinical Excellence. *One to One Interventions to Reduce the Transmission of Sexually Transmitted Infections (STIs) Including HIV, and to Reduce the Rate of Under 18 Conceptions, Especially Among Vulnerable and at Risk Groups.* Public Health Intervention Guidance 3. London: NICE, 2007. Available at: ℜ www.nice.org.uk/ (accessed 9 February 2011).

Royal College of Paediatrics and Child Health. *Child Protection Companion.* London: RCPCH, 2006. Available at: ℜ www.rcpch.ac.uk.

Royal College of Paediatrics and Child Health, in collaboration with the Royal College of Physicians of London, and its Faculty of Forensic and Legal Medicine. *The Physical Signs of Child Sexual Abuse. An Evidence-Based Review and Guidance for Best Practice.* London: RCPCH, 2008.

Skin and soft tissue infections

📖 see also Chapters 15, 57, 72, 88, 91, 102, 105, 106, 110

Introduction

The skin consists of the superficial epidermis and the deeper dermis (Fig. 38.1). Soft tissues consisting of adipose tissue, fascia and muscle lie beneath the skin. The skin forms an important barrier as part of the body's innate resistance to infection. Nevertheless infections of the skin and subcutaneous tissues do occur and are common in childhood. The skin and soft tissues can be infected by bacteria, viruses, fungi, and parasites.

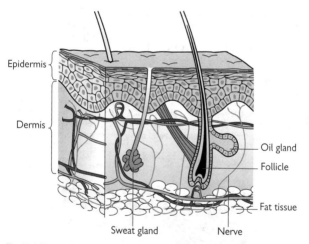

Epidermis

Dermis

Oil gland

Follicle

Fat tissue

Sweat gland   Nerve

Fig. 38.1 Human skin showing the epidermis, dermis, and subcutaneous tissue.

Bacterial infections

Cellulitis

Cellulitis is the term used to describe a bacterial infection of the dermis and subcutaneous tissues. It can occur on any part of the body although the arms and legs are probably the commonest sites. Cellulitis usually develops beneath an area of skin that has been broken or damaged. Cellulitis can vary in severity from a localized, self-limiting condition to a more extensive infection with toxic features.

Causative organisms
- *Staphylococcus aureus* (commonest)
- GAS (sometimes as coinfection with *S. aureus*)
- Rarely *Haemophilus influenzae*

Clinical features
- Red (rubor), painful (dolor), warm (calor), and swelling (turgor) of skin and subcutaneous tissues (the four classic signs of inflammation described by Celsus at around AD 0).
- Low grade fever.
- Toxic systemic features if extensive or progressive.
- Blue or purple tinge to cellulitis may suggest *H. influenzae* infection or beware necrotizing fasciitis (📖 p. 535).

Investigations
- Blood culture, FBC, and CRP if moderate or severe infection.

Treatment
- Mild cases treated with oral flucloxacillin.
- Moderate to severe cases treated with intravenous flucloxacillin ± benzyl penicillin or co-amoxiclav (has good activity against streptococcal and staphylococcal infection).

Impetigo

Impetigo is a superficial infection of the top layers of the epidermis. It is common in childhood and can occur on any part of the body although the face is particularly common in young children. Like cellulitis, it often develops at a site where the epidermis has been breached. The infection then develops as a result of invasion by the host's endogenous bacteria. Impetigo can be highly contagious and outbreaks have been reported.

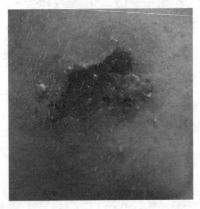

Fig. 38.2 Impetigo.

Causative organisms
- S. aureus—classically golden crusts
- GAS (less common)

Clinical features
- Superficial ulcer-like lesions, 0.5–6cm in diameter, usually with crusting, typically golden in colour.
- Early lesions may be vesicular.
- Non-tender.
- Can vary from single to multiple lesions all over body.
- Bullous form (consisting of big, round, fluid-filled blisters that burst leaving a ring-like lesion) can occur in infants and young children. Can look like cigarette burns—beware.

Investigations
- Skin swab

Treatment
- Mild cases can be treated with topical antibiotics, e.g. fusidic acid or mupirocin. There are increasing reports of topical fusidic acid resistance in skin infections.
- More extensive cases treated with oral flucloxacillin.
- Consider nasal mupirocin to eliminate nasal carriage of S. aureus, especially if recurrent or multiple cases.

Folliculitis and boils

Folliculitis is a localized infection of the hair follicles. It is quite common and tends to occur in patches, often where the hair follicles have been rubbed or damaged. It appears as multiple pimples or pustules at the sites of hair follicles. It is usually caused by S. aureus. Treatment is often not required. When it is, a topical antibiotic such as fusidic acid will usually suffice.

Boils (or furuncles) are small abscesses that develop in the hair follicles. Multiple, confluent boils are known as carbuncles. Again, boils and carbuncles are usually caused by S. aureus. They can be treated with oral flucloxacillin and/or by incision and drainage. Recurrent boils can be a marker of immune deficiency, especially neutrophil defects—although they virtually always are not!

Animal and human bites

Cutaneous and soft tissue infections can develop after bites by cats, dogs, and humans. In some cases it is advisable to prescribe prophylactic antibiotics after animal bites.

Causative organisms
- S. aureus, anaerobic cocci, and Bacteroides spp.
- GAS (human bites)
- Pasteurella multocida and Pseudomonas fluorescens (animal bites)

Treatment
- Prophylaxis with oral co-amoxiclav is recommended for cat and human bites and also for severe dog bites or dog bites that cannot be adequately cleaned and irrigated.

- Infected bites can be treated with oral co-amoxiclav.
- More severe infections should be treated with intravenous ceftriaxone/cefotaxime and metronidazole.

Staphylococcal scalded skin syndrome

Staphylococcal scalded skin syndrome is a toxin-mediated condition causing widespread desquamation of the skin. Staphylococci, often resident in the nares, release an exotoxin (exfoliatin), which damages linkage proteins in the superficial layers of the epidermis. Despite the dramatic appearance of the condition the skin in scalded skin syndrome usually heals quickly and without scarring.

Causative organism
- S. aureus

Clinical features
- Early lesions appear bullous.
- Followed by widespread shedding of the superficial layers of the skin, leaving raw red areas sometimes with serous discharge and later crusting.
- Lesions may be tender initially.
- Child is otherwise well.
- Children may have simultaneous impetiginous lesions, typically around the nose.

Investigations
- Nose swab

Treatment
- Intravenous flucloxacillin.
- Consider nasal mupirocin to eliminate nasal carriage of S. aureus.

Necrotizing fasciitis

Necrotizing fasciitis is an extensive infection of the deeper skin layers and soft tissues. It is caused by bacteria that can destroy the fascial layers of the subcutaneous tissues and hence allow the infection to spread. Necrotizing fasciitis is rare in children.

There are two types:
- **Type I necrotizing fasciitis: caused by polymicrobial infections** (Vibrio vulnificus, Clostridium perfringens, Bacteroides fragilis).
- **Type II necrotizing fasciitis: caused by** S. pyogenes infection or less commonly—MRSA. 30–50% of patients with S. pyogenes-associated necrotizing fasciitis develop streptococcal toxic shock syndrome. Pseudomonas is also an important cause, especially after trauma or burns, etc.

In children:
- Most cases of necrotizing fasciitis occur without an apparent preceding factor—may follow blunt trauma
- When a precipitating factor is present the most common factor is varicella infection, often on day 3 or 4 of rash.

Clinical features
- Extremely painful swelling of soft tissue, usually of a limb or the abdomen.
- Livid red/purple discolouration of skin, only as a late sign of necrosis.
- Fever and toxic features often present.

Investigations
- Blood culture, FBC, and CRP

Treatment
- Supportive.
- Multiple broad-spectrum intravenous antibiotics.
- Urgent surgical debridement based on clinical signs alone.

Viral infections

Chickenpox

Chickenpox (or varicella) is one of the common exanthemata of childhood. It is extremely contagious and almost all individuals are infected during childhood. Immunization is available but it is not currently on the routine UK schedule. Children with immune deficiency require protection from chickenpox. 📖 See p. 465.

Shingles

Shingles (or herpes zoster) is a skin condition caused by reactivation of the herpesvirus that causes chickenpox. It is moderately uncommon in childhood and, when it does occur, it can be a marker of immune deficiency if multidermatomal (📖 see Chapter 57, p. 465). Most children with shingles are in good health otherwise.

Molluscum contagiosum

Molluscum contagiosum is a skin infection caused by a poxvirus. It is quite common in childhood with up to 20% children being infected at some time. The individual skin lesions of molluscum contagiosum last for up to a couple of months but the lesions tend to propagate so an infection may persist for many months or even years before finally being eliminated by the immune system. Molluscum contagiosum appears to be more common and to last for longer in children with immune deficiency. Molluscum contagiosum is spread by direct contact or fomites. It is moderately contagious. 📖 See Chapter 88, p. 633.

Warts and verrucae

Warts are rough, raised skin lesions up to 0.5cm in diameter. They are common in childhood. They are most often found on the fingers but can affect any part of the body. Warts are caused by human papillomaviruses that cause proliferation of the upper layers of the skin at the site of the wart. Verrucae (or plantar warts) are viral warts on the soles of the feet that have been flattened and driven into the skin by pressure.

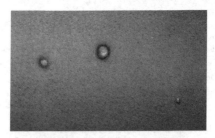

Fig. 38.3 Molluscum contagiosum.

Fungal infections

Tinea corporis (ringworm), tinea capitis (scalp ringworm), and tinea pedis (athlete's foot) are all fungal skin infections that can occur in childhood.

Clinical features
- Tinea corporis: large round scaly lesions, typically with a reddish border; lesions progress outwards with time, often leaving a pale centre of normal skin.
- Tinea capitis: papules or scaling lesions on the scalp that cause hairs to become brittle and broken; sometimes progress to form a boggy mass (a kerion).
- Tinea pedis: itchy scaling and cracking of the skin of the feet, particularly between the toes.

Parasites

Scabies
See Chapter 102, p. 697
  Scabies is an infestation of the skin caused by *Sarcoptes scabiei*, a parasitic mite. It is not uncommon in children. Scabies produces burrows and papules in the skin. The lesions are classically found in the interdigital spaces, wrists and ankles but, especially in young children, any area of skin can be affected. Scabies is extremely itchy so the lesions are typically accompanied by evidence of scratching.

Head lice
See Chapter 72, p. 542
Head lice (pediculosis) is a common childhood infestation of the scalp and hair. Head lice are small arthopods that can be seen on the hair and scalp. Nits are their empty egg cases and are attached to hair shafts.

Future research

- There is evidence of an increasing incidence of staphylococcal skin infections, but the cause is not clear.
- The use of fusidic acid cream for topical infections in an era of increasing fusidic acid resistance.

Further reading

Stevens DL, Bisno AL, Chambers HF, *et al*. Practice guidelines for the diagnosis and management of skin and soft-tissue infections. *Clin Infect Dis* 2005;**41**:1373–406.

Chapter 39

Toxic shock syndrome

📖 see also Chapters 36, 40, 105, 106

Toxic shock syndrome

- Toxic shock syndrome (TSS) is an acute febrile illness caused by Gram-positive bacteria (*Staphylococcus aureus*, *Streptococcus pyogenes*, and occasionally non-GAS) that rapidly progresses to shock with multiorgan failure.
- The capillary leak that underlies the disease results from intense T cell proliferation and cytokine release that is part of an inflammatory response initiated by bacterial protein exotoxins that act as superantigens.

Pathophysiology

- Superantigens are potent immunomodulatory proteins that stimulate T cells by directly binding class II molecules on antigen-presenting cells to the T cell receptor (Fig. 39.1).
- Unlike conventional antigens, superantigen stimulation is not major histocompatibility complex (MHC) class II restricted but is constrained in only a limited fashion by the specificity of the T cell receptor 'Vβ family' defined by the variable portion of the B chain of the T cell receptor (TCRVB).
- Superantigens stimulate a large proportion (up to 20%) of T cells resulting in intense immune activation and release of cytokines including TNFα, IL-1, IL-2 and interferon γ, which lead to the clinical features of TSS.

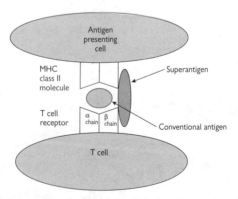

Fig. 39.1 Composite diagram contrasting T cell stimulation by a conventional antigen and a superantigen.

Incidence and aetiology

Streptococcal TSS

- *S. pyogenes*:
  - Gram-positive cocci
  - Form chains
  - Catalase negative
  - β-haemolytic colonies on blood agar
  - Lancefield typing (typing of the carbohydrate in the cell wall) identifies the organisms as GAS.
- Streptococcal TSS occurs in association with invasive *S. pyogenes* infections (isolation of the organism from a normally sterile site).
- Since the mid-1980s there have been increasing reports of streptococcal TSS around the world.
- The incidence of streptococcal TSS in industrialized countries is approximately 3.0 cases per 100 000.
  - The incidence in resource-poor countries appears to be at least three times higher.
- Streptococcal TSS can affect any age group:
  - Infants and the elderly are most at risk.
  - Approximately 20% of all cases of invasive *S. pyogenes* infections occur in children.

Staphylococcal TSS

- *S. aureus*:
  - Gram-positive cocci
  - Form clusters
  - Catalase positive
  - Coagulase positive.
- There are two types of staphylococcal TSS: menstrual and non-menstrual.

Menstrual staphylococcal toxic shock

- Accounts for 50–60% of adult cases of staphylococcal TSS.
- First described in 1980 in the USA in menstruating women using hyperabsorbable tampons.
- Incidence rates were as high as 12.3 per 100 000 in women of menstruating age.
- Incidence rates fell to 1 per 100 000 within 6 years of the removal of these tampons from the market, and continues at this rate today.
- Almost always associated with the superantigen toxic shock syndrome toxin-1 (TSST-1).

Non-menstrual staphylococcal toxic shock

- Accounts for nearly 50% of all cases of staphylococcal TSS.
- Surgical procedures and burns are important risk factors.

Clinical features

- Streptococcal TSS and staphylococcal TSS share similar clinical features including:
  - Fever
  - Diffuse, macular, erythematous, blanching ('sunburn') type rash, followed by desquamation after approximately 2 weeks (often as early as a few days in staphylococcal TSS)
  - Rapid progression to shock and multiorgan failure
  - Mucosal hyperaemia: non-purulent conjunctivitis; oropharyngeal changes including swollen lips or strawberry tongue; vaginal hyperaemia in the case of staphylococcal TSS.
- Approximately half of patients have hypotension at presentation and nearly all develop hypotension over the following 4 hours; subacute presentations in which patients deteriorate over days are rare.
- Other early signs suggesting capillary leak include postural hypotension, tachycardia, and increased capillary refill time.
- While it is not possible to reliably distinguish streptococcal from staphylococcal TSS from the clinical features alone, particularly early in the disease, there are some differences between the two syndromes (Table 39.1).

Table 39.1 Characteristic features of streptococcal and staphylococcal TSS

	Streptococcal TSS	**Staphylococcal TSS**
Mortality rate	30–60%	<3%
Positive blood cultures	60–80%	Low
Typical rash	Less common	Very common
Associations	Soft tissue infection	Tampon use
	Varicella infection	Surgical procedures
	NSAID	NSAID
		Burns
		Influenza infection

Streptococcal TSS

- Patients with streptococcal TSS may initially present with a flu-like prodromal illness with fever, myalgia, vomiting, and diarrhoea before their illness declares itself.
- Soft tissue infection is the most common associated focus of infection (>60% of cases).
  - Up to 75% of these soft tissue infections may progress to necrotizing fasciitis.

- Other associated clinical infections include empyema, septic arthritis, peritonitis, meningitis, tracheitis, endophthalmitis, and perihepatitis.
- Presents with bacteraemia alone without a clear focus in approximately 15% of cases.
- Neonatal streptococcal TSS is well-described.
  - In 75% of cases there is documented maternal vaginal carriage of S. pyogenes.

Necrotizing fasciitis
📖 See Chapter 38, p. 327
- 30–50% of patients with S. pyogenes associated necrotizing fasciitis develop streptococcal TSS.
- In children, most cases of necrotizing fasciitis occur without an apparent preceding factor.
- When a precipitating factor is present the most common factor is varicella infection.
  - Persistent fever or a new fever on day 3 or 4 of chickenpox should alert the clinician to the possibility of invasive S. pyogenes infection.
  - Blunt trauma is another risk factor in children.

Staphylococcal TSS

Menstrual staphylococcal TSS
- Starts within 2 days of the beginning or end of menses.
- Up to 30% of cases are recurrent.

Non-menstrual staphylococcal TSS
- Occurs in any age group and affects both sexes.
- Patients may only have a trivial cutaneous or subcutaneous (or undetected) infection as the focus of infection.
- In children the skin is the most common site of infection.
  - Other clinical syndromes include visceral abscesses, endocarditis, osteomyelitis, pyomyositis, mastitis, and peritonitis.
- Staphylococcal TSS has been associated with:
  - Surgical procedures: especially ear, nose and throat surgery and nasal packing
  - Postoperative wound infection and colonization: there may be no evidence of obvious inflammation of the wound
  - Burns: children are at particularly high risk; if TSS occurs it is usually in the first few days following the burn
  - Influenza infection: TSS occurring in children with influenza carries a high mortality rate
  - AIDS: recalcitrant desquamative syndrome
  - Chronic peritoneal dialysis
  - Childbirth.

Investigations and diagnosis

- Case definitions for both staphylococcal TSS and streptococcal TSS have been developed (Boxes 39.1 and 39.2).
  - The diagnostic criteria for TSS were designed as research criteria.
  - They have high specificity to identify established cases, but poor sensitivity, particularly early in the disease course.
  - Failure to meet these criteria should not delay a provisional diagnosis and the management strategies described below.

Investigations

- Patients with suspected TSS need adequate microbiological investigations including:
  - Blood cultures
  - Culture of any obviously infected sites as clinically indicated such as joint aspiration, pleural fluid aspiration
  - Culture of tampon and high vaginal swab in menstrual TSS.
- Patients with suspected TSS need investigating for the potential development of multiorgan failure including the following (these tests often need to be repeated):
  - Arterial blood gas
  - FBC
  - Creatinine, blood U&Es
  - Liver enzymes
  - Clotting profile including fibrinogen, D-dimers
  - Serum albumin
  - Creatinine phosphokinase
  - Chest radiograph.
- Establishing the presence of a tampon (and its prompt removal) is a crucial part of the examination and investigation of all post-menarche female patients with TSS.
- If the diagnosis of necrotizing fasciitis is not clear, several investigations may be useful including:
  - MRI
  - Frozen section biopsy specimens of suspected areas of tissue.
- However, if there is a strong suspicion of necrotizing fasciitis surgery should not be delayed.

Differential diagnosis

- Gram-negative septic shock
- Meningococcal sepsis
- Myocarditis
- Kawasaki disease
- Severe influenza
- Rocky Mountain spotted fever and other rickettsial infections
- Leptospirosis
- Measles
- Hantavirus

Box 39.1 Diagnostic criteria for streptococcal TSS

Streptococcal toxic shock syndrome—case definition
1. Isolation of GASi
   A. From a sterile site (definite case)
   B. From a non-sterile site (probable case)
2. Clinical signs of severity
   A. Hypotension
   AND
   B. Two or more of the following clinical and laboratory abnormalities:
       a. Fever (>38.5°C)
       b. Rash (diffuse macular erythema with subsequent desquamation)
       c. Renal impairment
       d. Coagulopathy (platelets <100 × 10^9 /l or disseminated intra-vascular coagulation)
       e. Liver enzyme abnormalities
       f. ARDS
       g. Extensive tissue necrosis (including necrotizing fasciitis)

Box 39.2 Diagnostic criteria for staphylococcal TSS

Staphylococcal toxic shock syndrome—case definition
1. Fever (>38.9°C)
2. Hypotension
3. Rash (diffuse macular rash with subsequent desquamation)
4. Involvement of three of the following organ systems:
   a. Liver (elevated transaminases)
   b. Blood (platelets <100 × 10^9/l)
   c. Renal (raised creatinine/urea or pyuria in absence of urinary tract infection)
   d. Mucous membranes (vaginal, conjunctival or oropharyngeal hyperaemia)
   e. Gastrointestinal (vomiting and profuse diarrhoea)
   f. Muscular (severe myalgia or raised creatinine phosphokinase)
   g. CNS (disorientation or alteration in consciousness without focal neurological signs)
5. Exclusion of the following illnesses by negative serology:
   a. Measles
   b. Leptospirosis
   c. Rocky Mountain spotted fever
6. Negative blood or cerebrospinal fluid cultures for organisms other than *S. aureus*
Probable case: 5/6 features, confirmed 6/6 including desquamation.

Management

There are four elements to the management of TSS:
- Supportive care
- Surgical intervention
- Correct antibiotic choice
- Adjunctive treatments:
  - Intravenous immunoglobulin
  - Clindamycin.

Supportive care
- As one of the defining features of TSS is the profound hypotension caused by toxin-mediated capillary leak, aggressive fluid replacement and the early use of inotropes is crucial.
- Renal support may also be required early; renal failure often precedes hypotension.
- Patients often require endotracheal intubation and ventilation, particularly when ARDS develops.

Surgical intervention
- Surgical intervention is particularly important in streptococcal TSS when there is soft tissue infection.
  - The mainstay of treatment in necrotizing fasciitis is debridement.
  - Wide debridement of non-viable tissue is critical and substantially improves outcome.
  - Surgical intervention is also important in establishing the diagnosis of necrotizing fasciitis.
- Surgical intervention is required less often in staphylococcal TSS.

Antibiotic therapy
- Empiric broad-spectrum antibiotics are required until streptococcal or staphylococcal aetiology is confirmed.
- Penicillin is the first line antibiotic of choice for streptococcal TSS.
- A β-lactamase resistant antibiotic such as flucloxacillin is the first choice for staphylococcal TSS.
- Flucloxacillin is also an effective anti-streptococcal antibiotic and should therefore be used when the aetiology is uncertain.
- Clindamycin is often also added acting as a protein synthesis inhibitor. Theoretical advantages of clindamycin include:
  - Inhibitory action on toxin production
  - Ability to potentiate phagocytosis
  - Post-antibiotic effect
  - Superior tissue penetration.
- Clindamycin should be added to the above standard treatment regimens rather than replace them.
  - Clindamycin is a bacteriostatic (not bactericidal) antibiotic.
- Vancomycin may need to replace flucloxacillin as empiric therapy if there is a significant likelihood of MRSA:
  - Hospital-acquired infection
  - In regions where susceptibility patterns suggest that there is a relatively high risk of community-acquired MRSA.

- Patients from communities with high rates of community-acquired MRSA infections.

IVIG therapy

- Studies suggest that streptococcal TSS may be a subgroup of sepsis where IVIG has a beneficial role.
  - There is only one randomized controlled trial of IVIG in streptococcal TSS. The trial was ceased prematurely because of slow patient enrolment.
  - The study found a trend towards improved survival at 28 days but did not find a significant difference in mortality.
  - An earlier observational historically controlled cohort study showed a significant difference in mortality at 30 days.
  - It is unlikely that another randomized controlled trial of IVIG will take place in either staphylococcal or streptococcal TSS.
  - Most experts recommend the use of IVIG in streptococcal TSS.
- The role of IVIG in staphylococcal TSS has been studied in even less detail.
  - Generally IVIG is not indicated because of the low mortality rate of staphylococcal TSS.
  - However, given that the pathogenesis of staphylococcal and streptococcal TSS is similar and that the superantigens produced by *S. aureus* and *S. pyogenes* share a common three-dimensional structure and mode of action, it seems likely that IVIG will also be beneficial in severe cases.
- There is no consensus on the dose of IVIG that should be given in TSS.
  - Suggested doses included in Table 39.2 are based on doses used in the randomized controlled trial of IVIG in streptococcal TSS and the higher single dose regimen proven of value in Kawasaki disease.

Table 39.2 Two suggested dosing regimens for IVIG in TSS

Regimen	Day 1	Day 2	Day 3
1	2g/kg	–	Repeat 2g/kg if patient remains unstable
2	1g/kg	0.5g/kg	0.5g/kg

Other factors in the management of patients with TSS

- Some studies have noted an association between the use of non-steroidal anti-inflammatory drugs (NSAIDs), necrotizing fasciitis, and streptococcal TSS.
- The underlying cause for this association may be:
  - NSAIDs mask fever and reduce pain and may therefore lead to delayed presentation
  - Inhibition of the normal feedback loop of prostaglandin on the production of TNFα by macrophages leads to an excess of cytokines that predisposes to TSS.

- NSAIDs should be avoided in patients with TSS.
- Some experts recommend generally avoiding NSAIDs in patients without a known source for their fever, and particularly in children with varicella (which is a predisposing factor for TSS).

Outcome

- The case fatality rate for streptococcal TSS ranges between 30% and 60%.
- There is high morbidity with streptococcal TSS, especially in cases of necrotizing fasciitis in which wide debridement, potentially with amputation, is performed.
- The case fatality rate for non-menstrual staphylococcal TSS is approximately 6% while that of menstrual TSS is <3%.

Prevention

Contact prophylaxis in streptococcal TSS
- The attack rate of streptococcal TSS in close contacts of patients with streptococcal TSS is higher than the attack rate in general population:
  - Data from Canada: secondary attack rate 294 per 100 000
  - Data from the USA: secondary attack rate 66 per 100 000.
- There is no evidence to suggest that contact prophylaxis is effective in preventing disease in contacts.
- The advantages of contact prophylaxis are potentially preventing disease in contacts and preventing transmission of virulent strains.
- The disadvantages of contact prophylaxis include the unnecessary use of antibiotics in most contacts and the risk of serious side effects including anaphylaxis.
- Expert opinion varies on the use of contact prophylaxis.
- Options for secondary prophylaxis following streptococcal TSS include penicillin plus rifampicin.

Prevention of recurrent menstrual staphylococcal TSS
- Patients who have had a first episode of staphylococcal TSS are at risk of recurrent episodes. Risk factors include:
  - Menstrual TSS, particularly in the first 6 months after the episode of TSS
  - Inadequate anti-staphylococcal antibiotic therapy
  - Inadequate antibody response to staphylococcal toxin.

Future research

- The changing epidemiology of both staphylococcal and streptococcal TSS is the subject of ongoing surveillance in many centres.
  - The problem of MRSA, both hospital and community acquired, is increasing.

- Despite the increasing rates of community-acquired MRSA and their association with severe soft tissue infections, there is currently no evidence to suggest that these organisms are more likely to cause TSS.
- Improved knowledge of the immunopathogenesis of superantigen-mediated disease may lead to the development of new therapeutic agents.

Further reading

Darenberg J, Ihendyane N, Sjolin J, et al. Intravenous immunoglobulin G therapy in streptococcal toxic shock syndrome: a European randomized, double-blind, placebo-controlled trial. *Clin Infect Dis* 2003;**37**:333–40.

Kaul R, McGeer A, Norrby-Teglund A, et al. Intravenous immunoglobulin therapy for streptococcal toxic shock syndrome—a comparative observational study. The Canadian Streptococcal Study Group. *Clin Infect Dis* 1999;**28**:800–7.

McCormick JK, Yarwood JM, Schlievert PM. Toxic shock syndrome and bacterial superantigens: an update. *Annu Rev Microbiol* 2001;**55**:77–104.

The Working Group on Severe Streptococcal Infections. Defining the group A streptococcal toxic shock syndrome: rationale and consensus definition. *JAMA* 1993;**269**:390–1.

Chapter 40

Trauma, bites, and burns

📖 see also Chapters 38, 39, 48, 105, 106

Bites

- The majority of bites are due to dogs (80–90%), cats (5–15%), humans (3–20%), and rats (under 2%), with other animals contributing a small percentage of the cases.
- Dog bites tend to be on the limbs, particularly on the arms, with up to 25% of bites being on the head and neck. Preschool children tend to have bites on their heads, as this part of the body is closer to the biting reach of the animal than in older children.
- The main locations of cat bites in about 60% of cases are on the arms, approximately 28% on the head and neck, and the rest mostly on the lower limbs.
- Human bites are found on the hand, arm, shoulder, and leg in male victims, and in addition, in females, bites may occur on the breast or genitalia. Many people bitten manage the bite without further consequences; this applies to an estimate 5 out of 6 people who are bitten.
- In over 70% of cases, people are bitten by animals known to them; children are at high risk on injury, with children <5 years of age being at highest risk, from provoking animals.

Incidence

- US data show that over 4.5 million Americans are bitten every year, 400 000 require treatment and about 20 die from their injuries, mostly by exsanguination. They account for 1% of visits to emergency departments in the UK, with young males being more often bitten by dogs.
- Infectious complications can occur from all types of bites. Infection is usually polymicrobial, with up to 173 types of bacteria being found in the oral cavity. Bites usually contain aerobic and anaerobic bacteria, with *Pasteurella*, *Streptococcus*, *Staphylococcus aureus*, and the anaerobes *Fusobacterium* and *Bacteroides* most commonly identified from animal bites.
- Cat bites and hand wounds are more likely to become infected.
- Bloodborne viral infections may also be transmitted via a bite, including hepatitis viruses and HIV.

Principles of management of bites

- The following features should be documented:
    - How and when did it occur? Is there any delay in presentation?
    - When did it happen and in what circumstances?

- Assessment of the wound.
- Cleaning and debriding the wound.
- Consideration of prophylactic antibiotics.
- Treatment of any infections.
- Appropriate tetanus pre-emptive measures.

History

A history must be taken that includes any bleeding tendency, underlying immunosuppression or deficiency in making a competent immune response. This includes a history of diabetes or steroid therapy, liver disease or functional asplenia.

Immunization status including tetanus status must be documented and if required, booster vaccines administered. The mechanism must be determined and the possibility of non-accidental injury considered; if there is concern, safe guarding procedures should be activated.

Examination

The location of the bite, its appearance, and if there is any associated damage to structures at the bite site, for example, tendons, nerves, joints, blood vessels, or involvement of any organs such as the eye, must be documented and acted upon.

The clenched fist also has the potential for the metapharyngeal space to be breached by a bite which can lead to osteomyelitis, septic arthritis, or tracking infections within synovial sheaths.

Cleaning the wound

Wound cleaning is mandatory in the management of any bite. The wound should be irrigated with water, pain relief given, and the bite examined.

The risk of infection is estimated to be greater than 1 in 10 cases if any of the following apply:
- Full thickness puncture
- Deep penetration
- Injury occurred over 24 hours ago
- Devitalised or dead tissues
- Hand or foot wounds
- Medical predisposing conditions
- Underlying injury to other structures other than skin.

Penetrating wounds on the distal aspects of limbs, such as the foot or hand are at higher risk of infection, especially if the wound comprises puncture-like lacerations, which inoculate organisms into deeper tissues.

Dirty wounds, i.e. those with debris or faecal material contaminating the wound, are also at higher risk of infection, and may require surgical debridement, along with wounds with extensive devitalized tissues.

Avoid primary closure in:
- Deep puncture wounds
- Infected wounds
- Dirty wounds
- Bites to the feet or hands (consult with the recognized expert in your area)
- Wounds >24 hours of age.

Prophylactic antibiotics
- The use of antibiotics is controversial.
- Suggested sites for the use of prophylactic antibiotic use include:
  - Joints, bone or tendons
  - Hand or foot bites
  - Cat bites
  - Devitalized or dead tissue, or heavily contaminated tissues
  - Deep puncture wounds
  - Immunosuppression.
- Erythromycin should NOT be used as *Pasteurella* is resistant to this antibiotic.
- Co-amoxiclav is the best antibiotic—give for 3 days as prophylaxis, 7–10 days for established secondary infection.

Insect bites

Incidence
Up to 100% of the population gets bitten by an insect every year, but the number of fatalities are small, comprising on average about 4 deaths per annum.

UK insects
The very few harmful arthropods of the UK comprise:
- Hymenoptera—bees (including bumble bees and honey bees), wasps (including hornets and yellow jackets)
- Diptera—mosquitoes, horseflies, stable flies, blackflies
- Siphonoptera—fleas (human, cat, dog)
- Scabies
- Bedbugs
- Phthiraptera—lice.

Management
The child should be assessed for any life-threatening conditions such as an anaphylactic reaction.

Small local reactions
- If a sting is in place, remove without squeezing it.
- If bitten by a tick, remove it with tweezers (do not burn it off as otherwise the skin may be burnt!). Consider sending for identification.
- Thoroughly wash the site with water and cold compresses can be applied (never put ice directly on a wound as otherwise cold thermal injury can take place) along with mild analgesia such as paracetamol.
- A mild potency hydrocortisone cream can be applied such as 1% strength but a lesser dose should be used on facial bites.
- Antihistamines may have a place to reduce swelling and irritation, especially a sedating one, should the irritation be disturbing sleep.

Large reactions
These are defined as extending beyond the site of the bite.
- Offer pain relief—usually simple analgesia is sufficient.

- A short course of antihistamines—non-sedating for day time use and a sedating one for night-time may be helpful to the patient.

Systemic reactions

Anaphylaxis is likely if there are features of these three categories:

- Sudden onset and rapid evolution of signs and symptoms
- An impact on A and/or B and/or C
- Cutaneous features and/or mucosal involvement (e.g. flushing, angioedema, urticaria).

Cutaneous features alone are not indicative of anaphylaxis; however, up to 20% of patients with anaphylactic reactions do NOT have a cutaneous manifestation.

Hence, consider if the reaction is a systemic one, especially if there are any of the following:

- Signs of airway difficulty or obstruction
- Increased respiratory effort
- Hypotension, marked pallor, collapse, chest pain.

Burns

The skin acts a barrier, having a role in the regulation of temperature and water loss from the body. Once breached, these functions may be reduced, and heat loss accompanied by fluid loss can occur. The tissues deeper to the skin may become accessible to colonization by cutaneous commensals as well as pathogenic bacteria.

Prophylactic antibiotics are not routinely recommended, as the normal flora may be disturbed and lead to infection with other pathogens including fungal infection. Burns commonly occur in children, varying from superficial scalds to full thickness and life-threatening conditions.

Initial management of a child with a burn

- The initial approach is A (airway), B (breathing) and C (circulation), D (disability), and E (exposure) as in the management of any potentially life-threatening condition.
- Heat that may cause inhalation injury such as upper airway obstruction is life threatening; hence a child whose voice has changed pitch or is unable to speak properly should be considered for emergency intubation.
- The majority of burns do not fall into this life-threatening group; however, a full history and explanation is required in all cases, as a small number of cases are due to non-accidental injury, and must be managed appropriately.
- The assessment of pain and its relief at the earliest stage possible is mandatory.
- Tetanus status must be assessed and appropriate treatment given accordingly (📖 see Chapter 108, p. 735).

Assessment of the burn

The depth, location and size of the burn are important features as these have a bearing on the healing process and the need for involvement of specialists, such as plastic burns surgeons and their teams.

Depth

Superficial burns (formerly known as first-degree burns) only affects the epidermis, but are nonetheless painful as cellular contents reach pain fibres in the dermis. An example of superficial burn is sunburn.

Partial thickness burns (formerly called second-degree burns) do extend into the dermis but do not obliterate structures such as hair follicles or sebaceous glands, whose lining within the dermis is epithelial tissue. Hence, regeneration of the burnt area comes from marginal growth *and* growth from the epithelial structures that go into the dermal tissues. This means that there may not necessarily be scarring, as the whole burn area can be regenerated from epithelial cells.

Blisters may appear with this type of burn and are painful, for the same reasons as seen in superficial burns.

Full thickness burns (formerly called third-degree burns) involves the dermis, so that structures such as the hair follicles and sebaceous glands are destroyed. As the pain receptors are also destroyed, this lesion tends to be painless in the affected area (note that there may be gradients of burns so that surrounding tissues may show partial thickness or superficial thickness burns.

Full thickness burns are associated with scarring and a poor cosmetic result unless plastic expertise is sought, as the deeper regenerative epithelial layers have been destroyed.

Location and size

Full thickness burns, fire injuries, and burns over 30% of surface area are more likely to become infected. Large burns—over 30%, also cause significant immunosuppression. Humoral, T cell, and neutrophil immune deficits have been reported.

For all ages, the following surface areas apply
- The anterior and posterior aspects of trunk = 26%
- The neck circumference = 2%
- The upper arm (humeral part) = 4%
- The forearm = 3%
- The dorsum of the hand = 1.5%
- The plantar aspect = 1.5%
- The dorsum of the feet = 1.75%
- The plantar aspect of the foot = 1.75%
- The genital area = 1%
- Each buttock = 2.5%

Management

As noted previously, attention is first paid to ABC and pain relief. Thereafter simple measures such as cooling the burns with tepid water (very cold water can cause hypothermia).

A simple non-adherent covering can be applied, such as clingfilm in the first instance so that the wound can be observed.

Complications

Infection is often a difficult diagnosis in children with burns as they usually have a high white cell count and CRP. Nearly all children with a serious burn have a high fever, often for a week or longer.

The classical signs of burn wound infection are local signs of inflammation, or a purulent exudate, with or without clinical signs of sepsis syndrome. A skin biopsy may be helpful in confirming the diagnosis and for culture. Early infection in the first two days is usually due to skin organisms, including GAS and *S. aureus*.

By around 1 week, most burns are colonized by Gram-negative organisms, including *Pseudomonas* and other Enterobacteriaceae. Later infections include those caused by *Candida*, *Aspergillus*, and other fungi. Later infections of nosocomial organisms have been reported. Inhalation pneumonitis can be complicated by severe pneumonia.

TSS is an uncommon complication but can be lethal if it is not recognized. It may occur in any size of burns including small burns. There will often not be the appearance of infection at the wound site but the symptoms of being unwell with the signs of erythema, vasodilation, tachycardia, tachypnoea, diarrhoea and 'toxic' appearance should raise the suspicion of this disorder.

Management

- Routine prophylactic systemic antibiotics are no longer used in burns units, or for burns treated and sent home.
- Careful dressing and use of topical antimicrobial agents are often used.
- Replacement immunoglobulin is now also no longer used.
- Systemic antibiotics are given only for clinical or proven sepsis. Use as narrow-spectrum as possible, with short treatment duration. Very narrow-spectrum penicillin-based antibiotics may be used in the first 2 days, but an agent active against *Pseudomonas* should be used after the first few days (e.g. piperacillin, tazobactam).
- Note that the pharmacokinetics of antibiotics may be altered in burns patients. Renal impairment is also common.

Future research

- Further studies to define the optimal topical antimicrobial agent and regimen.
- Improved clinical and laboratory tests to diagnose serious infections.

Further reading

Fleisher GR. The management of bite wounds. *N Eng J Med* 1999;**340**:138.

Rodgers GL, Mortensen J, Fisher MC, Lo A, Cresswell A, Long SS. Predictors of infectious complications after burn injuries in children. *Pediatr Inf Dis J* 2000;**19**:990–5.

Chapter 41

Travelling abroad with children

📖 see also Chapters 33, 34, 42

Introduction

When adults take children on trips they can worry too much, or they can be so relaxed as to overlook the dangers—it is tricky being a parent! The travel industry frequently underplays risks, indeed the whole idea of travel may be sold as an escape to a health-giving environment.

The outcome of a family trip overseas depends on:

- Destination and style of travel
- Pre-existing medical conditions
- Parental experience and knowledge
- Availability of safe equipment and safety equipment
- Parental willingness to consent to immunization and also—if appropriate—to comply with malaria prophylaxis
- Parental willingness to follow other precautions including bite prevention and sun protection.

Causes of ill health

It is difficult to study outcomes in travelling children. Broadly, patterns of disease in travelling families parallel those in the home environment, but with additional hazards and infection risks (such as swimming in *Schistosoma*-infected lakes and rivers). Travelling children, like other children, commonly ingest undesirable substances. In resource-poor countries ingestion is made more likely when, for example, fuel is stored in old cola bottles.

Trauma is also more likely where safety standards are different from at home, especially where conditions are less familiar and traffic is on the 'wrong' side of the road. Toddlers may fall off flat roofs or through insecure balustrades, or hazards may be highlighted in a language unfamiliar to the caring adults. Drowning is also a common cause of death. Adventure travel probably comes with increased risks of trauma; parents are well advised to book with companies with experience of child clients—so that safety equipment is age appropriate.

Motion sickness

This can be a huge challenge to travelling families. It is rare below the age of 2 years, and the peak age is between 3 and 12 years. Females are almost twice as susceptible as males (1.7:1). Hyoscine (Joy-rides, Kwells) is effective and fastest acting in preventing travel sickness but if more than one dose is given it causes dry mouth and drowsiness. The skin patches that release hyoscine over 72 hours are not recommended for children under 10 years. Antihistamines (cinnarizine, meclozine, and cyclizine) are better for multiple dosing but need to be started before the onset of symptoms; dosing starting the night before travel can work well. Ginger is also an effective antiemetic, even in the form of ginger biscuits.

Immunization and prophylaxis

- Travel immunizations are given in addition to routine childhood vaccines yet some parents resist immunization, even when travelling into regions where vaccine-preventable diseases are common. Routine childhood immunizations are especially important in travellers to regions where vaccine delivery or health infrastructure is poor.
- Information on which vaccines are needed for travelling from Europe is available on the NHS 'fit for travel' website (⌖ www.fitfortravel.nhs. uk).
- Those visiting friends and relations are at increased risk of infection compared with tourists. Children raised in resource-rich countries will be immunologically naïve compared with family members raised overseas, yet relatives may not see the need for bed nets or malaria prophylaxis.
- Commonly parents assume that vaccines provided free by the NHS are the most important ones, thus hepatitis A and typhoid are accepted whereas meningococcal ACWY may not be.
- There are some challenges in immunizing the very young. For example, there is a poor immune response to typhoid in children <18 months. Yellow fever vaccine is contraindicated in children <6 months and should be used with caution <9 months of age. It is probably wise to defer to a specialist travel practitioner if the family is travelling to a high-risk or remote destination or going on an extended trip.
- The BCG vaccine is recommended for those <16 years of age who are going to live or work with local people for more than three months in a country where the annual incidence of TB is 40/100 000 or greater.

Malaria

- Small children and also pregnant women are most likely to die if they contract malaria so families may need to be encouraged to rebook for safer destinations—until children are capable of reporting early symptoms. About 300 children are treated for malaria in Britain annually, which represents around half of the total paediatric reports for Europe. There is concern that prescribing antimalarials to small children may appear to sanction an unwise and risky trip into a highly malarious region.
- Malaria prevention means avoidance of bites:
  - Permethrin impregnation of cover-all clothes
  - An effective repellent applied frequently to any exposed skin
  - Permethrin impregnated bed nets.

- Bite prevention precautions may be difficult to apply in young children and a curfew—retiring to screened accommodation—at 6pm when mosquitoes are most voracious may be necessary yet difficult to enforce.
- Bite prevention is crucial and cover-all clothes (which can be proofed with permethrin) and 30–50% DEET applied to any skin that is left exposed is protective. Children should sleep under a permethrin-impregnated bed net if the bedroom is not mosquito-free. Applying DEET repeatedly to extensive areas of skin in infants is undesirable and unnecessary. Babies can be protected by cot-nets, and cover-all clothes.
- If parents are prepared to take adequate preventive measures and there are good reasons to travel into regions where there is a high risk of contracting malaria (i.e. much of sub-Saharan Africa) then a prescriber may offer mefloquine (Lariam) or Malarone (combination of atovaquone and proguanil) prophylaxis. Details of prophylaxis is given in the BNFC (⅍ www.bnfc.org).
- Advice on malaria areas and specific drugs is also given by the National Travel Health Network and Centre (⅍ www.nathnac.org) or the Fit for Travel website (⅍ www.fitfortravel.scot.nhs.uk).
- Mefloquine can be given (crushed or chopped) to any child weighing more than 5kg; it does not seem to cause the neuropsychiatric side effects that are reported in some adults. Weight is a better guide to dosing than age.
- Malarone paediatric tablets can be given for prophylaxis daily to children over 10kg and these tablets may also be crushed or mixed with food or a milky drink.
- Homoeopathic prophylaxis is contrary to homoeopathy theory and is not promoted by competent homoeopaths, nor should it be endorsed by paediatricians.
- Reminding parents about the prompt reporting of fever especially within 3 months of leaving a malarious region can also be life-saving.

Diarrhoeal disease

The commonest cause of **morbidity** in travelling children is diarrhoeal disease. Travel—or more specifically eating in restaurants and hotels—increases the risk of diarrhoea even in northern Europe and North America (attack rate in adults is in excess of 5%). During any trip to the Indian subcontinent and tropical Latin America the attack rate is probably >50% per trip. The risks in children, especially in the under 3s, are high and the consequences potentially graver. It is essential that parents understand oral rehydration (and local alternatives to oral rehydration solutions, e.g. fresh coconut water), and can recognize the clinical signs of dehydration. Some cautious advisers say travel to high-risk regions of diarrhoeal disease is foolhardy with young children, but risks depend on the preparedness of the parents.

Peel it, boil it, cook it or forget it is a useful guide to safe food. Ice-cream and hotel buffets are risky in regions where electricity is intermittent or hygiene standards are poor. Parents may find it helpful to know that a few minutes of a 'rolling boil' will kill most organisms including amoebic cysts. Iodination is an effective back-up and is unlikely to cause upset over a brief trip but will not kill *Cyclospora*.

Any persisting gastrointestinal symptoms on return should be investigated by sending stools on three different days with a request for microscopy for cysts and ova and stool culture.

Skin infections

In hot climates, young **skin** needs sun protection, even when bathing.

- There is a good range of clothes/swimwear and beach 'pods' with ultraviolet protection factor ratings.
- Any insect repellent should be applied 30–60 minutes after sunscreen.
- Beach shoes protect feet from coral, sea urchin spines, broken glass, and used hypodermics.
- Long, loose, 100% cotton clothes protect from sunburn, biters, scratches, and stings.
- There is a strong association between sunburn in childhood and skin cancer later.
- Heat stroke is a significant risk in small infants—especially in cars.
- Prickly heat or miliaria rubra is common especially in young infants; vitamin C is no help and antihistamines do not relieve symptoms since the mechanism is not histamine mediated. It settles when sweating is reduced by a few hours per day in an air-conditioned environment or by cooling under a fan. Secondary infection is common.
- Mobile youngsters sustain innumerable grazes and it is important especially in warm climates—for any wounds to be cleaned and covered to prevent sepsis. Creams tend to promote infection. Potassium permanganate, a good drying antiseptic, is available in many regions.
- Scratching mosquito bites is also a problem.

Atopic conditions

Atopic conditions can be unpredictable during travel. Often hay fever and asthma improve but stress and dry aircraft air may precipitate an asthma attack. Eczema should get no worse as long as moisturizers are applied liberally and there is no sensitivity to sunscreens. DEET repellent is unsuitable on broken skin. Acne may worsen or improve in increased sun exposure.

High-risk travellers

Immunocompromised children may need or choose to travel; their increased risks and issues include the following.

- Live vaccines: These should be avoided in immunocompromised children (except HIV-infected children with CD4 counts >15%). Otherwise full immunization as per travel schedules should be stressed (including influenza and hepatitis B).
- Emergency antibiotic course prescription: All immune suppressed travellers to resource-poor countries should be prescribed a supply

of an antibiotic such as ciprofloxacin or azithromycin, depending on resistance patterns at the destination country. They should be advised to have a low threshold for taking antibiotics for any diarrhoeal illness, other than mild watery diarrhoea.

HIV-infected children

- Families of HIV-infected children will need advice on the safe transport and storage of antiretrovirals during trips. They may also need advice about possible drug interactions with other medication.
- HIV-infected children can be given most travel vaccines when needed, except in those with very low CD4 T-cell counts: Inactivated typhoid, hepatitis B, rabies, hepatitis A, and meningococcal ACYW vaccines.
- However, there is insufficient evidence as to the safety of yellow fever vaccine in HIV-positive people.

Children with cancer

- Families should be strongly discouraged from travelling with immunocompromised children during the immediate **post-chemotherapy** or **radiotherapy** period, at least until the treatment course is complete, neutrophil counts have returned to normal, and the patient is not requiring transfusions.

Transplant recipients

- Traveller's diarrhoea may be associated with greater risk in a transplant recipient for reasons over and above the increased susceptibility to infection such as increased risk of compromised renal function from dehydration and altered absorption of post transplantation immunosuppressants.

Post-splenectomy patients

- Prior to travel, parents should ensure that splenectomized children are up to date with pneumococcal, *Haemophilus influenzae* type b, and meningococcal C vaccines according to prevailing guidelines. They should also consider meningococcal ACWY vaccination. A 'standby' course of a broad-spectrum antibiotic therapy such as co-amoxiclav, should be considered for children who may have limited access to emergency medical care during their travel.
- Asplenic children have a high risk of severe malaria. If travel to regions of high malaria transmission is unavoidable then asplenic travellers and those with thalassaemia and sickle cell disease should seek expert advice regarding malaria risk and prevention before travel. They must pay meticulous attention to bite prevention and adequate malaria prophylaxis must be taken.
- Parents of asplenic children should have a low threshold for seeking urgent medical advice if they experience an unexplained fever, whether or not presumptive antimicrobial therapy has been started.

Antibody-deficient children

- In travelling children who require replacement immunoglobulin for a congenital or acquired humoral immune deficiency, protection against travel-acquired infection is optimized by scheduling their dose close to departure. Vaccine efficacy is likely to be poor in children with immunoglobulin deficiency.

Drug interactions

- Antimalarials may interact with some antiretrovirals and transplant-related immunosuppressives. Chloroquine can increase serum levels of cyclosporin, and perhaps sirolimus and tacrolimus. Data are limited regarding other possible interactions between travel-associated drugs and antirejection drugs. The effect on cyclosporin levels of short courses of ciprofloxacin or azithromycin for travellers' diarrhoea is thought not to be a significant risk.

Less familiar 'tropical' infections reported to be of heightened risk to the immunocompromised are:

- Helminth infections: These may become overwhelming in the immunocompromised. *Strongyloides* infection may be especially disastrous so children should be advised against walking barefoot in tropical areas that might be contaminated with excreta.
- Leishmaniasis (both cutaneous and visceral) in atypical forms: This may be more frequently encountered in immunosuppressed patients. The most important personal protective measure in endemic regions is excluding minute biting sandflies by sleeping under an insecticide-treated bed or cot net.
- *Cyclospora* and *Cryptosporidium* infections can also be severe in the immunocompromised, so in endemic regions water should be boiled before drinking.

First aid kits

Large medical kits are seldom necessary; most drugs are available over-seas but paediatric preparations may be unpalatable, unobtainable, or unsafe (there have been deaths from contaminated paracetamol syrup in Bangladesh and Haiti); colourful dressings (which have 'magical' anal-gesic properties) may be difficult to find. Over-the-counter remedies may contain pharmaceutical mixtures or even counterfeit medicines. Parents might be encouraged to travel with a health guide.

Suggested minimal kit

- Insect repellent—up to 30% DEET can by used on children but use with long clothes reduces the amount that needs to be applied. Concerns about DEET toxicity are now largely discounted, with most reports due to accidental ingestion; sensible family advice therefore is to recommend wipes or a roll-on preparation and avoid prolonged use and application onto broken skin. If the travelling infant is too young for the parents to feel happy about using DEET, they possibly should not be taking the child to a high malaria risk setting.
- Sunscreen: Test for sensitivity before travel; so-called sunblocks reduce wavelengths causing sunburn without completely protecting from cancer-causing wavelength. It is probably better to apply SPF 15–25 and reapply frequently. Sun products need to be replenished annually too.
- Paracetamol and/or ibuprofen syrup: Pleasant, melt-in-the-mouth paracetamol (= acetaminophen) is available in the USA.
- Motion sickness preparation.

- Digital thermometer.
- Steri-Strips.
- Colourful pictorial sticking plasters.
- Drying antiseptics, e.g. Savlon Dry iodine spray.
- Mild to medium strength steroid cream for itching bites, jellyfish stings, and exacerbations of eczema
- Sometimes a broad-spectrum antibiotic such as amoxicillin.

Probably the most challenging time for children to travel is between the onset of independent mobility (often at 8–9 months) and the start of the age of reason with the onset of the ability to describe symptoms (from perhaps 3 years). With intelligent preparation, appropriate immunization, prophylaxis, and plenty of time, family travel need not have health implications. However, sometimes it is the duty of a doctor to point out that certain trips are perhaps just too hazardous to particular children and/or individuals of certain ages.

Future research

A systematic investigation of child illness among returning visitors to friends and family would form a useful addition to the literature.

Further reading

Wilson-Howarth J, Ellis M. Illness in expatriate families in Kathmandu, Nepal. *Travel Med Int* 1997;**15**:150–5.

Wilson-Howarth J, Ellis M, Denmark R. *From the Other Side: Anxieties and Misconceptions Amongst Expatriates in Nepal.* Proceedings of the First British Travel Health Conference, 20 February. London: BTHA, 1999.

Wilson-Howarth J, Ellis M. *Your Child Abroad: a Travel Health Guide.* UK: Bradt Travel Guides/USA: Globe Pequot, 2005.

The unwell child returning from abroad

📖 see also Chapters 33, 34, 41, 49, 54, 61, 67, 85, 104, 114, 115, 116, 117

Introduction

The number of families travelling abroad with their children has increased, exposing them to infections they would not normally encounter at home. The reason why most children travel to the tropics is to visit friends and relatives in their parents' country of origin. Often this means:

- They are less likely to seek pre-travel advice or take preventive measures
- They travel to rural areas for longer periods and have an increased risk of infections such as malaria, traveller's diarrhoea, enteric fever (typhoid or paratyphoid), and hepatitis A.
- They may delay seeking medical help when they return to their country of residence because of cultural and language barriers.

Sixty percent of children have an episode of illness during or after travel to the tropics, despite taking preventive measures:[1]

- Common symptoms are diarrhoea, abdominal pain, and fever (15%)
- Most episodes of illness occur during the overseas visit, rather than after return (median onset 7 days from start of the visit). For many infections children may have returned from abroad within the incubation period
- 52% of children are given medication because of these episodes but only 19% seek medical attention
- Although children are infrequent travellers to the tropics, those who do travel have an increased risk of infection compared with adults, especially for malaria, traveller's diarrhoea, and hepatitis A.

It is essential to take a travel history in all children presenting with fever. In febrile children who have recently travelled to the tropics, common infections (such as infectious mononucleosis or respiratory or urinary tract infections) are as common as tropical infections.

Children who present with fever after travel to the tropics need assessment for both common and tropical infections, especially malaria.

Common conditions

The most common reasons for seeking medical advice in returned travellers are fever, diarrhoea, respiratory tract illness, and skin lesions.

Fever

- The commonest tropical infections in children admitted to hospital with fever after travel to the tropics are malaria, diarrhoea, hepatitis, and typhoid (see Table 42.1).
- The usual European infections are as common as tropical infections.
- Antibiotic-resistant bacteria are more frequent in some countries and need to be considered. These include:
  - Community-acquired MRSA in USA
  - Penicillin-resistant pneumococci in Spain, Greece, USA
  - Carbapenem-resistant *Enterobacteriaceae* in India/Pakistan
  - Quinolone-resistant *Salmonella typhi* in India or Pakistan.

Table 42.1 Causes of fever in 229 children admitted to hospital after returning from the tropics (some children had more than one infection)[2]

Tropical		Universal		Other	
Malaria		Respiratory infection		Acute leukaemia	1
Vivax	30	Lower	27		
Falciparum	9	Upper	12		
Diarrhoea		Urinary tract infection	7	Systemic lupus	1
Traveller's[a]	21				
Bacterial	22				
Giardiasis	6				
Cryptosporidiosis	3				
Hepatitis	15	Cellulitis/ lymphadenitis	6	Kawasaki disease	1
Typhoid	8	Viral gastroenteritis	4	No diagnosis	69
Dengue	2	Meningococcal disease	2		
Pulmonary tuberculosis	2	Measles	1		
Rickettsial infection	1				

[a] Culture negative diarrhoea, beginning during travel.

Diarrhoea

- Traveller's diarrhoea is one of the commonest illnesses to affect people who travel to the tropics or subtropics. Young children have the highest risk of traveller diarrhoea. The clinical course in infants may be severe and protracted and very rarely some may develop a severe enteropathy, needing parenteral nutrition.
- Children admitted to hospital with traveller's diarrhoea are usually older and more likely to have bacterial and protozoal infections than local children admitted with gastroenteritis, who commonly have a viral infection.
- The organisms found in the stools of children with traveller's diarrhoea include *Campylobacter*, *Shigella*, *Salmonella* spp., enteropathogenic *Escherichia coli*, and *Cryptosporidia parvum*.
- Children who have been to resource-poor countries may return with intestinal parasites which can cause asymptomatic infections (such as helminths, *Giardia*, or *Entamoeba*).

Respiratory illness

Respiratory tract infections are common in children returning from abroad (see Table 42.1), but pulmonary tuberculosis needs to be considered as a cause.

Skin lesions

These can be discrete lesions (e.g. infected insect bites (common), cutaneous leishmaniasis and cutaneous larva migrans (rare)) or generalized rashes (dengue, measles).

Immigration

Recent immigrants may have special health needs, including children adopted from other countries. Infections to consider include hepatitis B and C, syphilis, human immunodeficiency virus infection, tuberculosis, and intestinal parasites.

Routine immunizations

Many children born abroad are likely to have received the following vaccines: BCG, diphtheria/polio/tetanus (DPT), oral polio, hepatitis B, and measles in the first year of life and a few may have received MMR (in a private clinic). Hib vaccine is now available in an increasing number of resource-poor countries. Overseas children are unlikely to have received pneumococcal, meningococcal C, or human papillomavirus vaccines.

Children arriving from areas experiencing long-term conflict may not have been immunized and are thus at risk of vaccine-preventable disease such as measles or diphtheria.

Epidemiology

In recent years an increase in international migration has resulted in more people living in countries where they were not born, but who may return to their country of origin at intervals.

In the UK, between 2003 and 2005, visits to tropical destinations increased by 28%. The number of visits made by travellers to friends and relatives has also increased.[3]

Imported infections were responsible for 1.3% of admissions to a paediatric ward.[4] However, deaths from imported infection are rare in children (0.15% for imported malaria).

In travellers returning from abroad the likely infections vary with the area visited. Malaria is one of the most common causes of fever among travellers returning from any region worldwide, especially Africa, whereas enteric fever is seen mostly in travellers returning from South Asia (see Table 42.2). Children account for 15–20% of imported malaria and 25–33% of imported enteric fever (typhoid and paratyphoid infection).

Table 42.2 Common causes of febrile illness in travellers returning from developing countries, by region visited[5]

Region	Illness
Caribbean	Dengue, infectious mononucleosis, enteric fever
Central America	Malaria, dengue, infectious mononucleosis
South America	Dengue, malaria, infectious mononucleosis
Sub-Saharan Africa	Malaria, Rickettsial infection
South Central Asia	Dengue, enteric fever, malaria
South East Asia	Dengue, malaria

Clinical presentation and differential diagnosis

The differential diagnosis should take into account a detailed travel history that includes:
- Exact regions visited
- Common diseases in the region at this time
- Traveller's activities while away
- Vaccines, antimalarials, and other preventive measures taken.

Many common bacterial and viral infections have short incubation periods and will have their onset either abroad or within the first 2 weeks of return.

Diseases with longer incubation periods, such as giardiasis, viral hepatitis, *Plasmodium vivax* malaria, and tuberculosis, can present weeks to months later.

Examination

Fever

Children with imported infections often present with non-specific symptoms (fever, lethargy, malaise). The pattern of fever is unreliable for predicting imported malaria in children as the 'classic' pattern occurs in less than a quarter of cases. Most children have no clinical focus of infection.

Hepatosplenomegaly

- The most helpful clinical findings are hepatomegaly, splenomegaly, and jaundice in children with malaria, hepatitis, and enteric fever.
- Splenomegaly is found in fewer than half of children with imported malaria.
- The combination of jaundice and fever is uncommon in young children with acute viral hepatitis. Children with this combination should be investigated to exclude malaria, enteric fever, infectious mononucleosis, or leptospirosis.

Diarrhoea

Although diarrhoea affects many people who travel to the tropics, other infections such as malaria, enteric fever, or pneumonia can also present with fever and diarrhoea and these should always be considered.

Rash

Skin problems may present as discrete lesions or a generalized rash.
Causes of discrete skin lesions include:
- Infected insect bites (often due to *S. aureus* infection)
- Cutaneous larva migrans
- Cutaneous leishmaniasis.
Causes of a generalized rash include:
- Maculopapular rash—measles, dengue
- Non-blanching rash—meningococcal disease or rickettsial infection.

Children with rickettsial infection may have an eschar (black scab) at the site of the infecting tick bite.

Investigations

Almost 50% of febrile children presenting to hospital after returning from the tropics have a treatable condition, and the most important is malaria. Children can die of untreated malaria.

The majority of diagnoses requiring treatment can be made using simple investigations:
- Stool microscopy and culture
- Blood film for malaria
- Chest X-ray
- Blood culture.

Children presenting with fever should be investigated as described in the NICE guideline 'Feverish illness in children' (ℜ www.nice.org.uk/CG047).

Febrile children who have travelled abroad in the preceding year should have the following investigations:
- FBC
- Blood film for malarial parasites
- Stool culture
- Chest X-ray.

For children who have travelled in the preceding month, a blood culture should also be taken (to look for enteric fever). Other investigations should be done as clinically indicated (e.g. LFTs).

All children presenting with fever who have travelled to a malarious area in the past 12 months should be investigated for malaria.
- The diagnosis of malaria is made by examination of thick and thin blood films or antigen test. Thick blood films are more sensitive, whereas thin films help to confirm the malaria species.
- Children with suspected malaria, who have a negative blood film, should have at least two repeat blood films, since the initial blood film may be negative in up to 7% of cases.

Thrombocytopenia is often present in children with malaria. A platelet count above 190×10^9/l had an NPV of 97% for malaria versus all other causes of fever.[6] WCC and CRP are generally unhelpful although these may be raised in malaria.

A markedly raised eosinophil count may indicate an invasive helminth infection or schistosomiasis. An elevated eosinophil count often indicates an asymptomatic helminth infection—think worms!

Management and treatment

Management and treatment depend on the differential diagnosis of the cause(s) of fever. If a child remains febrile but no diagnosis has been made it may be worth:
- Repeating initial investigations (blood film for malaria, chest X-ray, blood culture, LFTs)
- Checking serology for other infections (hepatitis, dengue, *Rickettsia*, EBV)
- Looking for non-infectious causes of fever (connective tissue disorder, Kawasaki disease, malignancy)
- Discussing the case with a paediatric infection specialist.

The treatment of specific infections is described elsewhere in the manual (e.g. malaria, hepatitis, enteric fever, and tuberculosis. 📖 See Chapters 18, 85, 113, 114).

Traveller's diarrhoea
- Traveller diarrhoea in children is often different from other forms of gastroenteritis.
- It is more likely to be due to bacterial and protozoal infections than viral infections. Traveller's diarrhoea is usually self-limiting; however, antibiotic treatment (depending on causative organism) may be needed.

Follow-up and outcome

Follow-up and outcome depend on which infection(s) are the cause(s) of fever. Most children recover well with timely, appropriate treatment.

Children travelling to the tropics often do not take preventive measures. This consultation may be a good opportunity to stress the need for malaria prophylaxis and travel vaccines for future visits. Only 3–15% of children with imported malaria have taken malaria prophylaxis and few children with imported infections have received pretravel vaccinations. Of children in the UK with malaria, 26% have previously been diagnosed with malaria, suggesting missed opportunities to educate families on malaria prevention.

Future research

- Studies of methods to improve uptake of malaria prophylaxis and travel vaccines.
- Improved surveillance of travel-associated infections to help identify at-risk groups and assess the effectiveness of public health interventions.

Key references

1 Newman-Klee C, D'Acremont V, Newman CJ, Gehri M, Genton B. Incidence and types of illness when travelling to the tropics: a prospective controlled study of children and their parents. *Am J Trop Med Hyg* 2007;**77**:764–9.

2 Riordan FA. Fever in the returned paediatric traveller. *Adv Exp Med Biol* 2009;**634**:217–30.

3 Health Protection Agency. Foreign travel associated illness, England, Wales, and Northern Ireland. 2007. http://www.hpa.org.uk/Publications/InfectiousDiseases/TravelHealth/0708Foreigntravelassociatedillness2007/ (Accessed 23 September 2010).

4 Riordan FAI, Tarlow MJ. Imported infections in East Birmingham children. *Postgrad Med J* 1998;**74**:36–7.

5 Freedman DO, Weld LH, Kozarsky PE, *et al.*, GeoSentinel Surveillance Network. Spectrum of disease and relation to place of exposure among ill returned travelers. *N Engl J Med* 2006;**354**:119–30.

6 West NS, Riordan FA. Fever in returned travellers: a prospective review of hospital admissions for a 2 1/2 year period. *Arch Dis Child* 2003;**88**:432–4.

Further reading

Hill DR, Ericsson CD, Pearson RD, *et al.* The practice of travel medicine: guidelines by the Infectious Diseases Society of America. *Clin Infect Dis* 2006;**43**:1499–539.

Ladhani S, Aibara RJ, Riordan FA, Shingadia D. Imported malaria in children: a review of clinical studies. *Lancet Infect Dis* 2007;**7**:349–57.

Chapter 43

Urinary tract infection

📖 see also Chapters 37, 69

Introduction

- *Definition*: UTI consists of bacteriuria in the presence of symptoms.
- UTI is a common bacterial infection that can affect infants and children. Approximately 10% of girls and 3% of boys will have had a UTI <16 years.
- Symptoms range from a mild cystitis to systemic symptoms such as fever, vomiting, failure to thrive, or irritability. Significant dehydration and electrolyte imbalance can be seen in infants in the first 3 months of life. UTI is therefore a frequent differential diagnosis in many children presenting in primary care and in the hospital setting.
- In most children, urinary infections are isolated acute infections from which they recover quickly.
- A small minority of children with UTI may have significant underlying pathology such as:
  • Congenital renal tract malformations, e.g. renal dysplasia and/or hydronephrosis or vesicoureteric reflux (VUR)
  • Renal scarring as a consequence of recurrent febrile UTIs.
- Asymptomatic bacteriuria: This is the presence of significant bacterial growth with or without pyuria in a child who is entirely well on direct questioning and clinical assessment. This needs no treatment or investigation.

Causative organisms

- The bacteria that cause urinary tract infections originate from gut flora.
- The ability of bacteria to cause urinary infections depends on host factors as well as bacterial virulence factors.
- Due to the presence of specific virulence factors that enable them to attack the uroepithelium, the most common type of bacteria causing urinary tract infections are uropathogenic *Escherichia coli* (UPEC), which account for 70–90% of community-acquired infections.
- UPEC have the ability to express adhesins, haemolysins, and other molecules, which makes them the most likely organisms to cause infection by inducing inflammation of the uroepithelium.

- Other bacteria, referred to as 'non-*E. coli*', can also cause UTI.
  - Examples are: *Klebsiella*, *Proteus mirabilis*, *Pseudomonas*, coagulase-negative staphylococci, streptococci (e.g. GBS), enterococci, *Staphylococcus aureus*, *Haemophilus influenzae*, 'fastidious' organisms.
  - These non-*E. coli* organisms often do not possess the virulence factors seen in UPEC. Their ability to cause urinary infections depends heavily on the presence of host factors: structural urinary tract abnormalities leading to urinary stasis; renal calculi, urinary catheters.
  - Therefore, one of the indications for investigating the urinary tract in children is the type of organism involved in the infection.

Epidemiology

- 1 in 10 girls and 1 in 30 boys will have had a UTI by the age of 16 years.
- The incidence of UTI in children less than 3 months of age is higher in boys, most probably reflecting a higher incidence of obstructive congenital urogenital abnormalities in males, e.g. posterior urethral valves. After this age, girls have a higher incidence of UTI: 2.1% of girls and 2.2% of boys will have had a UTI <2 years of age.
  - Children with UTI and congenital renal tract abnormalities are more likely to present with severe systemic illness and tend to present in infancy.
- Recurrence:
  - Children presenting in infancy have a higher rate of recurrence than those presenting later.
  - Girls are more likely to have recurrences of UTI.
  - The presence of dysfunctional bladder and/or chronic constipation increases the risk of recurrence of UTI.

Clinical presentation and differential diagnosis

- Infants and children presenting with unexplained fever of 38°C or higher should have a urine sample tested after 24 hours at the latest.
- Infants and children with symptoms and signs suggestive of urinary tract infection (UTI) should have a urine sample tested for infection.

Severity of illness varies and the clinical presentation can be classified into:
- 'Cystitis' or lower tract infection. The symptoms are confined to the bladder and typically consist of dysuria, frequency, incontinence, urgency of micturition, sometimes accompanied by haematuria.
- 'Acute pyelonephritis' or upper tract infection, which is defined by the presence of fever (≥38°C) or other systemic symptoms: loin pain, vomiting, failure to thrive or persistent irritability.
- In practice it is often not possible to make this differentiation in infants. It is advisable to assume that all UTIs in infants are upper tract in nature.

- The most common form of presentation of UTI in infants is with a non-specific fever (≥38°C) and vomiting.
- Babies <3 months of age can occasionally present with dehydration, hyponatraemia, and hyperkalaemia mimicking the findings in congenital adrenal hyperplasia.
- In boys, check whether there is a good urinary stream—'fountain'—as a poor stream may indicate bladder outlet abstruction.

Urine collection and testing

- Collecting an uncontaminated urine sample is one of the greatest challenges in diagnosing UTI in young children and indeed in clinical paediatrics!
- The gold standard is via suprapubic aspiration, but this is very rarely performed because:
  - It requires training and cannot be done in primary care
  - It is difficult to do in children >6 months
  - It is recommended that it should be performed under ultrasound guidance.
- Clean catch is the recommended method, in which the parents sit by the child, while giving lots of oral fluids.
  - If a clean catch sample is unobtainable a urine pad or urine bag can be used. Both methods run the major risk of contamination; there is some evidence that this can be minimized by changing the pad every 30 minutes.
- Urine testing:
  - In children ≥3 years, urine dipsticks with reagent strips for nitrite and leucocyte esterase are useful for the rapid diagnosis of UTI, which need to be confirmed by culture results.
  - Children <3 years should have urgent microscopy rather than urine dipstick for the rapid diagnosis of UTI.
  - Table 43.1 shows guidance on the interpretation of urine dipstick results to be used in children aged ≥3 years.
  - Table 43.2 shows guidance on the interpretation of urgent microscopy results.

Table 43.1 Interpretation of urine dipstick results in children ≥3 years old

Result	Significance
Both leucocyte esterase and nitrite are positive	The child should be regarded as having UTI and antibiotic treatment should be started. A urine sample should be sent for culture
Leucocyte esterase is negative and nitrite is positive	Antibiotic treatment should be started if the urine test was carried out on a fresh sample of urine. A urine sample should be sent for culture. Subsequent management will depend on the result of urine culture

Table 43.1 (Contd.)

Result	Significance
Leucocyte esterase is positive and nitrite is negative	A urine sample should be sent for microscopy and culture. Antibiotic treatment for UTI should not be started unless there is good clinical evidence of UTI (e.g. obvious urinary symptoms). Leucocyte esterase may be indicative of an infection outside the urinary tract which may need to be managed differently
If leucocyte esterase negative and nitrite negative	UTI is unlikely. Antibiotic treatment for UTI should not be started, and a urine sample should not be sent for culture. Other causes of illness should be explored

Table 43.2 Interpretation of urine microscopy results

Microscopy results	Pyuria positive[a]	Pyuria negative[a]
Bacteriuria positive	The infant or child should be regarded as having UTI	The infant or child should be regarded as having UTI
Bacteriuria negative	Antibiotic treatment should be started if clinically UTI	The infant or child should be regarded as not having UTI

[a]Pyuria is defined as ≥5 white cells/high power field.

The confirmed diagnosis is made by culture. Definition of UTI is a growth in urine of a single bacterial organism of more than 10^5 CFU/ml, however the evidence base for this threshold is weak. Although in most instances there is also pyuria (≥5 white cells/high power field) this may sometimes be absent. Any positive culture in a suprapubic aspiration sample should be regarded as a UTI.

Other dipstick abnormalities, for example proteinuria or haematuria bear no relationship to the likelihood of UTI.

Clinical assessment

- Infants <3 months with a suspected diagnosis of a UTI should be assessed by a paediatrician.
- The history and examination of all children with confirmed UTI should be recorded and should include the following:
  - Temperature
  - Hydration
  - History suggesting previous UTI or confirmed previous UTI
  - Recurrent fever of uncertain origin
  - Antenatally diagnosed renal abnormality
  - Family history of vesicoureteric reflux or renal disease
  - Constipation
  - Dysfunctional voiding including urine flow
  - Enlarged bladder
  - Abdominal mass

- Evidence of spinal lesion—check the back!
- Growth
- Blood pressure.

Management

Antibiotics

- Each paediatric unit should have its own local antibiotic policy based on local sensitivity data.
- The resistance of E. coli to amoxicillin is currently too high for this antibiotic to be recommended as a first-line antibacterial.
- Children with cystitis/lower tract symptoms can be treated with a 3-day course of antibiotics. A recent Cochrane review demonstrated no clear evidence of benefit from longer treatment courses.[1] Common and useful antibiotics are trimethoprim, nitrofurantoin (should not be used in acute pyelonephritis/upper tract UTI), and cefalexin.
- Children with acute pyelonephritis/upper tract infection should be treated with a 7–10-day course of oral antibiotics. There is little good evidence on the optimal duration of treatment for more severe pyelonephritis in children. The evidence that is available suggests that intravenous antibiotics given for 2–3 days until there is resolution of fever and systemic illness followed by a week's oral course of antibiotics has the same outcome as a 10-day intravenous antibiotic course.
  - Exceptions to the initiation of oral therapy include continued vomiting, evidence of circulatory shock, or the presence of potential obstruction such as hydronephrosis.
  - Continuing fever at the end of 48 hours in spite of suitable antibiotics should be investigated with a repeat urine culture and an ultrasound of the renal tract as urinary obstruction can be a cause for failure to respond to antibiotics.
- There is no need to check a post-treatment urine sample if the child is asymptomatic.
- There is no indication for the routine use of antibiotic prophylaxis after treatment of the acute infection.

Subsequent management

- Renal parenchymal defects are found in approximately 5% of children, if investigated after their first UTI.
  - From studies on prenatal scanning and postnatal follow-up these defects in boys are more likely to be congenital in origin (renal dysplasia).
  - Girls are more likely to acquire them through recurrent infections particularly in association with systemic symptoms.
- VUR is present in approximately a third of children with UTI.
  - There is a positive association of VUR and febrile UTI.
  - Although there is some association of VUR and renal parenchymal defects, VUR appears to be only a weak indicator.
  - These defects may be present in the absence of VUR.
  - Unfortunately, interventions in VUR in the form of either surgery or long-term antibiotic prophylaxis have not been shown in

randomized controlled studies to alter outcome in terms of both scarring prevention and in preventing further UTIs.
- Bladder dysfunction plays a key role in UTIs, and VUR can be a secondary effect. It is important, therefore, to make a clinical assessment of bladder function in children with UTIs.
- Long-term sequelae:
  - The risk of hypertension in children after UTI appears to be small and associated with more severe or bilateral scarring. Data from several sources give the incidence of hypertension in the adult population between 11% and 20%. The main cause for high blood pressure in late adolescence and adulthood in those who have a history of childhood UTI seems to be essential hypertension. Lifestyle factors also probably represent a much larger risk compared to UTI in the development of hypertension.
  - Similarly, the effect on renal function is more likely to be seen in cases where there has been a reduction of renal mass, seen in severe bilateral renal scarring, which is rare.

Investigation of the renal tract after UTI

- Current recommendations have moved away from investigating every child with a first UTI. There has also been a shift away from focusing on identifying VUR, although this remains an area of controversy. The current approach is to try to identify obstructive uropathy, severe renal scarring, and dysfunctional voiding.
- Investigations depend on the clinical features and are targeted to the minority of children with risk factors:
  - Children <6 months
  - Serious acute episode
  - Non-*E. coli* UTI
  - Clinical evidence of possible obstruction
  - Febrile infections
  - Recurrent UTIs.

Who needs investigation?
Some children will need investigation after **a first UTI** and these include:
- Children <6 months of age (Table 43.3).
- Children with an **atypical presentation**:
  - Seriously ill
  - Poor urine flow
  - Abdominal or bladder mass
  - Raised creatinine
  - Septicaemia
  - Failure to respond to treatment with suitable antibiotics within 48 hours
  - Infection with non-*E. coli* organisms.
- Children with **recurrent infections** also need investigation—recurrent UTI is defined as two or more UTIs where at least one has been an acute pyelonephritis/upper tract infection, or three or more episodes of cystitis/lower tract infection.

- In the UK, current investigation and management follows the NICE guidelines on UTI (www.nice.org.uk/CG54).[2] Protocols vary across Europe and local policies should be followed. The evidence base for all recommendations is still very good.
- The recommendations vary depending on age, clinical features, and recurrence.
- The main form of investigation is ultrasound, looking for features of possible obstruction (hydronephrosis/bladder abnormalities; see Tables 43.3–43.5).
- There is no need for routine micturating cystourethrogram (MCUG) in infants to look for VUR but an MCUG may be needed in a minority of cases where bladder dysfunction with or without outflow obstruction is suspected on ultrasound.
- A minority will also require a DMSA scan (if indicated it should be done around 6 months post UTI to avoid false positives).

Table 43.3 Recommended imaging schedule for infants <6 months

Test	Responds well to treatment within 48 hours	Atypical UTI[a]	Recurrent UTI[a]
Ultrasound during the acute infection	No	Yes[c]	Yes
Ultrasound within 6 weeks	Yes[b]	No	No
DMSA 4–6 months following the acute infection	No	Yes	Yes
MCUG	No	Yes	Yes

[a]See text for definition.

[b]If abnormal consider MCUG.

[c]In an infant or child with a non-*E. coli* UTI responding well to antibiotics and with no other features of atypical infection, the ultrasound can be requested on a non-urgent basis to take place within 6 weeks.

Copyright National Institute for Health and Clinical Excellence (NICE). CG54. *Urinary Tract Infections in Children (diagnosis, treatment and long term management)*. London: NICE, 2007. Available at: www.nice.org.uk/CG54.[2]

Table 43.4 Recommended imaging schedule for infants and children ≥6 months but <3 years

Test	Responds well to treatment within 48 hours	Atypical UTI[a]	Recurrent UTI[a]
Ultrasound during the acute infection	No	Yes[c]	No
Ultrasound within 6 weeks	No	No	Yes

Table 43.4 (Contd.)

Test	Responds well to treatment within 48 hours	Atypical UTI[a]	Recurrent UTI[a]
DMSA 4–6 months following the acute infection	No	Yes	Yes
MCUG	No	No[b]	No[b]

[a]See text for definition.

[b]While MCUG should not be performed routinely it should be considered if the following features are present: Dilatation on ultrasound; poor urine flow; non-*E. coli* infection; and family history of vesicoureteric reflux.

[c]In an infant or child with a non-*E. coli*-UTI, responding well to antibiotics and with no other features of atypical infection, the ultrasound can be requested on a non-urgent basis to take place within 6 weeks.

Copyright National Institute for Health and Clinical Excellence (NICE). CG54. *Urinary Tract Infections in Children (diagnosis, treatment and long term management)*. London: NICE, 2007. Available at: ✍ www.nice.org.uk/CG54.[2]

Table 43.5 Recommended imaging schedule for children ≥3 years

Test	Responds well to treatment within 48 hours	Atypical UTI[a]	Recurrent UTI[a]
Ultrasound during the acute infection	No	Yes[b,c]	No
Ultrasound within 6 weeks	No	No	Yes[b]
DMSA 4–6 months following the acute infection	No	No	Yes
MCUG	No	No	No

[a]See text for definition.

[b]Ultrasound in toilet-trained children should be performed with a full bladder with an estimate of bladder volume before and after micturition.

[c]In a child with a non-*E. coli* UTI, responding well to antibiotics and with no other features of atypical infection, the ultrasound can be requested on a non-urgent basis to take place within 6 weeks

Copyright National Institute for Health and Clinical Excellence (NICE). CG54. *Urinary Tract Infections in Children (diagnosis, treatment and long term management)*. London: NICE, 2007. Available at: ✍ www.nice.org.uk/CG54.[2]

Follow-up and outcome

The indications for follow-up are:
- Recurrent UTIs
- Renal parenchymal defects (unless unilateral and minor, provided no recurrent UTI or at risk of hypertension because of lifestyle factors or family history of hypertension, or chronic kidney disease)
- Children with bilateral renal abnormalities, impaired kidney function, hypertension, and/or proteinuria (in liaison with a paediatric nephrologist)
- Obstruction (in liaison with paediatric urologist).

Advice to parents/carers or to young people

- To seek medical help if symptoms do not settle within 48 hours of starting treatment or if the child gets worse.
- What symptoms to look out for in the future, particularly non-specific fevers and the need to collect a urine sample as well as seeking medical advice if they suspect a UTI.
- Preventive measures such as ensuring a good fluid intake, avoiding constipation and addressing any issues around bladder function.
- If renal tract investigations are needed these should be explained.
- It is helpful to have an advice leaflet to hand out with pictures, e.g. see the UTI information sheet at the Medicines for Children website (⅏ www.medicinesforchildren.org.uk).

Future research

- Further work on the rapid diagnosis of UTI (e.g. automated urine microscopy or the use of dipsticks stratified by age to help in the prompt diagnosis of UTI).
- Role that probiotics may play in the prevention of UTI.
- The advances already made in the understanding of virulence factors and host factors involved in UTI to be developed to ultimately arrive at alternative ways of treating urine infections.
- Large-scale, prospective study on the multiple factors involved in the long-term outcomes of children with UTI.

Key references

1 Michael M, Hodson EM, Craig JC, Martin S, Moyer VA. Short versus standard duration oral antibiotic therapy for acute urinary tract infection in children. *Cochrane Database of Systematic Reviews* 2003, Issue 1. Art. No.: CD003966. DOI: 10.1002/14651858.CD003966.
2 National Institute for Health and Clinical Excellence. Urinary Tract Infections in Children (diagnosis, treatment and long term management). Clinical guidance 54. London: NICE, 2007. Available at: ⅏ www.nice.org.uk/CG54.

Further reading

Goday G, Svanborg C. Urinary tract infections revisited. *Kidney Int* 2007;**71**:721–3.

Montini G, Rigon L, Zucchetta P, *et al.* On behalf of IRIS Group. Prophylaxis after first febrile urinary tract infection in children? A multicenter, randomized, controlled, noninferiority trial. *Pediatrics* 2008;**122**:1064–71.

Upper respiratory tract infections

📖 see also Chapters 28, 40, 65, 70, 77, 80, 89, 99, 106

Introduction

- *Definition*: URTIs are infectious diseases anatomically restricted to the upper respiratory tract including the nose, sinuses, ears, pharynx, and larynx.
- This chapter focuses on acute URTI including common cold, rhino-sinusitis, otitis media, pharyngitis/tonsillitis, and laryngitis/laryngo-tracheitis.
- URTI are generally uncomplicated, self-limiting diseases and in the great majority of cases do not require antibiotic treatment
- Unusual organisms should be considered in children from abroad.
- Immune deficiency should only be considered in children with:
  - Severe disease
  - Recurrent severe purulent URTI (e.g. otitis media, rhinosinusitis)
  - Serious complications.

Common cold

Causative organisms
- Most (95%) of episodes are caused by one of over 200 different viruses; the most frequent viruses are:
  - Rhinovirus
  - RSV
  - Adenovirus
  - (Para-)influenza virus
  - Corona virus
  - Human metapneumovirus (hMPV)
  - Bocavirus.
- Up to 2% may be complicated by bacterial superinfection.

Epidemiology
- URTI may constitute about 70% of primary care visits with a peak during the winter months.
- The frequency of episodes varies by age and the degree of daycare exposure.
- Between 1 and 10 episodes/year of URTI is usual with a peak between 6 months and 6 years of age. Thereafter 1–2 episodes/year occur mainly during the winter months.

Transmission and incubation period

- Viruses affecting the respiratory tract are primarily transmitted by droplets from human to human. Alternatively, infectious secretions can be spread by direct contact, especially via contaminated hands and fomites.
- The incubation period varies between:
  - 1 and 4 days (influenza virus, rhinovirus, corona virus)
  - 3 and 6 days (respiratory syncytial virus, parainfluenza virus, human metapneumovirus)
  - 2 and 10 days (adenovirus).

Clinical features and sequelae

- A common cold is characterized by varying combinations of the following signs and symptoms:
  - Nasal congestion due to mucosal hyperaemia, oedema
  - Clear, watery to viscous or purulent nasal discharge
  - Breathing or feeding difficulties, especially in young infants
  - Sore throat, cough
  - Fever, malaise, fatigue, loss of appetite, muscle aches, headache
  - Conjunctivitis.
- Within 7–14 days the patient gradually recovers without sequelae.

Diagnosis

- Based on clinical findings with no further investigations in uncomplicated cases. Naso-pharyngeal aspirates or swabs for various rapid antigen tests, culture, or PCR for both viral and bacterial organisms are used for research purposes only.
- The diagnostic value of bacterial organisms identified in nasopharyngeal secretions is limited due to the high rate of bacterial colonization of the respiratory mucosa.

Management and treatment

- Antibiotics are not indicated.
- Nasal decongestants to facilitate breathing and feeding. Locally administered isotonic saline is sufficient especially when mucosa is dry or with limited secretions. Local vasoconstrictive decongestants (e.g. xylometazoline hydrochloride, oxymetazoline) can be considered for children aged 6 years or older and should not be prolonged beyond 5 days to avoid the 'rebound phenomenon'.
- Antipyretics/analgesics (e.g. paracetamol, ibuprofen) to reduce fever.
- There is little evidence for 'immune system stimulating or enhancing' bacterial or herbal therapies, or vitamins or minerals.
- There is little evidence and even less plausibility for hot steam!
- Etheric oils or creams (e.g. mint, eucalyptus) may provide symptom relief, but should be used with caution due to potential irritability of the skin and eyes, and drying of mucous membranes.

Prevention

- Hand hygiene, in particular in healthcare institutions, to prevent nosocomial transmission.
- Respiratory hygiene, e.g. single use tissues for sneezing and removal of nasal secretions.
- Social distancing may reduce the spread of respiratory tract viruses.

- Disinfection of the patient's environment is not of proven benefit in the outpatient setting.
- Influenza vaccines are effective in preventing seasonal or pandemic Influenza. They are primarily indicated for children at risk of severe or complicated disease (e.g. patients with significant heart, lung, renal, liver or neuromuscular disease, immune-suppression, cystic fibrosis, and prematurely born infants).

Acute rhinosinusitis

Rhinitis is an infection of the nasal mucosa potentially associated with sinusitis, an infection of either maxillary, frontal, ethmoidal, or sphenoid mucosa with accumulation of (purulent) secretions in the respective cavities.

Causative organisms

- Rhinitis is caused by common cold viruses—primarily rhinoviruses.
- Bacterial superinfection occurs in less than 5%. Frequent causative bacterial organisms for sinusitis are:
  - *Streptococcus pneumoniae*, *Haemophilus influenzae* (mainly nontypable), *Moraxella catarrhalis* (together ~90%)
  - *Streptococcus pyogenes*, *Staphylococcus aureus*, anaerobic bacteria.

Epidemiology

The epidemiology of rhinosinusitis is identical to that of common cold. Maxillary and ethmoidal sinuses are present from birth. The sphenoid and frontal sinuses are developed by the age of 3–7 and 7–12 years, respectively.

Transmission and incubation period

- Identical with common cold.

Clinical features and sequelae

- Acute rhinosinusitis is generally a self-limiting disease with a duration of about 2–3 weeks. In addition to the nasal symptoms:
  - Tracking of purulent nasopharyngeal secretions at the back of the throat in patients with sinusitis may cause persistent cough (*syndrome déscendant*)
  - Increasing pressure of trapped pus in sinusitis may cause toothache or frontal or temporal headache.
- Potential important complications are:
  - (Peri-)orbital cellulitis
  - Dental abscesses
  - Cavernous sinus thrombosis
  - Frontal abscess, Pott's puffy tumour
  - Meningitis, intracranial empyema.

Diagnosis

- The diagnosis of rhinitis is based on its clinical features. Acute sinusitis may be diagnosed in patients with:
  - High fever, pronounced malaise, and purulent nasal secretions for more than 3 days.
- Worsening nasal secretions and/or cough after 5–7 days.
- Persisting nasal secretions and/or cough for more than 10 days.

- Conventional sinus radiographs demonstrate poor sensitivity, specificity, and positive predictive values, and are generally not recommended.
- The radiological method of choice is CT or MRI but both are very rarely indicated unless complications are suspected.
- Detection of the causative organism is best done on sinus aspirates, but is rarely needed.

Management and treatment

- There is limited evidence for any added value of antibiotics in the treatment of acute rhinosinusitis, unless the patient:
  - Is systemically very unwell
  - Has symptoms and signs suggestive of serious illness and/or complications
  - Is at high risk of serious complications due to pre-existing illness (e.g. patients with significant heart, lung, renal, liver or neuromuscular disease, immunosuppression, cystic fibrosis, and prematurely born infants).
- Bacterial superinfection cannot be inferred from:
  - The colour of nasal secretions
  - A duration of symptoms for longer then 7–14 days.
- Patients should be actively reassured that antibiotics:
  - Are not needed immediately
  - Are not expected to make a difference to symptoms
  - May have side effects (e.g. diarrhoea, vomiting, or rash).
- If indicated, oral antibiotics of choice for 7 days are:
  - Amoxicillin for uncomplicated illness, consider the following for severe infection or if no improvement on amoxicillin after 48 hours:
  - Clavulanate *or*
  - Cefuroxime *or*
  - Clindamycin.
- Unless clinical improvement is observed within 48 hours, the diagnosis and selected antibiotic should be reviewed.
- In purulent rhinitis, especially when unilateral, a nasal foreign body should be excluded by local inspection and be removed, if present.

Prevention

Identical with common cold.

Acute otitis media

AOM is an infection of the middle ear mucosa including the tympanic membrane mostly in combination with a common cold. The great majority of AOM cases are due to viral infections, especially influenza, RSV, and adenovirus.

Causative bacterial organisms

- ~90%: *Streptococcus pneumoniae*, *Haemophilus influenzae*
- ~10%: *Moraxella catarrhalis*, *Streptococcus pyogenes* (Lancefield group A β-haemolytic *streptococcus* (GABHS))

In addition to pneumococci and *Haemophilus* spp., *Staphylococcus aureus* and *Pseudomonas aeruginosa* are found in suppurative complications of AOM such as mastoiditis.

Epidemiology

- AOM is a frequent cause of paediatric primary care visits for sick children.
- By 3 years of age, over 80% of children have had at least one episode of AOM. By 7 years of age, 40% have six or more recurrences.

Transmission and incubation period

- Similar to common cold for viral causes. Bacterial AOM arises from proliferation of colonizing bacteria during viral disease.
- Risk factors for colonization with oto-pathogens are young age, crowding, attendance of daycare centres, viral upper respiratory tract infections, and siblings. Colonization is decreased by sanitation, conjugate vaccine, breastfeeding, and in the presence of a balanced nasopharyngeal flora.

Clinical features and sequelae

- AOM typically presents during or after a common cold with acute onset of fever, earache, irritability, vomiting, or acute otorrhoea not caused by external otitis.
- AOM is a self-limiting disease in 80% of children after 4 days.
- Potential important rare complications are mastoiditis, hearing loss, and meningitis.

Diagnosis

- Clinical diagnosis of AOM relies on visualization (otoscopy) and functional testing (pneumatic otoscopy, tympanometry, acoustic reflectometry) of patients with the signs and symptoms listed above.
- Otoscopy shows a highly inflamed, entirely red, undifferentiated, bulging tympanic membrane as an expression of a sometimes visible middle ear effusion, or a perforation with middle ear secretions in the ear canal. Functional testing demonstrates tympanic immobility.
- In contrast, acute otitis with effusion (AOE) will show an essentially non-inflamed eardrum with visible middle ear effusion as a result of reduced middle ear ventilation via the eustachian tube.
- While there is some degree of clinical overlap, paediatricians should make all efforts to distinguish the two entities as diagnostic uncertainty is a major reason for unnecessary antibiotic prescribing in developed countries, where infants and toddlers spend a mean of between 40 and 50 days of their life/year on antibiotics for the first two years of their life (detailed instructions available at the following websites: PedsEd (℞ http://pedsed.pitt.edu/) and UTMB (℞ www.utmb.edu/pedi_ed/AOM-otitis/default.htm).

Management and treatment

- No prescribing or delayed antibiotic prescribing strategies are now generally recommended in children. This includes immediate symptomatic therapy with regular antipyretics/analgesics, followed by clinical review 24–72 hours later with re-evaluation regarding potential antibiotic treatment.

- **The theoretical aims of antibiotic treatment may be amelioration and abbreviation of disease, prevention of complications, and eradication of oto-pathogens. Antibiotics do *not*:**
  - Reduce pain on day 1; a reduction of pain is observed on day 2–7. However, appropriate treatment with antipyretics/analgesic/anti-inflammatory controls pain without antibiotics
  - Prevent development of contralateral AOM
  - Accelerate resolution of middle ear fluid
  - Have a beneficial effect on hearing
  - Appear to be justified as an immediate treatment strategy for prevention of suppurative complications—this is because the number needed to treat to prevent one case of mastoiditis is over 4000, and the course of treated mastoiditis in developed countries is most commonly now benign
  - Reduce substantially the overall number of signs or symptoms but may cause side effects
  - Contribute to reduce the detrimental effects of increasing antibiotic resistance, if prescribed unnecessarily.
- Immediate antibiotic prescribing should still be considered for children:
  - <2 years with bilateral acute otitis media
  - With marked otorrhoea, not caused by external otitis
  - Who are systemically very unwell
  - With symptoms and signs suggestive of serious illness and/or complications (mastoiditis, abscess, intracranial complications) (but refer immediately to hospital!)
  - At high risk of serious complications because of pre-existing illness (e.g. significant heart, lung, renal, liver, or neuromuscular disease, immunosuppression, cystic fibrosis, prematurely born infants and toddlers)
  - Recurrent AOM.
- If indicated, the oral antibiotic of choice is amoxicillin. High dose amoxicillin should be used in areas with high rates of penicillin-resistant pneumococci. Because of the improved effectiveness of amoxicillin/clavulanate against *H. influenzae* and *M. catarrhalis*, amoxicillin-clavulanate (7:1), or cefuroxime axetil, may be used after 48 hours of treatment failure with amoxicillin (see local guidelines).
- Duration of antibiotic treatment for AOM is 5 (children ≥2 years) to 10 (children <2 years) days.
- In children with difficulties in oral antibiotic uptake, ceftriaxone once daily for 1–3 days IM or IV is an effective alternative.

Prevention

- Immunization with conjugated pneumococcal vaccines is the most effective strategy to prevent acute otitis media—in spite of the relatively weak effect (10–30%) in preventing AOM.
- Recurrent episodes may be best prevented by early immunization in infancy. Moreover, long-term low-dose daily amoxicillin has been reported to be efficient in a few case series. Once recurrent disease is established, tympanostomy tube placement is another treatment option.

- Other preventive measures such as reduction of risk factors of colonization and decrease of continuous use of pacifiers may be considered, but contribute comparatively little to preventing disease overall.

Tonsillo-pharyngitis

Tonsillo-pharyngitis (TP) is an infection of the tonsils and pharyngeal mucosa mostly during a common cold.

Causative organisms

- Viral causes are similar to the common cold apart from Epstein–Barr virus and Coxsackie herpangina, both of which cause severe pharyngitis.
- The major bacterial cause of TP is S. pyogenes (GABHS). In adolescents, Fusobacterium necrophorum (angina Plaut–Vincent) appears to be increasing.
- Other causes of acute pharyngitis include group C and G streptococci, Corynebacterium diphtheriae, Mycoplasma pneumoniae, and Chlamydia pneumoniae.

Epidemiology

- GABHS TP may occur at any age. However, it is rare in children <3 years and is primarily a disease of children 5–15 years of age.
- GAHBS tonsillitis usually occurs in winter and early spring.
- The incidence rate of post-streptococcal rheumatic fever is now less than 0.5 cases per 100 000 in resource-rich countries and 100–200 cases per 100 000 in resource-poor countries.

Transmission and incubation period

- Acute GABHS pharyngitis is transmitted by droplets from human to human.
- The incubation period is 2–4 days.
- Pharyngeal carriage does not appear to be infectious.

Clinical features and sequelae

- Features suggestive of GABHS as a causative agent are:
  - Sudden-onset sore throat
  - Pain on swallowing
  - Fever
  - Scarlet fever rash
  - Headache
  - Nausea, vomiting, and abdominal pain
  - Tonsillo-pharyngeal erythema (dark red)
  - Tonsillo-pharyngeal exudates
  - Soft palate petechiae ('doughnut' lesions)
  - Beefy, red, swollen uvula
  - Tender, enlarged anterior cervical nodes
  - Patient 5–15 years of age

- Presentation in winter or early spring (in temperate climates)
- History of exposure.
- Features suggestive of viral origin are:
  - Conjunctivitis
  - Rhinitis
  - Hoarseness
  - Cough
  - Diarrhoea
  - Characteristic exanthems.
- Duration of disease is on average 1 week.
- Purulent complications of bacterial pharyngitis (<1%) include:
  - Retropharyngeal abscess
  - Peritonsillar abscess (quinsy)
  - Lemierre's syndrome (peritonsillar abscess, jugular vein thrombosis, and septic pulmonary emboli in *Fusobacterium* infection).
- Non-purulent complications:
  - Scarlet fever: A rash caused by exotoxin released by GAHBS, appears 12–48 hours after onset of fever and lasts about 3–5 days. In contrast to the rash potentially caused by penicillins, it does not involve the perioral area and spares palms and soles.
  - Acute post-streptococcal glomerulonephritis occurs approximately 10 days after onset of streptococcal pharyngitis; most cases remain asymptomatic. If symptomatic, oedema, haematuria, proteinuria, and arterial hypertension prevail.
  - Rheumatic fever is a well-described inflammatory disease following GABHS pharyngitis. Cross-reactive antibodies are hypothesized to involve the heart, skin, joints, and brain. First-time attacks tend to occur 2–3 weeks after onset of GAHBS pharyngitis.
  - Poststreptococcal reactive arthritis tends to occur about 10 days after an episode of GABHS pharyngitis, does not respond well to acetylsalicylic acid and may involve any joint in a persistent manner. Arthritis of rheumatic fever tends occurs later (~14–21 days), responds well to acetylsalicylic acid, and only involves large joints in a migratory manner. However, it is not yet fully understood whether both entities are part of the same spectrum of disease.
  - Paediatric autoimmune neuropsychiatric disorder associated with streptococcus (PANDAS) should currently be considered as a hypothesis in need of verification.

Diagnosis

- Several scoring systems have been developed to predict bacterial TP. The four Centor criteria are probably most widely used:
  - Fever *and*
  - Tonsillar exudate *and*
  - Tender anterior cervical lymphadenopathy or lymphadenitis *and*
  - Absence of acute cough.
- A positive throat culture for GABHS in unwell patients of 3–15 years of age; the presence of 3–4 Centor criteria and the absence of signs and symptoms of viral disease increase the pretest probability to demonstrate an aetiological agent rather than colonization.

- Many GABHS rapid tests are commercially available. However, the specificity and sensitivity of these tests vary widely and should be locally compared with the results of blood agar plate cultures to estimate the positive and negative predictive values pertinent to the local population.
- In patients with features of viral disease (e.g. cough, rhinitis, almost normalized wellbeing following antipyretics), testing for GABHS should not be performed or, if done, the finding of GABHS on rapid test or culture should be interpreted with caution as regards to an aetiological role of concurrent disease.
- Urine tests to detect asymptomatic acute poststreptococcal glomerulonephritis are not recommended.

Management and treatment

- Effects of antibiotic treatment for GABHS TP are:
  - Reduction of the contagiousness from 6–14 days to 24 hours
  - Reduction of duration of symptoms by only 16 hours
  - Reduction of the rate of quinsy. However, given the small absolute risk, over 4000 children with tonsillitis have to be treated to prevent one case of quinsy.
  - Reduction of inflammatory complications with the same efficacy after several days (up to 9 days) of TP as compared with immediate treatment. These complications are now extremely rare in developed countries and are not a reason to prescribe antibiotics as the absolute risk reduction is also extremely small.
- No or delayed antibiotic treatment is generally recommended for TP.
- Immediate treatment may be considered if all four Centor criteria are present.
- A 10-day course of oral penicillin V still remains the treatment of choice in view of rheumatic fever prevention. However, compliance is known to be very low. Alternative regimens with similar effectiveness regarding bacterial eradication are high-dose amoxicillin twice daily or narrow-spectrum oral cephalosporins for 5 days. Erythromycin and clarithromycin are the macrolides of choice for patients with penicillin intolerance or allergy.
- A follow-up throat culture is not indicated.

Prevention

- A causal prevention is not available.
- Children may return to daycare or school after 24 hours of antibiotic treatment.
- GABHS rapid antigen tests of throat cultures or antibiotic prophylaxis are not indicated in asymptomatic contact persons.

Laryngotracheitis

Laryngotracheitis (croup syndrome) is a viral infection of the laryngeal and tracheal mucosa.

Causative organisms

- Identical with common cold. Most frequent are parainfluenza 3 and influenza viruses.

Epidemiology

- In the winter months, children between 6 months to 6 years are commonly affected. Most are <3 years of age.

Transmission and incubation period

- Identical with common cold.

Clinical features and sequelae

- Fever.
- Sudden onset of hoarse voice often at night.
- Pathognomonic 'seal-like' barking cough.
- Potentially rapid progression to stridor and sometimes pronounced dyspnoea.

Diagnosis

- Based on clinical features alone.
- Important differential diagnoses should be considered:
  - Foreign body aspiration (no fever, little improvement on croup treatment)
  - Diphtheria
  - Epiglottitis (severely ill child with muffled rather than hoarse voice)
  - Bacterial tracheitis (rare in children).

Management and treatment

- Close monitoring as progression to life-threatening disease may be rapid.
- Assurance of parents.
- Anti-inflammatory antipyretics
- Oral corticosteroids (e.g. dexamethasone 0.5 mg/kg single dose)
- Adrenaline nebulizer for severe dyspnoea (monitor for at least 4 hours for potential relapse (most within 1–2 hours).

Prevention

- Identical to common cold.

Further reading

Altamimi S, Khalil A, Khalaiwi KA, Milner R, Pusic MV, Al Othman MA. Short versus standard duration antibiotic therapy for acute streptococcal pharyngitis in children. *Cochrane Database Syst Rev* 2009;**1**:CD004872.

National Institute for Health and Clinical Excellence. *Prescribing of Antibiotics for Self Limiting Respiratory Tract Infections in Adults and Children in Primary Care.* Clinical guideline 69. London: National Institute for Health and Clinical Excellence. Available at: ♪ www.nice.org.uk/CG69.

Vergison A, Dagan R, Arguedas A, et al. Otitis media and its consequences: beyond the earache. *Lancet Infect Dis* 2010;**10**:195–203.

Zoonoses

📖 see also Chapters 54, 56, 67, 74, 82, 91, 98, 103, 111, 112, 114, 118

Introduction

Zoonoses are infections that are naturally transmitted from vertebrate animals to humans. Some zoonotic infections can be acquired from other humans, as well as from animals. For others, humans represent a dead-end host from whom ongoing transmission cannot occur. With the exception of a few infections in the former group most zoonoses are uncommon in children. There are around 2000 cases/year of notified zoonoses in adults and children in the UK.

Careful consideration of the likelihood of exposure should be done when assessing children in whom the differential diagnosis might include zoonoses. The possibility of a zoonotic infection must not be overlooked, but at the same time care must be taken not to over-investigate children for rare infections.

This chapter considers the most common and/or important zoonotic infections that might be seen in the UK and Western Europe: specialist advice or texts should be consulted where a diagnosis of a rare zoonosis acquired overseas is being considered. To make a diagnosis of zoonotic infection requires:
- Knowledge of the clinical manifestations of the diseases
- Understanding of the local epidemiology of zoonoses
- Identification of a detailed exposure history for the individual patient.

Causative organisms

The pattern of infections seen in different areas of the world depends on the types of animal to which humans may be exposed. Tables 45.1–45.3 summarize common and/or important zoonoses according to their likelihood of being encountered in Europe. In Western countries, most zoonoses are acquired from pets or other domesticated animals.

For a zoonosis to occur there has to be indirect or direct contact between the animal and child. Routes of transmission are:
- Direct skin contact, including via bites and scratches
- Ingestion of contaminated material in food or water
- Inhalation of contaminated material
- Transmission via an insect vector.

Clinical presentation

Descriptions of individual zoonotic infections are provided in the relevant disease-specific chapters in this book. However, a brief description of the main clinical features of individual infections is provided in Tables 45.1–45.3.

Commonest presentations of zoonotic infections are:
- Localized skin and soft tissue infections
- Gastrointestinal infections.

These infections are:
- Generally easy to diagnose, because the onset is acute, the incubation period is short, and the symptoms and signs are easy to identify.
- Often more common in young children because their curiosity and lack of understanding of hygiene place them at greater risk of exposure.

Less common presentations are:
- Multisystem disease with non-specific signs
- Pneumonia.

These infections are often more uncommon in children than adults, because children are less likely to be have been exposed. Infections are more difficult to diagnose because the possible clinical manifestations are protean, and there may be no clear exposure history to prompt consideration of the diagnosis.

Careful history taking is required to ensure that clues as to the possibility of zoonotic infection are not missed. Key points are:
- Pets—especially unusual pets
- History of any other contact with animals or their environment within the likely incubation period. This may require careful questioning around leisure pursuits, e.g. animal petting farms (and in the case of older children, possible occupational exposure)
- Travel history
- Ingestion of unusual foods
- Time of year may also be important, especially where insect vectors are involved.

Table 45.1 Zoonoses commonly acquired in the UK

Infection	Microorganisms	Animal source	Route(s) of transmission	Incubation period	Clinical presentation
Bacterial infection of animal bites	Pasteurella multocida Capnocytophaga Staphylococci, Anaerobes, etc. Infections are frequently polymicrobial)	Dogs, cats (most commonly)	Inoculation via bite	1–3 days	Skin and/or soft tissue infection
Cat scratch disease	Bartonella henselae	Cats and other animals	Inoculation via scratch or bite	3–10 days	Lymphadenopathy, fever
Dermatophytes	Wide variety of species, especially Microsporum spp. Trichophyton spp.	Various: mainly dogs, cats	Skin contact	1–2 weeks	Skin and hair infections
Toxocariasis	Toxocara canis, Toxocara cati	Dogs, cats	Ingestion of worm eggs excreted in dog and cat faeces	Variable: larvae remain viable indefinitely	Asymptomatic (most common); visceral larva migrans; ocular toxocariasis

(Continued)

Table 45.1 (Contd.)

Infection	Microorganisms	Animal source	Route(s) of transmission	Incubation period	Clinical presentation
Toxoplasmosis	*Toxoplasma gondii*	Cats	Ingestion of oocysts in cat faeces	5–20 days	Asymptomatic (most common); glandular fever-like illness; severe disseminated infection in immunocompromised patients
		Sheep, pigs, cattle	Ingestion of tissue cysts in raw or undercooked meat	10–23 days	
Gastrointestinal infections	*Campylobacter* spp. *Salmonella enterica* *E. coli* O157 *Cryptosporidium* *Giardia lamblia*	Wide range of animals and birds	Ingestion through direct contact with infected animals or consumption of contaminated food or water	Usually 2–5 days	Diarrhoea: may be complicated by systemic illness (especially in the very young or immunocompromised)

Table 45.2 Zoonoses infrequently acquired in the UK

Infection	Microorganisms	Animal source	Route(s) of transmission	Incubation period	Clinical presentation
Lyme disease	*Borrelia burgdorferi*	Deer, sheep, other animals	Tick bites	1–4 weeks	Cutaneous lesions (erythema migrans); systemic illness
Leptospirosis	*Leptospira* spp.	Rodents, ruminants	Contact with contaminated water, e.g. via mucous membranes or damaged skin	3–21 days	Systemic flu-like illness; bleeding, liver and kidney failure may follow 7–10 days later
Psittacosis	*Chlamydophila psittaci*	Birds	Inhalation	5–14 days	Atypical pneumonia
Q fever	*Coxiella burnetii*	Livestock, especially sheep, goats, and cattle	Inhalation	9–40 days	Atypical pneumonia; hepatitis
Hydatid disease	*Echinococcus granulosus*	Dogs	Ingestion of eggs in dog faeces		Ingestion of eggs excreted by dogs
Fish tank granuloma	*Mycobacterium marinum*	Fish	Direct contact with water from aquariums	At least 2–3 weeks	Granuloma at the site of entry; further granulomas may occur later along the path of lymphatic drainage

Table 45.3 Zoonoses rarely or never acquired in the UK, but may be imported

Infection	Microorganisms	Animal source	Route(s) of transmission	Incubation period	Clinical presentation
Rabies	Rabies virus	Any infected animal, especially cats, dogs, foxes, bats	Animal bite	1–4 weeks	Cutaneous lesions (erythema migrans); systemic illness
Tick-borne encephalitis	Tick-borne encephalitis virus (a flavivirus)	Small rodents	Tick bites	7–14 days	Biphasic: initial viraemic illness followed in 20–30% of patients by central nervous system disease 7–8 days later
Brucellosis	Brucella spp.	Cattle, goats, sheep, pigs	Usually by ingestion of unpasteurized milk or dairy products	5–30 days	Systemic illness
Avian influenza	Avian influenza viruses, e.g. H5N1	Poultry, water fowl	Direct contact	3–5 days	Influenza: may be severe
Anthrax	Bacillus anthracis	Livestock, wild animals	Usually by direct contact; inhalation or ingestion may occur	2 days to several weeks	Characteristic black-centred skin ulcer; systemic illness; pneumonia

Bovine tuberculosis	Mycobacterium bovis	Cattle	Ingestion of unpasteurized milk		Indistinguishable from infection with Mycobacterium tuberculosis
Cysticercosis	Taenia solium (pork tapeworm) Taenia saginata (beef tapeworm)	Cattle, pigs	Ingestion of meat	Around 10 days to establishment of intestinal infection	Intestinal tapeworm infection Neurocysticercosis (following T. solium)
Arboviruses, e.g. West Nile Virus	West Nile virus (a flavivirus)	Birds	Mosquito bites	3–14 days	Asymptomatic (80%); systemic illness which may be severe

Management and treatment

The management and treatment of zoonoses is disease-specific and is considered in individual chapters in this book. Guidance on the recognition, investigation, and management of zoonoses produced by the HPA may also be useful.

It is important to remember that some zoonoses are statutorily notifiable under veterinary and/or human legislation. The primary purpose of the notification system is to identify possible outbreaks and epidemics and initiate appropriate action as soon as possible. The large outbreak in the UK of E. coli O157 disease in children associated with visiting an animal petting farm is a salutary reminder of the potential for zoonotic infections to occur as large and/or serious outbreaks. It is recommended that any serious zoonotic infection that may be of public health importance should be notified via the HPA, even if it is not statutorily notifiable.

Prevention

General preventative measures:
- Good personal hygiene
- Avoid children having unsupervised contact with animals or their environment
- Ensure that pet cats and dogs are regularly wormed
- Protect damaged skin when having contact with animals or their environment
- Ensure that food is thoroughly cooked
- Avoid consuming unpasteurized milk or dairy products
- Avoid drinking water that may be contaminated with animal faeces.

Specific preventive measures will depend on the individual disease but may include:
- Immunization (rabies; tick-borne encephalitis)
- Antimicrobial prophylaxis (bites)
- Use of insect repellent (insect-borne infections).

Further reading

Colville J, Berryhill D. *Handbook of Zoonoses: Identification and Prevention.* St Louis: Mosby, 2007.

Health Protection Agency. *Guidelines for Investigation of Zoonotic Diseases.* 2009. Available at: www.hpa.org.uk/topics (accessed 23 September 2010).

Chapter 46

Adenovirus

📖 see also Chapters 11, 20, 27, 31, 44

Name and nature of organism

- Adenoviruses, so named because they were first isolated from adenoidal tissue surgically removed from children in 1953, infect most mammals, birds, and reptiles.
- Human adenoviruses (HAdV) are medium-sized (80–100nm), non-enveloped viruses with icosahedral symmetry, and easily visible on negative staining electron microscopy.
- The nucleocapsid is composed of 252 capsomers, with 12 vertices and seven surface proteins. The genome is linear, non-segmented, double-stranded DNA, encoding about 30 proteins.
- HAdV (family *Adenoviridae*, genus *Mastadenovirus*) are classified into seven subgenera (A–G).
- There are at least 54 immunologically distinct serotypes, differentiated by quantitative neutralization with hyperimmune sera.

Epidemiology

- Initially recognized as a cause of acute respiratory disease in children and young adults, HAdV are associated with a wide variety of clinical syndromes, from asymptomatic or mild infection, typical self-limiting respiratory, gastrointestinal, or ophthalmological illnesses, through to rarer severe and occasionally fatal disease.
- There is striking concordance between disease syndrome and serotype, although this is not absolute and there is some inconsistency between the serotype associations reported in the literature.
- HAdV are present all year round; respiratory infections show typical seasonality while gastrointestinal disease does not.
- Infection occurs at any age in children, typically from infancy to school age. Most children have had one form of HAdV infection by age 10 years.
- HAdV usually cause localized infections; generalized infection is commoner in immunocompromised patients.
- Outbreaks occur in young adults in institutions such as the army.

Transmission and incubation period

- HAdV are relatively stable to chemical or physical agents and adverse pH conditions, allowing prolonged survival outside the body, in water, and on fomites (such as doorknobs, hard surfaces, toys) for many hours.

- HAdV are highly contagious; there are very high levels of viral particles in secretions of infected individuals (10^{5-6} /ml in sputum or oral secretions) coupled with a very low infective dose (e.g. the inhalation of as few as five virions in droplet nuclei).
- Acquisition is via one of several routes: respiratory droplets, ingestion via faecal-oral route, contact—especially hand-to-eye transfer, water, e.g. inadequately chlorinated pools, and venereal.
- Route of acquisition can determine the disease syndrome caused, e.g. HAdV7 can cause severe lower respiratory tract infection if inhaled but mild gastrointestinal disease when introduced orally.
- Incubation period is also affected by route of acquisition, ranging from 2 to 14 days between inhalation and onset of respiratory illness, and 3 to 8 days between ingestion and gastrointestinal symptoms.
- Infections are lytic: the adenovirus enters epithelial cells and the replication cycle results in cytolysis, cytokine production, and induction of the host inflammatory response. Some HAdV serotypes cause cellular cytopathic effect with rounded, swollen cells.
- Chronic or latent infection frequently occurs but the exact mechanism is unknown. After recovery of illness or following asymptomatic infection, HAdV maintain latent persistent infections in tonsils, adenoids, and other lymphoid tissues, and can shed from the respiratory tract, stool, and urine for months to years. Shedding is especially prolonged in children and immunocompromised individuals.

Clinical features and sequelae

- HAdV infections are very common, most are asymptomatic. Symptomatic HAdV disease forms a wide variety of clinical syndromes, the majority of which involve the respiratory tract. There is striking, but not absolute, association between HAdV serotype and clinical syndrome (Table 46.1).

Table 46.1 Clinical syndromes of HAdV disease

Clinical syndrome	At risk	Associated serotypes
Pharyngitis	Infants	1, 2, 3, 5, 7
Pharyngoconjunctival fever	All	3, 4, 7
Acute respiratory disease	Boarding schools	4, 7, 14, 21
Pneumonia	Infants	1, 2, 3, 7, 14, 21, 30
Follicular conjunctivitis	All	3, 4, 11
Epidemic keratoconjunctivitis	All	8, 19, 37
Pertussis-like syndrome	Infants	5
Acute haemorrhaghic cystitis	Infants, older children	11, 21

(Continued)

Table 46.1 (*Contd.*)

Clinical syndrome	At risk	Associated serotypes
Acute infantile gastroenteritis	Infants	12, 18, 31, 40, 41
Mesenteric adenitis, intussusception	Infants	1, 2, 3, 5, 6
Hepatitis and multi-organ disease in immunocompromised patients	Any	5, 34, 35
Meningitis		3, 7

Respiratory

- Respiratory HAdV serotypes account for an estimated 5% of respiratory infections across all ages and about 10% of lower respiratory tract infections in childhood. Acute respiratory disease (ARD) typically presents with fever, non-specific upper respiratory symptoms of rhinorrhea, cough, and pharyngitis (may be exudative), usually lasting 3–5 days.
- Lower respiratory tract infections, including tracheobronchitis, bronchiolitis, and pneumonia, may mimic respiratory syncytial virus infection or influenza, although associated conjunctivitis is a clue to adenoviral aetiology. Pulmonary infiltrates are often diffuse and reticulonodular, but may be lobar.
- HAdV has been isolated from children with a whooping cough-like syndrome in the absence of *B. pertussis* infection, however whether HAdV are the aetiological agent remains unclear.
- Sporadically, severe disease such as necrotizing HAdV bronchiolitis occurs in previously healthy immunocompetent infants; bronchiolitis obliterans may then ensure. Fatal HAdV pneumonia, although rare, can occur in neonates infected by virulent serotypes.
- Non-pulmonary complications of respiratory HAdV infection include meningoencephalitis.
- Clusters of severe and occasionally fatal disease were seen in a number of US states in 2006–7, largely due to a new variant of HAdV 14 little seen before in children.

Gastrointestinal

- Ingested HAdV can cause gastroenteritis that is clinically indistinguishable from other causes such as rotavirus. HAdV serotypes are responsible for an estimated 10% of infantile gastroenteritis, typically in the second year of life when maternally derived humoral immunity has waned. Watery, non-bloody diarrhoea typically precedes vomiting and the infant can be symptomatic for 1–2 weeks.

- However, enteric HAdV serotypes replicate readily in human intestine and can be detected from asymptomatic individuals so their role in the setting of a diarrhoeal syndrome may not always be causal. Conversely, some serotypes (40, 41) are fastidious in culture and were termed 'noncultivatable' and evaded detection before newer methods became available.
- Intussusception can complicate HAdV gastroenteritis. Interestingly, up to 40% of infants with intussusception are positive for non-enteric serotypes from stool or mesenteric lymph nodes, and most have no evidence of infection with enteric strains (i.e. 40, 41).
- Mesenteric lymphadenitis or hyperirritable small bowel associated with non-enteric adenoviral infection has been postulated as a precursor to intussusception; the role of HAdV in this setting is unclear, and as most patients with intussusception have no evidence of HAdV infection, intussusception probably has multiple aetiologies.

Ocular

- Pharyngoconjunctival fever syndrome most often affects school-aged children and is highly contagious via respiratory secretions and contact with ocular secretions.
- Sporadic outbreaks occur in small groups, especially in the setting of inadequately chlorinated water such as private swimming pools or lakes, although confirming the water source of HAdV is often difficult.
- Fever, sore throat, coryza, and acute conjunctivitis are seen, with or without pharyngitis or a respiratory syndrome, and these may precede the eye signs: follicles in bulbar, and/or palpebral conjunctivae, typically with a mild granular appearance.
- Unilateral before progression to bilateral redness is typical, associated with mild (rarely severe) pain (indicating corneal involvement), photophobia, tearing, pruritus, and morning crusting for up to 5 days.
- In epidemic keratoconjunctivitis, severe follicular keratoconjunctivitis and palpebral oedema is typically granular and haemorrhagic conjunctivitis can develop.
- Visual haziness or impairment indicates keratitis or corneal inflammation and may persist for months to years.
- Preauricular lymphadenopathy (Parinaud's syndrome) is not common in ocular HAdV disease but when present is highly suggestive of HAdV.

Renal

- Haematuria may occur in the setting of nephritis (usually febrile) or haemorrhagic cystitis (typically not).
- Acute haemorrhagic cystitis usually affects children >5 years, especially immunosuppressed individuals (e.g. kidney or bone marrow transplant recipients, HIV infected).
- Boys are affected more often than girls.
- Grossly bloody urine usually lasts 3 days or so although associated, dysuria and frequency can be prolonged, especially in haematopoietic stem cell recipients.

Other
- Symptoms of HAdV in otherwise healthy individuals also include rash, malaise, and headache or frank encephalitis, hepatitis (sometimes with dramatically elevated transaminases), and myocarditis.

Immunocompromised patients
- Transplant recipients and those with primary and acquired immunodeficiency states are especially at risk of severe HAdV disease.
- T-cell immunodeficiency related to HIV infection has been associated with adenoviral infections, particularly in infants and children infected with HIV. Most often seen are pneumonitis and haemorrhagic cystitis, cholecystitis, and severe hepatitis.
- Pre-existing latent HAdV are reactivated during immunosuppression in paediatric recipients of solid organ transplants, with diffuse adenoviral infection of the allograft itself, and is a major problem in the rejection of transplanted hearts and lungs. Use of newer, more potent immunosuppressive regimens has increased the frequency of severe adenovirus infections.
- Haematopoietic stem cell transplant recipients are also prone to severe HAdV disease, risk factors including allogeneic stem cell transplantation, T-cell depletion and nonmyeloablative conditioning regimens, lymphopenia, young age, and graft versus host disease.
- Manifestations may vary but features include dyspnoea, dry cough, focal pulmonary signs of pneumonitis, haemorrhagic cystitis (usually uncomplicated haematuria), nephritis (fever, haematuria, flank pain, and worsening renal function), hepatitis/liver failure.
- Risk is highest during the acute post-transplantation period.
- Transplant outcomes include both allograft loss and recovery.
- Mortality rates associated with adenovirus infections among transplant recipients can be high.

Clusters of fatal disease in young adults
- Fatal disease may occur especially from HAdV 7, also 3 and 4.
- HAdV 14 has caused rare outbreaks of ARD since 1955; a notable cluster in certain US states over 14 months from May 2006 involved over 14 cases of which 40% of affected persons were hospitalized, almost half in intensive care, with a 5% overall mortality.

Diagnosis

- Diagnostic tests are now predominantly by molecular detection methods, being specific, sensitive and fast.
- PCR methods can be used on a variety of specimens (e.g. respiratory, tissue, urine, blood). Options include locally developed methods with broad or all subtype specificity, or commercial PCR kits with defined, narrower subtypes detected. Real-time PCR assays permit virus quantification, which is especially important in longitudinal monitoring of the immunocompromised.
- HAdV from stool are detectable through non-serotype specific enzyme immunoassay. Immunofluorescence techniques still have utility,

especially for rapid diagnosis out of hours and for direct examination of tissue specimens. These methods have superseded virus isolation in cell culture.
- Serology is rarely useful because seroreactivity to HAdV is common; by age 4 years, around half of all children have detectable titres.

Management and treatment

- Most adenoviral infections in the immunocompetent host are self-limiting and do not warrant specific therapy. However, HAdV keratitis is treated to preserve vision with early topical steroids administered under specialist ophthalmologic care. Severe adenoviral disease, especially in immunocompromised hosts, drives the search for effective therapies.
- Absence of T-cell–specific immunity appears to be a poor prognostic sign for recovery, regardless of antiviral therapy.
- Antiviral agents inhibiting viral DNA and protein synthesis have generally been ineffective against HAdV infection. Several drugs, such as ribavirin (which inhibits viral replication by inhibiting DNA and RNA synthesis in RSV), and cidofovir (a nucleotide analogue that selectively inhibits viral DNA production in CMV), have been used to treat HAdV infections, especially the immunocompromised, with variable success.
- Benefit of dual therapy with ribavirin and cidofovir has been documented in case series. Cidofovir therapy may result in complete clinical resolution in haematopoietic stem cell recipients, where virus can become undetectable without severe nephrotoxicity.
- Anecdotal reports of success with intravesical cidofovir against HAdV haemorrhagic cystitis may reduce the systemic toxicity. However, HAdV disease in immunosuppressed hosts are more likely to be disseminated rather than localized.
- Anecdotal success with intravenous antivirals combined with pooled IVIG is also reported.
- No available studies adequately address issues such as which syndromes are most likely to respond to treatment, which patients develop limiting haematological toxicity from ribavirin or nephrotoxicity from cidofovir.
- The development of improved adenovirus therapy still remains a challenge.

Prevention

- Infection control measures: in healthcare settings, effective isolation procedures, handwashing, and sterilization of instruments prevent nosocomial infection. This is particularly important in ophthalmology practice, where contact precautions must be robust. Hospitalized patients with HAdV pneumonia require both droplet and contact precautions. Any HAdV syndrome in a healthcare worker warrants exclusion from work until symptoms resolve.

- Vaccine: a live enteric-coated adenovirus vaccine against serotypes 4 and 7 was in production for two decades; it was limited to military use but with notable effect. When given orally, these serotypes induce effective humoral immunity without producing disease. No HAdV vaccines have since been developed.

Future research

- HAdV have great potential as vectors for vaccination and for gene therapy because they can be genetically altered *in vitro* without producing infectious, pathogenic viral offspring.
- The potential for gene therapy is based on a DNA segment that codes for an enzyme or protein product that corrects a human genetic defect being delivered to the host by an adenovirus vector.

Further reading

Russell WC. Adenoviruses: update on structure and function. *J Gen Virol* 2009;**90**:1–20.
Cody JJ, Douglas JT. Armed replicating adenoviruses for cancer virotherapy. *Cancer Gene Ther* 2009;**16**:473–88.
Marcos MA, Esperatti M, Torres A. Viral pneumonia. *Curr Opin Infect Dis* 2009;**22**:43–7.

Amoebiasis

📖 see also Chapters 22, 42

Name and nature of organism

Amoebiasis, caused by the protozoa *Entamoeba histolytica*, only occurs in humans and primates. *E. histolytica* is indistinguishable from the non-pathogenic *Entamoeba dispar* (described in 1978) and *Entamoeba moshkovskii*, (described in 1941) using conventional microscopy.

Recent molecular techniques have demonstrated that of these three species only *E. histolytica* definitely causes disease. Numerous other protozoa have been identified in human faecal samples; the majority are non-pathogenic but if identified are generally indicative of high rates of faecal contamination. Experienced laboratories can separate the majority of cysts of *E. histolytica/dispar* by light microscopy.

Epidemiology

- *E. histolytica/dispar* occur worldwide but the majority of cases are in developing countries or in travellers returning from these countries. The greatest disease burden occurs in Central America and western South America, West and South Africa, parts of the Middle East and the Indian subcontinent.
- Worldwide approximately 500 million people are infected with *E. histolytica/dispar*. The true incidence of asymptomatic carriage of *E. histolytica* is unclear and it is therefore difficult to determine an accurate incidence of true *E. histolytica* infections. Best estimates are that only 10% of infections are caused by *E. histolytica* (50 million cases), the rest by *E. dispar*.
- The incidence of paediatric amoebiasis is poorly documented. In the UK between 1992 and 2006 <10% of all cases reported to the HPA occurred in children <14 years. While uncommon in children under 5 years in Europe, this is not necessarily mirrored in resource-poor countries, from where case reports of colitis and amoebic liver abscesses in neonates have been reported.
- *E. histolytica*, spread by the faecal oral route, occurs most frequently where human waste is used as a fertilizer or contaminates water sources. Cysts can persist in damp environments such as soil for months and are resistant to conventional chlorination as well as gastric acid. Ingested cysts develop into trophozoites in the small intestine and then pass to the colon where they feed on luminal bacteria and partially digested food. The trophozoites divide by binary fission and form cysts that are passed in the stool completing the cycle. Trophozoites cannot survive outside the body.

Clinical features

Asymptomatic carriage

Asymptomatic carriage rates are lower than previously reported. In patients identified carrying *E. histolytica* probably 90% will remain asymptomatic and eliminate the organism without any treatment.

Intestinal disease

In follow-up studies of asymptomatic carriers over 1 year, 4–10% develop colitis, when the intestinal mucosa is breached. This can occur months or even years after infection. Usually there is a 1–3-week history of worsening diarrhoea progressing to dysentery. In 80% of patients this lasts for less than 4 weeks while in approximately 10%, gastrointestinal symptoms may persist for longer than a year (a third in some studies). Pain is common, occurring in up to 80%, but constitutional symptoms are uncommon: weight loss <50% and fever 10–30%.

Fulminant colitis with perforation is rare, occurring in 0.5% of cases, most frequently affecting the caecum and ascending colon. Those at most risk include the very young and old, the malnourished, pregnant women, and those receiving corticosteroids. Mortality from fulminant colitis with perforation was 40% but with early diagnosis and intervention has fallen to less than 3%. Abdominal pain, distension, and tenderness occur in the majority.

Systemic disease

The commonest systemic manifestation in amoebiasis is amoebic liver abscess (ALA), occurring in 0.5–1.5% of patients infected with *E. histolytica*; equal sex predominance in children in comparison with adults where 90% occurs in men.

The proportion of patients with ALA and concurrent or prior intestinal disease including dysentery is variable; quoted rates range from 30% to 60%. ALA can occur months to years after travel to an endemic area. In the majority of ALA cases the right lobe of the liver is involved (drainage of ascending colon and caecum), and 70% are single abscesses. ALA patients have:
- Fever and pain: 85–90%
- Weight loss: 30–50%
- Diarrhoea: 20–30%
- Cough: 10–30%
- Hepatomegaly: 30–50%
- Jaundice: 6–10%.

Symptoms are present for <10 days in 80% of patients. Reactive pleural effusions and a raised right hemidiaphragm are common but can signify rupture of the ALA through the diaphragm into the pleural space.

Very rarely disease disseminates further, either by rupture of the ALA or during intestinal perforation and peritonitis to the pericardium, genitourinary system, and brain.

Differential diagnosis

Intestinal disease

- 'Traveller's' diarrhoea
- Shigellosis, Salmonellosis, *Campylobacter* enteritis
- Entero-invasive and entero-haemorrhagic *Escherichia coli*
- Coeliac disease, tropical sprue
- Inflammatory bowel disease

Amoebic liver abscess

- Bacterial liver abscess
- Echinococcal cyst
- Primary or secondary liver malignancy

Investigation

A detailed travel history, often going back a number of years, is vital to suspect *E. histolytica* infections. The results of investigations need to be considered in the context of a patient's history.

Light microscopy

- Stool microscopy is the mainstay of diagnosis and screening of patients with intestinal disease. Detection of protozoal cysts in saline or Lugol's iodine-stained faeces is relatively straightforward, however, the differentiation between *Entamoeba* sp. and other intestinal flagellates species requires experience.
- If dysentery is present then fresh warm stool needs to be sent urgently for microscopy to look for trophozoites with ingested red blood cells, diagnostic of *E. histolytica*. If the sample is allowed to cool then *E. histolytica* trophozoites lose red blood cells and are impossible to separate from the trophozoites of *E. dispar/moshkovskii* and difficult to separate from cysts of *E. hartmanni* and *E. coli*.
- Microscopy of ALA fluid if available rarely identifies trophozoites but antigen detection has a high sensitivity and specificity.

Antigen detection

Possible on frozen stool or ALA abscess fluid samples <24 hours old. An ELISA based assay using a monoclonal antibody against the Gal/GalNAC-lectin specific to *E. histolytica* developed by TECH LAB, USA, is available in the UK, and has sensitivity and specificity exceeding 96% in amoebic dysentery and ALA (Figs 47.1 and 47.2).

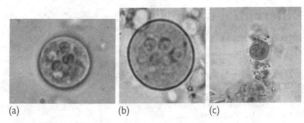

Fig. 47.1 Cysts of (a) *E. histolytica/dispar* (size range 10–15µm); (b) *E. coli* (size range 10–35µm); and (c) *E. hartmanni* (size range 5–10µm).
Source: ℗ www.cdc.gov.

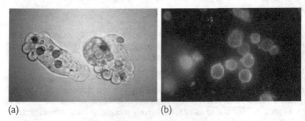

Fig. 47.2 *E. histolytica* trophozoites: (a) ingested red blood cells; (b) Fluorescein isothiocyanate (FITC) immunofluorescent antibody (IFA) staining.
Courtesy: Wendy Bailey, Liverpool School of Tropical Medicine.

Serology

More than 90% of patients who have had amoebiasis develop antibodies to *E. histolytica*, possibly lower in asymptomatic carriers. The serological tests available remain negative in *E. dispar/moshkovskii* carriers. In amoebic dysentery and ALA, serology is positive in 88% and 90–100% of patients, respectively. In acute ALA, serology may be initially negative if there is a very short history but becomes positive 2–4 weeks later. Antibody titres remain elevated for years even after successful treatment and therefore they have limited application in endemic countries where up to 30% of the population may be seropositive.

Endoscopy

Endoscopy in amoebic colitis may demonstrate non-specific findings but occasionally the pathognomonic finding of a flask-shaped ulcer can be seen. Endoscopy needs to be combined with histology and antigen detection methods.

Imaging

Plain chest and abdominal radiographs may reveal a raised hemidiaphragm or pleural effusion. Ultrasound, CT, and MRI can characterize liver lesions. Gallium scans can potentially differentiate between cold ALA and hot bacterial abscesses. Repeat scanning is sometimes useful to demonstrate resolution of liver lesions but complete resolution even with cure does not always occur or may be delayed.

Treatment

E. dispar and probably *E. moshkovskii* infections do not require treatment. All *E. histolytica* infections require intestinal luminal clearage with or without treatment for systemic/invasive disease. Where identification of *E. histolytica* from *E. dispar* and *E. moshkovskii* is not possible, luminal cidal treatments without confirmation are sometimes used with the risk of increasing drug resistance.

Asymptomatic intestinal disease

Diloxanide furoate
Side effects: flatulence, vomiting, urticaria, pruritus.

Paromomycin
Side effects: nausea and stomach cramps.

Nitazoxanide
Side effects: abdominal pain, diarrhoea, vomiting, headache, flatulence, fever, eye discoloration, rhinitis, discoloured urine.

Iodoquinol
Side effects: diarrhoea, dizziness, headache, nausea, vomiting, rectal itch, and stomach cramps.

Metronidazole is not effective therapy to remove luminal carriage; 50% fail to eliminate after a 10-day course.

Invasive bowel and systemic disease

Only rarely do patients with ALA require drainage. Resolution of fever occurs within 3–4 days after starting treatment. Perforation, peritonitis, and septicaemia are managed as in routine practice with the addition of metronidazole for 5 days.

Important: If the patient is critically unwell they need coverage for secondary sepsis from bowel flora.

Metronidazole
Side effects: gastrointestinal disturbances (including nausea and vomiting), taste disturbances, furred tongue, oral mucositis, anorexia.

Tinidazole
Side effects: same as metronidazole but fewer.

A recent Cochrane review concluded that tinidazole was superior to metronidazole; fewer treatment failures and side effects were noted but the quality of the studies was poor.

Probiotics

Recent small studies have demonstrated that the use of the probiotic *Saccharomyces boulardii* in resource-poor countries reduced the length of diarrhoea and cyst excretion in children. Large, better quality studies are required before probiotics are routinely added to treatment regimens.

Prevention

- Interruption of the faecal oral route.
- Improved sanitation.
- *E. histolytica* only occurs in primates including humans. A vaccine, if available would prevent disease; an area of possible future research.

Further reading

Fotedar R, Stark D, Beebe N, Marriott D, Ellis J, Harkness J. Laboratory diagnostic techniques for *Entamoeba* species. *Clin Microbiol Rev* 2007;**20**:511–32.

Gonzales ML, Dans LF, Martinez EG. Anti-amoebic drugs for treating amoebic colitis. *Cochrane Database Syst Rev* 2009;**15**:CD006085.

Pritt BS, Clark CG. Amebiasis. *Mayo Clin Proc* 2008;**83**:1154–9.

Solaymani-Mohammadi S, Petri W. Entamoeba histolytica *(Amebiasis)*. In: Long S, Pickering L, Prober C, eds. *Principles of Paediatric Infectious Diseases*, 3rd edn. Edinburgh: Churchill Livingstone, 2008:1236–40.

Anaerobic infections

📖 see also Chapters 22, 28, 38, 40, 44

Introduction

Anaerobic organisms are those which replicate preferentially at reduced oxygen tension (📖 see Definitions). Most clinical anaerobic infections in humans are caused by commensal bacteria from the skin and mucous membranes. These can cause serious infections in children in all body sites but are often related to entry of organisms from mucous membranes or gut, especially in chronic infection or immunocompromise. They are commonly found with other aerobic or anaerobic organisms in polymicrobial infections.

Nearly all anaerobic infections originate inside the host except for infections following bites or penetrating trauma, and those caused by *Clostridium* spp.

When to suspect anaerobic infection

- Infection at sites of anaerobic colonization, e.g. head and neck, abdomen, female genital tract.
- Possible spread from such sites, e.g. CNS infection from head and neck, aspiration pneumonia.
- Entry of external anaerobes, e.g. surgery, penetrating injury including human or animal bites, indwelling devices, e.g. shunts, tracheostomy.
- Host susceptibility, e.g. after splenectomy.

Mixed infections of aerobic and anaerobic organisms are more common than isolated anaerobic infections.

Microbiology

Definitions

Strict anaerobes only survive in conditions of reduced oxygen levels.
Microaerophilic organisms require small amounts of oxygen to replicate.
Facultative anaerobes can replicate in the presence or absence of oxygen.
Strict aerobes replicate only if oxygen is present.

Classification

The clinically important obligate anaerobic bacteria are listed below.

Gram-positive cocci

- *Peptostreptococcus* spp.

Gram-positive bacilli

- Spore-forming and non-spore-forming

Spore-forming

- *Clostridium*. spp.—the most important being *C. tetani*, *C. difficile*, *C. botulinum*, *C. perfringens*

Non-spore-forming

- *Actinomyces* spp., *Propionibacterium acnes*, *Propionibacterium propionicus*, *Bifidobacterium eriksoni*, *Bifidobacterium dentium*

Gram-negative cocci

- *Veillonella* spp.

Gram-negative rods

- *Bacteroides fragilis* group
- Other *Bacteroides*: *B. gracilis*, *B. ureolyticus*
- Pigmented *Prevotella* spp.
- Other *Prevotella* spp.
- *Fusobacterium* spp. including *F. nucleatum*, *F. necrophorum*

Clinical infections

Specific anaerobic conditions

Clostridial infection

For *C. tetani*, *C. difficile*, and *C. botulinum*, see Chapters 108, 60, and 52, respectively.

Actinomycosis

- *Actinomyces* spp. (most commonly *A. israelii*) may be part of the normal flora of the mouth, gastrointestinal tract, or vagina. Actinomycosis is a rare cause of sub-acute or chronic infection in children, which presents as lymphadenopathy that develops into 'woody' abscesses, which may form sinuses. Classically the sinuses drain yellow sulphur granules which are pathognomic. The child is usually afebrile and well, but with a chronic induration in the affected area that crosses tissue planes. Lesions may mimic chronic abscesses or malignancy, and the organism may resemble *Nocardia* spp.
- Abscesses may develop following extraction of carious teeth (cervical), oesophageal disruption (thoracic), or use of intrauterine devices (pelvic); they may also occur in the brain after bites. Treatment often involves surgical debridement but prolonged antibiotic therapy is essential (6–12 months of intravenous then oral penicillin is usual, or alternatively clindamycin or tetracyclines).

Anaerobic infections by body system

CNS infections

- Anaerobes can cause brain abscesses, subdural empyemas, epidural abscesses, and meningitis; they may also complicate intraventricular shunt infections. The usual sources of bacteria are head and neck infections originating in the adjacent ears, mastoids, sinuses, oropharynx, or teeth.
- **Shunt infections** can be caused by anaerobes. *Propionibacterium acnes*, a skin commensal, is a recognized organism. Shunts ending in the peritoneum may be infected by gastrointestinal organisms such as *Bacteroides fragilis*. Anaerobic shunt infections commonly result in milder fever and lower CSF white cell counts than aerobic infections.
- **Brain abscesses** are more likely to have an anaerobic component if they are secondary to sinusitis, acute or chronic otitis media, or mastoiditis. Anaerobes can also complicate the intracranial infection associated with Potts puffy tumour (severe frontal sinus abscess with osteomyelitis). Treatment of brain abscess is prolonged and difficult requiring neurosurgical input and medical management with long courses of antibiotics with good blood–brain barrier penetration. Bacteria generally grown from abscesses include the pigmented *Prevotella* spp., *Porphyromonas* spp., *Bacteroides* spp., *Fusobacterium* spp., *Peptostreptococcus* spp., and microaerophilic *Streptococcus* spp.
- **Meningitis** is rarely caused by anaerobic bacteria in children. It should always prompt the careful clinical examination of the child for a dermal sinus. There are case reports of anaerobic meningitis most commonly complicating an underlying head or neck infection—*Bacteroides fragilis* has been isolated from the CSF in children with a history of chronic otitis media, infected ventriculoperitoneal shunt, abdominal sepsis and an infected pilonidal sinus or midline dermoid cyst. *B. fragilis* meningitis carries high mortality and morbidity, with premature infants and neonates at particularly high risk. In children with associated risk factors, CSF and blood should be sent for anaerobic and aerobic culture.

Head and neck infections

Anaerobic organisms form part of the normal oropharyngeal flora and are often isolated in chronic infections of the head and neck.

- **Teeth**—anaerobic bacteria colonize the mouths of infants within the first few months of life, and greatly increase in numbers once teeth erupt. Bacteria in root canals of necrotic pulp and periapical lesions are predominantly anaerobic. It is common to find transient low level bacteraemia following tooth extraction in children (up to 65%), of which half the strains are anaerobes or micro-aerophilic streptococci. Organisms that predominate include *Prevotella* spp., *Porphyromonas* spp., *Fusobacterium* spp., and *Peptostreptococcus* spp.
- **Ears**—anaerobes are cultured in up to 10% of patients with acute otitis media, and 42% of those with effusions. Predominant species include Gram-positive cocci (*Peptostreptococcus* spp.) and anaerobic Gram-negative rods (*Prevotella* spp., *Porphyromonas* spp., *Bacteroides* spp., and *Fusobacterium* spp.).

- **Lemierre's disease** is the most severe manifestation of infection with *F. necrophorum*. This Gram-negative rod is found in the oropharynx as well as the gastrointestinal and female genital tracts. It can cause purulent and necrotic infections at various sites. Head and neck infections include pharyngitis, sinusitis, parotitis, dental and middle ear infections. Lemierre's disease comprises local septic thrombophlebitis of the jugular vein, bacteraemia, and possible distal septic metastases. Meningitis and osteolysis of the temporal bone or other long bones may also occur. The initial focus is usually the middle ear, but may be the pharynx or teeth. Anaerobic bacteraemia may also complicate thrombophlebitis of other veins.

- Diagnosis may prove difficult, as the disease is fairly rare, and cultures may be sterile or polymicrobial. The key is finding septic thrombophlebitis on ultrasound. Molecular analysis by PCR and sequencing may be necessary to identify *F. necrophorum* from samples, e.g. middle ear fluid, pus from abscess formation or CSF.

- Treatment is with antibiotics. In a recent review of 25 cases of Lemierre's, children were treated with a combination of high dose amoxicillin/clavulanate, metronidazole, and clindamycin and all made good recovery. Antibiotics should be given for 2–6 weeks minimum but may be needed for months if severe mastoiditis is present with slow recovery. Oral therapy can be given after clinical improvement and normalization of inflammatory markers. Mastoidectomy and anticoagulant therapy should also be considered. Mortality was >90% in the pre-antibiotic era but deaths are uncommon with good microbiological diagnosis, appropriate antibiotics, and intensive care.

- **Tonsils**—acute bacterial tonsillitis is usually caused by aerobic *Streptococcus* spp., but there is increasing evidence for the involvement of anaerobes in chronic tonsillitis and complications such as peritonsillar and retropharyngeal abscess and Vincent's angina—*Fusobacterium* spp., Gram-negative anaerobic bacilli, and *Peptostreptococcus* spp. have been isolated. Children who undergo tonsillectomy for recurrent chronic tonsillitis show a significant drop in the number of anaerobic bacteria in the oropharyngeal flora post-tonsillectomy.

Pleuropulmonary infections

- **Aspiration pneumonia**—aspiration of oropharyngeal secretions or gastric contents, and severe periodontal disease or abscess are the highest risk factors for developing anaerobic pleuropulmonary infections in children; tracheostomies also increase the risk of anaerobic infection. Complications include lung abscess or empyema. Predominant organisms include *Peptostreptococcus* spp., *Fusobacterium* spp., pigmented *Prevotella* spp., *Porphyromonas* spp., and *Bacteroides fragilis*. Microbiological diagnosis may be complicated by contamination of sputum samples by oropharyngeal organisms.

Intra-abdominal

- Anaerobic bacteria are part of the normal gastrointestinal flora. Peritonitis and abscess formation are the result of entry of enteric

bacteria into the peritoneal cavity. Perforated appendicitis resulting in peritonitis or periappendicular abscess is the most common cause in children. The most common organism isolated is *Escherichia coli*, but mixed cultures and anaerobes are frequently present, especially once an abscess has formed. *B. fragilis* is the most common anaerobe isolated, followed by *Peptostreptococcus* spp. and *Clostridium* spp.
- Therapy consists of surgical management and an antibiotic combination that covers both aerobes and anaerobes. Cefotaxime and metronidazole, or ampicillin with metronidazole and an aminoglycoside, have been shown to be effective.

Female genital tract
- Anaerobes are common in the genital tract in sexually active females. Infections that may be polymicrobial include bacterial vaginosis, soft tissue perineal and vulval abscesses, pelvic collections, intrauterine device-associated infections, and postoperative obstetric and gynaecological infections. Predominant bacteria include *Prevotella* spp., *Peptostreptococcus* spp., *Porphyromonas* spp., *Clostridium* spp., and *Actinomyces* spp.

Skin and soft tissue
- **Bite wounds** often contain anaerobic oral flora, including microaerophilic *Eikenella* spp. in human bites and *Pasteurella multocida* in animal bites.
- **Gas gangrene** is a deep-seated infection of the muscle caused by *C. perfringens* or *C. septicum*. It is extremely rare in children and is associated with underlying neutrophil dysfunction, bowel ischaemia or trauma . Non-specific symptoms include vomiting, diarrhoea, blood per rectum, severe abdominal pain, and an acute abdomen. Crepitus in muscles can sometimes be felt. Mortality is high, and survivors are more likely not to have abdominal involvement, to receive early parenteral antibiotics, have no underlying medical risk factors, and undergo surgical debridement. Hyperbaric oxygen may be useful.
- **Tropical ulcers** in children are most commonly caused by *Fusobacterium* spp.

Osteomyelitis and septic arthritis
- **Osteomyelitis** may be anaerobic in facial or cranial bones following local spread from soft tissue, or in long bones following trauma, haematogenous spread, or bone hypoxia secondary to sickle cell disease or vascular ischaemia. Infection is likely to be polymicrobial, and associated with anaerobic infection elsewhere in the body.
- **Septic arthritis** due to anaerobes is rare, but is more likely to be monomicrobial than osteomyelitis. It is usually due to haematogenous spread from anaerobic infection elsewhere in the body.
- **Diagnosis** requires tissue samples of bone or synovial pus. *Peptostreptococcus* and *Bacteroides* are the most common anaerobic organisms at all sites. *Fusobacterium* may complicate sickle cell disease, and *Clostridium* may be found with contamination after trauma.
- **Treatment** requires adequate surgical debridement or pus drainage, orthopaedic involvement, and antibiotic treatment with good bone or joint penetration.

Bacteraemia
- **Anaerobic bacteraemia** in children is rare, carries a high mortality and is usually associated with a localized infection and risk factors such as indwelling catheters or recent gastrointestinal or pelvic surgery. Children who have malignant disease, particularly leukaemia, chronic renal failure, decubitus ulcers, or a known immunodeficiency, are at increased risk of anaerobic bacteraemia. Infectious mononucleosis has also been reported to predispose to anaerobic bacteraemia. Neonates are at increased risk—anaerobic Gram-positive cocci sensitive to penicillin appear more commonly in the first few days of life and are associated with chorioamnionitis; anaerobic Gram-negative organisms appear later, are less sensitive to penicillins and may be associated with necrotizing enterocolitis. Routine culture for anaerobes in previously healthy children who do not present with possible anaerobic site of infection is not recommended as the yield is so low. The most commonly recovered organism from anaerobic blood cultures overall is *B. fragilis*.
- **Diagnosis**—blood cultures from children are often taken into single aerobic blood culture bottles. These require smaller quantities of blood than adult bottles. Some anaerobes will be isolated from these, but if there is a strong clinical suspicion of anaerobic infection, a separate anaerobic bottle should also be inoculated. This requires larger volumes of blood and may prove difficult in small patients or neonates.

General management

Management of anaerobic infections includes toxin neutralization, surgical debridement or drainage if appropriate, and antimicrobial therapy. Surgical involvement in cases of abscess formation, severe skin or bone/joint infection, or gastrointestinal infection is crucial. Other therapies, such as hyperbaric oxygen in order to improve tissue oxygenation may be useful, but lack evidence.

Antimicrobials

Antimicrobial sensitivities of anaerobes are rarely routinely tested and little is known about geographical and temporal variation. The *Bacteroides* group are best studied, as these are known to be virulent bacteria with mechanisms to evade antimicrobials. It is important to liaise with the local microbiology laboratory or regional/national anaerobic reference laboratory.

B. fragilis is largely resistant to penicillins but generally sensitive to penicillins with β-lactamase inhibitors. *B. fragilis* is sensitive to carbapenems and metronidazole, but resistant to many cephalosporins. There is currently sensitivity to clindamycin, although resistance is rapidly rising. The newer fluoroquinolones, such as moxifloxacin, have been approved by the US Food and Drug Administration (FDA) for use against skin infections that may contain anaerobes. Moxifloxacin has good *in vitro* activity against *Bacteroides*, although resistance is rising in the USA. Tigecycline is another recently approved antibiotic with good *in vitro* activity against *Bacteroides* and most other anaerobes, and little resistance known. *Fusobacterium* are largely sensitive to penicillins, penicillins with β-lactamase inhibitors and cephalosporins. *Prevotella* and *Porphyromonas* spp. have high resistance to penicillins, which may be overcome by the addition of a β-lactamase inhibitor. They are uniformly sensitive to carbapenems and metronidazole. The non-spore-forming Gram-positive bacilli, such as *Propionibacterium* and *Actinomyces*, are usually sensitive to penicillins, β-lactamase inhibitors, cephalosporins, and carbapenems. Most are resistant to metronidazole.

Gram-positive cocci, *Peptostreptococcus*, have variable resistance to penicillin, metronidazole and clindamycin, while retaining susceptibility to β-lactamase inhibitors and carbapenems. There is increasing resistance recognized to the newer fluoroquinolones.

Table 48.1 Treatment suggestion for anaerobic infection by clinical presentation

Clinical	Likely organism	Suggested antibiotic	Comments
Central nervous system			
Brain abscess	Mixed	Dependent on organism – if unknown metronidazole + cephalosporin or carbapenem	
Shunt infection	*Bacteroides fragilis*	Carbapenem + metronidazole, tigecycline	Largely resistant to penicillin
	Propionibacterium acnes	Penicillin +/- beta lactamase inhibitor, cephalosporin, carbapenem	
Anaerobic meningitis	*Bacteroides fragilis*	Carbapenem + metronidazole, or tigecycline	
	Clostridium perfringens	Penicillin or carbapenem or cephalosporin	
Head and neck			
Tooth abscess	Mixed	Co-amoxiclav or macrolide or metronidazole	Surgical drainage first line

(Continued)

Table 48.1 (*Contd.*)

Clinical	Likely Organism	Suggested Antibiotic	Comments
Chronic tonsillitis	*Fusobacterium*, gram negative anaerobic bacilli and *Peptostreptococcus*	Co-amoxiclav in chronic cases	May require beta-lactamase inhibitor after repeated use of penicillin
Lemmiere's disease	*F. necrophorum*	Co-amoxiclav or metronidazole or clindamycin	Usually needs to cover aerobic organisms as well
Chronic otitis media	Mixed	Co-amoxiclav, macrolide, metronidazole, clindamycin	May also need to cover *Pseudomonas spp.* if present. Surgical debridement may be necessary
Chronic sinusitis	Mixed	Co-amoxiclav, macrolide, metronidazole, clindamycin	
Pleuropulmonary			
Aspiration pneumonia	*Peptostreptococcus*, *Fusobacterium*, pigmented *Prevotella*, *Porphyromonas spp.* And *Bacteroides fragilis*	Co-amoxiclav or carbapenem or metronidazole	
Intra-abdominal			
Peritonitis and abscess	*E coli*, *B. fragilis*, *Peptostreptococcus*, *Clostridium*	Cefotaxime and metronidazole, or ampicillin and metronidazole and aminoglycoside	Surgical input essential
Female genital tract	*Prevotella spp.*, *Peptostreptococcus*, *Porphyromonas*, *Clostridium spp.* *Actinomyces spp.*	Doxycycline or macrolide and cephalosporin or clindamycin or metronidazole.	Covers aerobes, anaerobes and sexually transmitted pathogens
Skin and soft tissue			
Neonatal omphalitis	*Bacteroides* or *Prevotella*	Co-amoxiclav or metronidazole	
Acne	*Propionibacterium*	Tetracycline	

Table 48.1 (Contd.)

Clinical	Likely Organism	Suggested Antibiotic	Comments
Bites	*Eikenella* – human	Co-amoxiclav or clindamycin	
	Pasteurella multocida – animal		
Necrotizing fasciitis	Anaerobic cocci and *B. fragilis* + aerobes	Penicillin and aminoglycoside and metronidazole	
Gas gangrene	*Clostridium perfringens*	Penicillin or macrolide or clindamycin	
Bones and joints			
Septic arthritis	*Peptostreptococcus* or *Bacteroides*	Clindamycin	Surgical drainage important
Osteomyelitis	*Peptostreptococcus*, *Bacteroides*	Clindamycin	Surgical debridement important
	Fusobacterium (sickle cell)		
	Clostridium (trauma)		
Bacteraemia	*Bacteroides fragilis* most commonly	Co-amoxiclav, or carbapenem or metronidazole	Rising resistance to penicillin, local resistance patterns important

NB: Antibiotic choices may also need to cover aerobic organisms

Further reading

Brook I. Overview of anaerobic infections in children. *Pediatr Infect Dis J* 2009;**4**:3–9.

Hecht D. Anaerobes: Antibiotic resistance, clinical significance and the role of susceptibility testing. *Anaerobe* 2006;**12**:115–21.

Le Monnier A, Jamet A, Carbonnelle E, *et al. Fusobacterium necrophorum* middle ear infections in children and related complications. *Pediatr Infect Dis J* 2008;**27**:613–17.

Lemierre A. On certain septicaemias due to anaerobic organisms. *Lancet* 1936;**227**:701–3.

Chapter 49

Arboviruses

📖 see also Chapters 13, 41, 42

Introduction

Arboviruses are **ar**thropod-**bo**rne viruses. They cause disease in domestic and wild animals, and in humans they pose a threat to public health because of their epidemic and zoonotic potential. The vectors are species restricted and determine the geographical distribution and seasonality of each virus. Disease outbreaks caused by arboviruses are sporadic and unpredictable.

Arbovirus infection in humans may cause:

- Acute haemorrhagic fever
- CNS infection (encephalitis, aseptic meningitis, or myelitis)
- Acute polyarthropathy
- Non-specific febrile illness often with rash
- Perinatal illness.

Name and nature of organism

Arboviruses that cause human disease are members of three main virus families: the *Togaviridae* (genus *Alphavirus*), *Flaviviridae*, and *Bunyaviridae*. Most arboviruses have an RNA genome. Arboviral infections are mostly zoonotic involving a non-human primary vertebrate host and a primary arthropod vector. Viral replication in the arthropod vector (mosquitoes, ticks, or sandflies) is a prerequisite step before transmission to the next host.

Epidemiology, transmission, and incubation period

Humans and domestic animals become infected with arboviruses when they encroach on a natural focus of zoonotic infection or the virus escapes this focus via a secondary vector or vertebrate host. Humans are usually 'dead-end' hosts because they do not produce significant viraemia. Important exceptions are dengue, yellow fever, and chikungunya, where vectors spread disease from person to person.

Arboviral infections are vector dependent and usually seasonal; mosquito-borne infections occur during the wet seasons/summer. In tick-borne encephalitis (TBE) in central Europe, two peaks of activity of *Ixodes ricinus* have been observed: in May/June and in September/October. In colder regions of northern Europe and in mountain regions a single summer peak is detected. Cases of clinical illness occur more often at the extremes of age. Incubation periods of disease range from 1 to 18 days (Table 49.1).

In recent decades, the geographical distribution of disease caused by arboviruses has expanded. Outbreaks of West Nile fever have occurred in Europe, especially in the Mediterranean basin. Moreover, Crimean-Congo haemorrhagic fever (CCHF) is endemic in many European countries and serious outbreaks have occurred, particularly in the Balkans, Turkey, and Southern Federal Districts of Russia. In 2000, Rift Valley fever was reported for the first time outside the African continent, with cases being confirmed in Yemen and Saudi Arabia.

Dengue ranks as the most important mosquito-borne viral disease in the world. In the past 50 years, the incidence has increased 30-fold. An estimated 2.5 billion people live in over 100 endemic countries and areas where dengue viruses can be transmitted. Up to 50 million infections occur annually with 500 000 cases of dengue haemorrhagic fever and 22 000 deaths mainly among children. Prior to 1970, only nine countries had experienced cases of dengue haemorrhagic fever (DHF); since then the number has increased more than fourfold and continues to rise.

Japanese encephalitis is the most important cause of arboviral encephalitis with over 45 000 cases reported annually. Arboviruses are the most common causes of episodic encephalitis in the USA, with reported incidence of 0.2 per 100 000. However, these statistics may be misleading because most people bitten by arbovirus-infected insects do not develop clinical disease.

Table 49.1 Common arboviruses

Name	Human disease	Vector	Geographical distribution	Reservoir	Incubation (days)
Flaviviridae					
St Louis encephalitis	Encephalitis	Mosquito	Americas and Caribbean	Birds	4–14
West Nile fever	Encephalitis	Mosquito	Asia, Africa, Europe, Americas	Birds	5–15
Powassan	Encephalitis	Tick	North America and Asia		4–18
Japanese encephalitis	Encephalitis	Mosquito	Asia	Water birds	5–14
Tickborne encephalitis complex	Encephalitis	Tick. Occasional cases by ingestion of 'infected' cow or goat milk	Europe and Asia	Deer, rodents	7–14
Murray Valley encephalitis	Encephalitis	Mosquito	Australia and New Guinea		
Dengue fever	Febrile illness—may be biphasic with rash, haemorrhagic fever and shock	Mosquito	Tropical areas worldwide	N/A	4–7
Yellow fever	Febrile illness, hepatitis, haemorrhagic fever	Mosquito	Tropical areas of South America and Africa	N/A	3–6

Bunyaviridae				
Rift Valley fever	Febrile illness, ocular disease, meningoencephalitis, haemorrhagic fever	Mosquito infected blood and tissues Ingestion of 'infected' milk	Africa, Saudi Arabia, Yemen and Indian Ocean	Domestic and wild animals 2–6
Crimean-Congo haemorrhagic fever	Febrile illness, haemorrhagic fever	Tick, infected blood and tissues Ingestion of 'infected' milk	Africa, Europe and Asia	Domestic and wild animals, birds 1–13
California serogroup viruses	Encephalitis	Mosquito	Americas, Europe and Asia	Small mammals 5–15
Oropouche virus fever	Febrile illness	Midge	Central and South America	N/A 2–6
Hantavirus fevers	Haemorrhagic fever with renal syndrome or with cardiopulmonary syndrome	Aerosolized rodent excreta or rodent bites	Asia, Europe and Americas	
Toscana and Sicilian virus	Febrile illness Aseptic meningitis	Sandfly	Europe and Asia	
Togaviridae				
Chikungunya virus	Febrile illness, arthropathy, occasional meningoencephalitis	Mosquito	Africa, Asia and Europe	N/A 1–12

(Continued)

Table 49.1 (Contd.)

Name	Human disease	Vector	Geographical distribution	Reservoir	Incubation (days)
Eastern equine encephalitis virus	Encephalitis	Mosquito	Americas	Birds	3–10
Western equine encephalitis	Encephalitis	Mosquito	Americas	Birds	2–10
Venezuelan equine encephalitis	Encephalitis	Mosquito	Americas	Small mammals and horses	1–4
Mayaro virus	Febrile illness and arthropathy		Americas		1–12
Ross River virus	Febrile illness and arthropathy		Australia and Oceania		
O'nyong nyong virus	Febrile illness and arthropathy		Africa		
Sindbis virus	Febrile illness and arthropathy	Mosquito	Africa, Scandinavia, Northern Europe, Asia and Australia		
Reoviridae					
Colorado tick fever	Febrile illness—may be biphasic	Tick	North America and Asia		1–14
Rhabdoviridae					
Vesicular stomatitis virus		Sandfly and blackfly	Americas and Africa		

Clinical features and sequelae

The majority of arbovirus infections are asymptomatic or may result in a non-specific flu-like syndrome. Infections are characterized by viral replication in endothelial and macrophage/monocyte lineage cells inducing type 1 interferon production.

Onset may be insidious or sudden with fever, headache, myalgias, arthralgias, malaise, and occasionally prostration. Infection may, however, lead to secondary viraemia and subsequent infection of target organs. Which organs are targeted depends on the tropism of the virus. Access to the brain may be via infection of endothelial cells in the cerebral vasculature or invasion of the choroid plexus. Secondary viraemia can lead to haemorrhagic fever or encephalitis, with a fatal outcome or permanent neurological sequelae.

Only a very small proportion of infected children progress to overwhelming disease. Antibody-mediated immunity is important in controlling secondary viraemia and progression of disease. Recovery from disease relies on cell-mediated immunity.

Acute haemorrhagic fevers

Dengue has a wide spectrum of clinical presentations. Dengue fever and DHF are caused by four closely related virus serotypes (DEN 1–4). Each serotype is sufficiently different that there is no cross-protection and epidemics caused by multiple serotypes (hyperendemicity) can occur.

Infection produces sudden-onset fever, headache, retro-orbital pain, extremely painful myalgia (break bone fever), arthralgia, facial flushing/erythema/rash, nausea, and vomiting. The classic dengue fever lasts 2–7 days, with a biphasic fever pattern. It tends to be milder in children than adults. The white cell and platelet count may drop until the end of the febrile phase. The acute phase may last up to 1 week, with a prolonged convalescence characterized by weakness, malaise, and anorexia.

DHF is an immunopathological consequence of infection in a patient with serotype specific-immunity from a previous infection with a virus of another serotype. Immune enhancement leads to increased uptake of 'new' virus coated with pre-existing non-neutralizing antibody into macrophages via the Fc receptor. Virus replicates in macrophages leading to an increased virus load; in turn macrophages become activated and release inflammatory cytokines.

Disease is more severe in children and the presence of maternal antibody in infants may result in DHF even from a first infection with Dengue virus. Criteria for DHF include a haemorrhagic tendency (positive tourniquet test, spontaneous bruising, mucosal bleeding, injection site bleeding, epistaxis, haematemesis, bloody diarrhoea), thrombocytopenia (<100 000 platelets/μl) and organ involvement (massive gastrointestinal bleeding, acute liver failure, acute renal failure, encephalopathy or encephalitis, cardiomyopathy). Evidence of plasma leakage (haematocrit >20% higher than expected, pleural effusion, ascites, hypoproteinaemia) is an indication of progression to severe dengue/dengue shock syndrome.

Dengue shock syndrome is defined as DHF plus a weak rapid pulse, a narrow pulse pressure (<20mmHg), poor peripheral perfusion, and reduced level of consciousness. DHF is fatal in up to 30% of untreated cases. The key to survival is early diagnosis and active supportive care.

Yellow fever cases have increased over the past two decades due to declining population immunity to infection, deforestation, urbanization, population movements, and climate change. There are an estimated 200 000 cases of yellow fever, causing 30 000 deaths, worldwide each year. Once contracted, the virus incubates for 3–6 days, followed by infection that can occur in one or two phases.

The first, acute, phase usually causes fever, myalgia, prominent backache, headache, rigors, anorexia, nausea, and vomiting. Most patients improve and symptoms disappear after 3–4 days.

Around 15% of patients enter a second, more toxic phase within 24 hours of the initial remission. High fever returns and a multiorgan illness follows. The patient rapidly develops jaundice, renal impairment, abdominal pain, vomiting, and a bleeding diathesis. Half of the patients who enter the toxic phase die within 10–14 days, the rest recover without significant organ damage. Up to 50% of severely affected persons without treatment will die from yellow fever.

CCHF has the most extensive geographical distribution of the medically important tick-borne viral diseases. Onset of symptoms is sudden, with fever, myalgia (aching muscles), dizziness, neck pain and stiffness, backache, headache, photophobia, and acute confusion. Other clinical signs include tachycardia, lymphadenopathy, a petechial rash and mucosal bleeding. There is usually evidence of hepatitis. The severely ill may develop hepatorenal and pulmonary failure after the fifth day of illness. The mortality rate from CCHF is approximately 30%, with death occurring in the second week of illness. In those patients who recover, improvement generally begins on the ninth or tenth day after the onset of illness.

Acute polyarthropathy

Chikungunya virus has been responsible for an ongoing and rapidly moving outbreak in the past 6 years in the Indian Ocean, Europe, Asia, Oceania, and Africa. After infection with chikungunya virus, there is a silent incubation period lasting 2–4 days on average (range 1–12 days). Clinical onset is abrupt with high fever, headache, back pain, myalgia, and arthralgia; the latter can be intense, affecting mainly the extremities (ankles, wrists, phalanges) but also the large joints. Skin involvement is present in about 40–50% of cases, and consists of a pruriginous maculo-papular rash predominating on the thorax, facial oedema, or in children, a bullous rash with pronounced sloughing, and localized petechiae and bleeding gums. Erratic, relapsing, and incapacitating arthralgia is the hallmark of chikungunya, although it rarely affects children. It may persist for several months.

Neurological complications such as meningoencephalitis have been reported. Chikungunya virus has been isolated from two children with clinical signs of encephalitis and meningitis. Among 35 women who were ill with chikungunya at delivery in a recent outbreak, 30 delivered an infected newborn baby, of which 27 were severely affected. The possible risks of embryopathy, fetopathy, and late sequelae are unknown.

CNS infection

Tick born encephalitis (TBE) includes three subtypes: Western subtype, Far Eastern subtype and Siberian subtype. The number of human cases of TBE in all endemic regions of Europe has increased by almost 400% in the past 30 years; the risk areas have spread and new foci have been discovered. The incubation period of TBE is 7 days on average, but incubation of up to 28 days has been described. Approximately two-thirds of human TBE virus infections are asymptomatic.

TBE often has a biphasic clinical course. The first viraemic phase lasts 5 (range 2–10) days, and is associated with non-specific symptoms (fever, fatigue, headache, myalgia, nausea). This phase is followed by an asymptomatic interval lasting 7 (range 1–21) days, which precedes the second phase, when the CNS is involved (meningoencephalitis, myelitis, paralysis). The western European subtype is associated with milder disease, with 20–30% of patients experiencing the second phase, mortality rates of 0.5–2%, and severe neurological sequelae in up to 10% of patients. In children, the second phase of illness is usually limited to meningitis, whereas adults >40 years are at increased risk of developing encephalitis. The Far Eastern subtype is associated with a monophasic illness, with no asymptomatic interval preceding the onset of neurological disease, mortality rates of up to 20%, and higher rates of severe neurological sequelae.

Japanese encephalitis virus epidemics occur in late summer in temperate regions, but the infection is enzootic and occurs throughout the year in many tropical areas of Asia. The incubation period is 5–14 days. Onset of symptoms is usually sudden, with fever, headache and vomiting. The illness resolves in 5–7 days if there is no CNS involvement. The mortality in most outbreaks is <10%, but is higher in children and can exceed 30%. Neurological sequelae in patients who recover are reported in up to 30% of cases.

West Nile virus encephalitis has been the cause of recent outbreaks in North America and Europe. In humans it usually produces either asymptomatic infection or mild febrile disease with rash, arthritis, myalgias, weakness (a transient poliomyelitis-like 'acute flaccid paralysis' with acute respiratory involvement), lymphadenopathy, and meningoencephalitis. It can cause severe and fatal infection in <1% of infected patients due to neuroinvasive disease. There is some limited evidence of persistence.

Diagnosis

Arbovirus infection diagnosis is difficult because many other agents cause similar symptoms.

Laboratory diagnosis of human arboviral disease relies on rapid serologic assays such as IgM-capture ELISA (MAC-ELISA) and IgG ELISA soon after infection. Early in infection, IgM antibody is more specific, whereas later in infection, IgG antibody is more reactive.

Virus isolation and identification from serum, throat swab, CSF, and mosquito vectors is also possible. While PCR has been developed to identify a number of viral agents, such tests are not yet validated for routine rapid identification in the clinical setting.

Management and treatment

Early diagnosis in severe disease directly affects outcome. Treatment is supportive, including antibiotics for any secondary bacterial infections, aggressive management of haemorrhagic manifestations, multiorgan involvement, and neurological complications.

There are no effective antiviral drugs against arboviruses although ribavirin has been used with demonstrable benefit in a limited number of observational studies in CCHF. Chloroquine has been used in arbovirus polyarthritis with anecdotal benefits.

Prevention

Prevention methods include surveillance, vector control (aerial and house-to-house spraying), public education about reducing vector numbers and reducing vector exposure (insect repellents, bed nets, suitable clothing, low-risk outdoor activities, restricted travel to endemic areas), reservoir host control and the use of vaccines where available.

Human vaccines currently available include yellow fever, TBE, and Japanese encephalitis. Active research in dengue vaccine and chikungunya vaccine is promising.

Future research

- Emergence of arboviruses will continue to occur due to changes in ecological patterns, natural evolution of invertebrate vectors, vertebrate hosts, and the viruses themselves combined with rapid movement of people and animals on a global scale.
- Global warming will increase the geographical spread of arboviral infection and will need improved surveillance mechanisms.
- New data on viral replication offers substantial potential for the development of new drugs.

Further reading

Ahmed J. International network for capacity building for the control of emerging viral vector-borne zoonotic diseases: ARBO-ZOONET. *Euro Surveill* 2009;**14**:1–4.

Centers for Disease Control and Prevention, Division of Vector-Borne Infectious Diseases. *Information on Arboviral Encephalitides*. Available at: www.cdc.gov/ncidod/dvbid/Arbor/arbdet.htm (accessed 1 February 2011).

Powers AM. Overview of emerging arboviruses. *Future Virol* 2009;**4**:391–401.

World Health Organization (WHO) and the Special Programme for Research and Training in Tropical Diseases (TDR). *Dengue Guidelines for Diagnosis, Treatment, Prevention and Control*. 2009. Available at: www.cdc.gov/dengue/clinicalLab/index.html (accessed 1 February 2011).

Ascariasis

📖 see also Chapters 22, 35, 41, 42, 45

Infecting organism

- Ascariasis (also known as common roundworm or large roundworm infection) is caused by the nematode *Ascaris lumbricoides*.
- *A. lumbricoides* is a member of the soil-transmitted helminths.
- *A. lumbricoides* is white or yellow in colour and the largest of the round worms, ranging in size from 20–40cm in length and 0.5–0.6cm in width for females, and 12–25cm × 0.3–0.4 for males.
- *A. lumbricoides* almost exclusively inhabits humans with high specificity but can rarely infect pigs.

Life cycle

- Parasitic infection with *A. lumbricoides* occurs via ingestion of embryonated eggs. These are found in soil, human faeces and on contaminated food. Eggs can be spread by earthworms, insects, and burrowing animals, and can also become airborne, in wind-spread contaminated dust, which can be inhaled or swallowed by humans.
- There is little direct information on the interaction of *A. lumbricoides* larvae with humans; life cycle data come from experiments with mice.
- When *A. lumbricoides* eggs are swallowed, they pass into the intestine and hatch in the jejunum, releasing larvae measuring 50–70µm in length. The larvae enter the portal venous circulation via penetration of the small intestine wall, and migrate to the liver. They also circulate in the lymphatic system.
- The larvae travel via the venous circulation to the pulmonary circulation to the lungs, where they enter the bronchial tubes and penetrate the pulmonary capillaries to enter alveolar spaces. They then ascend into the trachea, and are swallowed, thus returning to the small intestine. They mature into adult worms, over 14–20 days, mate, and lay eggs.
- The cycle from ingestion to maturation take 18–42 days in humans. The adult parasite lives in the gut for 6–24 months.
- A female worm may contain up to 27 million eggs and can produce approximately 200 000 eggs per day. In the presence of male worms, the eggs are fertilized and therefore become infective. Eggs are discharged into faeces (approximately 9 weeks after initial ingestion of eggs) and incubate in the soil. Any fertilized eggs will then become infectious once they embryonate. *A. lumbricoides* eggs are resistant to environmental stresses.

Epidemiology

- Ascariasis is the most common infection caused by worms in humans and is endemic throughout the world.
- It is present in at least 150 countries worldwide, and more than 1.4 billion people (approx. a quarter of the population) are hosts to *A. lumbricoides*.
- Prevalence varies, but the highest frequencies are seen in tropical and subtropical areas, and particularly in developing nations (Box 50.1). The estimated prevalence across world regions is:
  - Asia and Oceania—75%
  - Africa and the Middle East—16.7%
  - South America, Central America, and the Caribbean—8.3%.
- Ascariasis is rare in the UK (80 cases per year on average)—most cases are likely to have been contracted abroad.

Box 50.1 General risk factors

- Crowded living conditions
- Low socio-economic class and poor sanitary conditions
- Malnourishment
- Living in regions where human faeces is utilized as fertilizer

---

- Children are particularly prone to ascariasis because of poorer hygiene habits than adults, and their tendency to put things in their mouths.
- The global prevalence in children is estimated to be up to 400 million. The most common age group infected is between 3 and 8 years old. The highest intensity of infection occurs in children harbouring other helminth infections (e.g. *Trichuris trichuria*, hookworm).
- Neonatal ascariasis can occur, probably as a result of transplacental infection.
- Around 50 million children are believed to have more severe nutritional morbidity due to high infection load. Young children are the most likely to have intestinal obstruction (85% of cases are reported in those aged 1–5 years).
- There are no racial or sexual biases associated with infection rates; however females are more susceptible to hepatobiliary and pancreatic ascariasis (HPA), and more often require biliary surgery, than males. HPA is less common in children.

Natural history and clinical presentation

The first sign of ascariasis is often excretion of a worm in the faeces, particularly in children in endemic areas. Symptoms of infection are dependent on the stage of development of the Ascaris, the site of the parasite, and the burden of worms involved.

Intestinal phase

- Ascariasis is often asymptomatic during mild infection, or can cause non-specific abdominal symptoms (nausea, vomiting, abdominal pain, diarrhoea, loss of appetite). Other symptoms may be: fever, coughing up worms, worms exiting the nose or mouth, weight loss, anal itching.
- *Intestinal obstruction:* Mature worms may form a bolus, causing intestinal obstruction (most often in the terminal ileum). Abdominal distension due to blockage is more common in children (85% of cases in children aged 1–5 years). Worms may become incarcerated, leading to obstructive pathology. The patient may have or rapidly develop sepsis, sepsis syndrome, and septic shock. The worm bolus may also cause **intussusception** or volvulus.
- Patients with obstruction often display abnormal vital signs (tachycardia, fever), and may vomit. Moderate to severe abdominal pain and tenderness can be either diffuse or localized, usually on the right side. The bolus may be apparent as a palpable mass. Increasing severity of symptoms is an indicator of progression of the obstruction, or **perforation**.

Migratory/larval phase

Worms may migrate to the lungs or biliary tract (see below), to the upper respiratory tract throat, (nose, lachrymal ducts, inner ear), eyes, vagina, kidneys, ureter, and bladder. Larval migration may cause: fever, convulsions, skin rash, conjunctivitis. A key feature is often **eosinophilia**. Death of worms in tissue leads to inflammation, necrosis, and abscess formation. Migrated larvae may enter the brain, spinal cord, and kidney tissue, but cannot survive, resulting in granuloma formation in these areas.

Pulmonary ascariasis

Migration of larvae into the lungs can cause pneumonitis, with associated asthma or wheeze, rales, cough, chest pain, blood-tinged sputum, shortness of breath. These signs may persist for several days. A large infestation can lead to **Löeffler pneumonia** (haemoptysis, transient eosinophilia, and lung infiltrates). Rarely a mature worm can migrate and obstruct the airway, causing respiratory distress.

Hepatobiliary and pancreatic ascariasis

Larvae can also migrate into the biliary tree, and then into the liver or pancreas; biliary tract, liver, and gallbladder blockage may result. Eggs or worm fragments deposited in the liver or biliary tract precipitate local reactions. Complications include:

- Acalculous cholecystitis (pain plus tenderness in upper right quadrant)

- Ascending cholangitis (often with fever, tachycardia, tachypnoea, jaundice, enlarged liver with severe pain, plus tenderness in upper right quadrant or diffuse)
- Appendicitis
- Biliary colic (associated with worms in ampullary orifice; occurs without fever or jaundice)
- Pancreatitis (vomiting likely, with pain plus tenderness of the epigastrium, upper left quadrant)
- Hepatic abscess (associated with intrahepatic duct blockage; tender, enlarged liver, pain plus tenderness in upper right quadrant)
- Gastric haemorrhage
- Peritonitis and/or peritoneal granulomatosis
- Meckel diverticulum inflammation
- Obstructive jaundice.

Chronic ascariasis is linked to malnutrition due to *malabsorption*. Children are particularly susceptible to protein, caloric, or vitamin A deficiency, resulting in physical and mental retardation syndromes, cognitive impairment, poor academic performance, and increased likelihood to catch other infectious diseases.

Mortality/morbidity

- The mortality rate with severe complications of infection may be up to 5%. Mortality is estimated at 10 000–100 000 deaths per year, of which the majority are children.
- The rate of complications ranges from 11% to 67%. Only a small percentage of infections cause serious pathology, but the sheer number of infected people mean this represents a substantial burden of clinical disease.
- Morbidity is proportional to the worm burden. Intestinal obstruction can occur with only four worms, but average worm burden is 59 worms for non-fatal cases, and 659 in fatal cases.

Diagnosis

- A stool sample is advised if the patient has non-specific gastrointestinal symptoms, and lives/has travelled within the last 1–2 years to an area where ascariasis is widespread.
- Presence of A. lumbricoides is usually diagnosed by microscopic examination confirming presence of eggs in a stool sample. Re-examination 3 weeks after treatment to check eggs and worms are eradicated is advised.
- Microscopy is performed using either a direct method (mixing stool with saline) or after concentrating the sample. Fertilized eggs are easier to identify than unfertilized eggs. It should be borne in mind that male-only infections are possible and then eggs are not present.

- Rarely the diagnosis may be made by study of adult worms that have been passed into the stool, coughed, or vomited out or even passed out of the nose.
- Microscopic examination of gastric contents may reveal larvae and/or eggs, and examination of sputum may reveal larvae.
- An FBC may show eosinophilia or anaemia, particularly during the phase of migration into the lungs.
- Signs of malnutrition are apparent in patients with a heavy burden of infection.
- Liver damage or low protein levels may be evident from LFTs.
- Imaging investigations, for the diagnostic imaging of complications of ascariasis include abdominal ultrasound, CT scanning, abdominal or chest radiography, or MRCP. HPA is often diagnosed by this method.
- Exploratory surgery may rarely be required, depending on infection site.

Differential diagnosis

Depending on symptoms displayed, this can include infection with *Trichuris*, appendicitis, malabsorption syndromes, asthma (for pulmonary ascariasis), pancreatitis, cholecystitis, cholelithiasis, and hypersensitivity pneumonitis.

Management

Anthelmintic chemotherapy

Oral anthelmintics are the first line of therapy to eradicate intestinal roundworms (Table 50.1). Symptoms usually disappear within 1 week of starting treatment. Two antihelmintics—mebendazole and piperazine—are currently licensed for use in the UK. Levamisole is also available, on a named-patient basis. (Note: antihelmintic drugs are not generally recommended in endemic areas with large worm burdens in patients with acute abdominal pain, because of the risk of precipitating complete bowel obstruction).

Table 50.1 Chemotherapeutic agents for treatment of ascariasis

Chemotherapeutic agent	Formulation	Dosage guidelines	UK paediatric licence
Mebendazole	100mg, chewable tablet	100mg, twice daily, for 3 days	Yes
Albendazole	400mg tablet	15mg/kg or 400mg in a single dose age 2+	No
		15mg/kg or 200mg in a single dose ages 1–2 years	

(*Continued*)

Table 50.1 (Contd.)

Chemotherapeutic agent	Formulation	Dosage guidelines	UK paediatric licence
Pyrantel pamoate	Oral suspension (250mg/5ml)	11mg/kg (up to max. of 1g per day) for 3 days	No
Piperazine	Syrup (750mg/5ml)	Single dose:	Yes
		<1 year: 0.8ml/kg (on doctor's advice only)	
		1–3 years: 10ml	
		4–5 years: 15ml	
		6–8 years: 20ml	
		9–12 years: 25ml	
		Dose repeated after 2 weeks	
Piperazine plus sennosides	Sachets of powder, containing 4g of piperazine phosphate BP, 300mg of standardized senna (equivalent to 15.3mg total sennosides), to be mixed into milk or water	Single dose in the morning:	Yes
		3 months to 1 year: 2.5ml	
		1–6 years: 5ml	
		6–18 years: contents of 1 sachet	
		Repeated at monthly intervals for up to 3 months	
Levamisole	50mg tablet	1 month to 18 years, at 2.5–3mg/kg (max. 150mg) in a single dose	No (named-patient basis only)

Benzimidazoles

This is the first-line treatment licensed in the UK, with reported efficacy of 76–95%. Mebendazole (along with albendazole) is a benzimidazole, and effectively kills intestinal worms via selective inhibition of glucose uptake in susceptible intestines. Due to teratogenic and tumorigenic potential, benzimidazoles are not licensed for use in children <2 years (and are not recommended for pregnant or lactating females).

- There are few adverse effects, since little drug is systemically absorbed (LFTs should be performed in individuals only with history of liver disease).
- Rarely side effects occur, mainly due to gastrointestinal intolerance: nausea, vomiting, abdominal pain, and diarrhoea.
- Very rarely, CNS symptoms occur: headache and dizziness.

- Other extremely rare adverse effects are rash (especially Stevens–Johnson syndrome, toxic epidermal necrolysis), agranulocytosis, angio-oedema, alopecia, and convulsions (in infants).

Although not licensed in the UK, administration of albendazole has been shown to have good tolerability, and efficacy in the treatment of ascariasis. Pyrantel pamoate is an acceptable alternative to benzimidazoles, but again unlicensed.

A systematic review and meta-analysis of current data on adults and children reported that single-dose oral albendazole, mebendazole, and pyrantel pamoate resulted in cure rates for infection with *A. lumbricoides* of 88% (557 patients), 95% (309 patients), and 88% (131 patients), respectively.[1] However, prolonged use of mebendazole in some parts of the world has led to reports of reduced efficacy suggesting possible emergence of resistance.

Piperazine

Piperazine is licensed for use in children aged between 3 months and 2 years, and is an effective alternative to mebendazole for adults. In children <3 months it may be advisable to delay treatment until they reach this age, where symptoms allow.

- Piperazine is recommended if partial intestinal obstruction occurs.
- Its acts by paralysing intestinal worms, and is therefore often given in combination with senna to aid in expulsion of worms. Piperazine dosing is by age and weight.
- Adverse effects are rare but include gastrointestinal disturbances (nausea, vomiting, colic, diarrhoea) and rarely allergic reactions (angioneurotic oedema and bronchospasm).
- Piperazine can cause neurotoxic reactions (cerebellar ataxia, clumsiness and gait abnormalities), and convulsions, usually at high doses or in people with severe renal insufficiency and epilepsy, and is therefore contraindicated in cases of renal disease, and epilepsy or other neurological disease.
- Note: Piperazine and pyrantel pamoate are antagonistic and therefore cannot be given concomitantly.

Levamisole

Levamisole is highly effective and is FDA approved, but not UK licensed and is only used on a named-patient basis if the other antihelmintics fail or are unsuitable, under specialist consultant guidance. Levamisole is a nicotinic acid antagonist, causing ascariatic paralysis.

- The main contraindications are known hypersensitivity or allergy to the drug, hepatic impairment, epilepsy, juvenile arthritis, and Sjögren's syndrome.
- Reported adverse effects are mainly abdominal pain and headache, but also include nausea, vomiting, diarrhoea and dizziness.

Care

In the case of acute abdominal symptoms, conservative treatment is first advised, with the antihelmintic to be administered after symptoms have subsided. Also, in the case of partial intestinal obstruction, before resorting to surgery, and in the absence of toxic signs (fever, tachycardia, vomiting, abdomen pain or an immobile, palpable mass) the following supporting care methods, administered using a nasogastric tube, may be effective:

• IV fluids, plus antibiotics, possibly with an anthelmintic
• Racine ± mineral oil plus a anthelmintic or Gastrografin.
• IV fluids possibly with an antispasmodic (alternatively may be given with saline enema).

Surgical procedures

In cases of intestinal or liver obstruction, or abdominal infection, surgical removal of the Ascaris may be needed (although very rarely in UK). In endemic regions, ascariasis is a major cause of several pathologies requiring surgery, including intestinal obstruction, appendicitis, volvulus, intussusception, ischemic bowel, hepatobiliary obstruction.

Management of complications

Pulmonary disease

Most cases do not require therapy. Bronchospasm can be managed with conventional therapy. Severe cases can be managed with systemic steroids and oxygen supplementation.

HPA

Aggressive antibiotic therapy for suspected infection and early direct removal of worms from hepatobiliary ducts, by endoscopic therapy, effectively combats HPA. Anthelmintics are then given, once abdominal symptoms improve.

Prognosis

• Most people recover from infection, without treatment.
• Treatment given for asymptomatic ascariasis gives an excellent prognosis (in some cases a repeat treatment is needed). This strategy significantly reduces complications of infection. Reinfection is common in endemic regions, and people may remain carriers of Ascaris.
• The prognosis in patients with bowel obstruction is generally good.

Prevention

• Prevention relies on improved sanitation, education of communities, and early chemotherapeutic intervention.
• Sanitary disposal of human waste, which can contain eggs, is important in preventing spread, but not affordable in many regions.
• In areas where human faeces are used as fertilizer, fruit and vegetables must be cooked where possible, or cleaned with iodine solution.
• Ascariasis is not spread directly person to person.
• Children should be taught to avoid putting things in their mouths, and to wash hands thoroughly.
• Preventive/routine deworming medication may be used for children in endemic/underdeveloped regions. Mass treatment of children every 6 months has been shown to improve health, cognitive, and educational

performance, and leads to weight gain. Screening is also beneficial for diagnosis and early treatment of asymptomatic carriers.
• The emerging resistance to benzimidazoles that has been reported may compromise universal prophylactic strategies—new classes of anthelmintics are required.

Future research

• Two broad-spectrum antiparasitic drugs, nitazoxanide and tribendimidine have yielded promising results. Further studies on the cost-benefits of different treatment strategies are underway.
• Vaccination against A. lumbricoides remains an ideal preventive method; however limited understanding of immunology of infection and lack of appropriate animal models currently bar the way to development.

Key reference

1 Keiser J, Utzinger J. Efficacy of current drugs against soil-transmitted helminth infections: systematic review and meta-analysis. *JAMA* 2008;**299**:1937–48.

Further reading

Bethony J, Brooker S, Albonico M, *et al.* Soil-transmitted helminth infections: ascariasis, trichuriasis, and hookworm. *Lancet* 2006;**367**:1521–32.

Massara, CL, Enk MJ. Treatment options in the management of *Ascaris lumbricoides*. *Expert Opin Pharmacother* 2004;**5**:529–39.

Chapter 51

Aspergillosis

📖 see also Chapters 2, 20, 23, 24, 27

Introduction

Aspergillosis encompasses a broad spectrum of diseases, from colonization and allergic hypersensitivity to invasive, necrotizing, and life-threatening infections.

Name and nature of organism

- Group of moulds: aerobic, spore-forming, catalase positive and thermophilic.
- Second to *Candida* organisms as cause of opportunistic fungal infections.
- Over 185 species (30–40 cause human disease).
- Commonest human pathogens:
  - *Aspergillus fumigatus*—causes over 70% human infections, can grow at >40°C
  - *Aspergillus flavus*—common in sinusitis, produces aflatoxin (toxin/carcinogen) which contaminates nuts
  - *Aspergillus niger*—main pathogen in otomycosis
  - *Aspergillus terreus*—resistant to amphotericin, important commercial uses, disseminates readily.
- Contaminate starchy foods, organic matter and farms/building sites.
- Used commercially in food, pharmaceutical production and as research organisms.
- Grow in fluffy white colonies on most mycological media.
- Produce septate hyphae with dichotomous 45° branching and tiny conidia spores (easily airborne, penetrate the lower respiratory tract)—beware hospital building work and immunocompromised children—a bad mix.
- Exhibit angiotropism and produce toxic metabolites that inhibit phagocytosis.

Epidemiology

- Ubiquitous worldwide, daily inhalation of hundreds of spores.
- Causes large fatal avian outbreaks (especially parrots/ducks).
- More prevalent in autumn/winter in Northern hemisphere.
- Affects all races, equal sex distribution, at any age.
- Most people are naturally immune.

Invasive disease
- Usually seen only if immunosuppressed (e.g. post transplant, on chemotherapy or steroids, functional neutrophil defects such as CGD, intravenous drug users, GVHD or graft rejection).
- Neutropenia for over 10 days is a major risk factor.
- Incidence varies by underlying condition.

Allergic disease
- High rates of positive *Aspergillus* skin tests in children with cystic fibrosis (50%) and asthma (25%) but only 1–2% develop allergic bronchopulmonary aspergillosis (ABPA).

Transmission and incubation period

- Spore transmission by inhalation or inoculation.
- Normal immune system usually eliminates spores.
- Respiratory tract is usual portal of entry and infection site.
- Increased disease risk if immunosuppressed, with possible auto-inoculation from previous colonization.
- Incubation depends on host factors and degree of exposure.

Clinical features and sequelae

See Tables 51.1 and 51.2.
- Persistent fever—high index of suspicion in continued febrile neutropenia—basis of empiric antifungals at around 5 days in most guidelines.
- May have features of underlying disease (e.g. clubbing in cystic fibrosis).
- Severity depends on immune status and site involved.
- Four main pulmonary diseases: aspergilloma, ABPA, invasive aspergillosis, and chronic necrotizing pulmonary aspergillosis (CNPA). Rarer hypersensitivity reactions include Malt worker's lung (extrinsic allergic alveolitis) and bronchocentric granulomatosis.
- Multiorgan infection occurs via haematogenous spread, with tissue infarction and necrosis.
- Can affect any organ (disseminated disease when two or more involved) e.g. lung, sinuses, brain, skin (around CVC), bone.
- 45–95% mortality.

Complications include:
- Major haemorrhage from erosion into pulmonary artery
- Pseudomembranous tracheobronchitis (airway occlusion from fungal and necrotic debris)
- DIC.

Worst prognosis if:
- Invasive aspergillosis in AIDS
- Severe invasive sinus disease post BMT—usually *A. fumigatus* or *A. flavus*
- Cerebral invasive disease—non-specific focal areas, may ring enhance

Table 51.1 Clinical manifestations of invasive disease

Diagnosis	Frequency and associated conditions/ risk factors	Symptoms and signs	Complications, morbidity, and mortality	Other facts
Localized invasive aspergillosis (pulmonary)	In up to 25% immunocompromised patients, e.g. long-term steroid use, neutropenia, post-haematological or solid organ transplant, chronic granulomatous disease, advanced stage AIDS, diabetes mellitus, severe sepsis	May be asymptomatic if severely immunocompromised Fever, cough, dyspnoea, tachypnoea, progressive hypoxaemia, pleural rub Occasionally haemoptysis or pneumothorax	Multifocal cavitating infiltrates Local extension into chest wall, brachial plexus, vertebral column or widespread dissemination Death from progressive respiratory failure or occlusive tracheobronchitis Often rapid progression, mortality 40–95%	90% of invasive cases are localised to lungs If responds to treatment still 50% chance of relapse with future immunosuppression
Multiorgan involvement (disseminated disease)	Occurs in 25% of initially localized cases Higher risk if more immunocompromised	Affects end organs (including kidneys, gastrointestinal tract, thyroid), soft tissue and bone Fever, chills, abscesses, thrombi, delirium, hepatic and renal failure, jaundice, abdominal pathology (pain, obstruction, haemorrhage)	DIC and shock Mortality rate high, depends on affected organs	

CNPA	Rare, although under-diagnosed. Seen in moderate immunosuppression (alcoholism, chronic steroid use), collagen-vascular disease, underlying lung pathology (e.g. chronic obstructive pulmonary disease), previous thoracic surgery	Subacute pneumonia unresponsive to antibiotics. Low-grade fever, malaise, weight loss, dyspnoea, signs of consolidation, may have haemoptysis	Cavitation of lung infiltrates, progressive respiratory failure. 40% mortality even in treated cases	Often treated empirically for TB before diagnosis. May only be detected post mortem
Endocarditis	After cardiac surgery (especially open heart) or on foreign material (e.g. prosthetic valve)	Murmur, fever, peripheral embolic events	Poor prognosis, 100% mortality without surgery. Consider lifelong oral prophylaxis (infection can recur on replaced prosthetic valve)	Aspergillus also causes pericarditis and myocarditis. Second commonest fungal cause
Invasive sinusitis	Rare. Commoner in tropics/subtropics. Immunocompromise not essential	Nasal discharge/epistaxis, fever, headaches/sinus tenderness. Dark nasal lesions, mucosal ulceration, necrotic nasal septum or turbinates. May have facial swelling	Spread to: • Sinus bones (osteomyelitis) • Brain (focal neurological signs, cavernous sinus thrombosis) • Eye (orbital cellulitis with diplopia and pain on lateral gaze, orbital apex syndrome with proptosis and sudden unilateral vision loss). Relapse risk if incomplete surgical evacuation	Often delayed diagnosis. Can be acute and fulminant or chronic and indolent

(Continued)

Table 51.1 (Contd.)

Diagnosis	Frequency and associated conditions/ risk factors	Symptoms and signs	Complications, morbidity, and mortality	Other facts
Cerebral	Seen in 5–40% of invasive cases Frequency highly dependent on underlying condition – BMT recipients at highest risk	Depend on severity of immunosuppression Raised ICP, hemiparesis, focal seizures, cranial nerve palsies (moderate immunocompromise) Generalized features with altered mental state and seizures (severe immunocompromise)	Commonly 100% mortality Beware of drug interactions between antifungals and anticonvulsants	Meningeal signs, papilloedema and fever uncommon
Endophthalmitis	Part of invasive disease in immunocompromised patients IV drug abusers may have ocular involvement alone	Pain, photophobia, visual loss Retinitis with infiltrates and haemorrhages, iridocyclitis, progressive vitreous involvement obscuring fundus	Retinal detachment/necrosis and blindness Often presents with coexisting endocarditis	Aspergillus also causes keratitis Always do an echocardiogram

Eumycetoma (maduromycosis)	70% affect the foot Risk factors: agricultural work, trauma, poor nutrition, walking barefoot, tropics/subtropics	Triad of tumefaction, sinus formation with purulent exudate and granulomata in subcutaneous tissues Usually painless, slowly progressive	Spread to muscle and bone causing deformity and loss of function with significant morbidity Occasionally spreads via blood or lymphatic system	No definitive treatment (combination of medical and surgical)
Cutaneous aspergillosis	Primary (surgical wounds, burns, vascular catheters) or secondary (disseminated from haematogenous spread) Seen in 5–10% of invasive disease	Red papules/nodules or haemorrhagic bullae, may be tender. Widespread lesions in disseminated disease Most commonly on head and limbs	Ulceration with necrotic crust, eschar formation Primary infection may become invasive if immunocompromised	Monitor cannulation sites carefully Secondary more common than primary

Table 51.2 Clinical manifestations of non-invasive disease

Diagnosis	Frequency and associated conditions/risk factors	Symptoms and signs	Complications, morbidity, and mortality	Other
ABPA	2–10% of patients with asthma and cystic fibrosis (excess mucus traps spores)	Cough and wheeze with worsening of previous respiratory symptoms	Relapsing and remitting course	Fleeting infiltrates on chest radiograph unresponsive to antibiotics
	Also in chronic eosinophilic pneumonia and bronchiolitis obliterans organising pneumonia	Fever, general malaise, haemoptysis, sputum production, dyspnoea, respiratory distress	Worsens asthma control, increasing steroid dependence	Hypersensitivity from fungal colonization causing persistent irritation
	Highly suspicious if central bronchiectasis in asthma	Can mimic asthma exacerbation or pneumonia	35% exacerbations are asymptomatic but still result in lung damage (e.g. bronchiectasis)	Commonly occurs with allergic fungal sinusitis
	Genetic predisposition if HLA DR2 positive (HLA DQ2 may be protective)		5 stages (I to V). Stage V is severest with progressive fibrosis and irreversible lung function decline	
Aspergilloma	10–20% of those with pre-existing cavitary disease (e.g. TB, cystic fibrosis, emphysema, sarcoidosis, PCP)	Often asymptomatic. Haemoptysis in 50%.	10% spontaneously resolve, 85% improve after surgery, 5% have lifelong illness	May be seen incidentally on CXR
	Can develop secondary to invasive disease	Also cough, fever, weight loss, general malaise. Usually have symptoms for over 3 months before presentation	Risk of chronic cavitary pulmonary aspergillosis if immunocompromised	Chronic infection from non-allergic colonization in pre-existing cavity
		Can occur in other cavities (e.g. sinuses)	Mortality depends on haemoptysis severity	

Allergic rhinosinusitis	Rare cause (<5% of those with chronic symptoms) More common if atopic disease, nasal polyps, previous nasal surgery	Chronic symptoms: postnasal discharge or purulent rhinorrhoea, nasal congestion, sinus tenderness, headaches Frequent relapses of symptoms	Risk of secondary bacterial infection (suspect if increasing pain) Rarely extends to adjacent areas (e.g. sudden vision loss secondary to nerve compression)	Type 1 hypersensitivity reaction Commonly in adolescents/young adults
Otomycosis (Singapore ear)	Accounts for 10% of all otitis externa After ear injury or instrumentation, bacterial infection, in humid climates	Otalgia, pruritus, ear discharge (grey-white thick debris containing hyphae), tinnitus Complain of ear feeling 'blocked'	Otitis media, tympanic membrane perforation, external auditory canal osteitis Can result in deafness	Treat with topical antifungals Do not need to be immunocompromised

- Bilateral diffuse lung disease
- Continued immunosuppression, persistent neutropenia, relapsed leukaemia
- Delayed/suboptimal therapy.

Diagnosis

High index of suspicion if fever in immunocompromised host does not respond to broad-spectrum antibiotics.

Remember:

- Serological tests unlikely to be positive if immunosuppressed
- Positive cultures from non-sterile sites (e.g. lung/sinus) may represent colonization, so correlate with clinical picture.

- Appropriate specimens: blood, urine, sputum, endotracheal secretions, CSF, sinus washout, BAL, synovial/pleural/peritoneal fluid, bone marrow, nails, hair, needle biopsy.
- Microscopy for fungi using Grocott's or Gomori methamine silver stain.
- Positive culture for definitive diagnosis:
  - Takes up to 4 weeks
  - Blood cultures rarely positive
  - Fungal media increases isolation chance.
- Galactomannan assay:
  - Galactomannan is a circulating antigen (*Aspergillus* cell wall component)
  - Detectable 5–8 days before clinical signs
  - Weekly levels used as screening tool or to assess treatment response
  - ELISA ± PCR (highest sensitivity from serum and brocho-alveolar lavage BAC)
  - Especially accurate in patients with haematological malignancies or transplants
  - False positives more common in children (with autoantibodies, other invasive mycoses, airway colonization, caspofungin/piperacillin/tazobactam use)
  - False negatives seen in non-neutropenic patients or those already on antifungal treatment/prophylaxis.
- Other assays include 1,3-B-glucan (another circulating antigen) and Limulus (endotoxin detection).
- Allergy investigations:
  - Skin prick tests (ABPA excluded if negative) and positive radioallergosorbent test (RAST)
  - Anti-*Aspergillus* antibodies (elevated precipitin levels)
  - IgE (often >1000 in ABPA, falls on steroid treatment, serial levels indicate progress).
- Imaging:
  - Chest radiograph useful in allergic and infective disease; *note:* chest CT findings often much more abnormal than X-ray—frequently surprising!
  - CT/MRI of involved area in invasive disease.

Specific findings

Aspergilloma:
- Usually in upper lobes
- CT: mass shifts within cavity when patient moves.

ABPA:
- Mucus: degenerating eosinophils and fungal hyphae
- Imaging: mucoid impaction with (perihilar) pulmonary infiltrates.

Allergic rhinosinusitis:
- Nasal discharge: fungal elements
- CT: central hyperattenuated areas within sinus cavity.

Invasive aspergillosis:
- Histology: acute inflammatory infiltrate, angioinvasion, tissue necrosis.
- Lung imaging: solitary or multiple nodules, cavitations, wedge-shaped pleural-based infarcts, diffuse alveolar infiltrates. Early CT shows 'halo' sign (haemorrhage around central necrotic nodule), with later 'air crescent' sign (as nodule cavitates)—much less common in children who usually show just dense focal consolidation.
- Sinus disease: fluid opacification on MRI, unilateral involvement of multiple sinuses, absent air–fluid levels and smooth thickened sinus lining on CT.
- If cerebral involvement, imaging may show infarction or abscess with ring enhancement.

Management and treatment

Invasive disease:
- Improve host defence systems by reducing/discontinuing immunosuppressants if possible, consider G-CSF if neutropenic.
- Better survival with earlier treatment so start empirical therapy as soon as clinically suspicious (e.g. no response to broad-spectrum antibiotics within 5 days).

Allergic disease:
- Complete fungal eradication is difficult so aim for symptom control

Consider:
- Surgical resection if localized non-responding disease
- Bronchial artery embolization for massive haemoptysis

Beware:
- Side effects when altering medicines (e.g. adrenal suppression after steroid use)
- Increased risk of surgical procedures in patients with already limited pulmonary function.

Antifungals
- Very limited PK data for most drugs in children.
- Limited direct comparison studies—almost no data on combination/ salvage therapy.

- Systemic antifungals are not indicated in non-allergic colonization.
- Only use combination therapy if treatment failure or continued progression on monotherapy.

Choices (Table 51.3)
Macrolides
- Amphotericin B:
  - Ambisome is widely used as first line therapy
  - Broad spectrum, effectiveness reduced by concomitant use of triazoles
  - Poor penetration into cavities
  - Nephrotoxic (especially in haematology and diabetic patients)—lipid preparations reduce risk of systematic reactions, hypokalaemia and renal impairment, but are more expensive.

Antifungal triazoles
- Affect CYP450 enzyme system so beware of drug interactions.
- Most are broad spectrum (fluconazole not active against *Aspergillus*).
- Voriconazole:
  - First line for invasive aspergillosis and salvage therapy for other fungal infections
  - Not effective against mucormycosis
  - Try to avoid in pregnancy (fetal risk)
  - Monitor levels in non-responders: may have low levels as pharmacokinetics very complex
  - Transient visual loss may be seen in children.
- Itraconazole:
  - Poor absorption in severely ill patients (altered gastric pH)
  - Useful if not tolerating standard antifungals.
- Posaconazole:
  - Doses not established in children <12 years
  - Better activity against zygomycosis/mucormycosis infections than other azoles
  - Only available in oral formulation.

Echinocandins
- Micafungin
- Caspofungin—use in refractory invasive aspergillosis or if intolerant to other therapies
- Narrow spectrum of activity, only use if confirmed diagnosis
- May worsen hepatic/renal dysfunction and myelosuppression
- Levels ↑ by ciclosporin, ↓ by carbamazepine, phenytoin, rifampicin, dexamethasone.

Table 51.3 Summary of treatment options in Aspergillosis by clinical disease

Diagnosis	Medical treatment	Surgical management
Aspergilloma	Only treat if symptomatic. Multiple cavities may need lifelong treatment Prolonged course of oral itraconazole produces some resolution in 60% (voriconazole as alternative)	Partial lung resection if massive haemoptysis (difficult if scarring or pleural adhesions)
ABPA	Aim to ↓ IgE levels to normal range for non-ABPA affected asthmatic patient. Restart treatment if levels rise to above twice that limit Oral corticosteroids (inhaled less effective), e.g. prolonged course of oral prednisolone If chronic or recurrent, use itraconazole for faster clinical and radiological resolution. Also facilitates steroid tapering, reducing total dose (alternatives = voriconazole, posaconazole) Case reports of new anti-IgE monoclonal antibody (omalizumab) to reduce inflammation	
Allergic sinusitis	Steroids and antifungals (topical nasal or systemic) reduce recurrence Immunotherapy If possible mucormycosis then start amphotericin or posaconazole as first line (voriconazole ineffective)	Endoscopic sinus surgery improves drainage if obstructive symptoms Resect nasal polyps Debridement of sinuses removes inciting fungal allergic mucin

(Continued)

Table 51.3 (Contd.)

Diagnosis	Medical treatment	Surgical management
Eye disease	Endophthalmitis: systemic and intravitreal antifungals Keratitis: topical and systemic (± intracameral) antifungals	May be needed in refractory disease—partial vitrectomy in endophthalmitis or keratoplasty in keratitis
Invasive aspergillosis	Intravenous voriconazole or liposomal amphotericin as first line (better tolerated and increased efficacy than amphotericin B deoxycholate) Add caspofungin in severe infections (other salvage therapies = amphotericin, posaconazole) Therapy usually for minimum of 4–12 weeks May benefit from adjuvant IFN-γ if not neutropenic (especially in CGD)	Resection of: • Localized disease with failed medical therapy • Infected cardiac valves or vegetations • Cerebral lesions • Necrotic sinus tissue • Cutaneous lesions • Areas of osteomyelitis or soft tissue infection • Lesions contiguous with heart or great vessels, involving chest wall or risk of pulmonary artery perforation • Any mass before starting intensive chemotherapy or immunosuppression
CNPA	Same first-line treatment as invasive aspergillosis (most evidence supports itraconazole use only because the other triazoles are newer) Oral treatments preferred as prolonged course of several months needed for clinical and radiographic resolution	Resect localized disease if failed medical treatment, especially if bleeding from necrotic area

Prevention

General precautions

- Careful use of immunosuppressants (including steroids).
- Education of patients at risk.
- Examine for chronic sinus colonization before transplant conditioning.
- Close attention to ventilation systems and during construction/ renovation work—conduct formal risk assessment before the builders start!

If immunocompromised or known hypersensitivity/allergy

- Care with invasive procedures, avoid skin trauma.
- Use laminar airflow, particulate air filtration and positive air pressure cubicles.
- Avoid high-risk environments (dusty areas, marshes/forests, compost heaps/rotting vegetation) and activities (gardening).

Prophylactic antifungals

- Posaconazole is sometimes recommended as first-line prophylaxis, especially in high-risk haematology patients with GVHD or neutropenia. Others include itraconazole (good in CGD) and micafungin.
- Voriconazole is used as secondary prophylaxis in previously treated patients needing further immunosuppression.
- Inhaled amphotericin B is useful post lung transplantation with positive sputum colonization or intranasally to control nasal colonization.

Future research

As medical advances lead to increased transplantation and longer stays on intensive care, more evidence is needed to support the best combination treatment regimens and how to treat refractory infections.

Further population studies including who benefits most from prophylaxis, susceptibility factors (e.g. defective mannose-binding lectin production) and resistance mechanisms will allow better targeted approaches to infection.

Further reading

Thomas L, Baggen L, Chisholm J, Sharland M. Diagnosis and treatment of aspergillosis in children. *Expert Rev Anti Infect Ther* 2009;**7**:461–72.

Walsh TJ, Anaissie EJ, Denning DW, *et al.* IDSA guidelines. Treatment of aspergillosis: clinical practice guidelines of the Infectious Diseases Society of America. *Clin Infect Dis* 2008;**46**:327–60 (Aspergillosis Patient Support. Contains information leaflets on prevention and common forms of infection). Available at: ℜ www.aspergillus.org.uk/newpatients/guides.php (accessed 1 February 2011).

Botulism

📖 see also Chapter 30

Name and nature of organism

- *Clostridium botulinum* is an anaerobic, spore-forming, Gram-positive bacillus.
- Ubiquitous organism with spores widely distributed in soil, dust, vegetables, silage, manure.
- Produces neurotoxins (types A–G); most cases due to types A, B or E (and rarely F).
- Toxin binds irreversibly to peripheral nerves and prevents acetylcholine release at the neuromuscular junction, leading to flaccid paralysis.

Epidemiology

- **Food-borne botulism** arises from contaminated foods that have been preserved under anaerobic conditions. Most cases are associated with home-preserved meats, fish and vegetables and canned products. There were 36 cases in the UK between 1980 and 2006, of which 27 occurred as an outbreak in 1989 due to hazelnut yoghurt contaminated with toxin-containing canned hazelnut flavouring. Sporadic cases have been associated with imported foods from southern and eastern Europe.
- **Wound botulism** occurs following contamination of wounds due to penetrating injuries and is most frequently seen in the context of injection drug use. There were >100 cases between 2002 and 2007.
- **Intestinal colonization botulism** occurs mostly in infants, especially <6 months of age, although a few cases have occurred in adults. Ingestion of spores from contaminated honey, dried formula milk, or the environment leads to germination, gut colonization and toxin production. There were eight cases in the UK between 1978 and 2007.

Transmission and incubation period

- **Food-borne botulism** is due to absorption of preformed toxin from the gastrointestinal tract. Timing of symptoms is dependent on the dose of toxin absorbed; typically, onset is 12–36 hours (median 24 hours) post-ingestion but can occur from 6 hours to 8 days after eating contaminated food.

- **Wound botulism** occurs after growth of the organism and production of toxin in contaminated wounds.
- **Intestinal colonization botulism** is due to intestinal colonization and production of toxin. It appears to occur particularly around the time of infant weaning, when the flora of the gastrointestinal tract is changing.
- Rare iatrogenic cases of botulism have occurred following use of botulinum toxin (Botox) in the USA.
- Aerosolized toxin is a potential route of infection following bioterrorism.

Clinical features and sequelae

- Neurological features are similar, irrespective of route of toxin entry.
- Botulism is characterized by an acute descending, symmetrical, flaccid paralysis, in the absence of fever and with no loss of sensory awareness.
- Cranial nerve palsies often predominate initially: double vision, extraocular weakness, ptosis, facial palsy, dysphagia, dysarthria.
- Weakness of neck, arms, and respiratory muscles usually follows; respiratory arrest can occur.
- The child is afebrile and well. Autonomic nervous system involvement leads to dry mouth, dilated pupils, cardiovascular changes and bladder involvement.
- Botulinum toxin does not cross the blood–brain barrier so mental status is unaffected.
- **Foodborne botulism** can be associated with gastrointestinal symptoms, such as nausea, vomiting, diarrhoea, and abdominal cramps, followed by constipation.
- **Intestinal colonization botulism** in infants may present with early constipation, followed by non-specific manifestations of intoxication, such as lethargy, failure to feed, hypotonia, drooling, and decreased crying.
- **Differential diagnoses** include myasthenia gravis, Guillain–Barré syndrome (this is an ascending paralysis whereas botulism is a descending paralysis; also Guillain–Barré syndrome is very rare in infants and has elevated CSF protein), tick paralysis, toxic exposure (carbon monoxide, ethanol, organophosphates, paralytic shellfish poisoning), poliomyelitis, CNS brainstem infections, stroke, and CNS mass lesions.

Diagnosis

- Diagnosis is by detection of botulinum toxin or isolation of the organism.
- Samples should be collected and sent to a National Reference Laboratory (in the UK discuss with HPA: call 0208 200 6868/4400;

24-hour service), including faeces (minimum 10g in sterile container), vomitus or gastric washings (minimum 10g in sterile container), serum (minimum 10ml, prior to administration of antitoxin).
- In infants, a rectal washout may be required to obtain a stool sample if constipated.
- Potentially contaminated food samples should be obtained as a matter of urgency and discussed with the HPA (as above).
- LP, edrophonium challenge, and brain imaging may be required to clarify diagnosis (the CSF and neuroimaging are normal in botulism).

Management and treatment

Foodborne botulism
- Specific antitoxin must be given as soon as possible—do not await diagnostic tests; in the UK this is available from the HPA.
- Repeat doses may be given within 24 hours if deterioration continues.
- No role for antibiotics.
- Supportive care including ventilation, hydration, and nutrition.

Wound botulism
- Surgical debridement is essential.
- Intravenous penicillin and metronidazole.
- Specific antitoxin (as above).

Intestinal colonization (infant) botulism
- Human-derived botulinum immunoglobulin (BabyBIG) should be obtained from the Infant Botulism Treatment and Prevention Programme, California, USA (℗ www.infantbotulism.org; discuss with on-call physician +1 510 231 7600).
- Antibiotics are contraindicated as they may further disturb gut flora and increase toxin production.
- Supportive care may be required for several weeks, with attention to airway protection, ventilation, treatment of secondary infection, management of constipation, and adequate nutrition. Mortality is very low with a prompt diagnosis and supportive care.
- Full recovery is possible due to growth of new nerve endings.

Prevention
- Proper handling and preservation of foods.
- Infants should not consume honey.
- In the UK, inform the HPA of suspected cases immediately so that other exposed individuals can be traced.

- Standard universal precautions (gloves, gowns, handwashing) should be employed for hospitalized cases.
- Person-to-person spread of botulism does not occur.

Further reading

Health Protection Agency. Botulism, Guidance, Clinical Management and Sampling. Last reviewed 2010. Available at: ℘ www.hpa.org.uk/webw/HPAweb&HPAwebStandard/HPAweb_C/1204012994953?p=1203928707354 (accessed 1 February 2011).

Brucellosis

📖 see also Chapters 33, 45

Introduction

Brucellosis is a highly transmissible zoonotic disease with infection occurring in cattle, sheep, pigs, goats, and humans. Brucellosis in humans is also known as Mediterranean fever, Malta, or undulant fever. It was a major cause of disease after the Crimean War and General Bruce identified the microorganism 30 years later. The disease remains the world's most common bacterial zoonosis, with over half a million new cases annually.

Name and nature of organism

- *Brucella* species are small Gram-negative facultative intracellular coccobacilli that localize within cells of the reticuloendothelial system. They do not possess flagellae, endospores, a capsule or native plasmids. The outer cell membrane has a dominant lipopolysaccharide component, which is the principal factor in determining virulence.
- There are six species within the genus *Brucella*: *B. abortus*, *B. melitensis*, *B. suis*, *B. ovis*, *B. canis*, and *B. neotomae*. Human infection is mainly caused by *B. melitensis*, *B. abortus*, and *B. suis*.

Epidemiology

- *Brucella* infection is widespread throughout the world and endemic areas include Eastern Europe, Asia, Africa, and Central and South America.
- The Middle East and the Central Asian republics have some of the highest reported incidences of the disease.
- In Europe brucellosis occurs in the Mediterranean basin, Northern Ireland and the Caucasian districts of Russia.

Transmission and incubation period

- Brucellosis is a zoonosis. The main reservoirs are cattle, sheep, goats, and swine. The organism is found in a number of wild animals.
- The incubation period for brucellosis varies depending on the type of organism, the route of transmission, and the infective dose. In approximately half the cases the incubation period is short, typically 5–30 days, but other cases can be up to 24 months.

Modes of transmission

- Inoculation through cuts, abrasions and mucosal membranes from infected animals and their secretions.
- Accidental self-inoculation by veterinarians performing vaccinations.
- Ingestion of raw milk, unpasteurized dairy products (e.g. goat's cheese) and raw or undercooked meat.
- Inhalation of infected aerosols in laboratories and abattoirs.
- Person-to-person transmission is rare. However, there is a risk associated with organ/tissue transplantation, sexual transmission, and mother-to-child transmission via breast milk.
- Brucellosis has been implicated as a possible bioterrorism agent, particularly in the aerosolized form.

Clinical features and sequelae

Acute brucellosis

In children, brucellosis is frequently a mild, self-limiting illness when caused by *B. abortus*. A more severe illness occurs with *B. melitensis*. A key element in the history is exposure to an infected animal or food. Symptoms are diverse and non-specific, usually occurring within 2–4 weeks of inoculation.

Symptoms

- Fever—undulant; rises and falls like a wave; very variable
- Weakness
- Excessive sweating
- Lethargy
- Anorexia
- Weight loss/failure to thrive
- Arthralgia
- Myalgia
- Abdominal pain
- Headache.

Clinical findings are often minimal but may include hepatosplenomegaly and lymphadenopathy.

Complications

- Osteoarticular: Common; monoarticular arthritis (usually of the knees, ankles and hips), spondylitis, osteomyelitis and sacroiliitis—looks like JIA because of systemic features.
- Genitourinary: Rare; orchiepididymitis, glomerulonephritis, and renal abscesses.
- Neurological: Rare; optic neuritis, peripheral neuropathies, chorea, radiculopathy, meningoencephalitis, stroke and intracranial haemorrhage.
- Cardiovascular: Rare; endocarditis, aortic and cerebral aneurysms.
- Pulmonary: Rare; pneumonitis and pleural empyema.
- Ocular: Common and often missed; uveitis.
- Mucocutaneous: Rare; erythematous papular lesions, purpura, dermal cysts, and Stevens–Johnson syndrome.

In pregnancy, brucellosis carries increased risk of abortion and intrauterine transmission.

Brucellosis can also cause longlasting (more than 12 months) or chronic symptoms that include recurrent fevers, myalgia, fatigue, depression, and arthralgias. This form is primarily caused by B. melitensis and is rare in children. Chronic, localizing infection occurs when there is a persistence of infection in an abscess or other specific area.

Natural history and prognosis

- Brucellosis can be a self-limiting disease with full recovery, however, some will go on to have a protracted debilitating condition for many years.
- With treatment the majority of people recover. Others relapse despite appropriate treatment due to the presence of sequestered organisms within macrophages because of resistant organisms.
- Brucellosis is rarely fatal. The reported case fatality rate is <2%. Mortality is usually due to endocarditis.

Diagnosis

- The Rose Bengal test, an agglutination test, is the standard screening test due to its high sensitivity but it has low specificity.
- Confirmatory tests involving ELISA, tube agglutination, or culture should always be performed following screening tests.
- The sensitivity and specificity of the confirmatory agglutination tests depend on the cut-off value used, and on the background level of reactive antibodies in the population.
- ELISA has high sensitivity but the specificity is less than that of the agglutination tests.
- Isolation of the organism from blood or bone marrow is the gold standard diagnostic test but culture is difficult as the organism is slow growing and culture is often negative in chronic disease.
- Bone marrow cultures have a high sensitivity, shorter culture time, and are useful in patients with previous antibiotic use.
- Brucella can also be cultured from pus, tissue samples, and cerebrospinal, pleural, joint, or ascitic fluid.
- Point of care testing kits are available which are currently under evaluation for use in the field.

Management and treatment

- Treatment can be difficult and involves antibiotic treatment with a combination of antibiotics. Different regimens being used involve aminoglycosides, tetracyclines, rifampicin, co-trimoxazole, and quinolones.[1]

- As *Brucella* is an intracellular organism it requires prolonged treatment and relapses occur.
- A systematic review and meta-analysis of randomized controlled trials concluded that the preferred treatment should be with dual or triple regimens including an aminoglycoside and that treatment of at least 6 weeks' duration is associated with a lower risk of relapse.[2]
- In adults and children aged ≥8 years, use doxycycline and gentamicin.
- Young children and pregnant women, co-trimoxazole has been recommended combined with rifampicin in a combination for 6 weeks.
- There is limited evidence to support these regimens.
- Brucellosis cases should be notified to the local public health authority.

Prevention

- Elimination of brucellosis in animals through vaccination, testing, and slaughter of infected herds and testing of milk.
- Occupational hygiene—education of clinical and laboratory staff as to the risks of brucellosis and appropriate management measures.
- Education of farmers and workers in slaughter houses, butchers, and abattoirs to reduce exposure.
- Food hygiene—pasteurize or boil milk and dairy products, cook meat properly.
- Control of organ and blood donation to prevent person-to-person transmission.

Future research

- Further understanding of the diseases pathogenesis by determination of the mechanisms by which *Brucella* enters cells and evades intracellular killing and the host immune system.
- The validation of rapid diagnostic technologies developed for identification of *Brucella* species in natural or bioterrorism-associated outbreaks and the identification of markers for disease severity, progression, and treatment response.
- The development of improved optimum treatment regimens and improved antibiotic delivery methods.

Key references

1 Franco MP, Mulder M, Gilman RH, Smits HL. Human brucellosis. *Lancet Infect Dis* 2007;**7**:775–86.
2 Skalsky K, Yahav D, Bishara J, Pitlik S, Leibovici L, Paul M. Treatment of human brucellosis: systematic review and meta-analysis of randomised controlled trials. *BMJ* 2008;**336**:701–4.

Campylobacter

see also Chapters 12, 22, 42, 45

Name and nature of organism

- Gram-negative, spiral, flagellated, microaerophilic motile rods.
- One of the most common infective bacterial causes of gastroenteritis in the world.
- Over 20 species and subspecies currently listed, several of which are pathogenic in humans.
- The *Campylobacter* species most frequently associated with human infection are: *C. jejuni*, *C. coli*, and less commonly *C. upsaliensis* and *C. fetus*; *C. lari* and *C. hyointestinalis* rarely cause disease—predominately affecting the immunocompromised host.
- *C. fetus* is a rare cause of invasive disease in the neonate.

Pathophysiology and immunity

The exact way *Campylobacter* causes diarrhoea is still incompletely understood. It mainly affects the colon where it is thought to cause diarrhoea through a number of mechanisms including:

- Production of enterotoxin
- Direct invasion of intestinal epithelial cells
- Induction of local inflammatory responses.

Increased susceptibility of HIV-infected individuals and patients with hypogammaglobulinaemia indicate a role for both humoral and cell mediated immunity. *Campylobacter*-specific IgG can be demonstrated following infection and have been shown to be protective against disease. *Campylobacter*-specific secretory and serum IgA are associated with protection against disease.

Epidemiology

In Europe

- Peak incidence in children <5 years and young adults (especially infants).
- Risk factors for infection include spending time on a farm, contact with raw meat, household pets (especially kittens and puppies), and travel to areas of high incidence.
- Most cases are sporadic, however, outbreaks do occur associated with an infected source of food, milk, or water.

- In temperate climates, seasonal variations in incidence have been demonstrated, with infection being more common in the late spring in the UK.
- There are around 50 000 cases a year reported in the UK, with nearly 10 000 cases seen in children. Recently a decline in cases in young children has been noted.

In the resource-poor setting

- Children <2 years old are most frequently affected.
- Asymptomatic carriage is more common.
- Infection in later life is rare, thought to be a result of immunity developed through frequent exposure in childhood.

Transmission and incubation period

- *Campylobacter* is a zoonotic infection.
- The incubation period ranges from 2 to 5 days but can be up to 11 days.
- Minimum infective dose is low: 500–800 organisms.
- Many animal hosts including domestic, wild and farm animals (particularly poultry).
- Transmission is thought to be most commonly via the oral route from contaminated food (especially chicken), unpasteurized milk, or water.
- Direct transmission from person to person is rare but has been reported. *C. fetus* infection of the newborn occurs, the source of the infection being the mother.

Clinical features

- *Campylobacter* infection can be asymptomatic. Disease is mostly intestinal but can also be extraintestinal. Common clinical features of gastrointestinal infection include:
  - Diarrhoea—can be profuse and watery with blood streaking, pus, and mucus
  - Abdominal cramps and pain—can be mistaken for appendicitis or intussusception
  - Vomiting—less common
  - Fever, malaise, headache.
- In most children this is a mild illness of 1–2 weeks, but a few children develop a severe picture mimicking inflammatory bowel disease. The infection can persist with chronic symptoms, or bacteraemia—especially in the immunocompromised host.
- Extraintestinal infection is rare but possible sites include meningitis, osteomyelitis and endocarditis. Severe invasive disease is more likely in the immunocompromised.
- *C. jejuni* infection of the newborn usually presents as intestinal infection whereas *C. fetus* more frequently presents as premature labour, sepsis or meningitis. Mortality is a rare but possible outcome, especially at the extremes of age or with immunocompromise.

Complications

Potential complications are mostly immunologically based and include:
- Guillain-Barré syndrome; *Campylobacter* infection is a common antecedent to Guillain–Barré syndrome and is thought to be related to lipo-oligosaccharides that mimic gangliosides, leading to autoimmune damage to peripheral nerves
- Miller–Fisher syndrome: variant of Guillain–Barré syndrome (ophthalmoplegia, ataxia, areflexia)
- In China outbreaks of severe acute motor axonal neuropathy occur—Chinese paralytic syndrome—with rapid onset of severe paralysis
- Reactive arthritis— in young men, around 2 weeks later, especially in the knees
- Reiter's syndrome (asymmetrical arthritis, urethritis, ophthalmitis)—HLA-B27 association
- Haemolytic-uraemic syndrome
- Erythema nodosum.

Investigation and diagnosis

- Dark field microscopy and Gram stain of stool—by recognition of characteristic morphology (spiral morphology and darting/spinning motion).
- More commonly isolated from stool by culture using selective media for *Campylobacter*, which suppresses the growth of normal flora. Species other than *C. jejuni* may be missed using this technique.
- Organisms can be isolated from blood cultures and other extraintestinal sites of infection.

Management and treatment

- Mainstay of treatment is supportive, ensuring adequate hydration, electrolyte replacement and analgesia if necessary.
- Antimotility agents should not be used.
- Antibiotics can be used for more severe or prolonged infection and infection in immunocompromised children.
- Antibiotics have been shown to shorten the duration of symptoms and excretion of *Campylobacter* when used early in infection.
- Macrolides (clarithromycin, azithromycin) are suitable first-line oral agents. *Campylobacter* is inherently resistant to penicillins and increasingly globally ciprofloxacin resistant.
- Ciprofloxacin is an alternative.
- Antibiotic treatment should be for 5–7 days for gastrointestinal infection.
- Antibiotic resistance is an issue and treatment of mild disease should be avoided to help limit the emergence of resistance.

- Aminoglycosides, clindamycin, meropenem, and imipenem are suitable first-line IV agents. For invasive infections, prolonged courses of antibiotics may be necessary.
- Once an isolated organism's specific antibiotic sensitivity is known antibiotic treatment should be adjusted accordingly.

Outcome

- Most infection is self-limiting with full resolution of symptoms.
- Relapse, chronic infection and carriage state can occur and are more likely if immunocompromised.
- Excretion of organisms has a mean duration of 16 days when not treated with antibiotics.
- Severe invasive infection is rare but most commonly occurs in the neonate or immunocompromised and has a high associated mortality.
- Reactive arthritis is usually self-limiting.

Prevention of further cases

Preventive measures include:
- Storing cooked and raw food separately
- Thorough cooking of potentially contaminated food
- Washing work surfaces and utensils following preparation of raw foods.
- Taking care when visiting farms, ensuring handwashing after contact with farm animals. Careful handwashing when handling domestic animals, especially young animals with diarrhoea.

Normal enteric precautions are usually sufficient to control person-to-person spread.

Future research

There is currently no vaccine for *Campylobacter* infection. Vaccine research is limited by the theoretical risk of Guillain–Barré syndrome. The *C. jejuni* genome was first sequenced in 2000.

Further reading

Janssen R, Krogfelt KA, Cawthraw SA, van Pelt W, Wagenaar JA, Owen RJ. Host-pathogen interactions in campylobacter infections: the host perspective. *Clin Microbiol Rev* 2008;**21**: 505–18.

Chapter 55

Candidiasis

📖 see also Chapters 6, 8, 19, 20, 23, 24, 29, 30

Name and nature of organism

- Due to infection with *Candida* spp.
- Over 200 species, but only 12 are of medical importance.
- Single-cell eukaryotic yeast that reproduces by asexual budding.
- *Candida* surface proteins mediate adhesion to epithelium, followed by invasion.

Epidemiology

- Superficial candidiasis is common and occurs worldwide.
- The vast majority of cases are caused by *Candida albicans*.
- Non-*albicans* species, such as *Candida parapsilosis*, *Candida glabrata*, *Candida krusei*, *Candida lusitaneae*, and *Candida tropicalis* may be isolated, especially in invasive disease or immunocompromised patients.
- *C. glabrata* is frequently resistant to fluconazole; *C. krusei* is invariably resistant to fluconazole.

Transmission and incubation period

- Part of commensal flora of mouth, gastrointestinal tract, vagina and skin in approximately 20% of individuals.
- Colonization increases with age and during pregnancy. Babies acquire their mother's *Candida* species.
- Alteration of host flora (e.g. following broad-spectrum antibiotics), immunosuppression, and illness predispose to yeast overgrowth and infection. Risk factors for invasion are prolonged neutropenia while reduced T cell numbers or function leads to severe mucosal disease.
- Can be acquired by person-to-person contact or from contaminated dummies, feeding bottles, etc. Can also be acquired from birds and mammals.
- Sexual transmission can occur.
- Incubation period variable and not well described, but probably 2–5 days.

Clinical features and sequelae

Oropharyngeal candidiasis
- White plaques on buccal and gingival mucosa, tongue and palate—difficult to scrape off.
- May also present with erythematous mucosa or angular stomatitis.
- Oral pain may lead to reduced oral intake.
- Dysphagia or pain on swallowing should prompt consideration of oesophageal candidiasis.

Oesophageal candidiasis
- Oropharyngeal candidiasis in combination with dysphagia or retrosternal pain on swallowing (highly predictive).
- Associated with underlying advanced HIV infection, chemotherapy, or other cause of immunosuppression.
- Differential diagnosis includes CMV and HSV oesophagitis, which may co-occur with *Candida*.

Skin infection
- Occurs in moist, occluded sites such as axillae and groins.
- Common in napkin area of infants, where it presents as a confluent erythematous rash with satellite lesions—can lead to skin breakdown.

Nail infection
- Chronic *Candida* paronychia is usually secondary to repeated, prolonged immersion of hands in water.
- Can cause onychomycosis with thickened, friable nails.
- Differential diagnosis is dermatophyte infection, which is more common.

Vulvovaginitis/cystitis
- Uncommon in prepubertal girls, in whom a non-infectious cause of vulvovaginitis is more likely.
- More common beyond puberty.
- Risk factors include underlying diabetes, pregnancy, HIV, use of antibiotics or oral contraceptive pill.
- Presents with vulvovaginal erythema, irritation, pruritus, pain on micturition and discharge (usually thick, white and curd-like but can be thin).
- Cystitis is associated with immunodeficiency, prematurity, prolonged catheterization and prolonged antibiotic courses—always check for upper renal tract invasion.

Chronic mucocutaneous candidiasis
- Rare immunodeficiency due to specific T cell defect.
- Chronic, severe onychomycosis and mucocutaneous candidiasis.
- Associated with autoimmune polyendocrinopathy type I and thymomas.
- Often requires chronic suppressive therapy with fluconazole or itraconazole.

Diagnosis

- Skin, oropharyngeal and vaginal swabs can be cultured on Sabouraud agar plates, with growth of characteristic yeast colonies in 1–2 days.
- Nail clippings should be examined by direct microscopy of wet mounts in potassium hydroxide, and cultured on Sabouraud agar plates.
- Isolation of *Candida* may represent colonization rather than infection.
- *C. albicans* produces a classical 'germ cell' form when incubated in human serum—used as a rapid, but not certain test to confirm *C. albicans* species—and therefore usually fluconazole sensitive.

Management and treatment

Oropharyngeal candidiasis

- Oral nystatin solution or miconazole gel.
- Treat for 48 hours beyond clinical resolution.
- Ensure sterilization of dummies and feeding bottles, especially in recurrent candidiasis.
- Severe, persistent or recurrent cases may require oral fluconazole and should prompt consideration of underlying immunodeficiency.

Oesophageal candidiasis

- Oral fluconazole for 7 days (or until symptoms resolved).
- Itraconazole should be used in fluconazole-refractory cases.

Napkin candidiasis

- Topical nystatin cream plus oral nystatin to prevent reinfection from gastrointestinal tract.
- Treat for 48 hours beyond clinical resolution.

Nail infection

- Ensure samples taken for culture to distinguish from dermatophyte infection.
- Infection associated with paronychia may respond to topical treatment with imidazole lotion, alternating with an antibacterial lotion.
- For nail plate infection, oral itraconazole appears most effective and may be used for 1 week per month for 2 months.

Vulvovaginal

- Topical clotrimazole pessary or 10% vaginal cream.
- Use of a steroid-containing preparation may reduce irritation.
- Single-dose oral fluconazole is an alternative.
- For severe disease, repeat oral fluconazole dose after 72 hours.
- Topical vaginal preparations may damage latex condoms—check and advise.

Prevention

- *Oropharyngeal candidiasis*: sterilization of dummies and teats; if breastfeeding, check for maternal nipple infection.
- *Napkin candidiasis*: Attention to hygiene and regular changing of nappies.
- *Vulvovaginal candidiasis*: If recurrent, may benefit from decolonization of gut, which may be source of infection; if sexually active, screen and treat partner for penile candidiasis.

Future research

- The changing burden of disease due to non-*albicans Candida* strains.
- Risk–benefit analysis of prophylactic prevention strategies.

Further reading

Clinical Effectiveness Group, British Association of Sexual Health and HIV. *United Kingdom National Guideline on the Management of Vulvovaginal Candidiasis*. London: BASHH, 2007. Available at: www.bashh.org/guidelines.

Pappas PG, Kauffman CA, Andes D, *et al.* Clinical practice guidelines for the management of candidiasis: Update by the Infectious Diseases Society of America. *Clin Infect Dis* 2009;**48**:503–35.

Roberts DT, Taylor WD, Boyle J. Guidelines for treatment of onychomycosis. *Br J Dermatol* 2003;**148**:402–10.

Chapter 56

Cat scratch disease

📖 see also Chapters 15, 45

Name and nature of organism

- The causative organism is *Bartonella henselae*.
- *B. henselae* is a Gram-negative coccobacillus that can also cause bacillary angiomatosis and bacillary peliosis hepatitis, reported mainly in patients with HIV.

Epidemiology

- Cat scratch disease is rare and occurs mainly during the autumn and winter. In the UK there are around 100 confirmed cases/year in all ages.
- It is most commonly seen in children and adolescents
- Cats are the common reservoir for *B. henselae* and in 90% of the cases there is a history of close contact with cats, frequently kittens. Up to half of all cats are infected at some time.

Transmission and incubation period

- Cat fleas (*Ctenocephalides felis*) transmit the microorganism between cats, but their role in transmission of *B. henselae* to humans has not been defined.
- Bacteraemia in cats associated with human disease is common.
- Cat scratch inoculates the microorganism in the human skin.
- No evidence of person-to-person transmission exists.
- It usually takes 7–12 days from the scratch to the appearance of the primary skin lesion.
- Lymphadenopathy occurs 5–50 days (median 12 days) from the appearance of the skin lesion.

Clinical features and sequelae

- In otherwise healthy people the most important clinical manifestation is lymphadenopathy involving the nodes that drain the site of inoculation (usually axillary, cervical, epitrochlear, or inguinal nodes) following scratches on the hands and arm.
- The appearance of lymphadenopathy is usually preceded by a red skin papule at the presumed site of inoculation.
- The skin that covers the involved nodes is tender, warm, and red.

- Fever and mild systemic symptoms occur in about a third of children.
- In normal children, most cases just get better with no treatment and usually no diagnosis is made either.
- Very rarely systemic spread occurs leading to PUO, with widespread lymphadenopathy and granulomatous lesions causing hepatosplenomegaly.
- Other very rare complications include a remarkably benign encephalopathy, aseptic meningitis, neuroretinitis, osteolytic lesions, pneumonia, erythema nodosum, thrombocytopenic purpura, relapsing bacteraemia, and endocarditis.
- Classically, but rarely, infection can cause Parinaud's oculoglandular syndrome, in which direct infection into the eye gives unilateral conjunctivitis and preauricular lymphadenopathy.
- Bacillary angiomatosis are multiple vascular skin lesions that are often papular. Bacillary peliosis are similar vascular granulomatous lesions in the liver and spleen. These are both seen only in people with significant immunocompromise—classically AIDS.

Diagnosis

- IFA or enzyme immunoassays (EIAs) are commercial tests for serum IgM and IgG antibodies to the pathogen. The IgM is not very useful and a rise in IgG titres is best.
- PCR testing of clinical specimens appears promising but is still mainly a research tool.
- A lymph node biopsy classically shows granuloma and cat scratch disease is one of the main diagnoses to consider. There are other diseases that produce a similar picture, including brucellosis and mycobacterial infections. The classic stain is the Warthin–Starry stain, which may show the organism.
- Inflammatory markers, CRP, and ESR are generally raised.

Management and treatment

- Most children just get better by themselves and reassurance is all that is usually required. In a normal child, spread and complications are very rare. Even when the rarer complications do occur a very good outcome is usually seen in previously normal children.
- As you would expect, response to antibiotics is limited. Azithromycin has been used with only a moderate benefit. There are no good clinical trials.
- Antibiotic treatment is recommended for patients with systemic disease and is mandatory for immunocompromised individuals.
- Macrolides, co-trimoxazole, rifampicin, ciprofloxacin, and parenteral gentamicin are all effective. The optimal duration of their administration is not known.

- In patients with severe or systemic disease (such as endocarditis) therapy should include the addition of intravenous gentamicin for a minimum of 2 weeks.
- In immunocompromised patients, longer durations of antimicrobial therapy may be appropriate (up to 3 months) to prevent relapse. This depends on the severity of the immunocompromise and specialist advice should be sought.
- Doxycycline or macrolides are effective for the treatment of bacillary angiomatosis and bacillary peliosis hepatitis. Treatment duration should be at least 2 weeks (cutaneous manifestations only) or at least 4 weeks for patients with visceral lesions.

Prevention

- Immunocompromised subjects should avoid close contact with cats completely or at a minimum stay away from cats that scratch or bite and are <1 year. For example, do not buy a kitten for a child with newly diagnosed leukaemia.
- Sites of cat scratches should be immediately washed.
- Treating cat flea infestations may reduce cat-to-cat transmission of *B. henselae*.
- Testing of cats for *B. henselae* infection is not recommended.

Future research

- More information on the prevalence of the different clinical manifestations and sequelae is required.
- Standardization of diagnostic PCR assays is needed for use in routine clinical practice.
- The risk–benefit balance of antibiotic therapy, the optimal drug, and duration are all still unclear.

Further reading

Florin TA, Zaoutis TE, Zaoutis LB. Beyond cat scratch disease: widening spectrum of *Bartonella henselae* infection. *Pediatrics* 2008;**121**:e1413–e25.

Maman E, Bickels J, Ephros M, *et al.* Musculoskeletal manifestations of cat scratch disease. *Clin Infect Dis* 2007;**45**:1535–40.

Schutze GE. Diagnosis and treatment of *Bartonella henselae* infections. *Pediatr Infect Dis J* 2000;**19**:1185–7.

Chicken pox—varicella zoster

see also Chapters 10, 34, 38

Name and nature of organism

- Varicella zoster virus is one of the eight herpesviruses known to infect humans.
- VZV is known by many names, including chickenpox virus, varicella virus, zoster virus, HHV-3.
- VZV virions are spherical and 150–200nm in diameter.
- VZV DNA is a single, linear, double-stranded molecule.
- The capsid is surrounded by a number of proteins that play a critical role in initiating the process of viral replication in infected cells.
- It is very susceptible to disinfectants.

Epidemiology

- Humans are the only source of infection.
- In Europe the primary infection occurs mainly during childhood (in the first 10 years of life) with a peak incidence during winter and early spring. In the tropics the attack rates are lower so there are more susceptible adults.
- Virtually all children in developed countries catch chicken pox at some time.
- Where routinely administered, vaccination has significantly modified varicella epidemiology, both reducing clinical disease and shifting the incidence to higher age groups, especially when vaccination is not universally taken up.
- In surveillance areas with high vaccine coverage, the rate of varicella disease decreased by approximately 85%.

Transmission and incubation period

- It is one of the most contagious infections—the household attack rate for non-immune individuals is around 90%.
- Humans are infected when the virus comes in contact with the mucosa of the upper respiratory tract or the conjunctiva.
- Person-to person transmission occurs by direct contact or airborne droplet spread followed by mucosal invasion. There is a primary viraemic phase, with uptake of the virus by the reticuloendothelial system, followed by a secondary viraemia to the

skin and mucosal surfaces. Normal cell-mediated immunity is critical for clearance. VZV develops latency in the dorsal root ganglion cells.

- *In utero* infection as a consequence of maternal infection during pregnancy is possible.
- Nosocomial transmission of varicella can be a problem on paediatric units.
- Children are contagious from 1 to 2 days before the onset of the rash until crusting of the lesions.
- Incubation period is between 10 and 21 days, but most children usually become ill around 14 days after a contact. This may be shorter in immunocompromised children or longer in subjects who have received VZIG.
- Varicella can develop between 1 and 16 days of life (usually between days 9 and 15) in infants born to mothers with active varicella around the time of delivery.
- Immunity is generally lifelong.

Clinical features

- Primary infection causes varicella (chicken pox). Asymptomatic primary infection is unusual, but because some cases are mild, they may not be recognized.
- Varicella is characterized by a generalized, pruritic rash of macules that develop into vesicles, then pustules, and finally crusts. A few lesions are classically umbilicated. The rash is seen mostly on the head and trunk.
- The rash appears in crops, with waves of new lesions occurring for 3–6 days. Most children have hundreds of spots, which heal mostly without scarring. The child is usually febrile.
- In normal children varicella is a mild disease that spontaneously resolves in about 1 week. Complications are rare. Each child in a family who catches varicella tends to develop sequentially worse disease. The last child to catch it is usually the sickest!
- Young infants, adolescents, and adults generally have a more severe disease with higher rates of complications.
- In immunocompromised children, including those with HIV or that have received long-term therapy with corticosteroids, progressive severe disseminated varicella can develop. It is characterized by high fever of long duration, continuing eruption of skin lesions and the progressive appearance of complications. In some case, despite adequate treatment, the disease can be fatal. Haemorrhagic varicella with bleeding into and around the lesions is also seen.

Complications

In a recent prospective study, severe complications were seen in around 1/100 000 children. The most common admissions to hospital were secondary bacterial skin infections with sepsis (usually GAS or staphylococcal infections), pneumonia, encephalitis, cerebellar ataxia, toxic shock, purpura fulminans, and necrotizing fasciitis.

Zoster—shingles

- Shingles is the reactivation of dormant VZV usually as a dermatomal vesicular rash in the distribution of 1–3 sensory dermatomes, frequently associated with local pain. There are few systemic symptoms and no systemic dissemination in immunocompetent individuals, but postherpetic neuralgia can persist for weeks to months after resolution of the rash.
- In immunocompromised patients, lesions can appear outside the primary site and the patient can have visceral complications.
- Patients at risk for developing recurrent varicella or disseminated herpes zoster include those with the following conditions: HIV, those receiving intermittent courses of high-dose corticosteroids (>2mg/kg of prednisone or equivalent) for treatment of asthma and other illnesses, congenital T lymphocyte defects, or chronic cutaneous or pulmonary disorders.
- Infection of the fetus during the first 20 weeks of gestation can cause fetal death or congenital varicella syndrome, mainly characterized by limb atrophy and scarring of the skin of the extremities. In some cases CNS and eye diseases can occur.
- Infection of the fetus during the second 20 weeks of pregnancy can cause unapparent fetal varicella with subsequent herpes zoster in early life without having had extrauterine varicella.
- In newborn infants varicella can be fatal if the mother develops the disease from 5 days before to 2 days after delivery. If varicella develops in the mother more than 5 days before delivery and the gestational age is ≥28 weeks, the child is likely to be protected by maternal specific IgG antibodies.

Diagnosis

- The diagnosis can usually be made based on the characteristic clinical picture without the need for laboratory tests.
- Rapid diagnostic tests (PCR, direct fluorescent antibody) are the diagnostic methods of choice if available. PCR has the highest sensitivity and real-time methods can distinguish vaccine strain from wild-type.
- VZV can be detected by PCR or isolated by culture from scrapings of a vesicle base during the first 3–4 days of eruption. Isolation from other sites is less sensitive.
- Determination of specific IgG antibody in serum can be useful to retrospectively confirm the diagnosis. These antibody tests may be false-negative and are not as reliable in immunocompromised people.
- Determination of specific IgM is not reliable for routine confirmation of acute infection, but positive results indicate current or recent VZV infection.

Management and treatment

- Simple supportive care is sufficient for the great majority of children. This includes fluids, antipyretics if required, and observation for possible complications. There is some evidence that more layers of clothing leads to more spots, so keeping children cool is sensible.
- There are several drugs available with activity against VZV. Aciclovir is the only drug active against VZV licensed for use in children. It has been used for a long time in children and is safe and well tolerated. Resistance is rare.
- Famciclovir and valaciclovir have been licensed for treatment of zoster in adults. No paediatric formulation is available for either medication, and insufficient data exist on the use or dose of these drugs in children to support therapeutic recommendations; they should only be used under specialist guidance.
- Considering the mild course of the disease, aciclovir treatment is not recommended in otherwise healthy children; studies have shown that aciclovir treatment produces a reduction of only around 1 day in fever and rash.
- Oral treatment can be used in children at risk of moderate to severe varicella:
  - Those >12 years of age
  - Children with chronic severe underlying cutaneous or respiratory diseases
  - Children receiving long-term salicylate therapy
  - Children on short, intermittent or aerosolized corticosteroid therapy.
- Some experts recommend oral aciclovir for secondary household cases in which the disease is more severe than in the primary case.
- Drug therapy is considered to be effective only if aciclovir is administered in the first 48 hours of disease because viral replication stops by 72 hours after onset of rash.
- In pregnant women, a 7-day course of oral acyclovir or valaciclovir may be considered if it can be started within 24 hours of rash onset—because there are limited data on aciclovir during pregnancy, specialist advice should be sought.
- Oral aciclovir is not recommended for those at high risk for complications and severe illness because of poor bioavailability; use IV aciclovir instead.
- IV aciclovir is used for the following scenarios:
  - In complicated cases, even if they occur in otherwise healthy children. However, the efficacy of the treatment and the optimal duration of therapy are not established.
  - Pregnant women with severe or prolonged disease may need IV aciclovir; specialist advice should be sought
  - Neonates, under the supervision of a specialist
  - Immunocompromised patients (oral valaciclovir has been used successfully for mild cases).
- Immunoglobulin preparations are not effective once the disease is established.

- Infections caused by aciclovir-resistant VZV strains, which generally are limited to immunocompromised hosts, should be treated with parenteral foscarnet.
- Salicylates or salicylate-containing products must not be administered to children with varicella because they may increase the risk of Reye's syndrome. To control fever, paracetamol can be used at usual doses. Salicylate therapy should be stopped in a child who is exposed to varicella.

Prevention

- In addition to standard cleanliness, airborne and contact precautions are recommended in medical facilities for children with varicella or herpes zoster until crusting of the skin lesions. This period can last up to 1 week (until all lesions have crusted over) for otherwise healthy subjects with mild disease or several weeks for immunocompromised children with severe disease.
- For exposed susceptible patients, airborne and contact precautions from 10 until 21 days after exposure to the index patient are indicated; these precautions should be maintained until 28 days after exposure for those who received VZIG or the usual IVIG.
- Airborne and contact precautions are recommended for neonates born to mothers with varicella and should be continued until 21 or 28 days of age if they received VZIG or IVIG. Infants with varicella embryopathy do not require isolation.
- For children managed in the community the following advice should be given:
  - Stay away from school or nursery and do not go on air travel until 6 days after the last spot has appeared
  - Avoid contact with people who are immunocompromised, pregnant women, and infants aged ≤4 weeks.
- For immunocompetent patients with localized zoster, contact precautions are indicated until all lesions are crusted. Immunocompromised patients who have zoster (localized or disseminated) and immunocompetent patients with disseminated zoster require airborne and contact precautions for the duration of illness.
- In case of exposure to VZV, chemoprophylaxis is not routinely indicated. Potential interventions for susceptible people exposed to a person with varicella include varicella vaccine administered 3–5 days after exposure and, when indicated (see below), VZIG (1 dose up to 96 hours after exposure) or, if VZIG is not available, IVIG (1 dose up to 96 hours after exposure).

Definition of significant exposure

- The Department of Health in the UK considers the presence of the following factors as indicative of significant exposure to varicella zoster virus:

- Type of VZV infection in index case: Contact with chickenpox, disseminated zoster, immunocompetent individuals with exposed lesions and immunosuppressed patients with localized zoster (because of greater viral shedding)
- Timing of exposure: exposure to index case between 48 hours before onset of rash until crusting of lesions; or day of onset of rash until crusting (for localized zoster)
- Closeness and duration of contact: residing in the same household, maternal/neonatal contact, contact in the same room for a significant period of time (15 minutes or more), face-to-face contact, hospitalized in the same paediatric ward or hospital room of a patient with varicella; close contact (i.e. touching or hugging) with a person with active herpes zoster lesions.

- Susceptibility in healthy people is determined by establishing a history of chicken pox or demonstrating IgG antibodies to VZV.
- In immunocompromised persons testing for VZV IgG antibodies is recommended regardless of their history of chickenpox.

Varicella zoster vaccine

- Varicella vaccine is the best option for prevention of VZV infection in immunocompetent people. It is a live-attenuated preparation of the serially propagated and attenuated wild Oka strain. Subcutaneous administration is recommended, although IM administration has been demonstrated to result in similar rates of seroconversion.
- The following patients should not receive varicella vaccine:
  - People who are receiving high doses of systemic corticosteroids (2 mg/kg per day or more of prednisone or its equivalent) for at least 14 days. The recommended interval between discontinuation of corticosteroid therapy and immunization with varicella vaccine is at least 1 month.
  - Children with impaired humoral immunity may be immunized, but VZV vaccine should not be administered to children with cellular immunodeficiency. Exceptions include children with acute lymphocytic leukaemia in continuous remission for at least 1 year, with a lymphocyte count >700 /μl and a platelet count >100 × 10^3/μl, and children with HIV infection in CDC class 1 or 2 with a stable CD4+ T lymphocyte percentage of ≥25%.
  - Pregnant women, because the possible effects on fetal development are unknown. On the contrary, varicella vaccine should be administered to nursing mothers who lack evidence of immunity. There is no evidence of excretion of vaccine strain in human milk or of transmission to infants who are breastfeeding.
  - Varicella vaccine should not be administered to people who have had anaphylactic-type reaction to any component of the vaccine, including gelatin and neomycin.
  - Otherwise healthy children with moderate or severe acute disease, with or without fever.
- An immunocompromised person or a pregnant mother in the same household is not a contraindication for immunization of a child.

- Varicella vaccine is safe and well tolerated. Adverse events, usually mild, occur in 5–35% of the cases in the first 42 days after vaccination (mainly between days 5 and 26). High fever is rare and it occurs with the same frequency as in children receiving placebo; 3–5% of vaccinated children develop a generalized varicella-like rash, which includes only 2–5 skin lesions, usually maculopapular rather than vesicular. Severe adverse events, such as anaphylaxis, encephalitis, ataxia, erythema multiforme, Steven–Johnson syndrome, pneumonia, thrombocytopenia, seizures, Guillain–Barré syndrome, and death have been reported but in most of the cases a causal association cannot be determined and/or the vaccine was immunocompromised.
- VZV vaccine has been associated with development of herpes zoster mainly in immunocompromised, but also in immunocompetent children. However, herpes zoster in immunized people may also result from natural varicella infection that occurred before or after immunization.
- Vaccine-associated virus transmission to contacts is rare and only in the case of a rash developing in the immunized person.
- The administration of varicella vaccine during the presymptomatic or prodromal stage of illness does not increase the risk of vaccine-associated adverse events or more severe natural disease.
- Varicella vaccine can be administered simultaneously with other recommended vaccines. If not administered at the same visit, the interval between administration of varicella vaccine and other live-attenuated vaccines (including, measles, mumps, rubella) should be at least 28 days.
- When the vaccine was approved, a single dose for individuals <13 years and two doses for older people were recommended. Because there are data that indicate that the administration of a single dose may be ineffective in preventing outbreaks, implementation of a routine two-dose vaccination programme is recommended in some countries (first dose at age 12–15 months and the second at least 3 months later).
- Children aged ≥13 years and adults should receive two doses 4–8 weeks apart.

Varicella zoster immunoglobulin

- VZIG should be given to susceptible people at high risk of developing severe disease with significant exposure to VZV:
  - Immunocompromised children
  - Susceptible pregnant women
  - Newborn infants whose mother had onset of varicella within 5 days before delivery or within 48 hours after delivery
  - Hospitalized premature infants (>28 weeks' gestation) whose mother lacks a reliable history of varicella or serological evidence of protection, hospitalized premature infant (<28 weeks' gestation or ≤1000g birthweight) regardless of maternal history of varicella or VZV serostatus.
- VZIG prophylaxis may be ineffective in preventing varicella in immunocopromised patients; careful monitoring and drug treatment at first sign of illness are recommended.

- Any patient to whom VZIG is administered to prevent varicella should subsequently receive varicella vaccine according to recommendations appropriate for their age, the first dose of vaccine should be given 3 months after VZIG administration. If VZIG has been given within 3 weeks of administering a live vaccine the vaccine should be repeated 3 months later.
- The currently available vaccine is more than 95% effective in preventing moderate or severe disease. Mild infections are prevented in 70–85% of the cases.
- Children who develop varicella, despite vaccination, usually have a very mild disease with <30 vesicles, low fever, and rapid recovery.
- Whether Reye's syndrome results from administration of salicylates after immunization for varicella in children is unknown. However, salicylates should be avoided for 6 weeks after administration of varicella vaccine.
- Duration of immunity is not established. Available data suggest that protection can last for at least 20 years. However, these data have been collected in a period with a significant circulation of wild-type VZV and, consequently, with a high probability of natural boosting in immunized people.
- Varicella vaccination is recommended for susceptible healthcare workers.

Future research

- Further studies on the changing epidemiology of varicella and herpes zoster in relation to the extended use of varicella vaccine in different countries are required.
- Efficacy and safety of varicella vaccination, especially when administered in the tetravalent form combined with measles, mumps, and rubella, should be evaluated with more data in children with chronic underlying disease.
- Post-marketing surveillance safety studies on the use of combined measles, mumps, rubella, and varicella vaccines as well as long-term evaluation of duration of immunity in the general population are required.

Further reading

American Academy of Pediatrics Committee on Infectious Diseases. Prevention of varicella: recommendations for use of varicella vaccines in children, including a recommendation for a routine 2-dose varicella immunization schedule. *Pediatrics* 2007;**120**:221–31.

Liese JG, Grote V, Rosenfeld E, Fischer R, Belohradsky BH, v Kries R. ESPID Varicella Study Group. The burden of varicella complications before the introduction of routine varicella caccination in Germany. *Pediatr Infect Dis J* 2008;**27**:119–24.

Reynolds MA, Watson BM, Plott-Adams KK, *et al.* Epidemiology of varicella hospitalizations in the United States, 1995–2005. *J Infect Dis* 2008;**197** Suppl 2:S120–6.

Chlamydia

📖 see also Chapters 11, 27, 30, 37

Name and nature of the organism

- *Chlamydiae* are obligate intracellular Gram-negative bacteria with a unique life cycle involving two forms, the extracellular, infectious elementary body (EB) and the intracellular, metabolically active reticulate body (RB). EBs attach to host cells and following uptake transform into metabolically active RBs, which replicate within cytoplasmic inclusions and at the end of the life cycle turn into infectious EBs. The life cycle is complete when EBs are released from the host cell and infect new cells.
- The most important human pathogens are *Chlamydia pneumoniae* and *Chlamydia trachomatis*. *Chlamydia psittaci* is the cause of an important zoonosis with occasional human infections reported.

C. trachomatis infection

Epidemiology

- There are two biovars, LGV and trachoma, which causes oculogenital diseases other than LGV. There are many serovars with specific clinical and epidemiological features:
  - Serovars A through C are the cause of trachoma
  - Serovars B and D to K cause genital and perinatal infections
  - Serovars L (1, 2, 3) cause LGV.
- Oculogenital serovars of *C. trachomatis* are the cause of the most prevalent STI in industrialized countries, causing urethritis in men, cervicitis and salpingitis in women, and inclusion conjunctivitis and pneumonia in infants.
- The highest rates of infection are found in sexually active young people; in the UK a national *C. trachomatis* screening programme found positive screens in 9.5% of women and 8.4% of men.
- Co-infection rates with other STIs are high.
- *C. trachomatis* is the commonest cause of ophthalmia neonatorum.
- Asymptomatic infection of the nasopharynx, conjunctivae, vagina, and rectum can be acquired at birth.
- Sexual abuse should be considered when *C. trachomatis* infection is diagnosed in children beyond infancy who have vaginal, urethral, or rectal chlamydial infection.
- LGV serovars are worldwide in distribution and are especially prevalent in tropical and subtropical areas. Recently, outbreaks of LGV have been reported among men who have sex with men.

- Trachoma, which is a scarring conjunctivitis, is the most common preventable cause of blindness in the world; poverty and lack of sanitation are risk factors.
- Pelvic inflammatory disease (PID) and tubal factor infertility are important long-term outcomes.

Transmission and incubation period

- Genital infection is sexually transmitted; reinfections are common.
- Up to 10% of infants born to mothers with active, untreated, chlamydial infection develop clinical conjunctivitis; symptoms develop 5–14 days after delivery.
- Around 5% of infants born to mothers with active, untreated, chlamydial infection may develop pneumonia; onset is usually 1–3 months after delivery.
- Perinatally acquired infections can persist for as long as 3 years.
- Infection is not known to be communicable in infants and children.
- The incubation period of *C. trachomatis* illness can significantly vary. One week is the mean period.
- LGV is infectious during active disease and perinatal transmission is rare.
- Trachoma can be spread from eye to eye; flies are a vector between humans.

Clinical features and sequelae

- Neonatal conjunctivitis:
  - Conjunctival injection, swollen eyelids
  - Eye discharge can vary from scanty mucoid to a copious purulent discharge
  - In contrast to trachoma, scars and pannus formation are rare.
- Pneumonia in infancy:
  - It is an afebrile disease with slow onset and benign course
  - Usually characterized by repetitive cough, tachypnoea, and rales
  - Hyperinflation often accompanies the interstitial infiltrates seen on chest radiographs, although wheezing is uncommon
  - Peripheral eosinophilia is a characteristic laboratory finding.
- Infection of the genital tract:
  - Wide spectrum of disease with 75% of women and many men being asymptomatic.
  - Symptoms, consisting of mucoid discharge and dysuria, are usually less acute than with gonorrhoeae.
  - Main clinical presentations are: urethritis, cervicitis, endometritis, salpingitis, proctitis.
  - Epididymitis occurs in males as well as Reiter's syndrome (arthritis, urethritis, and bilateral conjunctivitis).
  - Children who have been sexually abused may acquire vaginitis and rectal infections which are usually asymptomatic.
  - In postpubertal females, *C. trachomatis* can cause PID, which can present with perihepatitis and ascites (Fitz–Hugh–Curtis syndrome).
  - Recurrent or chronic salpingitis can lead to ectopic pregnancy or (tubal factor) infertility.

- LGV is a chronic disease characterized by:
  - Initial ulcerative lesion of the genitalia
  - The second stage is characterized by unilateral tender and suppurative inguinal or femoral lymphadenitis with enlarging, painful buboes.
  - In the tertiary stage, rectovaginal fistulas and strictures can be seen.
- Trachoma is the consequence of repeated and chronic infections:
  - The initial infection is a follicular conjunctivitis, which may result in scarring and entropion (eyelid turning inward)
  - Chronic trauma to the cornea (abrasions by eye lashes) causes neovascularization and scarring of the cornea.

Diagnosis

Laboratory diagnosis

- Specimens—adequate samples for direct detection should contain columnar epithelial cells, which need to be transported in special media if cell culture is to be performed.
- Direct fluorescent antibody (DFA) test—high sensitivity for good quality (i.e. large number of epithelial cells present) conjunctival and male urethral specimens.
- Cell culture—gold standard, labour intensive, and not widely available.
- Nucleic acid amplification tests (NAATs) are highly sensitive for the detection of genital infections; non-invasive testing is possible (urine and self-collected vaginal swabs).
- In cases with medicolegal implications (i.e. sexual abuse of children or rape) only direct detection by isolation of *C. trachomatis* in cell culture or detection by a NAAT (with confirmation by a second NAAT using a different target) is acceptable.

Disease specific management

- Ocular trachoma is usually diagnosed clinically in countries with endemic infection:
  - Two out of four criteria should be present: (1) lymphoid follicles on upper tarsal conjunctivae; (2) typical conjunctival scarring; (3) vascular pannus; (4) limbal follicles
  - Confirmation by culture, staining or NAAT during active stage of disease
  - Serological tests are not helpful due to high seroprevalence in endemic populations.
- Neonatal pneumonia due to *C. trachomatis* can be suspected when the chest radiograph shows interstitial infiltrates and hyperinflation and blood cell count demonstrates eosinophilia ($\geq$0.3–0.4 × 10^9/l); culture of nasopharyngeal swab specimens confirms the diagnosis; an acute microimmunofluorescent serum titre of *C. trachomatis*-specific IgM may be elevated ($\geq$1:32).
- LGV can be diagnosed by culture or a positive NAAT from a specimen aspirated from a bubo or by serological testing.
- Diagnosis of genitourinary chlamydial disease should prompt investigation for other STIs, including syphilis, gonorrhoea, and HIV infection.
- When an infant has been infected, it is recommended to evaluate the mother for chlamydial as well as other STIs.

Management and treatment

- Neonatal conjunctivitis and pneumonia:
  - Topical treatment of chlamydial conjunctivitis is ineffective and unnecessary.
  - Oral macrolides are the drug of choice for conjunctivitis and/or pneumonia—erythromycin for 14 days or azithromycin for 5 days.
  - Because efficacy is only 80%, follow-up is recommended and a second course can be necessary.
  - If erythromycin is used, the risk of development of hypertrophic pyloric stenosis has to be taken into account in infants <6 weeks. The risk of hypertrophic pyloric stenosis may be lower with azithromycin.
- Uncomplicated genital infections are treated as follows:
  - Children: macrolide (erythromycin 7–14 days; may use azithromycin as a single dose in children >8 years or in those who weigh at least 45kg).
  - Adolescents: macrolide, doxycycline, or a quinolone for 7 days.
  - Doxycycline and quinolones are contraindicated during pregnancy.
- Trachoma can be treated by either the topical or the oral route.
  - Mild cases are usually treated with topical tetracycline or erythromycin ointment given twice a day for 2 months or twice a day for the first 5 days of the month for 6 consecutive months.
  - Oral erythromycin or doxycycline (for children aged ≥8 years) for 40 days are administered in the most severe cases.
  - A simple and effective alternative is represented by mass treatment to all residents of a village with a single dose of azithromycin.
  - Treatment is aimed at treating individuals with active infection and reducing infection load in endemic communities, but will not reverse scarring
- LGV is treated with:
  - Doxycycline (patients ≥8 years) for 21 days
  - Erythromycin base (patients <9 years) for 21 days.
- A diagnosis of *C. trachomatis* infection in an infant should prompt treatment of the mother and her sexual partner(s).
- Repeat testing (preferably by culture) is recommended 3 weeks after treatment in pregnant women.

Prevention

- Pregnant women at high risk of *C. trachomatis* infection (i.e. women aged <25 years and those with multiple sexual partners) should be targeted for testing the presence of *C. trachomatis*.
- Prophylaxis of infants born to infected mothers (who are at high risk of infection) is not usually recommended because its efficacy is not known. They should be treated if infection develops.
- Sexually active adolescents and young adult women aged <25 years should be tested at least annually for *C. trachomatis* infection during gynaecological visits, even if no symptoms are present or barrier contraception is reported; education on reducing transmission (e.g. condom use) is an essential part of prevention programmes.

- In areas that are endemic for trachoma, the WHO implements the SAFE approach: **s**urgery, **a**ntibiotics, **f**ace washing, and **e**nvironmental improvement. Azithromycin once or twice a year or topical tetracycline twice daily for 6 weeks has been effective in treating large populations.
- Non-specific preventive measures for LGV include education, condom use and case reporting.

Future research
- The role of maternal chlamydial infection in prematurity and in perinatal death.
- Standardized diagnostic tests for different infections caused by *C. trachomatis* have to be identified.
- More data are required on tolerability and efficacy of newer oral macrolide antibiotics, such as azithromycin, roxithromycin, or clarithromycin for chlamydial infections in neonates.
- Efforts to find a vaccine for *C. trachomatis* are ongoing.

C. psittaci infection

Epidemiology
- The major reservoir of *C. psittaci* are birds, especially pigeons, parrots and turkeys.
- The term psittacosis commonly is used for the human disease, although the term ornithosis more accurately describes the potential for all birds, not just psittacine birds, to spread this infection.
- Disease due to *C. psittaci* is worldwide distributed and tends to occur sporadically in any season.
- 48 cases of psittacosis were reported in the UK in 2009.
- The main risk factor is exposure to birds, but up to 20% of infected patients have no history of exposure.
- Infection is rare in children.

Transmission and incubation period
- Healthy and sick birds may harbour and transmit the organism, usually via aerosols from faecal dust or nasal secretions. Excretion of *C. psittaci* can be intermittent or persistent for weeks or months.
- Those exposed to infected animals (e.g. workers at poultry farms, pet shops, pet owners) are at high risk of infection.
- The incubation period is between 5 and 21 days.

Clinical features and sequelae
- Psittacosis is an acute febrile respiratory infection with high fever, non-productive cough, headache, and malaise. Severe interstitial pneumonia can occur, particularly in the immunocompromised. This is a difficult diagnosis to think of, unless one asks specifically about pets!
- Rare complications are pericarditis, myocarditis, endocarditis, hepatitis, and encephalitis.

Diagnosis

- Traditionally diagnosis has been confirmed by demonstrating a fourfold increase in IgG antibody titre determined by complement fixation testing between acute and convalescent specimens obtained 2–3 weeks apart.
- In addition to fourfold increase in IgG titre, a single micro immunofluorescence (MIF) IgM titre of 1:32 or greater confirm a suspected case.
- MIF IgM tests may be false-negative early during the acute illness.
- Isolation of the agent from the respiratory tract can only be performed in a reference laboratory due to the potential biohazard.

Management and treatment

- Standard isolation precautions are recommended.
- Tetracyclines are the drugs of choice, except for children younger than 9 years.
- Macrolides (erythromycin, azithromycin, clarithromycin) are the alternatives for children younger than 9 years of age (<12 years in the UK).
- In severely ill patients use IV doxycycline.
- Treatment should be administered for at least 10–14 days after defervescence.

Future research

- There is an urgent need for information and for awareness campaigns directed at professional healthcare workers and the general public.
- Implementation of new diagnostic methods in medical laboratories is an important area of research.

C. pneumoniae infection

Epidemiology

- All isolates of *C. pneumoniae* appear to be closely related serologically.
- The proportion of community-acquired pneumonias associated with *C. pneumoniae* ranges from 2% to 19% varying with geography, age group examined and diagnostic methods used.
- First infections are especially common between the ages of 5 and 15 years.
- Infection and reinfections are common because the period of immunity after a single infection is short.
- There is no evidence of seasonality.

Transmission and incubation period

- *C. pneumoniae* is transmitted from person to person through respiratory secretions.
- Spread of infection is enhanced by close proximity.
- The mean incubation period is 21 days.
- Nasopharyngeal shedding can occur for up to 6 months after acute disease.

Clinical features and sequelae

- There are no characteristic clinical features that distinguish *C. pneumoniae* from other common respiratory pathogens.
- Patients may be asymptomatic or mildly to moderately ill with upper and/or lower respiratory tract involvement.
- Pneumonia is the most important disease and it usually presents with mild constitutional symptoms including low-grade fever, malaise, headache, cough, pulmonary rales, and non-exudative pharyngitis.
- Illness can be prolonged and cough can persist 2–6 weeks with a biphasic course.
- Wheezing is a common clinical manifestation in children; *C. pneumoniae* has also been associated with exacerbations of chronic asthma.
- Coinfection of *C. pneumoniae* with other respiratory pathogens is common.
- The reported association of *C. pneumoniae* infection with the development of atherosclerosis and cardiovascular disease remains controversial.

Diagnosis

- Specific diagnosis is based on isolation of the organism by culture or positive NAAT; specimen types include posterior nasopharynx swabs, sputum, and BAL fluid.
- The MIF antibody test is currently considered the best serological test. A fourfold increase in IgG titre or an IgM titre ≥1:16 is considered indicative of acute infection.
- Specific IgM antibodies appear 2–3 weeks following primary infection and specific IgG antibodies peak after 6–8 weeks.
- Many children with culture or NAAT documented infection do not have detectable antibodies by MIF tests.
- Immunohistochemistry can be used to detect *C. pneumoniae* in tissue specimens, but it requires skill and control antibodies in order to avoid false-positive results.

Management and treatment

- Macrolides are the drugs of choice in paediatrics.
- Tetracycline, doxycycline, or quinolones are also effective but can only be administered in older patients.
- A 5-day course of azithromycin was shown to be effective in eradicating *C. pneumoniae* from the nasopharynx in 80% of children with pneumonia.
- Treatment may need to be continued for several weeks in some patients to reduce the risk of failure or recurrences.

Prevention

- Standard precautions are recommended.

Future research

- The association between *C. pneumoniae* and exacerbations of chronic asthma needs to be further clarified.
- The role of *C. pneumoniae* in other chronic inflammatory diseases requires more research.

- The optimal duration of antimicrobial treatment should be determined by well-designed clinical trials.

Further reading

Beeckman DS, Vanrompay DC. Zoonotic Chlamydophila psittaci infections from a clinical perspective. *Clin Microbiol Infect* 2009;**15**:11–17.

Blasi F, Tarsia P, Aliberti S. Chlamydophila pneumoniae. *Clin Microbiol Infect* 2009;**15**:29–35.

Crosse BA. Psittacosis: a clinical review. *J Infect* 1990;**21**:251–9.

Darville T. *Chlamydia trachomatis* infections in neonates and young children. *Semin Pediatr Infect Dis* 2005;**16**:235–44.

Miller KE. Diagnosis and treatment of *Chlamydia trachomatis* infection. *Am Fam Physician* 2006;**73**:1411–16.

Principi N, Esposito S. Emerging role of *Mycoplasma pneumoniae* and *Chlamydia pneumoniae* in paediatric respiratory tract infections. *Lancet Infect Dis* 2001;**1**:334–44.

Principi N, Esposito S, Blasi F, Allegra L, Mowgli Study Group. Role of *Mycoplasma pneumoniae* and *Chlamydia pneumoniae* in children with community-acquired lower respiratory tract infections. *Clin Infect Dis* 2001;**32**:1281–9.

Cholera

📖 see also Chapters 12, 42

Name and nature of organism

- Cholera is a bacterial infection of humans caused by *Vibrio cholerae*, a Gram-negative bacillus divided into >100 serogroups.
- In most areas where cholera is endemic, *V. cholerae* serogroup 01, biotype El Tor, serotype Ogawa or Inaba, is the principal pathogen, with serogroup 0139 responsible for infection in some areas of south Asia. Other serogroups may cause diarrhoea, but not the clinical or epidemiological pattern of cholera.
- The infective dose of cholera is relatively high (10^2–10^{10} organisms) and infectivity is increased in achlorhydria and chronic gastritis. The principal pathogenic factor is the polypeptide cholera endotoxin, comprising two subunits, A and B.
- The B subunit attaches to the epithelial cells, and 'allows' entry of the A subunit into the cells. The A subunit 'switches on' cyclic AMP, resulting in the efflux of water, bicarbonate and electrolytes, and the clinical dehydration and electrolyte imbalance that characterises cholera.
- In 2000 the full genome of *Vibrio cholerae* was characterized, and the location of the genes coding for the A (ct x A) and B (ct x B) toxin sub-units determined. An understanding of the toxin genes has enabled the development of improved cholera vaccines.

Epidemiology

- Pandemics of cholera have been described throughout history. The current pandemic (*V. cholerae* 01, El Tor) began in 1961 in Indonesia, and spread through south and east Asia, the Middle East, and in the 1970s into Africa, and, finally, in 1990 to Latin America. In 1993 a new serogroup, *V. cholerae* 0139 was reported in southern India, and has been responsible for outbreaks in Bangladesh and Thailand.
- Cholera is a faecal-oral disease, and occurs where sanitation and water supplies are inadequate, particularly in the poorer areas of the world, and in refugee and complex emergencies, like the Haitian earthquake disaster. Vibrios can survive for long periods in aquatic environments, and so provide a reservoir of infection when public health infrastructure is compromised. The El Tor biotype has an improved environmental survival compared to classical, and a

higher asymptomatic carrier:case ratio, which has contributed to its displacement of the classic biotype.

- Current areas where cholera continues to be endemic are parts of south Asia including India and Bangladesh, and much of sub-Saharan Africa. Large scale epidemics, often with high mortality, have occurred in the past decade among Rwandan refugees in the Democratic Republic of Congo, in southern Sudan, Angola and Somalia, and, in 2009, in Zimbabwe.

- While cholera is not of immediate public health importance in Europe, migration from sub-Saharan Africa, and south Asia, and particularly asylum seekers from areas of current conflict such as the Horn of Africa and Congo, make the importation of cholera a possibility.

- Since 2004, several cases of life-threatening cholera, including at least one death, have been reported in travellers returning to Europe from well-known resort areas in Kenya and Thailand. In England and Wales 41 laboratory confirmed cases of cholera were reported in 2007, and 37 in 2006.

Transmission and incubation period

- Transmission may occur directly through infected water, or in food contaminated by infected water or by asymptomatic carriers. Shellfish from contaminated environments have been responsible for outbreaks, as have vegetables irrigated or 'cleaned' with contaminated water.

- The latter has been associated with at least one outbreak from airline food!

- While symptomatic cases are the major cause of secondary cases in epidemic situations with crowding and poor hygiene, asymptomatic carriers are also a significant source for transmission.

- The incubation for symptomatic disease is usually 1–3 days, with a range of a few hours to 5 days. The incubation period may be shorter with a high ingested dose.

Clinical features and sequelae

- In most people, cholera is a mild typical gastroenteritic illness. Severe cholera is characterized by the abrupt onset of profuse watery diarrhoea, vomiting, and loss of electrolytes, resulting in dehydration which may be hyper or hyponatraemic, along with hypokalaemia and metabolic acidosis.

- In severe cases, without rapid and appropriate rehydration and correction of electrolyte imbalance, death can result very quickly from hypovolaemic shock and associated metabolic complications.

Diagnosis

- In endemic areas or in epidemics, cholera will be diagnosed clinically, and laboratory confirmation will only be required to guide public health measures.
- For suspected imported cases, routine laboratories will be able to diagnose *V. cholerae* from stool specimens or rectal swabs. Stools are cultured on selective media, and suspect colonies tested for agglutination with 01 antisera. Samples from possible 0139 cases would require referral to a reference laboratory.

Management and treatment

- Rapid and appropriate rehydration is the principal management intervention in cholera.
- For infants <1 year, the UNICEF guidelines are to give 100ml/kg over 6 hours (30ml/kg in the first hour, then 70ml/kg over the next 5 hours). For older children, 100ml/kg over 3 hours (30ml/kg within the first half hour, then 70ml/kg in the next 2.5 hours).
- In moderately dehydrated cases, oral rehydration requirements in the first 4 hours will range from 400 to 600ml in infants <1 year to 1–2l in children aged <5 years.
- While in the UK standard oral rehydration salts (Dioralyte, Electrolade) would be used, WHO and UNICEF now recommend a reduced osmolarity solution (Na 75mmol/l, glucose 75mmol/l, and K 20mmol/l), which has been shown to shorten the period of diarrhoea and reduce stool volume in cholera.
- A modified ORS solution, ReSoMal, has been developed for use in severely malnourished children with diarrhoea, but its efficacy in cholera has not been established.
- Appropriate antibiotics can reduce the volume and duration of cholera diarrhoea, and the excretion of cholera vibrios. In children aged <12 years, current WHO guidelines are a 3-day course of erythromycin, though recent studies have shown the efficacy of a single (20mg/kg) dose of azithromycin. For older children and adults, a 3-day course of doxycycline is recommended. Family contacts of the index case may also be given antibiotics.
- Isolation strategies for cases will be different between industrialized, and low-income countries. Imported cases will need to be barrier nursed, with strict hygiene precautions until the diarrhoea settles. Where epidemics occur in refugee camps or crowded urban slums, locally appropriate strategies will be needed to isolate or cohort patients to reduce the risk of transmission.

Prevention

- Cholera is a notifiable disease in the UK, and suspected cases should be notified to the local health protection unit immediately for follow-up of contacts and public health management.
- In resource-poor countries, emergency public health measures will be necessary to improve sanitation, control polluted water supplies, and improve hygiene at the household level by safe water storage, provision of soap, and appropriate education and information.
- Two oral cholera vaccines have been developed; whole cell/B subunit vaccine, available as Dukoral in the UK, and a recombinant vaccine, which has not been widely accepted. Dukoral, given as two doses 6 weeks apart (and an additional dose in 2–6-year-old children), gives up to 2 years' protection.
- Because the risk of exposure to cholera is low for normal travel and tourism in the tropics, immunization is recommended only for those to be considered at high risk, in particular health workers going to relief or disaster zones, and travellers with remote itineraries in cholera endemic areas. Dukoral does not give protection against *V. cholerae* 0139.
- In complex emergencies there may be a role for mass oral vaccination used pre-emptively in cholera risk areas, but standard public health activities to improve sanitation and water supplies would be the priority.
- In industrialized countries, an awareness of the possibility of cholera in returning tourists or new immigrants from cholera endemic areas is essential with the increasing level of international travel.
- While secondary transmission would be unlikely, identification of imported cases would raise the possibility of the diagnosis in returnees from similar areas.

Future research

- Continuing work on cholera genome to gain understanding of regulatory genes and relationship to environmental triggers.
- Epidemiological studies to investigate further the role of oral cholera vaccines in large-scale, complex emergencies.
- Public health studies to improve cholera control in low-income countries.

Further reading

Parment PA. Cholera should be considered as a risk for travelers returning to industrialized countries. *Travel Med Infect Dis* 2005;**3**:161–3.

Sack DA, Sack RB, Nair GB, Siddique AK. Cholera. *Lancet* 2004;**363**:223–33.

Tarantola A, Quatresous I, Paquet C. Risk and control of imported cholera in a high-income country. *Lancet Infect Dis* 2008;**8**:270–1.

Clostridium difficile infection

📖 see also Chapters 12, 17

Nature and name of organism

- *Clostridium difficile* is the most common cause of nosocomial and antibiotic-associated diarrhoea in adults and is an emerging cause of childhood diarrhoea.
- *C. difficile* is a Gram-positive, spore-forming bacillus.
- It is a commensal bacterium of the human intestine, and is carried asymptomatically in up to half of all normal neonates and approximately 3% of persons aged >2 years.
- *C. difficile* exists in an extracolonic spore form which is heat-resistant (thus allowing survival in healthcare settings for a prolonged period of time), acid resistant (thus permitting safe passage through the stomach), and antibiotic resistant.
- *C. difficile* returns to its vegetative state within the colon, where it is able to produce toxins that mediate disease.
- *C. difficile* produces two main toxins: toxin A ('enterotoxin') and toxin B ('cytotoxin'); a third toxin has also been identified (binary toxin) associated with a hypervirulent strain (📖 see Epidemiology, p. 489).

Transmission, incubation, and pathogenesis

- Transmission of *C. difficile* occurs by the faecal-oral route.
  - Reservoirs of *C. difficile* may be endogenous or environmental
  - *C. difficile* is highly transmissible via fomites and readily colonizes all hospital surfaces. Outbreaks in daycare settings have also been described.
- Once *C. difficile* has been acquired, colonization of the large bowel ensues. Interruption of the normal colonic flora by broad-spectrum antibiotics leads to increased susceptibility to colonization.
- The incubation period is unknown.
  - Clinical disease usually occurs 4–10 days after initiation of antibiotic therapy, although may occur up to 10 weeks after antibiotic therapy.
- *C. difficile* disease is caused by the action of the two toxins released by *C. difficile*.

Toxin A

- Toxin A is believed to be more important in the pathogenesis of *C. difficile* disease than toxin B.
- Toxin A binds to carbohydrate receptors on enterocytes that facilitate entry into the cell.
- Cellular damage leads to mucosal injury, inflammation, and secretion of fluid into the colon.
- Toxin A also appears to have an effect on neutrophil activation and recruitment.

Toxin B

Although Toxin B is a more potent toxin, it appears to play a role in disease once the intestinal mucosa is damaged by toxin A.

Binary toxin

- Binary toxin is only produced by the hypervirulent strain of *C. difficile* known as NAP1/B1/027.
- The role of this toxin is not well understood, but like all binary toxins (such as those produced by *Bacillus anthracis* and *Clostridium perfringens*), the toxin has two components: an enzymatic component and a membrane-altering component.

Pathological changes

- Adherent raised yellow and white plaques are seen on an inflamed mucosa; with progression of disease these plaques enlarge and coalesce (Fig. 60.1).
- Histologically, there is a neutrophilic infiltrate with colonic glands that are distended with mucin; the typical description is that of a volcanic eruption of neutrophils out of the mucosa into the lumen.

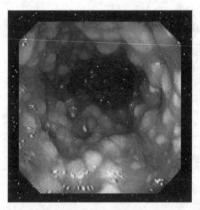

Fig. 60.1 Characteristic endoscopic findings of pseudomembranous colitis: raised pale plaques are seen on an inflamed mucosa. (Reproduced with the permission of D. M. Martin, from ℘ www.endoatlas.com/).

Epidemiology

- The organism was first identified in 1935 in the stool from healthy neonates, and was established as a cause of antibiotic associated diarrhoea in 1978.
- Infection with *C. difficile* is a nosocomial disease, although cases of community acquired *C. difficile* infection are increasingly being described, particularly in younger adults.
- The disease occurs only rarely without exposure to antibiotics and other drugs that alter the micro-ecology of the gut.

Burden of disease caused by *C. difficile*

- *C. difficile* associated infections became a major healthcare associated infection in the last decade:
  - *C. difficile*-associated disease reports doubled from 82 000 cases in 1996 to 178 000 cases in 2003 in the USA
  - In England, *C. difficile* as a reported cause of death increased nearly sevenfold between 1999 and 2006.
- *C. difficile* infections appear to be increasing in severity with many countries reporting:
  - Increased length of hospital stay, costs, colectomy and mortality in adults due to *C. difficile* infection.

C. difficile infections in children

- The true burden of disease in children has not been well documented because of variability in case definitions.
- However, as in adults, rates of *C. difficile* seem to be rising in children.
  - In a study of inpatients at 22 freestanding children's hospitals in the USA the annual incidence of *C. difficile*-associated disease increased from 2.6 to 4.0 cases per 1000 admissions between 2001 and 2006.
- There is currently no evidence to suggest that severity of disease is increasing in children.
- *C. difficile* has a specific epidemiology in the paediatric population:
  - Between 13% and 70% of infants may be asymptomatically colonized.
  - Colonization rates drop to approximately 6% in the second year of life.
  - Colonization rates in children aged >2 years are the same as for those in adults (approximately 3%).
- The reason for high colonization rates in neonates and infants is not clear. There is no association between colonization in infants and *C. difficile* disease. This may be due to a relative absence of receptors for toxin A on immature enterocytes. Infants with asymptomatic colonisation may be a reservoir for transmission to others.

Risk factors for *C. difficile* infection

Antibiotics

- Broad spectrum antibiotic use is the major risk factor for infection with *C. difficile*.
- Although clindamycin has traditionally been associated with *C. difficile* infection, any broad spectrum antibiotic can potentially lead to colonization with *C. difficile*.

- The most important antibiotics include:
  - Clindamycin
  - Cephalosporins
  - Quinolones.

Severe illness and complex chronic conditions

Chronic underlying medical conditions have been shown to be a risk factor for *C. difficile* infection in children, and this association is most likely related to increased exposure to both *C. difficile* and prolonged antibiotic therapy.

Hypervirulent strain: NAP1/B1/027

- This epidemic strain (North American Pulsed Field type 1/polymerase chain reaction ribotype 027) was first described in the 1980s following outbreaks in a number of North American states.
- This strain is considered to be hypervirulent for the following reasons:
  - Increased production of toxins A and B
  - Fluoroquinolone resistance
  - Production of binary toxin.
- This strain has been associated with severe disease in adults and children; it has also been associated with disease in older children without recent exposure to healthcare facilities or antibiotics.

Clinical features and sequelae

The clinical manifestations of *C. difficile* range from asymptomatic carriage to a fulminant colitis that can be fatal.

Spectrum of clinical disease

Asymptomatic carrier

- Most common in neonates.
- Also occurs in hospitalized patients (up to 20%) and patients in long-term care facilities (up to 50%).

C. difficile diarrhoea

- Watery diarrhoea.
- The diarrhoea is typically profuse and frequent (up to 15 times per day), but may follow a more mild course.
- Associated lower abdominal pain and tenderness, and fever.

Pseudomembranous colitis

- Systemic toxicity.
- May have passage of mucous and blood.

Fulminant colitis

- Severe abdominal pain, fever, hypovolaemia.
- In some children there may be marked abdominal distension but minimal diarrhoea.
- Can progress to toxic megacolon, bowel perforation, peritonitis, and eventual death.
- Mortality rates range from 3.8% in children to 16% in adults.

Relapse and reinfection
- Relapse is a common problem, occurring in 10–25% of initial treated cases.
- Occurs days to weeks after the initial episode, and is of similar or greater severity than the initial attack.
- Multiple relapses may occur.

Clinical disease in children <2 years of age
- Severe disease does occasionally occur in infants, especially in infants with a comorbid condition such as Hirschsprung's disease.
- The belief that infection with *C. difficile* is uncommon in young children has been challenged by recent data, perhaps because of the emergence of the NAP1/B1/ /027 strain.
- *C. difficile* as an emerging cause of community-acquired diarrhoea in the outpatient setting has been described.
- However, until further data are available, testing for *C. difficile* in children <2 years should generally be discouraged.

Diagnosis

- The diagnosis of *C. difficile* infection requires clinical suspicion and stool detection of *C. difficile* and its **toxin** (see below).
- Isolation of *C. difficile* without toxin may just represent normal bowel colonization.
- WCC can be useful for determining severity:
  - A peripheral WCC >15 000cells/mm^3 is indicative of greater severity of disease.
- Radiology (abdominal X-ray, CT) is usually not required unless there is concern about toxic megacolon.

Diagnostic difficulties in children
- Because of the high rates of asymptomatic colonization in infants, diagnostic strategies in young children are different from those in adults and older children.
- Children aged less than one year:
  - Routine testing for *C. difficile* should be restricted
  - Exceptions include patients with Hirschsprung's disease and immunocompromised/neutropenic patients.
- In children aged 1–2 years:
  - Routine testing should be discouraged
  - Careful clinical correlation is required (that is, at a minimum the patient should have diarrhoea and recent antibiotic exposure)
  - Other more common gastrointestinal pathogens that cause diarrhoea (for example rotavirus) should first be excluded.
  - Formed stool specimens should not be tested.
- Children aged >2 years can be tested in the same manner as older children and adults.
- It is not necessary to re-test after cessation of therapy unless there is return of symptoms.

Choice of diagnostic testing method for *C. difficile*

- A number of methods are available for detection of *C. difficile* in stool (Table 60.1); broadly there are two approaches:
  - Detection of the toxin (cytotoxicity assay, EIA, NAAT)
  - Detection of the organism (culture, common antigen testing).
- Toxin detection tests are preferred over organism detection tests. Tests that detect presence of the organism have the potential to yield false-positive results (up to 25%) because isolates may be non-toxigenic strains
- Toxin EIA testing is more commonly used than the cytoxicity assay.
  - Although the gold standard for the diagnosis of *C. difficile* infection has traditionally been the cytotoxicity assay, most diagnostic laboratories use an EIA to detect the presence of toxin because this assay is considerably less labour intensive and less expensive.
- There is increasing use of NAAT for detection of toxin B.

Table 60.1 Comparison of diagnostic tests for *C.difficile*

Method	Methodology	Sensitivity	Specificity	Turn-around time	Comments
Cytotoxicity assay	Two-step test: A portion of the filtrate is incubated directly onto a set of mammalian fibroblast monolayers and another is pre-incubated with antitoxin	80–85%	99%	24–48 hours	Has traditionally been the gold standard test
	A positive test is defined as presence of cytopathic effect in the first monolayer and absence of the cytopathic effect in the second				
	The characteristic cytopathic effect of *C. difficile* toxin is a rounded, asteroid-like cytotoxicity				
Toxin enzyme immunoassay	Direct stool EIA test for toxin A and/or B (detection of both toxins preferred)	50–70%	98–99%	1–2 hours	Numerous commercial kits are available

Table 60.1 (Contd.)

Method	Methodology	Sensitivity	Specificity	Turnaround time	Comments
Nucleic acid detection	Detection of a region within the toxin B gene	Not determined	>99%	~3 hours	Majority of strains produce toxins A and B, or toxin B only (only rarely do they produce toxin A only) FDA approved commercial systems are available
C. difficile culture	Specialized media required such as CCFA Colonies have a ground glass appearance and fluoresce yellow-green under UV light	>95%	>99%	48–72 hours	Testing that relies solely on culture has the potential to yield false positive results, therefore, it is recommended to supplement the test with a back-up testing method to identify toxin production Culture is required for epidemiological surveillance for typing
Common antigen testing		84–89%	90–98%	1–2 hours	This test is generally not recommended because false-positive results occur as a result of detection of non-toxigenic strains and as a result of cross-reactivity with other gut organisms

Management and treatment

The management of *C. difficile* infection involves the following steps:

1. Stop the offending antibiotic, or change the antibiotic to an agent that is less likely to predispose to *C. difficile* infection (if possible within the clinical scenario); such agents include aminoglycosides, macrolides, vancomycin.
2. Initiate appropriate infection control measures.
3. Commence antibiotic treatment against *C. difficile*, choosing antibiotic and dose based on the severity and whether this is a first episode or a relapse.

- Consider surgical consultation in severe disease.

Antibiotic choice

- Both metronidazole and vancomycin are effective against *C. difficile*.
- Metronidazole can be given orally or IV, but the oral route is preferred unless contraindicated (for example, ileus).
- Vancomycin is only effective if given orally.
- Vancomycin should be considered a second-line agent because of the potential risk of promoting vancomycin-resistant organisms.
- Although there is evidence that supports the use of vancomycin as a first-line agent in sicker adult patients, there is currently no evidence to support its use as first-line treatment in children.
- Other antibiotics such as nitazoxanide, teicoplanin, and rifampicin have also been used.

Experts differ in their treatment regimen; a suggested approach is the use of oral metronidazole for 10 days as standard first-line therapy. Severe disease with marked colitis or toxic megacolon is usually treated with IV metronidazole and oral vancomycin.

Surgery

- Surgery is required very rarely in children with *C. difficile* infection (in <1%) as compared with adults (approximately 2%).
- Surgery can be life-saving in the setting of severe disease such as bowel perforation with peritonitis and toxic megacolon.
- The most commonly performed surgical procedure is total colectomy with preservation of the rectum and ileostomy.

Intravenous immunoglobulin

- There is currently no convincing evidence to support the use of IVIG in the treatment of *C. difficile* infection.

Probiotics

- There is currently no convincing evidence to support the use of probiotics in the treatment of *C. difficile* infection.

Prevention and control

Prevention of *C. difficile* infection in the healthcare setting cannot be emphasized enough, and careful adherence to infection control policies is paramount in the control of this organism.

Prevention

Antibiotic choice

● Studies have shown that targeted restriction of antibiotics in healthcare facilities can lead to a rapid reduction in *C. difficile* both to prevent and during outbreaks (including clindamycin, quinolones, and cephalosporins).

Hand hygiene

● The mechanical effect of washing hands vigorously with soap and water is more effective in removing the spores of *C. difficile* than the use of alcohol-based products.

Environmental decontamination

● Thorough cleaning of hospital rooms of patients with *C. difficile* infection is very important in limiting spread of this organism.
● Because the spores of *C. difficile* are resistant to many hospital-grade disinfectants, the use of hyperchlorite solutions is indicated (more than 5000ppm available chlorine).

Future research

● Phase I clinical vaccine trials of *C. difficile* toxoid vaccines have shown promising result, including one trial in a small number of patients with recurrent *C. difficile* infection.
● The optimal testing and decontamination/cleaning regimens have not yet been defined.
● The risk–benefit analysis of restricting broad-spectrum antibiotic use needs further analysis. In many UK hospitals there has been a remarkable reduction in cephalosporin and quinolone use even in centres with low rates of *C. difficile* disease.

Further reading

Benson L, Song X, Campos J, Singh N. Changing epidemiology of *Clostridium difficile*–associated disease in children. *Infect Cont Hosp Epidemiol* 2007;**28**:1233–5.

Bryant K, McDonald LC. *Clostridium difficile* infections in children. *Pediatr Infect Dis J* 2009;**28**:145–6.

Kim J, Smathers SA, Prasad P, Leckerman KH, Coffin S, Zaoutis T. Epidemiological features of *Clostyridium difficile*-associated disease among inpatients at children's hospitals in the United States, 2001–2006. *Pediatrics* 2008;**122**:1266–70.

Cryptosporidiosis

📖 see also Chapters 19, 20, 21

Name and nature of organism

- A gastroenteritis-like illness that is self-limiting in immunocompetent individuals.
- Caused by a protozoan parasite that infects the epithelial cells.
- Most human infections are due to *Cryptosporidium parvum* or *Cryptosporidium hominis*.
- Infection with unusual species and genotypes can occur.

Epidemiology

- Infection occurs worldwide in adults and children, commonly in young children.
- Prevalence of infection is higher in developing countries.
- Outbreaks have followed failure of domestic water purification.
- Outbreaks can occur in institutions.
- <10 oocysts are required to cause infection.
- There are around 4000 reported cases/year in the UK overall.

Transmission

- Infection occurs following ingestion of oocysts, which are shed in human or animal faeces, or via contaminated water, food, or on fomites.
- Oocysts release sporozoites, which invade epithelial cells and form trophozoites. Trophozoites then sexually or asexually reproduce and produce more oocytes.
- Symptoms occur up to 14 days after ingestion of oocysts.
- Oocysts may be shed for 1–15 days after the resolution of symptoms.

Clinical features and sequelae

- Infection mainly affects the small intestine, but can be spread throughout the gastrointestinal tract.
- Asymptomatic infection can occur.
- Invasion of the luminal enterocyte border leads to villous atrophy, blunting, crypt cell hyperplasia, and mononuclear cell infiltration of the lamina propria.

- Watery diarrhoea, abdominal pain, nausea, and vomiting are the commonest features.
- Fever, anorexia, and fatigue can occur.
- Infection is usually self-limiting, lasting 10 days to 3 weeks.
- Weight loss and failure to thrive may be severe particularly in malnourished children.
- Seronegative reactive arthritis has been reported.
- Persistent and severe infection can occur in immunocompromised patients.
- Infection outside the gastrointestinal tract is rare in immunocompetent individuals.
- Biliary and pancreatic infection can lead to complications such as sclerosing cholangitis and pancreatitis in the immunosuppressed. Infection in the biliary tree can act as a reservoir leading to reinfection.
- Pneumatosis cystoides intestinalis, in which gas-containing cysts develop in the bowel wall, can occur in advanced HIV infection.
- Respiratory involvement and sinusitis have been reported in the immunocompromised, but the mechanism of infection is unclear.

Diagnosis

- Microscopic examination of stool specimens for oocysts, but infection cannot be excluded by analysing one stool sample only.
- Enzyme immunoassays and immunochromatological tests are available to test for the presence of oocyst wall antigens.
- Improved sensitivity is obtained using immunomagnetic staining.
- PCR also gives better sensitivity and ability to type different species.
- Oocysts can be seen on gut biopsy specimens.

Management and treatment

- Symptomatic treatment with rehydration therapy as required.
- Drug treatment is of limited benefit. There is no curative treatment.
- Several drugs have been tested in clinical trials, including nitazoxanide, paromomycin, rifabutin, several macrolides (azithromycin, clarithromycin, and spiramycin) and administration of bovine hyperimmune colostrums, but a Cochrane review of trials found insufficient evidence that any drug is able to reduce or cure the symptoms of Cryptosporidium infection or to effectively kill the organism among immunocompromised patients.[1]
- A 3-day course of nitazoxanide has been shown to reduce duration of diarrhoea and the parasite load in HIV-negative children, but with no effect in HIV-positive children.[2]
- In the immunocompromised patient the infection responds when the immune system recovers. Low CD4+ lymphocyte counts are associated with fulminant disease.
- Relapses of infection can occur if the infection has not been completely cleared.

Prevention

- Water supplies must be well maintained and protected against environmental contamination.
- Attention to personal hygiene is the key to preventing person-to-person spread.
- Infected people should be excluded from work, school, or other institutions until 48 hours after the diarrhoea has subsided.
- Oocysts are resistant to many commonly used disinfectants including chlorine.
- Immunocompromised patients may be advised to boil all water for drinking.

Future research

- Use of protease inhibitors in highly active ART (HAART) for HIV may have a beneficial effect in the treatment of cryptosporidiosis, above the effect on immune reconstitution, by inhibiting parasite development.
- *C. parvum* relies on inosine 5′-monophosphate dehydrogenase (IMPDH) to produce guanine nucleotides, and is highly susceptible to IMPDH inhibition. Both ribavirin and mycophenolic acid inhibit IMPDH and have been shown to have dose-dependent effect on *C. parvum* development and therefore may be of potential benefit.

Further reading

Abubakar I, Aliyu SH, Arumugam C, Usman NK, Hunter PR. Treatment of cryptosporidiosis in immunocompromised individuals: systematic review and meta-analysis. *Br J Pharmacol* 2007;**63**:387–93.

Amadi B, Mwiya M, Musuku J, *et al.* Effect of nitazoxamide on morbidity and mortality in Zambian children with cryptosporidiosis; a randomised trial. *Lancet* 2002;**360**:1375–80.

Chalmers RM, Davies AP. Minireview: Clinical cryptosporidiosis. *Experiment Parasitol* 2009;**10**:1016.

Cytomegalovirus

📖 see also Chapters 10, 15, 19, 20, 31

Name and nature of organism

- CMV is a human herpesvirus (HHV-5) of the *Betaherpesvirinae* subfamily.
- It is a large, enveloped, double-stranded DNA virus.
- Primary infection is followed by latency established primarily in cells of the myeloid lineage.
- In cell culture, infected cells swell up (cyto—cells, megalo—increase size, virus).

Epidemiology

- CMV is ubiquitous. Seropositivity increases with age and varies within and between populations. A higher prevalence is generally described in populations with lower socioeconomic status. The majority of children in resource-poor countries are seropositive by 1 year of age, with a slower, more gradual, increase in acquisition over time in developed countries (around 25% seropositivity by 1 year of age).
- The prolonged excretion of high levels of virus observed during the early years of childhood (whether congenitally or postnatally acquired) is thought to be a major contributor to spread of CMV infection in the developed world, particularly in the daycare setting.
- Seropositivity in pregnant women in the UK is around 60%. Congenital infection is reported in around 3/1000 live births in the UK. CMV is now the commonest congenital infection in Europe.

Transmission and incubation period

- Transmission is only from human to human and is most commonly via urine and saliva, although CMV may be detectable in many other body fluids.
- The median duration of excretion of CMV in urine in those infected congenitally/postnatally is around 4 years and 95% of congenitally infected babies are still excreting virus at 1 year of age.
- Congenital infection is thought to be transmitted from maternal blood via the placenta and is 40 times more common following primary infection in the mother during pregnancy than in those who have serological evidence of previous CMV infection.

- Perinatal/postnatal acquisition may be through cervical secretions during transition through the birth canal but is more commonly due to ingestion of infected breast milk. Rates of transmission are higher in premature and low birthweight neonates and in those fed fresh breast milk as opposed to frozen or pasteurized milk.
- Infection via blood transfusion was common prior to the routine use of leucodepleted and CMV-negative blood in high-risk subjects.
- Incubation has been predicted to be around 4–8 weeks based on studies in the settings of perinatal, post-transplant, and blood transfusion-acquired infection.
- In the case of congenital infection it is uncertain whether there is a maternal incubation followed by fetal incubation period, which has implications for diagnostic timing of amniotic fluid.

Clinical features and sequelae

Congenital

- Congenitally infected infants are broadly categorized into those who are symptomatic or asymptomatic at birth. Around 90% of babies with congenital CMV are asymptomatic at birth and the major concern in these babies is the 5–10% risk of developing hearing loss during the preschool years.
- Around 10% of infected babies have symptoms of CMV disease at birth, with classic features of thrombocytopenia, blueberry muffin rash, petechiae, IUGR, microcephaly, hepatosplenomegaly, and hepatitis/jaundice. Other CNS features are also common along with ocular abnormalities including chorioretinitis, optic atrophy, and strabismus.
- Sensorineural hearing loss (SNHL) is one of the most common manifestations of congenital CMV infection. It can be unilateral or bilateral, fluctuates and is progressive up to around 7 years of age. Half of babies with SNHL and CMV infection identified at birth will have no other clinical findings of CMV. SNHL may, however, be delayed in onset in around 30% and progressive in 50% of cases. SNHL is therefore reported by 5 years of age in around 35% of those with symptoms at birth and about 10% of those babies with no disease noted at birth. Overall CMV probably contributes to 25% of all SNHL.
- Long-term neurological disability (excluding SNHL) is reported in around 50% of those with and <5% of those without symptoms identified at birth.

Postnatal

- Postnatal disease is now most commonly seen in VLBW infants on neonatal units, who received CMV-infected breast milk from their mothers. It presents as pneumonitis, hepatitis, hepatosplenomegaly, lymphadenopathy, gastrointestinal disease, thrombocytopenia, and a sepsis-like syndrome.
- Long-term sequelae in these babies do not, according to current literature, seem attributable to CMV infection.

Immunocompromised children

- Immunocompromised patients (usually bone marrow or organ transplant) present with generalized systemic symptoms (often referred to as CMV syndrome) or organ-specific disease (including hepatic, pulmonary, and gastrointestinal manifestations, and occasionally CMV encephalitis). In the transplant group, CMV can also have indirect effects on outcomes such as graft rejection, and risks of other opportunistic infections.

Diagnosis

Direct methods

- Direct tissue culture of body fluids has traditionally been the gold standard for identifying infection; confirmation of a positive result may take up to 3 weeks.
- Methods utilizing immunofluorescent or immunoperoxidase-labelled monoclonal antibodies directed against the early antigen of CMV, and PCR identifying sequences within the CMV genome offer a rapid alternative with similar sensitivity and specificity to standard tissue culture.
- Urine or saliva are positive in up to 100% of infected individuals (although intermittent detection has been reported) and remain the diagnostic samples of choice for congenital infection.
- Isolation of CMV from a specimen acquired within the first 3 weeks of life is necessary to discriminate between congenitally and postnatally acquired infection.
- Blood PCR is only positive for CMV in around 80% of babies with CMV disease at birth. Recent data would suggest that blood samples should be taken within the first 10–14 days of life to completely exclude postnatal infection.
- Detection and quantification of virus in blood (using PCR or methods detecting presence of CMV antigen) is important for monitoring and detecting CMV viral load early in the transplant setting. Most children are now screened weekly post-transplantation by serial blood CMV PCR.
- Identification of CMV by PCR in amniotic fluid may establish whether antenatal transmission has occurred. Samples should ideally be acquired at least 7 weeks after maternal symptoms (if present) and after 21 weeks' gestation to minimize false-negative reports.
- Dried blood spots (Guthrie card) taken shortly after birth may be used retrospectively to confirm the presence of congenital CMV using PCR. Blood viral load is always lower than urine and saliva. The sensitivity and specificity of this method currently varies widely between laboratories depending on the extraction methods used, amount of starting material, and the part of CMV genome being amplified. If dried blood spots are negative on testing for CMV PCR, congenital CMV is not excluded.

Serology

- Serology is of limited use in those under 1 year of age but may be helpful as a first step in diagnosis in older children. IgM measurement may indicate primary infection but is only positive in around 70% of congenitally infected infants; false positive results are not uncommon, particularly during pregnancy.
- The use of IgG avidity is helpful in identifying primary infection in adults, particularly during pregnancy, but there are no published data on CMV IgG antibody maturation in younger children. High-avidity (stickiness/efficacy) IgG shows the presence of a more mature immune response. This implies an established infection that was not recently acquired.

Management and treatment

- Congenitally infected babies should be fully evaluated for signs of disseminated and CNS disease.
- Baseline investigations should include FBC, liver function, ophthalmologic review and formal audiological assessment. Cranial ultrasound, carried out by a skilled operator, is probably sufficient in the assessment of an asymptomatic baby with confirmed congenital CMV infection. MRI often gives additional information and can be helpful in providing more detailed assessment of those with mild ultrasound abnormalities or who have more symptomatic disease.
- In the UK, it is currently recommended that babies who are congenitally infected with CMV, without signs of disease, have 6-monthly hearing assessments for the first year of life, then annual checks until school age.
- In any symptomatic baby ophthalmic follow-up should probably continue for the first 1–2 years of life as late-onset eye disease has been reported.
- Antiviral treatment with the nucleoside analogue ganciclovir given twice daily IV for 6 weeks has been shown to decrease progression of SNHL and improve neurodevelopmental outcome in those with CNS disease if started early in neonatal life. The oral prodrug, valganciclovir (VGCV), is currently being evaluated in large studies. A randomized study comparing 6 weeks to 6 months of VGCV in babies with symptomatic congenital CMV disease will help to determine the optimum duration of therapy. In the UK the only clear indication for treatment in congenital CMV infection is currently symptomatic CNS disease.
- There are very limited pharmacokinetic data on ganciclovir and VGCV in premature infants and older children. Drug levels may be helpful in management, and should be performed in all children with treatment failure.
- There is at present no clear evidence for the use of antiviral treatment in postnatally infected neonates. Treatment may, however, be considered in those with severe liver disease or pneumonitis where other conditions have been excluded and the risk of treatment is balanced by the severity of disease.

- In transplant recipients and other immunocompromised children CMV infection and disease should be screened for regularly, and pre-emptive therapy started if a positive blood CMV PCR is found according to local protocols, in order to prevent the significant morbidity and mortality associated with CMV in these groups. Alternatively CMV prophylaxis should be commenced and continued until the child is considered at lower risk of CMV disease.
- Side effects of standard antiviral drugs are significant and the risks and benefits of treatment need to be discussed with families. The commonest side effects relate to bone marrow suppression (mainly neutropenia), which usually reverses on termination of therapy. The theoretical risk of longer-term side effects identified in ganciclovir and VGCV animal models, which include carcinogenicity and impaired fertility, are not fully evaluated in the clinical setting—no evidence has been found in limited follow-up studies.

Prevention

- Advice to CMV-seronegative pregnant women to avoid contact with potentially infected secretions in younger children has been shown to decrease transmission in the research setting. However, in most countries women are not offered routine antenatal serological screening for CMV, as it is currently of unproven benefit for the widespread prevention of CMV disease in neonates.
- Antiviral treatment may also prevent hearing deterioration and lead to improved neurological function at 2 years of age.
- Early detection of congenital CMV infection and enhanced hearing follow-up may enable early audiological input to maximize hearing in the prelinguistic stage.
- Preventive strategies using antiviral agents in the post-transplant period have significantly decreased morbidity and mortality attributable to CMV in this patient group.
- An effective vaccine against CMV does not currently exist, although a number of vaccine candidates are currently undergoing clinical trials.
- Randomized antenatal studies are underway of both valaciclovir and immunoglobulin in pregnant women with primary infection aiming to reduce vertical transmission.

Further reading

Dollard S, Grosse S, Ross D. New estimates of the prevalence of neurological and sensory sequelae and mortality associated with congenital cytomegalovirus infection. *Rev Med Virol* 2007;**17**:355–63.

Fowler K, Boppana S. Congenital cytomegalovirus (CMV) infection and hearing deficit. *J Clin Virol* 2006;**35**:226–31.

Hamprecht K, Maschmann J, Jahn G, Poets CF,Goelz R. Cytomegalovirus transmission to preterm infants during lactation. *J Clin Virol* 2008;**41**:198–205.

Knipe DM, Howley PM, Griffin DE, Lamb RA, Martin MA, Roizman B, eds. *Fields Virology*, 5th edn. Philadelphia: Lippincott Williams & Wilkins, 2007 pp. 2701–72.

Revello M, Gerna G. Diagnosis and management of human cytomegalovirus infection in the mother, fetus, and newborn infant. *Clin Microbiol Rev* 2002;**15**:680–715.

Schleiss M, McVoy M. Overview of congenitally and perinatally acquired cytomegalovirus infections: recent advances in antiviral therapy. *Expert Rev Antiviral Ther* 2004;**2**:389–403.

Snydman DR. The case for cytomegalovirus prophylaxis in solid organ transplantation. *Rev Med Virol* 2006;**16**:289–95.

The European Congenital CMV Initiative. Available at: ℘ www.ecci.ac.uk (accessed September 2010).

Diphtheria

📖 see also Chapters 13, 35, 42, 44

Name and nature of organism

- An illness that may involve the respiratory tract caused primarily by toxigenic strains of *Corynebacterium diphtheriae*, a Gram-positive, non-spore-forming pleomorphic rod.
- Main toxin is an exotoxin that consists of an active A domain and a binding B domain, which facilitates entry of toxin A into the cell. The A subunit inhibits protein synthesis, which has pathological consequences for many cell types.
- Non-toxigenic strains of *C. diphtheriae* can cause respiratory tract infections as well as (more rarely) cases of endocarditis or other forms of invasive disease.

Epidemiology

- Epidemiology has been markedly altered by the advent of vaccination in developed countries.
- In resource-poor countries, diphtheria remains a serious problem, with major outbreaks occurring in Africa, Latin America, and Asia; in addition, states of the former Soviet Union have been reporting large outbreaks since the 1990s, only controlled by widespread immunization of both adult and child populations.
- Humans are the sole reservoir of *C. diphtheriae*.
- Spread of the organism is mostly from respiratory droplets or contact with skin lesions.
- Peak season for respiratory disease is autumn and winter in the Northern Hemisphere.
- Incubation period is 2–7 days.
- Unimmunized individuals are more prone to severe disease. However, even immunized persons may become asymptomatic carriers or have mild disease. Therefore, infection control precautions need to be taken even with immunized individuals who have been exposed to an index case.
- Isolation of index cases is very important, as is informing local public health officials.
- Droplet precautions should be used with any patient with suspected diphtheria or carriers with pharyngeal diphtheria, until confirmation of negative cultures after antibiotic therapy has been completed. Contact precautions are recommended for patients with cutaneous diphtheria.
- For close contacts, the following steps are recommended:
  1. Surveillance for 7 days,
  2. Attempt to culture the organism from the oropharynx

3. Initiation of antimicrobial prophylaxis with erythromycin or benzathine penicillin G. Those with positive cultures should be treated for 10 days with erythromycin as the first-line treatment of choice.

Clinical features and sequelae

- Early symptoms of pharyngeal diphtheria are generally non-specific. Fever is not a major feature of the disease even though patients frequently appear toxic and with cardiovascular instability during the illness.
- Early on, the pharynx may appear slightly injected; within one to two days, patches of exudate appear and may form a leathery looking membrane covering the oropharynx. This membrane is highly adherent; attempts to remove it will result in bleeding.
- The neck may appear swollen and indurated, with enlargements of the anterior cervical lymph nodes (so-called 'bull neck appearance').
- Major risk of this infection is respiratory failure due to obstruction of the upper airway, which may require surgical intervention. Pneumonia and lower tract obstruction may also occur, presumably if the membrane gets dislodged accidentally.
- Although clinical toxicity is not uncommon, bacteraemia is rare with toxigenic isolates.
- Toxin-mediated secondary damage to other organs may occur, especially the myocardium (myocarditis/cardiomyopathy is a leading cause of death due to arrhythmias and heart failure), the kidneys (proteinuria), and the peripheral nervous system (peripheral neuropathy, motor more than sensory, generally several days to weeks after the onset of infection). Many of these symptoms have been ascribed to the effects of the diphtheria toxin.
- It is important to remember that primary sites other than the oropharynx may be involved: respiratory tract, conjunctivae, and vaginal infections have all been reported.

Diagnosis

- In the past, when more cases occurred in developed countries, even relatively inexperienced clinicians quickly became quite adept at making the diagnosis based on history and clinical examination alone. In the current era, few physicians in developed world settings have encountered patients with diphtheria and thus the diagnosis is most reliably and accurately made by laboratory methods.
- Specimens should be obtained for culture from the appropriate site(s): oropharynx, nose, skin or other mucosal site. Ideally, material from below the membrane or the membrane itself should be submitted for culture, as these materials have the highest yield. Alerting the laboratory of the possibility of diphtheria is critical, as the organism requires special medium for growth.

Management and treatment

- For patients with respiratory diphtheria, there is a substantial risk of rapid decompensation. For this reason, the mainstay of therapy for respiratory diphtheria is the administration of antidiphtheria antitoxin (from equine sources) by IV infusion when cases are suspected, even prior to bacteriological confirmation. This treatment is not without risks, as allergic reactions to horse proteins are not uncommon; skin testing for sensitivity to equine proteins is generally recommended.
- Antimicrobial therapy should also be administered. Generally, erythromycin or penicillin G for 14 days is recommended. While treatment with antibiotics probably reduces toxin production, helps to eradicate the organism, and reduces carriage, it is not a substitute for antitoxin therapy and is an adjunctive therapy.
- Disease does not necessarily confer long-lasting immunity; therefore convalescent patients should receive active immunization.
- Immunization of previously unimmunized asymptomatic carriers is recommended; for others who have been immunized but have not received a booster within 5 years, a booster should be administered as well.
- In general, two follow-up cultures are recommended following completion of therapy to confirm eradication. Should either of these cultures be positive, a new 14-day course of appropriate therapy should be initiated.

Prevention

- The mainstay of prevention is through active immunization with diphtheria toxoid-containing vaccines.
- Interestingly, although few would doubt the efficacy of active immunization, there has never been a carefully controlled diphtheria vaccine clinical trial demonstrating effectiveness.
- While several recently developed vaccines contain diphtheria toxoid (e.g. in the form of CRM_{197} protein), these vaccines should not be viewed as substitutes for diphtheria immunization.

Further reading

Belko J, Wessel DL, Malley R. Endocarditis due to *Corynebacterium diphtheriae*: A case report and review of the literature. *Pediatr Infect Dis J* 2000;**19**:159–63.

Golaz A, Hardy IR, Strebel P, *et al.* Epidemic diphtheria in the newly independent states of the former Soviet Union: implications for diphtheria control in the United States. *J Infect Dis* 2000;**181** Suppl 1:S237–43.

Mortimer EA, Wharton M. Diphtheria Toxoid. In: *Vaccines* 3rd ed. Plotkin SA, Orenstein WO, Eds. Chapter 9. Elsevier 1999. Philadelphia. pp. 140–57.

Wagner KS, Stickings P, White JM, *et al.* A review of the international issues surrounding the availability and demand for diphtheria antitoxin for therapeutic use. *Vaccine* 2009;**28**:14–20.

Chapter 64

Enteroviruses and parechoviruses

📖 see also Chapters 10, 14, 29, 30, 71

Introduction

- The enteroviruses are a genus of non-enveloped virus within the picornavirus family of small RNA viruses ('picorna' = pico (small) RNA).
- In addition to enteroviruses, there are eight other picornavirus genera, of which four cause human disease: cardioviruses, hepatitis A virus, kobuviruses, and parechoviruses.
- This chapter focuses on diseases caused by enteroviruses and parechoviruses, which were historically considered to be subtypes of enterovirus.
- Enteroviruses are RNA viruses with a single-stranded genome of approximately 7kb. The positive-sense genome can direct translation straight from its genetic material, and the viral RNA is capable of acting as infective material in isolation.

Name and nature of organism

- The translation machinery of infected cells is hijacked such that protein synthesis becomes almost entirely dedicated to viral protein synthesis. The viral RNA encodes four structural capsid proteins and seven non-structural proteins; the capsid proteins define the virus serotype.
- Historically, enteroviruses were classified into four groups based on patterns of pathogenesis in animal models: Coxsackie A, Coxsackie B, polioviruses, and echoviruses. However, the original schema does not correlate well with biological properties in humans, or with recent information on sequence data.
- A more recent classification (see http://ictvonline.org) defines ten enterovirus species, including seven human pathogens (Table 64.1). New enteroviruses are named with sequential numbers (onwards from enterovirus EV68); some of these may represent horizontal transfers from non-human hosts. Echoviruses 22 and 23 are now assigned to the parechovirus genus.
- The seven enterovirus species found in humans are:
  - Human enterovirus A (HEV-A)—which includes some Coxsackie A virus subtypes and enterovirus 71
  - HEV-B—which includes all Coxsackie B viruses, all echoviruses, Coxsackie A9 and enteroviruses 69 and 73
  - HEV-C—which includes some Coxsackie A viruses and polioviruses 1-3 (see Chapter 97)

- HEV-D—which includes several newer enteroviruses, e.g. 68 and 70[1]
- Human rhinovirus A, B and C including over 100 serotypes.

Table 64.1 Classification of enteroviruses

Species	Subtypes	Notes on clinical manifestations
HEV-A	Coxsackieviruses A2–8, A10, A12, A14, A16	Typically cause mild upper respiratory tract infections, including conjunctivitis, herpangina, pharyngitis. A16, A10, A5 associated with HFMD
	EV 71, 76, 89–91	EV 71—causes HFMD, with fatal rhomboencephalitis in some cases
HEV-B	57 types in total	
	Coxsackie B viruses 1–6	Pharyngitis often the presenting feature.
	All Echovirus types	Severe disease is associated with focal pneumonitis, meningitis (B5), pleurodynia (B3 and B5) and myocarditis and pericarditis (B5)
	Coxsackie A9	Rarely cause fatal illness, but hepatic necrosis is seen with some echoviruses; echovirus E3 is associated with wandering myoclonus; E6 with myocarditis; E9 is one of the most prevalent enteroviruses, commonly causing a febrile illness with a petechial exanthem or aseptic meningitis. Coxsackie A9 is associated with meningitis
	EV 69, 73–75, 77–8, 100–1	
HEV-C	14 types	
	Coxsackie A viruses (A1, 11, 13, 17, 19–22, 24)	A24 associated with haemorrhagic conjunctivitis
	Poliovirus types PV 1–3	Poliovirus infection is mostly asymptomatic but can cause meningitis and acute flaccid paralysis; 📖 see Chapter 97
HEV-D	3 types – EV 68, 70, 94	EV 68—respiratory illness
		EV 70—epidemic haemorrhagic conjunctivitis
		EV 94—flaccid paralysis
HRV-A/B/C	>100 serotypes	Most common human infection—common cold; also croup, bronchiolitis, pneumonia, asthma trigger

Enteroviruses infecting humans are grouped into five species as above by sequence homology in the VP1 capsid region; HFMD, hand-foot-and-mouth disease.

Epidemiology

Human enteroviruses A–D

- Humans are the only natural hosts for most members of the enterovirus family, including polioviruses, coxsackieviruses, and echoviruses. There is a worldwide distribution of enteroviral disease.
- Enteroviral infections are typically associated with outbreaks in summer and autumn in temperate regions, but with year-round infection in tropical areas. Children have a far higher burden of symptomatic infection than adults.
- Enteroviruses are widely prevalent; they may be responsible for more human viral infections than any other virus family. Among them, enteroviruses follow rhinoviruses as the most frequent cause of viral infection worldwide.
- Prevalence studies indicate that some subtypes are stable whereas others fluctuate in prevalence, with epidemics occurring when a virus moves back in to a non-immune population. Enterovirus 71, for example, has been associated with outbreaks with considerable morbidity and mortality, particularly in the Far East. Particular subtypes are often clinically apparently absent for decades, then suddenly produce new outbreaks.

Transmission and incubation period

- Enteroviruses are stable for several days at room temperature, and are resistant to alcohol-based cleaning products. They are inactivated rapidly by heat (>56°C) and dilute chlorine-based products.
- Spread is primarily faecal-oral, but nosocomial transmission on fomites is described and transmission is higher with overcrowding and poor hygiene.
- The incubation period for most infections is 3–10 days. Transmission is difficult to break because patients shed virus before they are symptomatic and asymptomatic shedding can continue from the throat (for weeks) and the stool (for months) after infection.

Natural history of infection

- Enteroviral infections show a biphasic course. Initial infection following oral entry leads to local invasion of the pharynx and alimentary tract before invasion of local lymph nodes. There is a period of minor viraemia which may be associated with non-specific mild symptoms. Following haematological spread, virus is taken up at secondary infection targets. Congenital infection may occur this way.
- Organ involvement and symptoms in the second phase of infection are determined by the tropism of the enterovirus. For example, following the primary viraemia, infections with a neurotropic virus manifest with CNS symptoms. Following viral replication in the target organs there is a second period of major viraemia (days 3–7).

- Virus is typically cleared by an antibody response, levels of virus starting to decrease after about 7 days.
- Immunopathology—cellular damage is thought to have both a viral cytopathic and a host immunopathological component although the relative contribution of each remains unclear.
- *In vitro* infection of cell cultures and murine models provide evidence for a strong role for cytopathic effects in neurological damage, pancreatitis, and in myocarditis.
- The adaptive immune system is thought to be important in control of enteroviral infection. A humoral response is associated with viral clearance, but the CD8$^+$ T cell response may contribute to long-term inflammatory damage following encephalitis.
- Murine models indicate that activation of the innate immune system via pattern recognition molecules such as TLR3 is also important.

Clinical features and sequelae

- Enteroviruses cause numerous infections in humans, and are associated with a wide range of clinical presentations including HFMD (📖 see Chapter 71), herpangina, pleurodynia, meningitis, and encephalitis.
- Most infections are self-limiting and mild, but with no effective treatment; serious, sometimes fatal enteroviral disease continues to pose a serious problem.
- Symptoms are wide-ranging, reflecting the particular viral subtype. There is considerable overlap among the non-polio enteroviruses.

Conditions associated with all non-polio enteroviruses

- Asymptomatic infection—serological studies indicate that there is a high level of unrecognized infection; overall approximately 50% of infections are asymptomatic, rising to 90% for some, such as Coxsackie A16 in those <5 years.
- Non-specific febrile illness—this is the most common manifestation of echoviral or Coxsackie infections, with abrupt onset of fever with headache. Sore throat, without any observable inflammation, and conjunctivitis may be present.
  - Enteroviruses are probably one of the commonest causes of admission to hospital in young infants with a fever. The clinical picture is typically 'viral' with minor URTI symptoms, mild vomiting and loose stools, irritability, and minor macular rash; recovery usually occurs within a week.
- Gastrointestinal symptoms are common; this is unsurprising given the tropism of enteroviruses for the gut.
  - Typical symptoms include diarrhoea, vomiting, constipation and abdominal pain, but in most cases gastrointestinal symptoms form only part of the illness. Rarely, more serious sequelae occur, including intussusception, hepatitis, pancreatitis, and peritonitis.
- Skin exanthems—enteroviruses cause a range of exanthems: macular, maculopapular, petechial, or morbilliform. Large blotchy papules are often seen in babies, around 10–20 on the trunk and body.

Neurological manifestations

- Meningitis is the most common neurological manifestation, most often diagnosed in young babies. The most commonly identified subtypes causing meningitis are Coxsackie B viruses (particularly B5), echoviruses and Coxsackie A9.
  - There are no clinical findings that reliably distinguish enteroviral from bacterial meningitis, although enterovirus CSF commonly has proportionately lower neutrophils, higher lymphocytes, slightly raised protein, but a normal glucose.
  - Enteroviral isolation from CSF is more likely in patients with a greater CSF leucocytosis.
  - Enteroviral meningitis is generally self-limiting, with resolution of symptoms within 1–2 weeks.
  - Although the prognosis is much better than for bacterial meningitis, follow-up studies of developmental outcome suggest that a mild impairment may be seen in a small proportion of patients.
  - Appropriate advice for parents is that their child has had meningitis, that the great majority of children after viral meningitis are completely normal, but some more subtle effects on school learning cannot be ruled out. Long-term routine clinic follow-up is not warranted in the absence of clinical concerns, but early referral to a psychologist for detailed assessment may be useful if the child has any schooling difficulties years later.

Encephalitis—enterovirus 71

- This subtype has been associated with epidemics of severe disease, with high rates of brainstem encephalitis (rhomboencephalitis) and death, from neurogenic pulmonary oedema and vasomotor collapse.
- Many infections are mild, or cause a HFMD illness, and the proportion causing severe neurological disease varies between outbreaks. There have been recent outbreaks of severe disease in the Far East, including Taiwan and China. Long-term neurological morbidity is very high after EV71 encephalitis and cardiopulmonary failure.

Flaccid paralysis

- The tropism of poliovirus for the anterior horn cells explains the paralysis seen in polio infections. Rarely, non-polio enterovirus infections cause paralysis, with enterovirus 71 being the most common cause.

Conditions associated with HEV-A

- Herpangina: There is a painful vesicular, blistering eruption on the oral mucosa towards the rear of the palate and around the tonsillar fauces. It is typical of Coxsackie A virus infection.
- HFMD—📖 see Chapter 71.

Conditions associated with HEV-B

- Pharyngitis—HEV-B infections often present with an abrupt-onset sore throat with fever. The pharynx is typically injected and sometimes exudative.

- Pleurodynia (Bornholm disease)—this is an epidemic disease with fever and acute inflamed, painful intercostal muscles. Spasmodic, sometimes severe pain is experienced in the upper chest or abdomen lasting minutes to hours, exacerbated by deep inspiration. There may be associated muscle tenderness. Children may also experience anorexia, nausea, vomiting, headache and sore throat.
  - The course may be biphasic, with episodic pains recurring after the initial febrile episode, lasting a couple of weeks overall.
  - Although many enteroviruses have been described as causing pleurodynia, HEV-B viruses are the most common, particularly Coxsackie B3 and B5.
- Myopericarditis—though many enteroviral types have been occasionally implicated, Coxsackie B viruses (especially B5) and echoviruses are the most common causes of myocarditis.
  - Manifestations range from arrhythmia to ventricular failure and death. In neonates disease can be particularly severe. Active young teenagers can develop acute chest pain or heart failure and may be diagnosed late.
- Enterovirus infection and diabetes—susceptibility to type 1 diabetes is known to have a strong genetic component, manifested particularly as HLA gene polymorphisms, but there is also an environmental component, widely believed to be an infectious trigger of autoimmunity to pancreatic β cells.
  - Enteroviruses, particularly coxsackievirus B4, have long been suspected of acting as such a precipitant. Although several studies have identified genomic enteroviral RNA in the blood of patients with type 1 diabetes, as yet there is not convincing evidence of a direct link between enteroviral infection and diabetes onset.

Conditions associated with HEV-C and HEV-D

- Common cold—coxsackievirus A21 (HEV-C) causes a mild, afebrile, coryzal illness
- Haemorrhagic conjunctivitis—both EV-70 (HEV-D) and coxsackievirus A24 (HEV-C) cause epidemics of haemorrhagic conjunctivitis.
  - The illness is spread by direct inoculation to the eye rather than by haematogenous spread following oral entry. Eye pain, photophobia, blurred vision, and erythematous congestion are seen. Resolution by day 7 is typical.

Neonatal disease

- Neonatal disease may occur transplacentally during maternal viraemia, or by oral inoculation during labour or in the neonatal period. There is often a history of recent maternal viral illness.
- Most neonatal infections are not clinically significant but a minority cause very severe sepsis-like illness resembling disseminated HSV disease.
- Other cases resemble bacterial sepsis at presentation, with fever, poor feeding, abdominal distension, irritability, rash and hypotonia. Blood indices include neutrophilia and thrombocytopenia, although with typically lower CRP than in bacterial sepsis.

- Respiratory, gastrointestinal, hepatic, cardiac, and CNS complications can follow, and in meningoencephalitis, CSF pleocytosis does not always develop, although white matter changes are generally seen on cranial imaging.
  - A worse prognosis is associated with prematurity, maternal illness at time of birth, onset of symptoms during the first week of life and absence of transplacental transfer of maternal antibody. Death is more common in babies with acute hepatic failure and coagulopathy, particularly if myocarditis is also present. Long-term sequelae are more common in those with encephalitis.
  - Echovirus E11 and coxsackieviruses B2–B5 are most often responsible for symptomatic infection, with B4 associated with more severe disease.

Diagnosis

- RT-PCR is now the most commonly used diagnostic tool, and is replacing the use of immunofluorescence testing after virus isolation by culture.
- Stool and upper respiratory tract secretions provide useful samples for enteroviral detection. CSF, vesicle fluid, pericardial fluid, myocardial biopsy, and blood can also be tested. As enteroviruses may be shed in the stool for many weeks post-infection, caution should be exercised in interpreting positive stool enterovirus PCR results.
- The usefulness of serological tests for enteroviruses is limited by the heterogeneity of the antibody response, which is subtype-specific. Serology is rarely helpful as a screening tool.

Management and treatment

- Enteroviral infections are generally self-limiting and require no specific treatment other than supportive care. However, although there is a need for specific antiviral treatment of severe disease, there is currently very limited evidence to support the use of any available treatment.
- IVIG use is controversial. In some countries, for instance Taiwan, where there have been large outbreaks of severe enterovirus encephalitis, IVIG is recommended for treatment of severe enteroviral infection. There is little evidence to support this approach. There are a number of case reports that support the use of IVIG in combination with pleconaril (see below) in enteroviral meningoencephalitis for immunosuppressed patients, particularly those with low immunoglobulin levels. IVIG has also been used for treatment of neonatal enteroviral infection, again without good substantiating evidence.
- Pleconaril (Picovir) is one of a number of antivirals that targets the relatively conserved VP1 capsid protein and blocks the unfolding of RNA. It has good *in vitro* activity against enterovirus, and good oral

bioavailability but despite initial promise, clinical experience showed only a modest effect in adult meningitis and no effect in a small RCT in infants. The drug is not currently available, but a trial in enteroviral disease is ongoing.

- Interferon β—In a small trial of adult patients with dilated cardiomyopathy and persistent myocardial viral replication by enterovirus or adenovirus, a 6-month course of interferon β was associated with enteroviral clearance in all patients, and haemodynamic improvement in 14 of 22 patients. A larger randomized, placebo-controlled study was then started. However, there are no paediatric data on the role of interferon β.

Prevention

- Continued clinical and laboratory surveillance of enteroviral disease is required so that appropriate measures can be implemented early in outbreaks of severe disease, as seen, for instance, in Singapore with EV71, where early reporting from childcare centres of HFMD led to local actions to contain further spread, including closure and cleaning.

Future research

- Virus biology: It is unclear why some enterovirus types are more pathogenic.
- Virus epidemiology and surveillance: The significant impact of outbreaks of EV71 in the Far East emphasizes the importance of understanding the epidemiology so that future epidemics can be anticipated.
- New drugs: The usefulness of pleconaril is still being investigated in a CASG phase II trial of infants with enteroviral sepsis syndrome (see: 🔖 www.clinicaltrials.gov).

Parechoviruses

- Parechoviruses are a recently described genus of picornavirus. Six types cause human disease: human parechovirus 1 to 6 (HPeV1–6). Types 1 and 2 were previously known as echovirus 22 and 23 respectively, but were reassigned to a new genus based on RNA sequence and *in vitro* cytopathology studies. Following this, the four additional types were described.
- Severe sepsis-like syndrome is characteristic of neonatal parechovirus infection, clinically similar to severe enteroviral infection and can require intensive care. High fever, marked CNS irritability and seizures (especially with HPeV1), and a rash or generalized redness can be presenting features.
- The CRP typically remains low. Although CSF pleocytosis rarely develops, meningoencephalitis is common, and white matter changes

are commonly evident on cranial imaging. Neurodevelopmental outcome can be poor.

- Unlike enterovirus infection, myocarditis is not seen. There have been several outbreaks on neonatal units of necrotizing enterocolitis and pneumonia in association with HPeV1.
- HPeV1 causes clinically apparent infections in early childhood after the protective effect of maternal antibody has waned, with a median age at infection of 18 months, particularly in late summer to early winter; almost all adults have antibodies against HPeV1 (infections with other parechovirus types are less common).
- Mild gastrointestinal and respiratory symptoms are most common. Although rare, severe disease has been described, for instance an outbreak where six patients developed flaccid paralysis. Myocarditis and encephalitis have also been described.
- Diagnosis is best made by RT-PCR from stool, respiratory samples or CSF using HPeV-specific primers, or by virus isolation. As with neonatal enterovirus infection, treatment of serious disease with IVIG has been tried, although further data are needed to support this approach.

Further reading

Joki-Korpela P, Hyypi T. Parechoviruses, a novel group of human picornaviruses. *Ann Med*, 2001;**33**:466–71.

Tebruegge M, Curtis N. Enterovirus infections in neonates. *Semin Fetal Neonatal Med* 2009;**14**:222–7.

Epstein–Barr virus

📖 see also Chapters 15, 44

Name and nature of the organism

- EBV is one of the human herpesviruses (HHV-4).
- EBV is named after Anthony Epstein and Yvonne Barr, who discovered the virus in 1964 in cells cultured from tumour specimens sent to them from Uganda by Denis Burkitt. Burkitt postulated that there might be an infective component to the tumours he was treating (Burkitt's lymphoma) and he was right!
- EBV most commonly infects B lymphocytes but, rarely, is also capable of infecting squamous epithelial cells, smooth muscle cells, T cells, natural killer cells, plasma cells, and follicular dendritic cells.
- EBV is the most common cause of infectious mononucleosis. Other pathogens causing similar symptoms include cytomegalovirus (CMV), newly acquired HIV and *Toxoplasma gondii*.
- In addition to endemic Burkitt's lymphoma, EBV is implicated in certain types of Hodgkin's and non-Hodgkin's lymphomas, undifferentiated nasopharyngeal carcinoma (NPC), and a proportion of gastric carcinomas. These cancers affect several hundred thousand persons per year worldwide. EBV is often claimed to be associated with chronic fatigue syndrome (CFS), but there is little evidence to support this.
- EBV exhibits a lifelong latent infection in healthy carriers harbouring EBV in B memory lymphocytes where no virus or viral products are expressed.
- Infectious virus is present in the saliva but replication of both the virus and infected B cells expressing viral products is usually controlled by antibody, natural killer and T cell responses in healthy individuals.
- In acute infection up to 20% of all circulating B cells may be infected.
- In immunocompromised patients (congenital or acquired) reactivation of EBV may lead to severe symptomatic infection or B cell lymphomas. EBV is associated with post-transplant lymphoproliferative disorder (PTLD), which may be either polyclonal or true malignant lymphoma.
- In X-linked lymphoproliferative disease (Duncan's syndrome) affected boys may develop overwhelming illness with EBV.

Epidemiology

- EBV occurs worldwide but the occurrence of the EBV-associated tumours, endemic Burkitt's lymphoma and undifferentiated nasopharyngeal carcinoma have distinct geographical patterns. Endemic Burkitt's lymphoma occurs in areas with holoendemic malaria while NPC is most common in Southern China.

- Humans are the only source.
- More than 90% of the population will have been infected by the virus in childhood, when it is most often asymptomatic. Infection during adolescence is much more likely to cause infectious mononucleosis (glandular fever).
- No seasonal pattern is documented.

Transmission and incubation period

- Transmission is by close personal contact with healthy asymptomatic carriers and spread is via saliva: 'the kissing disease'. Infectious mononucleosis is common in adolescents—typically spreading in schools or colleges.
- The virus is viable in saliva for several hours outside the body but transmission via fomites is unknown.
- The virus can also be isolated from blood, genital tract secretions, CSF and breast milk, although these are not thought to play a role in transmission.
- The incubation period is 4–7 weeks but the person will remain infected and infectious indefinitely after the symptoms have completely disappeared, in the same way as a normal healthy asymptomatic carrier.

Clinical features and sequelae

- The spectrum of disease is very wide, ranging from asymptomatic, through typical glandular fever to (very rarely) severe, prolonged and occasionally fatal illness.
- Infectious mononucleosis (glandular fever) is typically associated with fever, exudative pharyngitis, cervical lymphadenopathy, headache, hepatosplenomegaly, and malaise.
- Hepatitis is relatively common.
- A non-specific maculopapular rash is seen in up to 10% of cases.
- Palatal petechiae may be observed.
- In acute EBV, facial oedema/fullness is seen across the nasal area.
- Apparently normal young children can develop a severe illness with high fever, widespread marked lymphadenopathy, and hepatosplenomegaly.
- If amoxycillin or ampicillin is given, many cases will develop a florid rash.
- CNS complications include aseptic meningitis, encephalitis, and Guillain–Barré syndrome. These are usually only seen in severe cases.
- Rare complications include autoimmune haemolytic anaemia, thrombocytopenia, haemophagocytic syndromes, splenic rupture, orchitis, and myocarditis.
- Infectious mononucleosis doubles the subsequent risk of contracting multiple sclerosis and Hodgkin's disease, but a causal relationship in either case has not been established.

- In boys (classically aged 3–5 years) who develop an increasingly severe IM picture with worsening hepatitis, encephalopathy, and marrow failure urgently consider the possibility of X-linked lymphoproliferative syndrome (Duncan's syndrome) due to a defect in the *SAP* gene.

Diagnosis

- Usually based on typical clinical features.
- The blood picture shows a lymphocytosis with atypical lymphocytes.
- The most common serological test is based on the heterophile antibody test, (monospot or Paul Bunnell), in which the infected plasma agglutinates sheep erythrocytes. This test is specific but not sensitive. False-negative results occur in up to 25% in the first week, 5–10% in the second week, and 5% in the third. The antibody may not appear until the second or third week of illness, and in some, particularly young children, may not appear at all.
- More useful is specific EBV serology. IgM antiviral capsid antigen (VCA) or anti-early antigen (EA) is useful to identify recent infection whereas a positive IgG anti-VCA indicates past infection. Serum antibody against EBV nuclear antigen (EBNA) is only present weeks or months after the initial infection, so a positive anti-EBNA antibody test will exclude very recent infection. A negative anti-EBNA with a high positive IgG anti-VCA is indicative of recent infection.
- EBV viral load determined by quantative PCR is now commonly used routinely post transplantation to detect early signs of EBV reactivation and disease and prevention of PTLD.
- Differential diagnoses include;
  - Other viral causes (such as CMV or toxoplasmosis) especially in heterophile-negative patients.
  - HIV, which can mimic similar signs.
  - Acute leukaemia. The blood results of EBV and leukaemia may be confused. A bone marrow examination may be necessary for clarification.
  - Other causes of pharyngitis (*Streptococcus*, diphtheria, and respiratory viruses).

Management and treatment

- Infectious mononucleosis is generally self-limiting and therefore only supportive and/or symptomatic treatments are used. Antipyretics and simple anti-inflammatory medications may reduce fever and pain.
- Antibiotics are not recommended. If they are used, ampicillin and amoxycillin should be avoided as they are likely to produce a rash.
- Steroids have been effectively used for severe disease or massive pharyngeal swelling compromising the airway of the patient, however, a Cochrane review concluded that there was insufficient evidence to recommend steroid treatment for symptom control in simple glandular fever.

- Aciclovir may reduce initial viral shedding although there is little evidence to support its use. The antiviral agent valaciclovir may be of some use in reducing the EBV viral load and decreasing the severity of symptoms.
- Rest is important during the acute phase. Contact sports should be avoided until the patient is fully recovered and the spleen no longer palpable to avoid splenic rupture.

Prevention

- There is no vaccine currently available, although recent phase II trials of a recombinant subunit vaccine indicated that infectious mononucleosis can be prevented but not EBV infection itself.
- Patients with a recent primary EBV infection should not give blood.
- Affected individuals do not need to be isolated and there is no quarantine time.

Future research

- The prevalence of EBV-related cancers worldwide warrants work on laboratory assays to both detect and quantify the infection, which can be used as a tumour marker to support the clinical management of patients. International efforts are underway to establish a standard by which to calibrate EBV DNA measurement.
- The development of EBV vaccines to prevent or modify infection continues to progress as does the development of immunotherapeutic strategies for treatment of EBV tumours themselves.
- Gene expression profiling and proteomics aims to identify patterns of viral and human gene expression to correlate with diagnosis, prognosis, and response to therapy.

Further reading

Candy B, Hotopf M. Steroids for symptom control in infectious mononucleosis. *Cochrane Database Syst Rev* 2006;(**3**):CD004402.

Gulley ML, Tang W. Laboratory assays for Epstein–Barr virus-related disease. *J Mol Diagn* 2008;**10**:2799–2.

Katz BZ, Shiraishi Y, Mears CJ, Binns HJ, Taylor R. Chronic fatigue syndrome after infectious mononucleosis in adolescents. *Pediatrics* 2009;**124**:1899–3.

Sokal EM, Hoppenbrouwers K, Vandermeulen C, *et al.* Recombinant gp350 vaccine for infectious mononucleosis: a phase 2, randomized, double-blind, placebo-controlled trial to evaluate the safety, immunogenicity, and efficacy of an Epstein-Barr virus vaccine in healthy young adults. *J Infect Dis* 2007;**196**:17495–3.

Young LS, Rickinson AB. Epstein-Barr virus: 40 years on. *Nat Rev Cancer* 2004;**4**:7576–8.

Escherichia coli diarrhoea

📖 see also Chapters 12, 16, 22

Name and nature of organism

Escherichia coli is a Gram-negative motile bacillus of the *Enterobacteriaceae* (enteric bacteria) family. *E. coli* is part of the normal flora resident in the intestines of humans and other animals; they are usually harmless commensals. *E. coli* can be subdivided on the basis of variation in the lipopolysaccharide (O), flagella (H), or capsule (K) antigens.

Specific isolates of *E. coli* carry particular virulence genes, either on the chromosome or plasmids, which give them the capacity to cause various disease syndromes. *E. coli* that cause diarrhoea are grouped by the mechanism by which they cause disease in humans:

- Enteropathogenic (EPEC)
- Enterotoxigenic (ETEC) a common cause of traveller's diarrhoea
- Enteroinvasive (EIEC)
- Enterohaemorrhagic (EHEC) (sometimes also referred to as verocytotoxigenic *E. coli* (VTEC) or *E. coli* O157)
- Entero-aggregative (EAggEC).

Clinical features

The dominant features are of profuse **diarrhoea** (watery or bloody depending on the specific *E. coli* type) and **abdominal pain**/cramping. Other symptoms could include: fever; nausea with or without vomiting; rigors; anorexia; headache; myalgia; and bloating.

Diarrhoea may lead to complications, most commonly:

- Dehydration, renal failure, haemorrhagic colitis, seizures
- Haemolytic uraemic syndrome (EHEC)
- Thrombotic thrombocytopaenic purpura.

Diagnosis

- Stool microscopy and culture is insufficient for the specific diagnosis in most instances.
- *E. coli* is part of the normal intestinal flora and is easily grown from faeces. Pathogenic strains are not easily differentiated from commensal ones.
- The detection of EHEC (usually *E. coli* O157) is routinely carried out in microbiology laboratories. EHEC can be distinguished from normal *E. coli* because of its inability to ferment sorbitol, unlike other *E. coli*. Suspected isolates are confirmed as *E.coli* and serotyped to check if they are O157 or one of the other common serotypes such as O26.

- Infection with EHEC *E. coli* O157 results in persistent high levels of antibodies to the O157 LPS antigen. Detection of these antibodies may be useful to provide retrospective evidence of exposure or recovery from acute infection.

Management and treatment

- Most patients recover with supportive measures alone and do not require hospitalization.
- Dehydration and electrolyte imbalances should be corrected.
- Antibiotics should be reserved for cases that are severe, chronic, and/or with septicaemia.
- Antimicrobial resistance is common in these bacteria. Treatment should be guided by antimicrobial sensitivity testing. Co-trimoxazole, azithromycin, or ciprofloxacin may be considered if the organism is susceptible.
- The use of antibiotics in treating *E. coli* O157 is a risk factor for developing HUS and should be avoided.

Prevention

Travellers to low-income countries should be careful about where they eat, ideally only consuming hot food and drinks or bottled water, avoiding salads, and peeling their own fruit ('Cook it, boil it, peel it, or leave it').

Antibiotic prophylaxis for travellers is not recommended because of concerns about drug toxicity and the potential encouragement of resistance.

Future research

- Treatment options in EHEC, and strategies to reduce morbidity and mortality from HUS.
- Further evaluation of ETEC vaccinations (currently undergoing phase III/IV trials worldwide).

Further reading

Orth D, Grif K, Zimmerhackl LB, Würzner R. Prevention and treatment of enterohaemorrhagic *Escherichia coli* infections in humans. *Expert Rev Anti Infect Ther* 2008;**6**:101–8.

Safdar N, Said A, Gangnon RE, Maki DG. Risk of hemolytic uremic syndrome after antibiotic treatment of *Escherichia coli* O157:H7 enteritis: a meta-analysis. *JAMA* 2002;**288**:996–1001.

Giardiasis

📖 see also Chapters 21, 22, 42

Name and nature of organism

- *Giardia* organisms are a group of pear-shaped, flagellated protozoans. They have a ventral disc by which they attach to the duodenum and upper small intestine. They have two forms: the disease causing trophozoite, and the encysted form, which is transmittable in faeces.
- *Giardia duodenalis* (= *lamblia* = *intestinalis*) is the species found in humans, and also described in other mammals, birds, and reptiles.
- *Giardia* are one of the most primitive eukaryote cells.
- Ribosomal RNA analysis suggests that *Giardia* forms an evolutionary link from around 2 billion years ago at the divergence between prokaryotes and eukaryotes—really a very old infection!

Epidemiology

- *Giardia* is a ubiquitous organism that is found worldwide.
- The incidence and intensity of infection is greatest where sanitation and safe water supply is inadequate.
- Serological surveys have shown that adults in urban areas in developed countries have a seroprevalence of 18–24%, while in rural areas in resource-poor countries this is over 50%.
- In high-prevalence areas children acquire infection early, reaching adult levels of seroprevalence by 6 months of age.
- Children excrete *Giardia* episodically and are often asymptomatic.
- In Europe and America travellers returning from the Tropics account for at least half of all patients presenting with *Giardia*.
- In the UK there are around 500 reported cases/year in children, with the highest rates seen in the 1–4 year-age group (13/100 000 per year).

Transmission and incubation period

- Giardiasis is spread by faecal-oral contamination.
- Infected people excrete cysts, which can survive for months in moist soil or water.
- The cysts can survive the chlorine levels in treated drinking water and in cold mountain streams.
- The cysts are killed by cooking, but contaminated raw or undercooked foods can be a source of infection.
- There can also be direct person to person contact from contaminated hands, which leads to increased prevalence in daycare and institutional settings. Carers changing nappies are at increased risk.

- Sexual transmission can occur through oral/anal sexual practices.
- Ingestion of between 10 and 100 cysts is required to cause infection in humans.
- After ingestion the host's gastric acid causes excystation and each cyst produces two trophozoites.
- The trophozoites migrate to the duodenum and proximal jejunum where they attach to the mucosa by the adhesive ventral disc. They reproduce by binary fission or a very evolutionary basic form of sex. Multiplication is encouraged by the presence of bile, carbohydrate, and low oxygen concentration.
- Symptoms develop 1–2 weeks after ingestion, median around 7–10 days.
- Diarrhoea is thought to be caused by a number of mechanisms:
  • Direct physical injury of the mucosa
  • Formation of a physical barrier between the gut epithelium and the intestinal lumen.
  • Release of parasitic products such as proteinases or lectin
  • Mucosal inflammation associated with T cell activation and cytokine release.
  • Associated bacterial overgrowth
  • Bile salt depletion.
- Some trophozoites transform to cysts and pass into the faeces to complete the life cycle.

Clinical features and sequelae

- Common symptoms are: nausea, vomiting, flatulence, abdominal cramps, diarrhoea, and weight loss.
- In contrast to bacterial or viral diarrhoea, the onset of the diarrhoea may be more gradual and relatively mild.
- Symptoms last 2–4 weeks and without treatment most resolve spontaneously.
- 10–20% of people develop chronic infection with persistent loose stool, steatorrhoea, malaise and depression.
- Chronic giardiasis in children can present with weight loss or failure to thrive with malabsorption. There is no blood or mucus in the stool.
- Patients can present with reactive arthritis or an urticarial rash as part of a hypersensitivity reaction.
- Malnourished children have a high incidence of *Giardia* and other intestinal parasites. There is an association between frequent episodes of giardiasis, and stunting and cognitive impairment.
- Children with hypogammaglobulinaemia are at increased risk of disease and are more difficult to treat than those with normal immunity.
- T cell abnormality does not seem to increase susceptibility. In patients with HIV, *Giardia* rates are the same or lower than in the background population. This contrasts with the much higher rates of *Cryptosporidium* infection seen in patients with HIV and other T cell deficiencies.

Diagnosis

- The diagnosis is made by finding *Giardia* cysts or trophozoites in stool. Cyst excretion is intermittent. Trophozoites are only seen in diarrhoeal stool, but cysts can be found in asymptomatic carriers.
- Examination of a single stool has a sensitivity of 50–70%; with serial examination of three stools, sensitivities up to 90% can be achieved.
- Higher yields can be obtained from duodenal biopsy or aspiration.
- Stool examination is labour intensive and operator dependent.
- ELISA tests for *Giardia* antigen in stool are reliable, with a higher sensitivity than microscopy for a single sample, and allow rapid screening of large numbers of samples.
- Serological tests in plasma are insensitive for the diagnosis of disease.
- PCR techniques have also been developed for detection of *Giardia* in stool.
- However, in high-prevalence, resource-poor countries, microscopy continues to be the most readily available investigation and also allows detection of other intestinal parasites.
- Endoscopy is rarely necessary for routine diagnosis, but if it is to be done as part of investigations for malabsorption, samples should be collected to look for trophozoites.
- Apart from the presence of the trophozoites, the mucosal histology may show varying degrees of villous atrophy, crypt hyperplasia or inflammation with polymorphonuclear leucocytes or eosinophils.
- Malabsorption can occur despite normal light microscopy findings.
- *Giardia* does not invade the mucosa so eosinophilia or leucocytosis are not seen in peripheral blood.

Management

- The drug for which there is most experience is metronidazole, given orally once daily for three days.
- Treatment can be repeated if the infection is not eradicated.
- Tinidazole has a similar efficacy to metronidazole (70–100% eradication) and the advantage of single dose administration.
- Albendazole and mebendazole have lower reported efficacy (50–100%) but the advantage of covering for other intestinal parasites.
- Immunocompromised patients may require a longer course of treatment and specialist advice is recommended.

Prevention

- Safe disposal and treatment of faecal matter to prevent contamination of food and water are the mainstay of prevention. The fact that *Giardia* is still seen in countries with sophisticated sanitation shows that these measures will not eradicate the organism completely but will considerably reduce the prevalence and intensity of infection.

- Breast milk from mothers in endemic countries contains *Giardia*-specific IgA and exclusive breastfeeding does delay the appearance of infection in infants.
- Mass school-based treatment programmes are appropriate in high-prevalence areas, and are of benefit both for the individual child and for the wider community by reducing transmission rates. Drugs with both antihelmintic and antiprotozoan activity, such as albendazole and nitazoxanide, are valuable as many children will have multiple parasites.
- Vitamin A and zinc supplementation, given separately or together, reduce the frequency of *Giardia* infections in children.
- Returning travellers and migrants from high-prevalence countries contribute up to 85% of symptomatic disease in developed countries. Screening and treating migrants from high-prevalence countries may help to further reduce the incidence in developed countries.
- Simple handwashing is an important control measure in institutional settings.

Future research

- Despite extensive study of *Giardia* infection in mouse models and to a lesser degree in human *in vitro* systems, the most important antigens in inducing immunity are still unclear and may vary in different geographical regions.
- There are as yet no obvious candidate antigens for a human vaccine.
- A few animal studies on the induction of immunity have shown successful induction of specific immunoglobulin but without clinically significant protection from infection.
- It seems unlikely that an effective vaccine will be developed in the immediate future.
- Better implementation of known effective preventive measures will continue to be the most important factor in disease control.

Further reading

Chandy E, McCarthy J. *What is the Most Appropriate Treatment for* Giardiasis? Available at: ℬ www.ichrc.org (accessed 14 October 2010).

Farthing MJ. New perspectives in giardiasis. *J Med Microbiol* 1992;**37**:1–2.

Faubert G. Immune response to *Giardia duodenalis*. *Clin Microbiol Rev* 2000;**13**:35–54.

Gonococcal infection

📖 see also Chapters 11, 30, 31, 37

Name and nature of organism

- *Neisseria gonorrhoeae* is an intracellular Gram-negative diplococcal bacterium.

Epidemiology

- Gonorrhoea is the second most common bacterial STI in the UK.
- Humans are the only reservoir of infection.
- The source of the organism is the exudate/secretions from an infected mucosal surface.
- Childhood infection occurs as two distinct clinical entities:
  - Newborn infants
  - Children and adolescents.
- Infection in prepubertal children is commonly the result of child sexual abuse.
- The highest incidence of infection is in females aged 16–19 years.
- It is difficult to obtain data on younger adolescents due to asymptomatic infection and reluctance to access healthcare services.
- The highest rates of infection are in urban areas (e.g. London) and in black ethnic minority populations.
- Gonococcal infection often coexists with *Chlamydia trachomatis* infection.

Transmission

- Transmission is due to direct inoculation of infected secretions from one mucous membrane to another.
- The risk of acquiring infection varies between 20% and 50% after a single episode of vaginal intercourse.
- Infection of the newborn results from passage through the birth canal of an infected mother, although infection after caesarean delivery has been documented.
- Prematurity and prolonged rupture of membranes increase the risk of the neonate acquiring the infection.
- Infection in children and adolescents occurs through sexual contact.
- Reinfection with the same strain is common as protective immunity does not develop.

Incubation period

- Incubation is usually 2–7 days.
- Incubation in the neonate is often <3 days but occasionally symptoms do not develop until 2–3 weeks after delivery.

Period of infectivity

- Infectivity lasts for as long as no treatment is given and the discharge continues.
- Infectivity may occur with no or minimal symptoms, especially in females.
- In adults without treatment, infectivity can continue for 3–6 months.

Clinical features and sequelae

Newborn infants

- Prominent eyelid oedema followed by chemosis.
- Discharge is initially watery but progresses to become mucopurulent.
- It can be unilateral or bilateral.
- Corneal ulceration, perforation, and blindness can occur without treatment.
- Scalp abscesses can occur with the use of fetal monitoring in an infected mother.
- Rarely disseminated disease can occur, resulting in septic arthritis or meningitis.

Children and adolescents

- Involves mucous membranes exposed to sexual contact, e.g. genital tract, urethra, pharynx, and rectum.
- The clinical spectrum varies from asymptomatic infection (less common in prepubertal children) through vaginitis, urethritis, or cervicitis with discharge to pelvic inflammatory disease, epididymitis, and perihepatitis.
- Disseminated gonococcal infection occurs rarely and can result in septic arthritis and skin lesions—classically necrotic pustules on an upper limb with polyarthralgia or arthritis.
- The most significant long-term sequelae is salpingitis, leading to female infertility.
- An intact complement system is required to eradicate the organism.

Diagnosis

- Microscopic examination, Gram stain, and culture of exudate from a swab is the gold standard.
- When culturing samples from non-sterile mucosal surfaces, a culture medium that inhibits growth of normal flora and non-pathogenic *Neisseria* species must be used.

- NAATs are available but should be confirmed using culture.
- NAATs have good sensitivity and specificity for urine samples, male urethral, and endocervical specimens.
- Culture confirmation is essential in child sexual abuse cases for medicolegal purposes.
- Identification of *N. gonorrhoeae* should lead to screening for other STIs.

Management

- Antimicrobial resistance patterns are continuously changing.
- Surveillance systems are in place and it is important to understand local resistance patterns.
- Current recommendations involve using third-generation cephalosporins.

Newborn infants

- For an asymptomatic infant born to a clinically infected mother:
  - Use ceftriaxone or cefotaxime as a single dose.
- For uncomplicated ophthalmia neonatorum:
  - Topical treatment alone is inadequate
  - Use ceftriaxone as a single dose if not jaundiced
  - If jaundiced consider cefotaxime as a single dose or in a divided dose regimen
  - Irrigate the eyes well with saline several times a day until the purulent discharge subsides.
- If there is evidence of scalp abscess or septic arthritis, treatment should be continued for 7 days.
- For gonococcal meningitis treatment should be 10–14 days.
- It is important to consider the possibility of coexistent *Chlamydia* infection.
- Investigation and treatment of the mother should be done through specialists in genitourinary medicine.

Children and adolescents

- For uncomplicated infection:
  - Ceftriaxone or cefotaxime as a single dose
  Or
  - Cefixime orally for children >12 years.
- Disseminated infection should be treated for 7 days:
  - Treatment can be switched to oral after 24–48 hours if suitable agent available.
- Involve genitourinary medicine specialists to instigate contact tracing if appropriate.
- Consider child sexual abuse at any age but in particular for prepubertal children.
- Consider treating for *Chlamydia*.

Prevention of further cases

Newborn infants

- Where incidence of gonorrhoea is high, antimicrobial eye drops have been used routinely after birth. 1% silver nitrate has been used historically, with erythromycin, or tetracycline used more recently.
- In low-prevalence areas, screening of high-risk pregnant women should be offered.

Children and adolescents

- Children require protection from adults who seek underage sex.
- Adolescents require sex education and accessible health services.
- Contact tracing by genitourinary medicine specialist prevents further spread.

Further research

- The most cost-effective management of multiresistant gonococcal disease is yet to be determined.
- The role of routine antimicrobial eye drops in very high prevalence areas needs to be reinvestigated.

Further reading

British Association for Sexual Health and HIV. *National Guideline on the Treatment of Gonorrhoea in Adults*. 2005. Available at: www.bashh.org/documents/116/116.pdf (accessed 12 July 2009).

Health Protection Agency. *GRASP (The Gonococcal Resistance to Antimicrobials Surveillance Programme)—Report*. Trends in antimicrobial resistant gonorrhoea. 2008. Available at: www.hpa.org.uk.

McDonald N, Mailman T, Desai S. Gonococcal infections in newborns and adolescents. In: Finn A, Pollard AJ, eds. *Hot Topics in Infection and Immunity in Children IV. Adv Exp Med Biol* 2008;**609**:108–30. New York: Springer.

Woods CR. Gonococcal infection in neonates and young children. *Semin Pediatr Infect Dis* 2005;**16**:258–70.

Gram-negative bacteria

📖 see also Chapters 12, 20, 22, 30, 36, 104, 114

Name and nature of the organisms

These bacteria fall into two categories:
- *Enterobacteriaceae* (coliforms): Bacteria whose natural habitat is the gastrointestinal tract of humans and other animals.
- Non-fermentative bacteria: Bacteria whose natural habitats are principally the environment inside and outside hospital. Most important species are:
  - *Pseudomonas* species, especially *P. aeruginosa*
  - *Acinetobacter* species, especially *A. baumanii*
  - *Burkholderia cepacia* complex (Bcc)
  - *Stenotrophomonas maltophilia*.

Enterobacteriaceae

These can be considered in three groups:
- Species that are common commensals of the human gastrointestinal tract, and are common opportunistic community- and hospital-acquired pathogens, e.g. *Escherichia coli*, *Proteus mirabilis*.
- Species that are uncommon gastrointestinal commensals of healthy individuals, and are seen mainly as hospital-acquired pathogens, e.g. *Enterobacter*, *Klebsiella*, *Serratia* species.
- Strains that are unequivocal gastrointestinal pathogens, e.g. *Salmonella*, *Shigella*, *Yersinia* species; enteropathogenic strains of *E. coli*.

Epidemiology
- Almost all children are asymptomatic carriers of one or more strains of *E. coli* in the gastrointestinal tract. *Proteus* is a common commensal.
- For species that are more common in hospitalized patients, antibiotic exposure, duration of hospitalization, invasive medical procedures, and serious underlying disease are important risk factors.
- *Salmonella enterica* subspp. Typhi and Paratyphi, and *Shigella* spp., are human pathogens. Other gastrointestinal pathogens, including other salmonellae and *E. coli* O157 are also frequently carried by animals.

Transmission and incubation period

- Outside the neonatal period most *E. coli* infections are endogenous. Neonatal *E. coli* infections are acquired via mother-to-infant transmission.
- Without control measures all *Enterobacteriaceae* can readily spread in hospitals by direct or indirect person-to-person transmission: the hands of healthcare workers are an especially important route of spread.
- Gastrointestinal pathogens may be spread directly from person to person or animal to person via the faecal-oral route, or indirectly via contaminated food or water.
- Incubation periods vary according to the type of infection, the size of inoculum and route of entry into body: typically 1–5 days for exogenous infections.

Clinical features and sequelae

Infections in vulnerable patients can occur at almost any anatomical site.

Urinary tract infection

- *E. coli* and *Proteus* are the commonest causes of UTI.
- Other species also cause UTI, especially in children with recurrent infections, urinary tract abnormalities or those who are catheterized.

Gastrointestinal infections

- Strains of *E. coli* that are enteropathogens include:
  - Enteropathogenic *E. coli*—causes diarrhoea in infants
  - Enteroinvasive *E. coli*—causes dysenteric illness
  - Verotoxin-producing *E. coli*—causes diarrhoea (often bloody). Sequelae include HUS
  - Enterotoxigenic *E. coli*—causes traveller's diarrhoea.
- *Shigella sonnei* accounts for most cases of shigellosis in Europe: usually mild and self-limiting (other *Shigella* species cause more serious illness). Complications include convulsions and changes in mental status (usually self-limiting).
- Non-typhoidal serovars of *S. enterica* are the second commonest cause of bacterial gastroenteritis (after *Campylobacter*): complications include bacteraemia (infants and the immunocompromised are at increased risk); prolonged convalescent excretion of *Salmonella*.
- *S. enterica* subspecies Typhi and Paratyphi cause a systemic infection (enteric fever), often with little or no gastrointestinal upset.
- Any *Enterobacteriaceae* colonizing the gastrointestinal tract can be opportunistic pathogens in intra-abdominal infections, e.g. appendicitis, intra-abdominal abscesses.

Meningitis

- Meningitis caused by *Enterobacteriaceae* has a poor prognosis.
- *E. coli* is second only to GBS as a cause of neonatal meningitis; *Serratia* is an important cause of nosocomial meningitis on neonatal units.
- Rare outside infancy, except post neurosurgery (especially shunt-associated meningitis).

Respiratory tract infections

- Most important as a cause of ventilator-associated pneumonia.

Intravascular device-related infections
Septicaemia
- *Enterobacteriaceae* are the commonest causes of Gram-negative septicaemia.
- May be secondary to a local focus of infection (e.g. UTI).
- Primary septicaemia occurs in patients who are neutropenic or premature: the gastrointestinal tract is presumably the source of infection.

Diagnosis
- Culture of samples from the suspected site of infection is the mainstay of diagnosis of these infections.

Management and treatment
- β-lactam antibiotics are a mainstay of treatment. However β-lactamase production is common: different species produce different types of β-lactamase.[1]
  - *E. coli* and *Klebsiella* typically produce β-lactamases that confer resistance to amoxicillin, but co-amoxiclav and cephalosporins remain active.
  - *Enterobacter* and *Serratia* can produce cephalosporinases that confer resistance to cephalosporins and co-amoxiclav, as well as amoxicillin. Production of these enzymes may be induced by exposure to β-lactams: therefore isolates that appear sensitive on initial testing may become resistant during treatment.
  - Extended-spectrum β-lactamases (ESBL) are becoming increasingly common in species such as *E. coli* and *Klebsiella* that have previously been relatively antibiotic-sensitive. These enzymes confer resistance to penicillins and cephalosporins, and often coincide with resistance to other antibiotic classes, including aminoglycosides and fluoroquinolones.
  - Carbapenems are the β-lactamase class that has most reliable activity against *Enterobacteriaceae*, but carbapenemase-producing strains are emerging: treatment options for such strains are limited to a few older, more toxic antibiotics, e.g. colistin.
- Trimethoprim and nitrofurantoin are useful for UTIs, although *Proteus* species are always resistant to nitrofurantoin.
- For more serious infections, aminoglycosides, often in combination with a β-lactam antibiotic, are used.
- Fluoroquinolones (e.g. ciprofloxacin) are also useful, especially for treating gastrointestinal infections and infections with antibiotic-resistant *Enterobacteriaceae*: however, increasing resistance is a problem.

Prevention
- Prevention of transmission of *Enterobacteriaceae* in hospitals:
  - General hygiene
  - Care of invasive medical devices, e.g. intravascular devices, endotracheal tubes
  - Antibiotic stewardship

- Isolation of patients in high-risk situations (e.g. *Serratia* on neonatal units, antibiotic-resistant strains, gastrointestinal pathogens).
- Prevention of gastrointestinal infections in the community:
  - General hygiene, food hygiene
  - Care during contact with animals, e.g. animal petting farms
  - Exclusion of symptomatic children from school or nursery.

Non-fermentative Gram-negative bacteria

Epidemiology

- Opportunistic human pathogens, especially in hospitalized patients. Important risk factors for infection include:
  - Antibiotic exposure
  - Intensive and high-dependency care
  - Cystic fibrosis, neutropenia, burns.
- Hospital outbreaks can occur, especially on NICUs or PICUs.
- Some species, e.g. *P. aeruginosa* and Bcc are important pathogens in cystic fibrosis outside hospital.

Transmission

- Direct or indirect person-to-person transmission in hospitals.
- Bacteria also found in the hospital environment, especially moist settings (e.g. taps, sinks, ventilator equipment); *Acinetobacter* also found in dust.
- Routes of acquisition of bacteria outside hospital are poorly understood.

Clinical features and sequelae

Infections in vulnerable patients can occur at any anatomical site.

Urinary tract infection

- Especially in children with recurrent infections, urinary tract abnormalities or who are catheterized.

Respiratory tract infections

- Ventilator-associated pneumonia.
- Lower respiratory tract colonization and infection in cystic fibrosis and bronchiectasis.

Skin and soft tissue infections

- Infections with *P. aeruginosa* range from mild folliculitis to serious infections such as cellulitis, malignant otitis externa.
  - Infections in the presence of neutropenia can be fulminant or intractable.
- Important pathogens in patients with non-surgical wounds, especially burns (especially *P. aeruginosa*, *Acinetobacter*).

Intravascular device-related infections

Septicaemia

- May be secondary to a local focus of infection (e.g. urinary tract).
- Primary septicaemia occurs in those with neutropenia, prematurity.
- *P. aeruginosa* is particularly serious, with a high mortality rate.

Management and treatment

All of these bacteria are usually resistant to common antibiotics.

- *P. aeruginosa* is usually sensitive to:
  - Third-generation cephalosporins (e.g. ceftazidime) or anti-pseudomonal penicillins (piperacillin, ticarcillin)
  - Aminoglycosides: tobramycin more active than gentamicin *in vitro*, and often preferred for cystic fibrosis treatment
  - Carbapenems (meropenem, imipenem, doripenem, but **not** ertapenem)
  - Fluoroquinolones (e.g. ciprofloxacin)
  - Polymyxins
- Resistance to all of these agents may occur: most common with carbapenems and fluoroquinolones.
- Antibiotic sensitivities of *Acinetobacter* species are unpredictable: pathogenic strains often multiply antibiotic resistance. Carbapenems are the most reliable antibiotics.
- *S. maltophilia* is highly antibiotic-resistant. Strains may appear sensitive to anti-pseudomonal antibiotics *in vitro*, but clinical response to these agents is usually poor: co-trimoxazole is the most reliable antibiotic; ticarcillin + clavulanic acid (Timentin) is another option.
- Bcc also multiply antibiotic resistant: combinations of two or more agents generally used, based on results of sensitivity testing.

Prevention

- General hygiene, care of invasive medical devices, e.g. intravascular devices, endotracheal tubes
- Antibiotic stewardship
- Isolation of patients in high-risk situations (e.g. neonatal units, PICUs, cystic fibrosis clinics).

Future research

Increasing antibiotic resistance in Gram-negative bacteria means that development of new antibiotics is a major priority. The pipeline of novel antibiotics active against Gram-negative bacteria is extremely worryingly empty!

The role of colonization and prediction of subsequent invasive disease needs further study, especially in neonatal units. There is going to be a difficult balance between preserving carbapenamase antibiotics and empiric treatment of septic children colonized with ESBL organisms. Improved risk-based algorithms will be required.

Serious Gram-negative bacterial infections are still associated with high rates of mortality and morbidity: further research into the optimal management of these conditions is needed.

Vaccines to protect against some Gram-negative bacteria are at various stages of development. Further work is required to test these, and to better understand immune mechanisms to facilitate development of new vaccine technologies.

Key reference

1 Thomson KS. ESBL, AmpC, and carbapenemase issues. *J Clin Microbiol* 2010;**48**:1019–25.

Haemophilus influenzae

📖 see also Chapters 5, 27, 28, 29, 44

Name and nature of organism

- *Haemophilus influenzae* is a small, non-motile Gram-negative coccobacillus and is an important cause of invasive bacterial infections in children and adults.
- *H. influenzae* can be differentiated according to its capsular polysaccharide composition into six serotypes (a to f).
- *H. influenzae* serotype b (Hib) possesses a polyribosyl ribitol phosphate (PRP) polysaccharide capsule, which is the major virulence factor for the organism, and protects the organism from phagocytosis.
- *H. influenzae* strains that lack a polysaccharide capsule are classified as non-encapsulated.

Epidemiology

- Currently, Hib causes an estimated three million cases of serious disease and 400 000 deaths annually worldwide
- Prior to the introduction of routine vaccination, Hib was responsible for over 90% of invasive *H. influenzae* infections in young children.
- Children <5 years were at highest risk from Hib disease, with the peak incidence in the second half of the first year of life, when protective maternal antibodies waned.
- Asplenia, sickle cell disease, malignancy, and antibody deficiency syndromes are associated with an increased risk of developing invasive Hib disease.
- In children <5 years, other risk factors for invasive Hib disease include low socioeconomic status, lack of breastfeeding in infancy, and regular nursery or daycare attendance.
- Infections due to other *H. influenzae* serotypes and non-encapsulated *H. influenzae* are rare and summarized at the end of the chapter.

Hib conjugate vaccine

- The Hib conjugate vaccine induces both antibody production and immunological memory, and is highly effective in preventing invasive Hib disease.
- In the UK, the introduction of the Hib conjugate vaccine into the infant immunization programme at 2, 3, and 4 months of age in October 1992 led to a rapid decline in the incidence of invasive Hib disease across all age groups, through a combination of direct and indirect (herd immunity) protection.
- There is no evidence that other *Haemophilus* serotypes or other pathogens have replaced Hib as a cause of serious bacterial infections in children after the introduction of routine Hib immunization.

- Between 1999 and 2002, the number of cases increased, particularly in children <5 years, which led to the introduction of a 6-month booster campaign in 2003 and the subsequent introduction of a routine 12-month booster dose into the infant immunization programme.
- In 2009, there were only 37 cases in all age groups in England and Wales, including 6 in infants, 4 among 1–4 year-olds and 27 in adults.

Transmission

- Humans are the only known reservoirs for Hib.
- In the pre-vaccine era, children <5 years of age were the primary reservoirs of Hib, with nasopharyngeal colonization rates of 3–9%.
- Because the Hib conjugate vaccine also reduces carriage, vaccinated children are rarely colonized; instead, older children and adults are more likely to harbour the organism and may now act as primary reservoirs for ongoing transmission of Hib to susceptible individuals.
- Person-to-person transmission occurs through respiratory droplet spread, but may be acquired through contact with infected respiratory secretions.
- Carriers of Hib are infectious as long as organisms are present in the nasopharynx, which may be for a prolonged period even without nasal discharge.
- Second episodes of invasive Hib disease in the same individual are extremely rare, with only four cases reported in the UK since 1992.
- In the pre-vaccine era, household (mainly <5 year-olds and immunocompromised individuals) and daycare contacts had a higher risk of developing invasive Hib disease than the general population, although the risk was much higher in the former group; there are no studies on secondary infections after the introduction of routine Hib immunization.

Incubation period

- The incubation period is not known; however, susceptible individuals usually develop disease within 7 days of exposure to Hib.

Clinical features

- Children with invasive Hib disease may develop a range of clinical manifestations, particularly meningitis, septicaemia, and epiglottitis.
- The introduction of the Hib conjugate vaccine has altered the epidemiology and clinical presentation of invasive Hib disease in children such that the median age at Hib disease has shifted from 6–12 months to 2–3 years and meningitis (which used to account for 60–75% of cases in the prevaccine era) now accounts for around 25%, while bacteraemia now accounts for 50% of cases; the proportion of cases presenting with epiglottitis and other invasive infections remains at ~15% and ~10%, respectively.
- **Meningitis** due to Hib is clinically indistinguishable from other causes of bacterial meningitis; symptoms of meningitis include fever,

headache, photophobia, stiff neck, vomiting, and decreased mental status; severe cases may present with convulsions and coma; infants (<1 year) usually present with non-specific symptoms such as fever, vomiting, refusal to feed, and irritability, but severe cases may develop hypotonia, bulging fontanelle, a high-pitched cry, and convulsions; in industrialized countries, Hib meningitis has a mortality of ~5% but may be as high as 40% in resource-poor countries. In addition, 10–15% of survivors will develop severe long-term complications (e.g. cerebral palsy, hydrocephalus, epilepsy, blindness, sensorineural deafness) and a further 15–20% will have minor long-term sequelae (e.g. partial deafness, behavioural and learning difficulties, speech and language problems).
- **Epiglottitis** is a life-threatening condition that is caused by infection of the epiglottis, aryepiglottis, and arytenoids; it usually occurs in children aged 2–7 years, who present very acutely with a short history of high fever, tachypnoea, inspiratory stridor, and excessive drooling.
- Other less common clinical manifestations of Hib disease include pneumonia, cellulitis, septic arthritis, osteomyelitis, and pericarditis.

Diagnosis

- Epiglottitis is usually diagnosed clinically, but Hib may be isolated from blood cultures if taken prior to administering antibiotics.
- Diagnosis relies on isolation of *H. influenzae* from a normally sterile site (e.g. CSF, blood, joint or pleural aspirate, etc.) in a child with clinical symptoms and signs of infection.
- *H. influenzae* serotype can be confirmed by PCR; in the UK, this usually requires submitting the isolate to the HPA Respiratory and Systemic Infections Laboratory.
- Rapid antigen tests for Hib are available but rarely used.

Management and treatment

- Epiglottitis is an acute medical emergency; children presenting with acute airway obstruction usually require immediate intubation and ventilation.
- Third-generation IV cephalosporins, including cefotaxime and ceftriaxone, are the empirical treatment of choice for suspected invasive bacterial infections and are highly effective against all *H. influenzae*, including Hib.
- Adjuvant dexamethasone, especially if given before or with the first dose of antibiotic, will reduce the risk of long-term sequelae, including sensorineural hearing loss (SNHL), in patients with Hib meningitis.

Prevention

- The Hib conjugate vaccine remains the most effective measure for preventing invasive Hib disease.

- By reducing carriage, it also helps reduce transmission to susceptible individuals of all ages, thus providing herd protection.
- All children should be immunized in infancy (three doses in the first 6 months of life) and receive a booster dose at around 12 months of age.
- Unimmunized children >1 year would be sufficiently protected with one dose of the Hib conjugate vaccine.
- Rifampicin remains the prophylactic antibiotic therapy of choice among contacts of a case of invasive Hib disease because it can eradicate nasopharyngeal carriage in >95% of recipients, is well tolerated, and has an excellent safety profile.
- Treatment courses of quinolones and azithromycin may be suitable alternatives.
- Among index cases, treatment with >2 days of intravenous cephalosporins should eradicate nasopharyngeal carriage; however, patients treated with shorter courses or those treated with other antibiotics should receive rifampicin prophylaxis before hospital discharge in order to eradicate carriage.
- Children who develop invasive Hib disease, particularly if <2 years old, should have Hib antibodies checked after recovering from infection in order to ensure adequate protection against future Hib infections.
- Children with Hib antibody concentrations <1µg/ml or whose antibody concentrations cannot be measured should receive a dose of Hib vaccine after recovering from the infection, irrespective of their previous vaccination history.
- The local health protection unit should be informed of all cases of Hib in order to initiate contact tracing.
- All household contacts, including pregnant women, should be offered chemoprophylaxis if there is a vulnerable individual (an immunosuppressed or asplenic person of any age or a child <10 years, irrespective of vaccination status) in the household.
- All unimmunized and partially immunized children in the household should complete their primary immunization.
- Families of children attending the same preschool or primary school as the patient should be informed to seek medical advice if their child becomes unwell.

Invasive infections due to other *H. influenzae*

- Non-encapsulated *H. influenzae* commonly colonize humans and are a well-recognized cause of otitis media and sinusitis in healthy children, but are rarely responsible for invasive infections.
- Following the introduction of routine Hib immunization, infections due to non-type b *H. influenzae* have become relatively more important and account for ~80% of all invasive *H. influenzae* cases in children.
- In 2009, there were 82 cases of invasive non-type b *H. influenzae* disease in children <15 years in England and Wales, mainly due to non-encapsulated serotypes (71 cases).

- In the first week of life, the incidence of invasive non-encapsulated *H. influenzae* infections is 10 times higher than that for Hib and is associated with septicaemia in the mother, increased complications during labour, preterm delivery, a fulminant course of infection, and high case fatality, particularly among premature infants.
- After the neonatal period, invasive non-encapsulated *H. influenzae* infections are relatively rare and usually occur in children with underlying medical conditions (40–70%), particularly immunodeficiency; the case fatality rate is significantly higher than Hib, particularly in the first 6 months of life.
- Invasive infections due to other capsulated *H. influenzae* (a, c, d, and f) are extremely rare and mainly due to serotype f (~75%); they, too, usually occur in immunocompromised children.

Future research

- The duration of long-term protection provided by the Hib conjugate vaccines remains uncertain—in particular, there are concerns that because the Hib conjugate vaccine is so effective in reducing carriage, there will be fewer opportunities for natural boosting of immunity in children which may result in waning of protective Hib antibody concentrations, as has recently been shown in adults.
- The reduction in carriage of Hib in vaccinated children could also open an ecological niche and encourage colonization by other potentially pathogenic organisms, including non-b encapsulated and non-encapsulated *H. influenzae*, emphasizing the importance of continued long-term surveillance of invasive *H. influenzae* infections across all age groups.
- Further studies are also needed to define more clearly the risk factors, clinical presentation, and outcome of invasive non-type b *H. influenzae* infections in children.

Further reading

Heath PT, Booy R, Azzopardi HJ, *et al.* Non-type b *Haemophilus influenzae* disease: clinical and epidemiologic characteristics in the *Haemophilus influenzae* type b vaccine era. Pediatr Infect Dis J 2001;**20**:300–5.

Ladhani S, Slack MP, Heys M, White J, Ramsay ME. Fall in *Haemophilus influenzae* serotype b (Hib) disease following implementation of a booster campaign. Arch Dis Child 2008;**93**:665–9.

Ladhani S, Neely F, Heath PT, *et al.* Recommendations for the prevention of secondary haemophilus influenzae type b (Hib) disease. J Infect 2009;**58**:3–14.

Chapter 71

Hand, foot, and mouth disease

📖 see also Chapters 34, 64

Name and nature of organism

- HFMD is caused by enteroviruses, mainly coxsackieviruses A16 and A5 but others including A10, B1, B3, and enterovirus 71 have been implicated. Coxsackie A16 and enterovirus 71 are most commonly associated with epidemics.
- Enteroviruses are member of the *Picornovirus* family; small (*pico*) non-enveloped RNA viruses. Humans are the only known hosts of enteroviruses.

Epidemiology

- HFMD is common in children especially those aged 1–4 years. It has not been described in neonates or adults >65 years.
- Worldwide disease is endemic and occurs sporadically and in epidemics, especially in preschool childcare establishments.
- There is a bimodal seasonal pattern, with the disease being most common in summer and late autumn/early winter.

Transmission and incubation period

- Transmission is either by faecal-oral route or droplet spread from nasal secretions.
- Incubation period is 3–6 days.

Clinical features and sequelae

- Mild pyrexia usually precedes the illness by 3–5 days.
- Non-tender macular or vesicular lesions 4–8mm across tongue and buccal mucosa.
- 75% of cases develop a rash, usually 1 day after mouth lesions. The rash lasts about a week and can be tender vesicular, maculopapular, or pustular in morphology (4–8mm in size). The rash is more commonly present on the hands than on the feet and the dorsal surfaces are more commonly affected than the palms and soles. The rash can also develop on the buttocks, trunk, genitalia, face, and limbs.

- Classically vesicles are seen along the sides of the fingers, which is virtually diagnostic of HFMD.
- Rare features include the neurological complications of aseptic meningitis and encephalitis.
- Epidemic HFMD seen in Australia, Malaysia, Japan, Taiwan, Hong Kong and Singapore is associated with enterovirus 71. These epidemics are associated with a large number of children with HFMD developing rapid clinical deterioration with cardiopulmonary failure, pulmonary haemorrhage, or CNS involvement.

Diagnosis

- HFMD is typically a clinical diagnosis and no tests are required.
- Virus can be cultured from lesions or stool if required.

Management and treatment

- As HFMD is mild and self-limiting, symptomatic treatment is all that is usually required.

Prevention

- Children should be 'isolated' until the rash has settled. The virus may continue to be shed in stool for weeks after the infection; however, it is not practical to isolate them after the symptoms have settled.
- Strict personal hygiene should be encouraged and sharing of cups, cutlery, etc. should be prohibited.

Further reading

Frydenberg A, Starr M. Hand, foot and mouth disease. *Aust Fam Phys* 2003;**32**:594–5.

Chapter 72

Head lice (pediculosis)

see also Chapters 3, 21

Name and nature of organism

- Head lice (*Pediculus humanus capitis*) are arthropods.
- Humans are the only known host. The lice almost exclusively live on the scalp and attach to the hair-shafts by means of specialized claws.
- The parasites feed on scalp blood, accessed by piercing the skin. Without a blood meal (i.e. after leaving the host) head lice usually die within 2–3 days, but can rarely survive a few days longer.
- The adult head louse has a lifespan of approximately 1 month.
- During adult life the female lays between 5 and 10 eggs each day, which are attached to the hair shafts.
- Nymphs emerge from the eggs after 6–10 days, develop through several nymphal stages and become adults after about 10 days.
- Adult lice are approximately 1–3mm in size. Eggs measure approximately 0.8–1mm, but are still visible to the naked eye.
- Technically, 'nits' are empty egg cases (not unhatched eggs).

Epidemiology

- Recent large-scale epidemiological data are scarce.
- The most recent regional studies in the UK have reported prevalences between 2% and 10% among school-aged children. The prevalence is highest in preschool and early primary school children.
- Infestation of family members (most frequently siblings) of the index case is common.

Transmission

- Head lice are wingless insects and cannot fly or jump.
- Transmission predominately occurs via close physical contact (head-to-head).
- There is limited evidence that transmission can also occur via fomites (e.g. combs, hair accessories, hats and clothing).

Clinical features and sequelae

- Many infestations are asymptomatic.
- Pruritus affecting the scalp is the most common, and frequently the only, symptom reported. Pruritus tends to occur within 2–6 weeks

during the first infestation, but considerably earlier during subsequent infestations (often within 1–2 days). It is thought that this phenomenon is based on a delayed-type hypersensitivity reaction.
- Other potential signs include localized erythema and urticaria, as well as postauricular and cervical lymphadenopathy.
- Secondary bacterial infection (most commonly with *Staphylococcus aureus*) may occur.
- Head lice infestation can cause considerable distress to affected children and their families. Related bullying, social stigmatization and exclusion from school can have a significant impact on the child's emotional and psychological wellbeing.

Diagnosis

- The diagnosis of active head lice infestation is based on the detection of live lice.
- The entire scalp should be combed thoroughly with a detection comb (finer toothed than a conventional comb); wetting of the hair or use of hair conditioner can facilitate this process. The comb should be inspected for the presence of live lice after each pass, which may be aided by the use of a magnifying glass.
- Eggs should also be searched for, although their presence does not confirm active infestation. Viable eggs are tan- or brown-coloured, while hatched eggs are white or opaque. Eggs further than a few inches away from the scalp are unlikely to be viable, as new eggs are laid close to the scalp.
- Eggs should not be confused with dandruff; the latter is easily removed with a comb, whereas eggs stick firmly to the hair shafts.

Management and treatment

General principles

- Treatment should only be initiated when live lice are identified.
- The entire family of an index case should be screened; all affected individuals need to be treated to break the cycle of reinfestation.
- General household 'decontamination' measures (e.g. furniture and carpets) are unnecessary, as lice cannot survive for long periods without host contact. However, lice have been reported to migrate onto bedlinen, towels, and clothes. Although potential reinfestation from these sources continues to be debated, it may be advisable to change and wash these items regularly during the treatment phase. Machine laundering at 50°C or above is effective for decontaminating fabrics.

Pediculocidal treatment

• Four 'conventional' pediculocidal agents (which are essentially neurotoxic insecticides) are licensed for the treatment of head lice in the UK: malathion (Derbac-M®, Quellada M®) permethrin (Lyclear®), phenothrin, and carbaryl. However, the production of the latter two agents has been discontinued in the UK. There are no reports of neurotoxic side effects in patients when treatment is applied correctly. All preparations are available over the counter. Various formulations are available; lotions and liquid formulations are more effective than shampoos.

• Before the mid-1990s all 'conventional' pediculocides showed efficacies in excess of 80% in clinical trials. In the past decade, several studies have reported a considerable decline in the efficacy of these agents. Subsequently, *in vitro* studies have documented the emergence of resistance in the parasite population (based on genetic changes). Although a considerable proportion of 'treatment failures' are thought to be due to incorrect use of treatment and reinfestation rather than resistance, it is recommended to use a different class of pediculocide for re-treatment (note: permethrin and phenothrin both belong to the class of pyrethroids).

• Recently, two new preparations for the treatment of head lice have been licensed—a dimeticone-based solution (Hedrin®) and a solution containing isopropyl myristate/cyclomethicone (Full Marks Solution®). Unlike 'conventional' pediculocides, their pediculocidal action is not based on neurotoxic effects, but is thought be due to disruption of the water balance in lice. Early trials assessing these new preparations reported cure rates between 70% and 82%.

• Pediculocidal treatment has to be applied on two occasions seven days apart, as all agents primarily kill nymphs and adult lice, while their ovicidal activity is relatively poor. This time gap allows surviving eggs to hatch; new nymphs are then killed by the second application.

• The hair should be re-examined 2–3 days after the second application to detect any remaining lice (note: treatment will not remove eggs). If live lice are detected treatment should be repeated with another class of agents.

Alternative forms of treatment

• Wet combing, based purely on the mechanical removal of lice, is a potential alternative to treatment with pediculocides. Most studies reported cure rates ranging between 50% and 75% with this approach. A number of different louse and nit combs, as well as combined kits, are commercially available (e.g. the Bug Buster Kit—available on NHS prescription). Combs used for wet combing are even finer toothed than regular combs and detection combs. Any shampoo or conditioner can be used for this process, as these merely act as lubricants. Wet combing sessions (lasting for >30 minutes) should be carried out every 3 days for 14 days (i.e. five sessions in total). Although labour-intensive compared to pediculocidal treatment, there are no potential side effects and there are some data to suggest that many parents favour this approach over pediculocidal treatment when offered the choice.

- There is no convincing evidence that 'natural treatments' traditionally used in some cultures (e.g. herbal remedies, vinegar, alcohol, mayonnaise) are effective; some of these 'treatments' are potentially dangerous (e.g. petroleum, kerosene).

Prevention

- There are no effective strategies to prevent head lice infestation. Head lice have no preference for 'clean' or 'dirty', 'short' or 'long' hair. Also, contrary to common belief, the risk of head lice infestation is not related to social status.
- Although there is little evidence for this route of transmission—sharing of combs, brushes, and hair accessories with individuals known to have head lice should be avoided.
- Exclusion from school is not justified; however, prompt treatment should be encouraged.

Further research

- Knowledge about local resistance patterns within the parasite population may potentially aid in improving treatment success rates.
- Although the mode of action of dimeticone- and isopropyl myristate/cyclomethicone-based preparations makes the development of resistance relatively unlikely, this aspect requires close monitoring.
- All currently available treatment options are associated with considerable failure rates. Outside study conditions, treatment success rates are likely to be even lower. Therefore, novel agents and treatment methods should be actively investigated. Studies investigating oral ivermectin have shown promising results, but further data are needed.

Further reading

Mumcuoglu KY, Barker SC, Burgess IE, *et al*. International guidelines for effective control of head louse infestations. *J Drugs Dermatol* 2007;**6**:409–14.

Parasiticidal preparations. In: *The British National Formulary for Children*. London: BMJ Publishing Group, the Royal Pharmaceutical Society & the Royal College of Paediatrics and Child Health. Section 13.10.4; pp. 724–6.

The National Library for Health. NHS Clinical Knowledge Summaries: Head lice (clinical topic). Available at: http://cks.library.nhs.uk/head_lice (accessed 23 September 2010).

Tebruegge M, Runnacles J. Is wet combing effective in children with pediculosis capitis infestation? *Arch Dis Child* 2007;**92**:818–20.

Tebruegge M, Pantazidou A, Curtis N. What's bugging you? An update on head lice infestation. *Arch Dis Child Educ Pract Ed* 2010 (in press). doi: 10.1136/adc.2009.178038.

Chapter 73

Helicobacter pylori

see also Chapters 12, 13, 22

Name and nature of organism

- Gastric spiral organisms have been described in humans and other mammals throughout the past century, typically in association with gastritis and peptic ulcer disease.
- A gastric *Campylobacter*-like organism was first isolated in 1984, initially named *Campylobacter pyloridis*, then *Campylobacter pylori*.
- The genus *Helicobacter* was created in 1989, with *H. pylori* defined as the type species.
- *H. pylori* is a Gram-negative spiral organism that colonizes gastric mucosa. It preferentially colonizes the gastric antrum although it may also be found throughout the stomach. It is non-invasive.
- It occupies an inhospitable niche, at a site free from other bacterial colonization, where it has to survive for very long periods at low pH. It is predominantly found within and immediately beneath the gastric mucous layer, where there is less acid than in the gastric lumen, and little proteolytic enzyme activity.

Epidemiology

- This is one of the most common chronic bacterial infections of humankind, affecting over 50% of the world's population.
- There are major differences in incidence in populations worldwide; prevalence increases with age. Age-related prevalence rates vary from 40% in 50 year olds in the UK to 85% by 2 years of age in resource-poor countries.
- There has been a decreasing incidence of *H. pylori* colonization in successive generations of children, particularly from developed countries. There is a sharp fall in prevalence in those aged <50 years, which corresponds to individuals born after the second world war. Subsequent studies in the UK and other developed countries have revealed successive falls in adult *H. pylori* prevalence over recent decades.
- In all communities there is a strong association between *H. pylori* colonization and low socioeconomic status, particularly with determinants of early childhood living conditions.

Transmission and incubation period

- Transmission is almost certainly by direct person-to-person spread, with close personal contact being essential.
- The organism has been cultured from vomitus and faeces; isolated reports have identified bacteria and DNA from the oral cavity.
- Bacterial DNA has been detected in biofilms in water storage systems, but there is no good evidence to support the existence of environmental or animal reservoirs.
- The striking feature of *H. pylori*-associated upper gastrointestinal disease is the very long duration of colonization before the disease state develops. Typically colonization occurs in childhood, but disease appears in adult life after decades of colonization/infection.

Clinical features and sequelae

- Childhood acquisition is usually clinically silent.
- Children should only be tested for *H. pylori* if they have clinical evidence of gastritis or duodenal ulcer disease—not for mild recurrent abdominal pain.
- Colonization always causes gastritis. Gastritis alone does not cause symptoms.
- *H. pylori* is the major cause of duodenal ulceration worldwide.[1] Approximately 0.5% of the adult UK population (around 300 000 people, 20% of all general practice work load) are on long-term acid suppression because of peptic ulcer-related disease. The key underlying cause of this morbidity is *H. pylori* infection.
- Infection only rarely leads to duodenal ulceration in childhood. The proportion of infected individuals who develop duodenal ulceration increase with age, and by mid-adult life up to 10% of infected people in developed countries may have peptic ulceration.
- The pathogenesis of *H. pylori*-associated duodenal ulceration is incompletely understood, although certain bacterial genotypes are associated with disease expression.
- While it seems likely that these virulence determinants are associated with the development of disease, many subjects with apparently pathogenic strains of *H. pylori* within their stomachs remain symptom free, and many ulcer patients harbour 'non-pathogenic' isolates.
- Long-term *H. pylori* colonization is a risk factor for the development of gastric carcinoma in adult life. Infection has also been shown to cause very rare gastric mucosal B-cell non-Hodgkin lymphomas (MALTomas).
- There is no good evidence for a link between *H. pylori* and recurrent abdominal pain in childhood. Diagnosis of *H. pylori* should not form part of the investigation of abdominal pain in childhood unless duodenal ulceration is suspected.
- Iron deficiency: There is evidence that refractory iron deficiency anaemia may be associated with childhood *H. pylori* in some populations, and that eradication of *H. pylori* may improve response to iron therapy, but results of studies are inconsistent.[2]

Diagnosis

- Culture or histology from endoscopically obtained biopsies is the diagnostic gold standard. Endoscopy also establishes whether a duodenal ulcer is present. Gastric mucosal biopsies are cultured on selective enriched media, in a microaerobic atmosphere, at 37°C, for 5 days. Success has also been reported from research projects culturing samples obtained from string tests, vomitus, and occasionally faeces.
- Serology: Measurement of specific IgG by ELISA is a reliable diagnostic test, suitable for primary diagnosis in older children and adults. It may be unreliable in younger children (<10 years) and almost certainly unreliable among the <5s. It is not useful to check eradication or reinfection, as specific IgG levels may remain positive for 6–12 months after clearance of infection.
- Urea breath tests are widely used for non-invasive diagnosis of *H. pylori* in childhood, with sensitivities and specificities of over 95%. Both radio (^{14}C) and stable isotope (^{13}C) versions exist; they rely on ingestion of a labelled dose of urea, followed by breath collection 30–45 minutes later. A rise in isotopic ratio of the label (^{13}C or ^{14}C) in expired breath indicates gastric urease activity, which in humans is diagnostic of *H. pylori* colonization.
- Faecal *H. pylori* antigen can be detected by ELISA and is a reliable diagnostic test in children.
- Both faecal antigen ELISA and urea breath tests are suitable means of checking eradication and reinfection.

Management and treatment

- Only children with evidence of gastric or duodenal ulcer disease, lymphoma, atrophic gastritis, and a confirmed diagnosis of *H. pylori* should be treated.
- There is no good evidence to support treating children with no symptoms, recurrent abdominal pain, or a family history of ulcer disease and positive *Helicobacter* serology.
- There are not enough randomized controlled treatment trials in children.
- The organism is relatively protected from the host immune response, therefore intensive eradication therapy is required.
- The ability of small surviving inoculates to recolonize means that the emergence of antibiotic resistant strains is very likely. It is therefore important to ensure that when treatment is offered, complete courses are given, appropriate protocols that account for common local resistance patterns are followed, and treatment is reserved for those patients who will benefit from eradication.
- First-line therapies include two antibiotics combined with a proton pump inhibitor for 1–2 weeks. In children, treatment is usually given for 2 weeks, although it is not clear whether the higher eradication rates outweigh the increased side effects and poorer compliance.
- In children, two antibiotics out of metronidazole, clarithromycin, and amoxicillin are used, along with omeprazole.

- Antibiotic resistance is significant. The limited data suggest resistance rates of around 50% for metronidazole and 10% for clarithromycin across Europe. Check country-specific protocols.
- In older children and adults, the same antibiotic regimens are used, but lansoprazole usually replaces omeprazole.
- Poor compliance is associated with a high risk of persistent infection that becomes increasingly difficult to eradicate with further courses of therapy.
- Second-line therapies for eradication failure include colloidal bismuth subcitrate in combination with two antibiotics and a proton pump inhibitor. There may also be a role for ranitidine bismuth subcitrate in combination with two antibiotics. The duration of second-line therapy varies, but is usually for at least 2 weeks.
- Eradication should be confirmed by urea breath test or faecal ELISA 4 weeks after treatment has been completed.
- Patients with peptic ulceration and persistent *H. pylori* infection after second-line therapy require ongoing treatment. Ideally, they should be referred to a specialist centre for isolation of the infecting strain of *H. pylori* and antibiotic sensitivity testing, before embarking on further targeted treatment, which may include sequential antibiotic therapy, including tetracyclines in older children and adults. They should remain on proton pump inhibitors until their *H. pylori* infection is eradicated.
- Reinfection is unusual in those aged >5 years in developed countries. It is not known how common reinfection after eradication is in resource-poor countries, but rates may be very high.

Prevention

- There is no good evidence that the systemic and local immune response seen in *H. pylori* colonization either leads to eradication of the organism or protects against recolonization after treatment. Vaccines have been developed in animal models but are unlikely to be used in humans in the foreseeable future.
- There are no consistent data to support the use of pro or prebiotics to protect against *H. pylori* colonization.
- This may be a disappearing infection in many populations in developed countries—the 'disappearing cohort effect' has been explained above. This could be due to changes in early living conditions, relating to raised standards of living throughout the community.

Future research

- A more detailed understanding of pathogenesis and disease expression is being developed year on year.
- The role of the host immune response in regulating chronic infection, and the influence of chronic, often decades long, gastric inflammation on mucosal immune regulation are important to our understanding of all gastrointestinal inflammatory disease.

- The evolution of the *H. pylori* genome that occurs over decades within one stomach may also influence disease outcome.

Key references

1 Marshall BJ, Goodwin CS, Warren JR, *et al.* Prospective double blind trial of duodenal ulcer relapse rate after eradication of *Campylobacter pylori. Lancet* 1988;**ii**:1439–42.
2 Campbell DI, Thomas JE. *Helicobacter pylori* infection in paediatric practice. *Arch Dis Child Ed Pract* 2005;**90**:ep25–ep30.

Helminthiases

📖 see also Chapters 22, 42, 45

Overview

Helminthiases (parasitic worm infections) are the most common infections in people living in poverty in low- and middle-income countries. This chapter will focus on those causing multisystem disease.

- More than one billion people are affected worldwide, with children often suffering the severest disease because they experience the highest intensity infections, i.e. on average they harbour the largest number of worms in any age group.
- Helminths frequently establish long-standing infections in children and the resulting chronic inflammation and malnutrition can produce deficits in growth, physical development, and physical fitness.
- In some cases, chronic helminth infections produce intellectual and cognitive deficits so that helminthiases also adversely affect childhood learning and education, and ultimately economic development.
- Helminths that cause multisystem disease often exert their effects through larval stages or eggs that migrate through human tissues. The unique inflammatory response to such tissue-invasive organisms usually results in host elevations in IgE and tissue and peripheral blood eosinophils. Therefore, eosinophilia is often a hallmark of infectious helminthiases causing multisystem disease.
- Some but not all tissue-invasive helminths release eggs into the gastrointestinal tract so that many of the diseases discussed here would have negative fecal examinations. Instead, a serological analysis that measures parasite-specific antibodies is often required for diagnostic confirmation.

The major helminthiases discussed here are cysticercosis, hydatid disease, schistosomiasis, strongyloidiasis, toxocariasis, and trichinellosis.

Cysticercosis

Causative organisms

- Cysticercosis is an infection of the muscles, brain, and eye caused by the larval stages of the pork tapeworm, *Taenia solium*.
- When the infection occurs in the brain it is sometimes referred to as neurocysticercosis.

Epidemiology

- Cysticercosis is endemic in low- and middle-income countries where pigs are allowed to feed on human faeces (Fig. 74.1).

- Humans acquire the pork tapeworm, *T. solium*, by consuming uncooked or poorly cooked pork containing the larval stages. The resulting adult tapeworm produces few if any symptoms in the gastrointestinal tract.
- Individuals infected with the pork tapeworm shed eggs, which can be accidentally ingested by other humans. Cysticercosis therefore results when humans inadvertently substitute for the pig in the parasite's life cycle.
- Endemic and hyperendemic areas:
  - Latin America, especially Mexico (and 40 000–160 000 cases the in USA)
  - Eastern Europe
  - Sub-Saharan Africa, especially Burundi and elsewhere in eastern and southern Africa, as well as Cameroon
  - India, China, elsewhere in Southeast Asia.

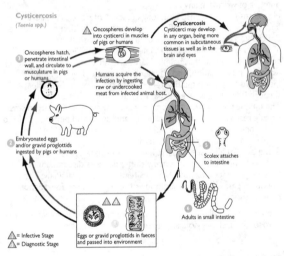

Fig. 74.1 Life cycle of *Taenia solium* and cysticercosis.

(From the Public Health Image Library of the US Centers for Disease Control and Prevention, ♪ http://phil.cdc.gov.)

Transmission and incubation period

- Accidental ingestion of *T. solium* eggs.
- Close personal contact with a tapeworm carrier or food handler.
- Eggs hatch following ingestion release oncospheres that enter muscles, brain, eye, establishing space-occupying lesions within 2–3 months.

Clinical features and sequelae
- Neurocysticercosis—active disease:
    - Single or multiple cysts
    - Neuroimaging reveals ring of inflammation
    - Generalized tonic clonic seizures
    - Partial seizures with generalization
    - Cerebral oedema and encephalitis with multiple cysts
    - Elevated intracranial pressure—rare.
- Calcified cysts of inactive disease—some controversy whether active cysts may also be calcified.
- Other forms:
    - Ventricular and subarachnoid neurocysticercosis
    - Ocular cysticercosis—altered vision or ptosis
    - Muscle involvement.

Diagnosis
- Neuroimaging:
    - 0.5–2.0cm cysts on CT or MRI
    - Presence of scolex (head) pathognomonic
    - Surrounded by oedema and inflammation seen with CT with contrast and/or MRI.
- Confirmatory serodiagnosis: Enzyme-linked immunotransfer blot for detecting anti-cysticercal antibodies.
- Resolution of multiple intracranial lesions on therapy or spontaneous resolution of single, small lesion.

Management and treatment
- Anticonvulsant therapy:
    - Antiepileptic drugs
    - Continue anticonvulsants with calcifications.
- Corticosteroids to reduce inflammation if required.
- Anthelmintics:
    - Not always required with single, resolving ring-enhancing lesion— albendazole or praziquantel.

Prevention
- Sanitation, animal husbandry, meat inspection.
- Veterinary vaccine to prevent transmission to people.

Hydatid disease

Causative organisms
- Cystic echinococcosis
- Larval tapeworm infection
- *Echinococcus granulosus*

Epidemiology
- Enzootic infection of dogs and sheep:
    - Dogs shedding tapeworm eggs ingested by sheep.

- Geographical distribution:
  - South America (especially Chile, Argentina, Uruguay, Andean region)
  - Mediterranean (especially Turkey)
  - Central Asia and South-Central former Soviet republics
  - China (especially western China, e.g. Tibet, Xinjiang provinces)
  - Selected areas in Africa
  - Australia
  - North America, sporadic cases among Inuit, also Arizona and New Mexico.
- High rates among indigenous populations.

Transmission and incubation period
- Accidental ingestion of eggs.
- Several year incubation before detectable cyst appears in the viscera.

Clinical features and sequelae
- Single hydatid cyst in most cases.
- Liver (two-thirds of cases)—hepatic enlargement in right upper quadrant, pain, nausea, vomiting, cyst leakage with allergic manifestations.
- Lungs (one-fourth of cases)—leakage of cyst fluid—chest pain, cough, dyspnoea.
- Other organs including the brain, kidney, spleen.
- Geographical variation in organ location.

Diagnosis
- Radiographic imaging (CT, MRI, ultrasound)
- Fluid-filled cysts
- Sometimes daughter cysts—internal septations noted on radiographs
- Confirmatory serology

Management and treatment
- PAIR:
  - Puncture using ultrasound guidance
  - Aspiration of liquid
  - Injection of scolocidal agent (ethanol, hypertonic saline)
  - Reaspiration.
- Albendazole:
  - Drug treatment used as adjunct with PAIR
  - Monitor liver function and blood cell counts with prolonged use.
- Surgical removal.

Schistosomiasis

Causative organisms
- Urinary and urogenital schistosomiasis
  - *Schistosoma haematobium*

- Intestinal and biliary schistosomiasis
  - *Schistosoma mansoni*
  - *Schistosoma japonicum*
  - *Schistosoma mekongi*

Epidemiology

- 200 million infections worldwide.
- 90% of cases in sub-Saharan Africa.
- Urinary and urogenital schistosomaisis—*S. haematobium*:
  - Two-thirds of cases worldwide
  - Most in sub-Saharan Africa, some cases in Egypt and Middle East
  - Waterborne infection transmitted from *Bulinus* snails (Fig. 74.2)
  - Highest intensity infections in children, adolescents, young adults
  - Important reproductive health problem for young women.
- Intestinal and biliary schistosomiasis—*S. mansoni*:
  - One-third of cases worldwide
  - Most in sub-Saharan Africa, some cases in Egypt and Middle East
  - Only form of schistosomiasis in the Americas, two to seven million cases, mostly in Brazil
  - Transmitted from *Biomphalaria* snails (Fig. 74.2)
  - Highest intensity infections in children, adolescents, young adults.
- Intestinal and biliary schistosomiasis—*S. japonicum* and *S. mekongi*:
  - One million cases
  - Most in China and Philippines (*S. japonicum*)
  - *S. japonicum* transmitted by *Oncomelania* snails (Fig. 74.2)
  - Highest intensity infections in children, adolescents, young adults.

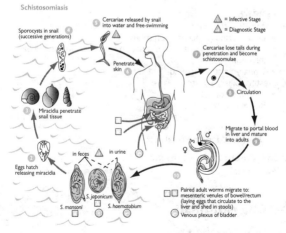

Fig. 74.2 Life cycle of human schistosomes and schistosomiasis.

(From the Public Health Image Library of the US Centers for Disease Control and Prevention, http://phil.cdc.gov.)

Transmission and incubation period
- Freshwater contact with cercariae.
- Direct skin penetration by cercariae (Fig. 74.2).

Clinical features and sequelae
- Clinical manifestations caused by inflammation and granulomas elicited by the parasite eggs in the host tissues.
- Acute schistosomiasis—Katayama fever:
  - Heavy exposure to *S. japonicum* and *S. mansoni* infection
  - 1–2 months after exposure to cercariae
  - Fever, chills, cough, headaches
  - Lymphadenopathy, hepatosplenomegaly, eosinophilia
  - Transverse myelitis in returning travellers (rare).
- Chronic schistosomiasis:
  - Urinary/urogenital schistosomiasis caused by *S. haematobium*
  - Impaired child development and anaemia
  - Haematuria, dysuria, increased frequency
  - Hydroureter, hydronephrosis
  - Renal failure
  - Squamous cell carcinoma of the bladder
  - Female genital schistosomiasis—increased risk of HIV/AIDS.
- Intestinal/biliary schistosomiasis caused by *S. mansoni*, *S. japonicum*, *S. mekongi*:
  - Impaired child development
  - Fatigue, abdominal pain, diarrhoea, bloody diarrhoea
  - Symmer's pipestem (periportal) fibrosis of the liver
  - Hepatosplenomegaly, oesophageal varices.

Diagnosis
- Urinary schistosomiasis:
  - Eggs in urine (concentration required)
  - Serological tests (may not distinguish between current and past infection)
  - Urinary tract ultrasound.
- Intestinal/biliary schistosomiasis:
  - Eggs in stool
  - Rectal biopsy for eggs
  - Serological tests (may not distinguish between current and past infection)
  - Ultrasound for periportal fibrosis.

Management and treatment
- Praziquantel

Strongyloidiasis

Causative organisms
- *Strongyloides stercoralis* is the major species.
- Only major helminth to replicate in human host (in association with hyperinfection).

Epidemiology

- Strongyloidiasis is a soil-transmitted helminthiasis (Fig. 74.3).
- Approximately 30–100 million cases worldwide, with highest rates in low- and middle-income countries, especially tropical regions of the Americas, Southeast Asia, and sub-Saharan Africa
- Foci also present in the USA (Appalachia), southern (Spain and southwest France) and eastern Europe, Japan, and Australia.

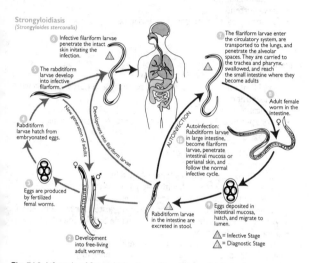

Fig. 74.3 Life cycle of *Strongyloides stercoralis* and strongyloidiasis.

(From the Public Health Image Library of the US Centers for Disease Control and Prevention, ℅ http://phil.cdc.gov.)

Transmission and incubation period

- Larvae in the soil penetrate through skin (similar to human hookworm infection).
- Migratory route through human tissues to reach the intestine unclear or controversial.
- Larvae can migrate through human tissues through the process of autoinfection with clinical manifestations sometimes appearing after years or decades.

Clinical features and sequelae

- Chronic strongyloidiasis:
  - Enteritis
  - Diarrhoea or diarrhoea alternating with constipation
  - Inflammatory bowel disease

- Urticaria
- Larva currens (subcutaneous larval migration in skin).
- *Strongyloides* hyperinfection:
  - In association with steroids used for treatment of other chronic conditions such as cancer, autoimmune disease, but also HTLV-1 (not so much HIV) and other underlying conditions
  - Severe diarrhoea
  - Ulcerative intestinal disease
  - Bronchopneumonitis
  - Larva currens
  - Secondary bacteraemias and bacterial meningitis
  - High mortality rate.

Diagnosis
- Detection of larvae (not eggs) in stool:
  - Often requires multiple stool exams
  - Amplification techniques: nutrient blood agar cultures, Baermann concentration.
- Serological testing—ELISA:
  - Poor specificity in patients coinfected with other helminths (endemic areas).

Management and treatment
- Ivermectin:
  - Safety in young children (<15kg) not established
  - Taken on empty stomach with water (opposite for albendazole)
  - Prolonged or repeated therapy for hyperinfection
  - Combining with albendazole has been suggested for hyperinfection
  - Veterinary formulations for patients unable to take orally
  - Taper steroids in hyperinfection.
- Alternative drugs: albendazole and thiabendazole.
- Antibiotics for bacteraemia and/or bacterial meningitis.

Toxocariasis

Causative organisms
- The canine roundworm *Toxocara canis*
- The feline roundworm *Toxocara cati*, also other zoonotic ascarids
- Larval migrans syndromes associated with eosinophilia and other sequelae

Epidemiology
- The most common helminth infections in the USA and Europe.
- High rates of infection among African American populations living in poverty.
- High rates of infection in Puerto Rico and among some Hispanic American populations.
- Endemic to Eastern Europe.

- Endemic to Brazil, Nigeria, and presumably other low- and middle-income countries.

Transmission and incubation period
- Accidental ingestion of *Toxocara* eggs (Fig. 74.4).
- Environmental contamination of sandboxes and playgrounds.
- Coinfections with toxoplasmosis.

Clinical features and sequelae
- Visceral larva migrans (VLM):
  - Very young children and toddlers 1–4 years of age
  - Loeffler's pneumonitis—wheezing and asthma
  - Hepatitis—hepatomegaly
  - Lymphadenitis
  - Cerebritis—seizures
  - Eosinophilia.
- Ocular larva migrans (OLM):
  - Older children and adolescents
  - Larval tracks and granuloma on the retina
  - Retinitis or endophthalmitis
  - Strabismus.
- Covert toxocariasis:
  - Asymptomatic or partial features of VLM
  - Eosinophilia, wheezing, abdominal pain.

Diagnosis
- VLM or covert toxocariasis—ELISA, high sensitivity and specificity, eosinophilia, elevated IgE and IgG.
- OLM—clinical diagnosis (low sensitivity of ELISA for OLM).

Management and treatment
- Covert toxocariasis or VLM sometimes self-limited.
- All three forms can be treated with albendazole.
- Corticosteroids sometimes helpful.
- OLM frequently requires additional surgical management.

Trichinellosis

Causative organisms
- *Trichinella spiralis* (worldwide) but at lest eight other geographically restricted species including *Trichinella britovi* in Eurasia, *Trichinella nativa* in the Arctic.

Epidemiology
- Worldwide distribution.
- Incidence has declined in North America except among the Inuit in the Canadian Arctic and infections among hunters who consume bears.
- European outbreaks have occurred, and the disease is still relatively common in eastern Europe.

Transmission and incubation period
- Occurs by ingestion of contaminated meat.
- Uncooked or undercooked pork for *T. spiralis* and other species.
- Incubation period of days to weeks before the enteral phase begins.

Clinical features and sequelae
- First, enteral phase, lasting days to weeks:
  - Diarrhoea, nausea, vomiting
- Second, parenteral phase (muscle phase):
  - Fever
  - Periorbital oedema
  - Muscle pain and myositis
  - Carditis and ECG changes
  - Neurotrichinellosis—meningoencephalitis (fewer than a quarter cases)
  - Eosinophilia.

Diagnosis
- Clinical diagnosis and epidemiological history
- Elevated creatine phosphokinase (CPK), LDH
- ECG changes
- Confirmatory serological tests
- Muscle biopsy

Management and treatment
- Analgesics/antipyretics
- Bed rest
- Monitor cardiac function
- Corticosteroids
- Albendazole 400mg orally twice daily × 8–14 days

Prevention
- Prolonged freezing or cooking of pork and other meats.

Cutaneous larva migrans (CLM)

- Caused by cat or dog hookworms—classically *Ancylostoma braziliense*. Larvae survive from dog faeces on beaches of Asia, Central and South America and Caribbean.
- In humans larvae penetrate the skin, but cannot migrate further. They migrate within the skin with a serpiginous track at a rate of 0.5–1cm/day for around 1 week causing itching and a local allergic reaction.
- Most commonly seen on feet or buttocks.
- Can be treated with topical thiabendazole, or oral albendazole. Does not cause systemic disease and larvae die at around 2 weeks anyway.

Future research

There is an urgent need for further large clinical trials to determine the most cost-effective treatment of most helminthiases in children.

Improved pharmacokinetic studies of anthelminthic drugs in young children. Developments of anthelminthic vaccines.

Further reading

Hotez PJ. *Forgotten People, Forgotten Diseases: The Neglected Tropical Diseases and their Impact on Global Health and Development*. Washington DC: ASM Press, 2008:218.

Hotez PJ. Neglected infections of poverty in the United States of America. *PLoS Neglect Tropical Dis* 2008;**2**:e256.

Hotez PJ. Mass drug administration and the integrated control of the world's high prevalence neglected tropical diseases. *Clin Pharmacol Therap* 2009;**85**:659–64.

Hotez PJ, Fenwick A, Savioli L, Molyneux DH. Rescuing the 'bottom billion' through neglected tropical disease control. *Lancet* 2009;**373**:1570–4.

Hepatitis B

📖 see also Chapters 4, 18, 76

Name and nature of infecting organism

- Hepatitis B virus (HBV) is a global health problem and can cause a wide spectrum of liver disorders including acute hepatitis, fulminant hepatitis, chronic hepatitis, liver cirrhosis, or hepatocellular carcinoma (HCC).
- HBV is a prototype member of the *Hepadnaviridae* family.
- The virus contains a partially double-stranded DNA, DNA polymerase with reverse transcriptase activity and hepatitis B core antigen (HBcAg), all surrounded by hepatitis B surface antigen (HBsAg).
- Eight genotypes of HBV have been defined (A–H), and each genotype has a unique geographical distribution. Infection with different genotypes may have different clinical course and outcomes.

Epidemiology

- HBV has a worldwide distribution. An estimated two billion people (a third of the world's population) have serological evidence of HBV infection, with an estimated 400 million people chronically infected with the virus.
- HBV is the tenth leading cause of death worldwide causing up to one million deaths a year.
- High prevalence regions include sub-Saharan Africa, most of Asia, and the Pacific islands. Low prevalence regions include most of western Europe and North America.

Transmission and incubation period

- The incubation period for acute infection ranges from 40 to 160 days, with an average of 90 days. Evidence of viraemia has been demonstrated as early as 6 days.
- Humans are the only natural reservoir of HBV.
- The main routes of transmission are parenteral or percutaneous exposure to infected blood or other body fluids such as semen, saliva contaminated with blood, or cervical secretions:
  • Sexual transmission (vaginal or anal intercourse)

- Sharing of needles or other equipment by injecting drug users
- Needle stick injuries
- Perinatal transmission from mother to child
- Human bites (rare).
- In areas of high prevalence, infection is acquired mostly by perinatal transmission from mother to child, although it may also occur by horizontal transmission between young children.
- In low-endemicity countries, most infections are acquired in adulthood by sexual transmission or sharing of blood-contaminated needles and equipment by IV drug users.
- Transmission through breastfeeding is extremely rare and mothers with hepatitis B are advised that it is safe to breastfeed their babies.
- The risk of developing chronic infection depends on the age at which the infection is acquired. Chronic infection occurs in 90% of those infected at birth, in 20–50% of those infected between the ages of 1 and 5 years, in 6–10% of those infected >5 years of age and <5% at older ages.

Clinical features and sequelae

Acute infection

- Hepatitis without jaundice is the predominant clinical presentation of acute hepatitis B infection (90% children, 50–70% adults).
- Most cases are asymptomatic or subclinical.
- Symptomatic acute hepatitis B is mostly a disease of older children and adults (33–50%). It produces typical illness in only 5–15% of children between 1 and 5 years of age while newborns generally do not develop any symptoms at all.
- Rarely (<1%) acute hepatitis B infection has a fulminant presentation. Newborns infected vertically from an anti-HBe-antibody positive mother appear to have a higher risk to develop fulminant hepatitis B infection at the age of 2–4 months.
- Blood tests: Liver enzymes especially transaminases are markedly elevated. HBsAg is the first marker to appear in the blood. Hepatitis B envelope antigen (HBeAg) may appear early but is usually cleared rapidly. Hepatitis B core IgM (IgM anti-HBc) is a helpful marker in the diagnosis of acute hepatitis B.
- In acute hepatitis B, HBsAg clears and its antibody (anti-HBs) appears within 6 months of disease onset. The seroconversion from HBeAg to anti-HBe-antibodies is associated with a reduction in the viral load and is the first step towards clearance of infection. Virus elimination is characterized by clearance of HBsAg and production of anti-HBs antibodies.

Chronic infection

- Chronic hepatitis B infection is defined as persistence of HBsAg in the serum for 6 months or longer. Children who are HBeAg positive are highly infectious carriers, whereas those who are HBeAg negative (usually anti-HBe positive) have a lower risk of transmission.
- Children with chronic hepatitis B infection are usually asymptomatic, unless complications such as cirrhosis or hepatocellular carcinoma arise.
- Occasionally extrahepatic manifestations such as papular acrodermatitis, lymphadenopathy, and nephrotic syndrome related to membranous glomerulonephritis occur. These manifestations are more often seen in children.
- Chronic hepatitis B has three phases, which are dependant on serum HBeAg and HBV DNA status:
  1. *Immune-tolerant phase* with high viral replication: HBeAg positive, high HBV DNA levels and normal level of aminotransferases. This pattern is mainly seen in children infected at birth who are usually asymptomatic. However, some children proceed to the next phase.
  2. *Immune-active phase* with elevated aminotransferases and marked inflammation, which may develop into fibrosis. Most individuals with a sudden elevation of aminotransferases undergo spontaneous seroconversion, where HBeAg becomes negative and anti-HBe develops. Most of these patients have no or mild non-specific symptoms. Most individuals who demonstrate this HBeAg seroconversion enter the third phase.
  3. *Inactive carrier state* with normalization of aminotransferases, a reduction in HBV DNA and improvement in hepatic inflammation.

Cirrhosis and HCC

For people with chronic hepatitis B, 15–25% progress to cirrhosis or HCC over a period of several decades. Progression to cirrhosis is favoured by high HBV viral load and presence of fibrosis on liver biopsy. HCC can also occur in the absence of cirrhosis. Seropositivity for HBsAg is one of the most important risk factors for the development of HCC. In areas of high endemicity of hepatitis B, more than 95% of HCC are HBsAg seropositive. The prognosis of childhood HCC is grave.

Diagnosis

Diagnosis is dependent on serology. Serological testing for hepatitis B antibodies and antigens indicates whether the child has acute or chronic HBV infection, is a high or low infectivity carrier, has natural immunity or immunity from vaccination. Table 75.1 summarizes the interpretation of serological tests in hepatitis B.

Table 75.1 Interpretation of serological test results for HBV

Status	Anti-HBc	Anti-HBc IgM	HBsAg	Anti-HBs	HBeAg	Anti-HBe
Acute infection	+	+	+	−	+/−	+/−
Chronic infection (high infectivity)	+	−	+	−	+	−
Chronic infection (low infectivity)	+	−	+	−	−	+
Recovery (natural immunity)	+	−	−	+/−	−	+/−
Immunity (after vaccination)	−	−	−	+	−	−

Management and treatment

- Most children with chronic hepatitis B in areas of low endemicity are either new migrants or vaccine failures. They should be referred to a specialist paediatric centre so that all the family may be supported, counselled, screened, and immunized. Annual review should include hepatitis B serology and hepatitis B DNA viral load, LFTs, α-fetoprotein, and abdominal ultrasound. This will detect evidence of seroconversion, progressive liver disease and/or HCC, and allow consideration of antiviral therapy.
- The incidence of HCC in children with chronic hepatitis B is low. There is no evidence to suggest that annual screening (with α-fetoprotein levels and abdominal ultrasound) is cost-effective or that it alters the natural course of the disease.

Antiviral treatment

- The goal of antiviral therapy for chronic hepatitis B is to eradicate HBV and prevent complications by shortening the duration of liver inflammation. However, available therapies have a limited effect on viral eradication, so the goal of the current antiviral treatment is to:
  - Reduce viral replication
  - Minimize the liver injury and related consequences of active viral replication
  - Reduce infectivity.
- Children with chronic hepatitis B often have mild or asymptomatic disease with minimal ALT elevations, despite often remarkably high levels of circulating HBV DNA (the immunotolerant phase of infection). Antiviral therapy in this group is usually ineffective.
- Consensus guidelines for treatment of chronic hepatitis B in children have not been established.
- HBV genotyping is not used to influence treatment decisions.

- Treatment involves interferons (IFN-alfa) or nucleoside analogues such as lamivudine. There is no uniform policy regarding the first-line agent and its duration in children. Drug resistance is a major problem.
- In children with active disease (ALT more than twice the upper limit of normal and active histology) both IFN-alfa and lamivudine have been shown to be effective in inducing loss of HBeAg, normalization of serum ALT levels, and improvements in liver histology. The best tool for evaluation of the need for treatment remains the liver biopsy. When to perform a biopsy is not always clear.
- IFN-alfa is given subcutaneously three times a week for 6 months. IFN is limited by its side effect profile although children tolerate treatment better than adults. The main side effects are fever, flu-like symptoms, and bone marrow suppression. IFN is contraindicated in children with decompensated liver disease, cytopenia, severe renal or cardiac disorders, and autoimmune disease.
- Lamivudine is well tolerated. The most significant limitation of lamivudine is the development of viral resistance with prolonged use. Hence long-term therapy in children should not be started without very careful assessment of the need for therapy.
- Children should ideally be treated in clinical trials. Treatment options will improve for children over time.

Prevention

- Public health measures for reducing transmission of HBV include: public information about the modes of transmission, promotion of safe sex, needle exchange programmes, and screening of high-risk groups (including pregnant women).
- Universal precautions should prevent exposure to blood or body fluids in healthcare settings.

Vaccination

- Many countries around the world have introduced universal immunization against HBV in their national schedule. In Europe 44 out of 52 WHO member states have introduced the vaccine. The UK is an area of low endemicity and has adopted a policy of selective immunisation of high risk groups combined with universal antenatal screening.
- HBV vaccine is recommended as pre-exposure prophylaxis in:
  • Injecting drug users and their children
  • Homosexual men
  • Individuals who change partners regularly
  • Close household family contacts of carriers of hepatitis B
  • Families adopting children from high or intermediate prevalence of HBV
  • Foster carers
  • Haemophiliacs and other children receiving regular blood or blood products and their carers

- Children with chronic liver disease or chronic renal failure including those on haemodialysis
- Healthcare workers who have direct contact with blood, blood stained body fluids, or patients tissues
- People travelling to areas of high or intermediate prevalence of hepatitis B
- Inmates of custodial institutions
- Staff and children with learning difficulties in residential homes.
- Primary immunization is three doses at 0, 1, and 6 months. Individuals at continuing risk of infection should be offered a single booster once only, 5 years after the primary course. Measurement of anti-HBs is not required either before or after this dose. The route of immunization is IM (not in the buttocks). The dose varies according to the manufacturer but is lower in children.

Infants born to hepatitis B-infected women

- Postexposure vaccination is recommended for babies born to infected mothers (HBsAg positive). These babies should be given an accelerated course of four doses of the vaccine (0, 1, 2, and 12 months).
- Babies born to highly infectious mothers (HBsAg plus no HBe antibody) should also receive hepatitis B immunoglobulin (HBIG) within 24 hours of birth, together with active immunization with an accelerated course of vaccination.
- Infants should be tested for HBsAg at 1 year of age. This testing can be carried out at the same time as the fourth dose of vaccine is given and will identify those who may have become chronically infected with hepatitis B. These infected infants need referral for specialist assessment and management.
- A single booster dose of hepatitis B vaccine should be given with the preschool booster immunizations (age 4–5 years). This will also provide the opportunity to check whether the child was properly followed up in infancy.

Other postexposure prophylaxis

Any individual potentially exposed to hepatitis B infected blood or body fluids should be offered protection against hepatitis with HBV vaccine with or without HBIG. See *Immunisation Against Infectious Diseases.*[2]

A common occurrence is a child receiving an injury from a needle found on the ground. In these circumstances a course of HBV immunization is started but immunoglobulin is not given. It is considered that immunization should be given within 7 days of exposure if it is going to give protection against the needle stick injury.

Future research

- Antiviral resistance is a major emerging problem in the management of patients with chronic HBV. Combination therapy with multiple agents would be a logical approach but has not been found to be superior to monotherapy so far.

- Adefovir, tenofovir, telbivudine, and entecavir, the newer antivirals, seem effective in adults. Studies in children are underway.

Further reading

Davison S, Boxall EH. Infective disorders of the liver. In: Deirdre K, ed. *Diseases of the Liver and Biliary System in Children*, 3rd edn. Oxford: Wiley-Blackwell, 2008.

Hepatitis B. In; *Immunisation Against Infectious Disease.*, 3rd edn. London: Department of Health. Available at: ℗ www.immunisation.nhs.uk (accessed 1 February 2011).

Public Health Laboratory Service Hepatitis subcommittee. Exposure to hepatitis B virus: guidance on post-exposure prophylaxis. *CDR Rev* 1992;**2**:R97–101.

Shah U, Kelly D, Chang MH, et al. Management of chronic hepatitis B in children. *J Pediatr Gastroenterol Nutr* 2009;**48**:399–404.

Hepatitis C

📖 see also Chapters 4, 18, 75

Name and nature of the organism

- Hepatitis C causes a viral inflammation of the liver affecting all age groups. In susceptible individuals it may progress to chronic liver disease, cirrhosis of the liver or, rarely, HCC. This progression is slow and complications are rarely seen in children.
- HCV is an enveloped single-stranded RNA virus, a member of the genus *Hepacivirus* in the family *Flaviviridae*.
- HCV is highly heterogeneous and widely divergent genetic strains can be identified. HCV can be classified into six distinct genotypes (GTs) and each genotype can be classified into numerous subtypes.

Epidemiology

- HCV is a global problem. Approximately 2–3% of the world's population are chronically infected with HCV.
- An estimated 200 000 people in the UK have chronic HCV infection—50% of whom are unaware that they carry the virus. There are variations in prevalence between different groups (0.04% in blood donors, 1% in people attending genitourinary clinics and up to 50% in IV drug users).
- Disease prevalence is low (<1%) in northern Europe, Australia, and Canada; intermediate (about 1%) in most of Europe, and USA and high (≥5–10%) in countries in Africa, Latin America, and Central and Southeast Asia. It is especially high in Egypt with a prevalence of 20%.
- The distribution of the six HCV genotypes varies between geographical regions. Genotype GT1 is most common in Europe; GT4 is seen in Egypt and many parts of Middle East and Africa.
- GT1 and 3 are common in injecting drug users in the UK.

Transmission and incubation period

- The most common mode of acquisition of HCV for children in the UK is perinatal transmission from an infected mother. The risk of vertical transmission is low (0–8%) but increases if the mother has a high level

of HCV RNA in blood, is co-infected with HIV or has early rupture of membranes.
- Children adopted from abroad are also at risk of HCV infection.
- Infection from HCV containing blood products is almost 100% efficient. This was the most important mode of HCV transmission for children until blood donors started to be screened for HCV in the UK in September 1991. Many haemophiliac patients were infected with HCV before plasma inactivation became standard in 1985.
- The most common route of infection in adults in the UK is through sharing contaminated needles during recreational injecting drug use. Other modes of transmission are by transfusion of unscreened blood products, tattooing, body piercing and acupuncture under unsterile conditions.
- The risk of transmission of HCV though a needle stick injury is around 3%, and depends on the level of viraemia (amount of HCV RNA in the blood).
- Sexual transmission is not an efficient means of transmission. The risk is <5% in monogamous relationships.
- Transmission through breastfeeding is extremely rare and mothers with hepatitis C may breastfeed their babies.
- The incubation period from exposure to antibody production is 8–9 weeks (range 2–26 weeks).

Clinical features and sequelae

- **Acute hepatitis C** infection is very rare in childhood.
- **Chronic hepatitis C** infection can be defined as persistently detectable serum HCV RNA for >6 months in children >2 years of age with or without derangement of LFTs. For younger children, chronic hepatitis C infection can be defined as hepatitis C RNA positivity for >2 years.
  - Chronic hepatitis C develops in 90% of vertically infected infants compared to 60–80% of older children infected by blood products.
  - Most children with chronic hepatitis C are asymptomatic. Hepatitis C in children seems to be a milder disease than in adults. Children with chronic hepatitis C have normal growth and generally do not show clinical signs of chronic liver disease.
- **Long term sequelae**: There is a slow progression to hepatic fibrosis with age. Fibrosis due to hepatitis C is usually mild in children but progressive disease may develop in up to 30%. The levels of aminotransferases do not correlate with clinical severity. After 20–30 years approximately 50% develop progressive liver disease and 20% develop cirrhosis.
- Risk factors for rapid progression are: older age at infection; male gender; heavy alcohol consumption; co-infection with HIV or hepatitis B and immunosuppression.

Diagnosis

- *ELISA for antibody to HCV*: Serological testing for antibodies to HCV by enzyme immunoassay is the primary screening test. HCV antibodies are usually detectible by ELISA 12 weeks after exposure to the virus.
- Screening tests are prone to false-positive results especially when testing a low-prevalence population.
- *Polymerase chain reaction (PCR) for HCV RNA*: This is a confirmatory test, and is used to follow up a positive HCV antibody test. If positive this is evidence of current or ongoing hepatitis C infection.
- *Recombinant immunoblot assay*: If the patient is HCV antibody positive but HCV PCR negative a supplemental test with recombinant immunoblot assay (RIBA) is performed to confirm the presence of HCV antibodies.
- In some cases, HCV antibodies may not be detectable even after 6 months of infection. In these cases HCV PCR testing is used to diagnose infection.
- An HCV antibody result is not reliable in immunosuppressed patients (HIV, antibody deficient, etc.) and these children should be tested for HCV RNA by PCR.
- HCV RNA levels are used for monitoring patients on HCV treatment to assess their response to treatment. Presently, the lower limits of detection of the virus by commercial kits range from 15 to 50 IU/ml.

Management and treatment

- Children with chronic hepatitis C should be referred to a paediatric specialist for information, counselling, family support, assessment, and treatment where appropriate.
- Annual reviews for these children include HCV RNA, LFTs, abdominal ultrasound, and α-fetoprotein (for the early detection of HCC).
- Liver biopsy is the best method to assess the severity of liver damage in patients with hepatitis C, but the availability of effective antiviral treatment means that this is required less often.

Antiviral therapy

- Effective antiviral therapy against hepatitis C is now available for children.
- The main aim of treatment in hepatitis C is to achieve a sustained viral response (SVR), defined as undetectable serum HCV RNA 24 weeks after completion of therapy. SVR should prevent progression of the disease.
- Combination therapy with pegylated interferon (subcutaneously three times weekly) and oral ribavirin is a safe, generally well tolerated, and reasonably effective treatment of childhood chronic hepatitis C. SVR is significantly higher in children with GT2 or 3 (80–84%) as compared with GT1 (45%).

- Common side effects of HCV treatment include: influenza-like symptoms and gastrointestinal complaints (fever, headache, anorexia, vomiting, abdominal pain, myalgia, and nausea).
- The duration of combination therapy depends upon the HCV genotype; 12 months for GT1 infections and 6 months for GT2 and 3 infections.

Management of HCV-positive mothers during pregnancy

- Elective caesarean section or breastfeeding has no demonstrable effect on transmission rates of hepatitis C, unless the mother is also HIV positive. If the mother is HCV antibody positive but HCV RNA negative, she should have a normal delivery and be encouraged to breastfeed her infant.
- If the mother is HCV antibody and HCV RNA persistently positive there is a risk of transmission to the baby although it is still low (0–8%). The risk of transmission increases in the presence of high maternal HCV viral load, early rupture of membranes, and presence of HIV. In these cases, caesarean section may be considered although there is insufficient evidence to recommend it.

Needlestick injury

- Following a needle stick injury from a known HCV RNA positive patient, the recipient should be tested for HCV RNA at 6 weeks. If negative, repeat testing for HCV RNA and for HCV antibody can be performed at 12 weeks. If these too are negative, a final test for HCV antibody at 6 months should be done to rule out viral transmission.

Prevention

- Hepatitis C testing should be offered to high-risk groups and also to those with unexplained jaundice and abnormal LFTs.
- If hepatitis C is diagnosed, testing of offspring, close household contact(s), or sexual contacts should be considered.
- Universal precautions should be taken in all healthcare settings to reduce the possibility of exposure to infected blood. These precautions are particularly important on renal dialysis units.
- Routine antenatal screening for hepatitis C is carried out in some countries with high prevalence. In the UK it is not recommended as part of the national antenatal screening programme, but is undertaken in some high-risk areas.
- No vaccine is available for HCV.

Future developments

- The long-term natural history of infection acquired at or before birth or in childhood is not clearly defined, and the reasons why in some individuals the disease progresses more rapidly than in others are not fully understood. Polymorphisms of interleukin-28B may affect clearance of HCV.

- Newer drugs for hepatitis C are in development. Protease inhibitors (telaprevir, boceprevir) are in phase III clinical trials. Polymerase inhibitors are in phase II and III clinical trials in adults. Monotherapy may lead to drug resistance and children should be treated within the context of clinical trials wherever possible.
- Modifications to the existing regimens such as the newer ribavirin (such as taribavirin), modified interferons (such as albuferon) and weight-based ribavirin dosage may be made available in future.

Further reading

Iorio R, Giannattasio A, Sepe A, Terracciano LM, Vecchione R, Vegnente A. Chronic hepatitis C in childhood: An 18-year experience. *Clin Infect Dis* 2005;**41**:1431–7.

Kelly D. Viral hepatitis B and C in children. *J R Soc Med* 2006;**99**:353–7.

Tajiri H, Inui A, Kiyohara Y, *et al.* Peginterferon alpha-2b and ribavirin for the treatment of chronic hepatitis C in Japanese pediatric and young adult patients: a survey of the Japan Society of Pediatric Hepatology. *Eur J Gastroenterol Hepatol* 2009;**21**:1256–60.

Chapter 77

Herpes simplex virus 1 and 2

📖 see also Chapters 4, 10, 11, 14, 20, 30, 31, 34, 38

Name and nature of the organisms

- Human HSV types 1 and 2 (HSV-1 and HSV-2) are part of the family of the Human Herpesviruses (of which they are the first two members: HHV-1 and HHV-2). They are enveloped, doubled-stranded DNA viruses that grow readily in culture, producing characteristic cytopathic effects. Like the other members of the Human Herpesviruses family, they persist lifelong in the body by remaining latent in nerve and ganglial cells with potential for episodes of reactivation.
- HSV-1 infections usually involve the face and skin above the waist and present in childhood.
- HSV-2 infections involve the genitalia and skin below the waist in sexually active adolescents, and are responsible for the majority of neonatal infections.

Neonatal infection

Epidemiology

- Neonatal infections are mostly caused by HSV-2 (50–75% of cases).
- The reported incidence differs widely between developed countries with reported rates of 1:3000–1:20 000 in the USA to 1:60 000 in the UK. Genital infections with HSV are increasing in the UK and neonatal infections are expected to become more prevalent.
- Infection is more likely to occur in premature infants as they do not benefit from passive maternal antibody transfer.

Transmission and incubation period

- Neonatal infection is usually transmitted from mother to child through viral shedding from the birth canal during delivery (85%).
- Transplacental infection is rare (~5%) and infection via an orolabial lesion from medical personnel or a family member is uncommon (~10%).
- Maternal primary infection with HSV at the time of delivery has the highest risk of transmission (25–57%) compared with recurrent maternal genital HSV (2%).

- Three-quarters of infected infants are born to women with asymptomatic shedding with no history or clinical findings of HSV during pregnancy or delivery.
- Other risk factors known to influence HSV transmission include:
  - Lack of maternal antibody
  - Increasing duration of rupture of membranes
  - Breeching of mucocutaneous barriers (e.g. use of scalp electrodes)
  - Mode of delivery (vaginal versus caesarean in women with active shedding of HSV at delivery).
- The incubation period for neonatal HSV is 1–6 days; disease is secondary to viraemic spread.
- Recent data suggest that some neonates with severe HSV disease may have a rare form of primary immunodeficiency in their toll-like receptor pathway.

Clinical features and sequelae

The clinical presentation in neonates can be classified into three distinct forms with different outcomes (Table 77.1):
- Skin-eye-mouth (SEM) disease
- Disseminated disease with or without CNS involvement
- CNS disease.

Table 77.1 Clinical characteristics of the three main presentations of neonatal HSV (percentages for sequelae and mortality in children treated with high-dose aciclovir)

Type of Disease	SEM	Disseminated	CNS
Frequency	45%	25%	30%
Symptoms	Vesicles on skin/mouth—scalp (sites of minor trauma) or conjunctivitis/keratitis	Sepsis-like Hepatitis/DIC Thrombocytopenia Pneumonitis ± CNS involvement Skin lesions ±	Lethargy Fever Convulsions—focal CT/MRI abnormal
Age of onset	5–14 days	5–10 days	2–4 weeks
Sequelae	1–5%	15–30%	50%
Mortality	0–1%	30–50%	15%

- Clinicians should suspect disseminated HSV infection in the septic infant presenting late in the first week or in the second week of life.
- Sequelae are high in CNS disease, even despite treatment with high-dose aciclovir.

- Relapses of SEM disease frequently occur in the first few months of life and can progress to CNS disease if these are not adequately treated.
- 20% of patients with ≥3 recurrences have their neurological outcome affected.

Diagnosis

- Clinicians should suspect disseminated HSV infection in the septic infant especially those with negative bacterial cultures, raised transaminases, a coagulopathy, and no clinical improvement on antibiotics.
- Patients with signs and symptoms of possible neonatal HSV infection should undergo a full screen including:
  - Scrapping of the base of the vesicles if present.
  - Surface skin swabs, nasopharynx, mouth, conjunctiva (pooled), and rectal swabs for viral culture.
  - FBC, LFTs, and clotting screen.
  - CSF for cell analysis and HSV PCR.
  - CT or MRI (better) of the brain should be considered in patients with CNS disease (+ EEG if CNS disease is suspected—temporal lobe spike and wave).
  - Ophthalmological review to exclude HSV retinitis.
- Identification and typing of the virus from a scrapping of the base of a vesicle can be done rapidly with PCR methods, immunofluorescence or direct antibody (EIA or ELISA) testing.
- Viral isolation by cell culture has historically been the mainstay of diagnosis, with characteristic cytopathic effects observed after 24–72 hours.
- HSV-DNA PCR can be performed on a variety of specimens and is now the diagnostic method of choice to diagnose CNS involvement.

Management and treatment

- Neonates with HSV infection should be treated with high-dose IV aciclovir. Recommended duration of therapy is 14 days for SEM disease and 21 days for disseminated and CNS disease.
- A repeat CSF HSV PCR is recommended at the end of the course of therapy in patients with CNS involvement to confirm clearance of the virus.

Prevention

During pregnancy

- Suppressive treatment from 36 weeks of gestation onwards is recommended by some experts to reduce the emergence of lesions around the time of delivery and the need for caesarean section. However, this approach reduces but does not completely eliminate asymptomatic shedding and its efficacy and safety in pregnant women has not been clearly established.

At delivery

- Caesarean section should be performed in women with prodromal symptoms or active lesions of genital HSV at the time of delivery. It should be performed within 4–6 hours from the rupture of membranes.

Studies have shown that neonatal transmission greatly decreases (but is not completely eliminated) using this approach.
- Asymptomatic neonates born to mothers with a *primary* genital lesion, either vaginally or by caesarean section with risk factors (rupture of membranes >6 hours prior to delivery; fetal scalp electrodes; chorioamnionitis; cervicitis), should receive a full diagnostic evaluation for HSV if there is no serological evidence of past maternal infection. Treatment with IV aciclovir should be initiated until the evidence of active infection has been ruled out.
- Asymptomatic neonates born vaginally to a mother with a *recurrent* genital infection can have HSV surface swabs (nasopharynx, mouth) taken at 24–48 hours to rule out active replication of the virus and should be monitored clinically at regular intervals in the first few weeks of life.

After SEM disease
- SEM disease often recurs and may progress to CNS infection if left untreated in the first few months of life. There is limited evidence that daily oral aciclovir prophylaxis given to infants for a period of 6–12 months after SEM disease reduces the incidence of these recurrences.
- Similar 'flares' may be seen after CNS disease with recurrent episodes of irritability and seizures. The role of long-term aciclovir prophylaxis is unclear.

Childhood infection

Epidemiology
- Most primary infections in children beyond the neonatal period are caused by HSV-1, whereas HSV-2 infection occurs in adolescents after the onset of sexual activity.
- Prevalence of HSV-1 seropositivity in children varies according to the geographical location and social class status. In the UK, the presence of HSV-1 antibodies reaches 50–75% by adulthood.
- The vast majority of primary infections in children are asymptomatic. In a study of 4000 children with HSV-1 seropositivity, only 12% had evident signs of primary infection.
- The virus remains latent for life (HSV-1 trigeminal ganglia: HSV-2 sacral sensory neural ganglia) with possible episodes of reactivation and neural axonal spread ('cold sores' or genital herpes) and periods of asymptomatic shedding.

Transmission and incubation period
- Transmission of HSV-1 occurs through mucocutaneous contact, often with asymptomatic children who are shedding the virus.
- Patients with primary gingivostomatitis shed the virus for ≥1 week.
- Patients with recurrent symptoms shed the virus for a shorted duration of 3–4 days.
- The incubation period is 2 days to 2 weeks.

Clinical features and sequelae

Gingivostomatitis

- Classical presentation of HSV-1.
- Occurs in 25–30% of children with primary infection.
- Prodromal symptoms include fever, nausea, malaise and anorexia.
- This is followed by the appearance of numerous vesicles, which break down rapidly to enlarging erythematous lesions with central ulcerations covered by yellow-grey membranes.
- Lesions are painful and may coalesce.
- Main clinical problem is dehydration, rarely needs hospital admission.
- Areas involved may include the buccal mucosa, tongue, posterior pharynx, and gingiva. Commonly satellite lesions are seen on the skin around the mouth.
- Healing occurs in 10–21 days.

Herpes labialis ('cold sores')

- Following primary infection, one-third of patients have episodes of viral reactivation consisting of orolabial lesions at the outer edge of the vermillion border.
- Fever or non-specific stressors can trigger episodes, which are usually preceded by a tingling or pain sensation at the site.
- Episodes last for 4–5 days, though HSV shedding is detected by PCR in between acute episodes.

Keratoconjunctivitis

- Follows auto-inoculation in a child with gingivostomatitis or herpes labialis.
- The episode presents with acute onset of pain, photophobia, and excessive lacrimation.
- This is followed by chemosis and periorbital oedema.
- The infection leads to corneal ulceration with pathognomonic branching dendritic lesions of the cornea and blurred vision.
- Resolution of the episode takes up to 4 weeks.
- Recurrent infections may lead to corneal opacification and corneal blindness.

Herpetic whitlow (herpetic paronychia)

- Result of auto-inoculation in children with orofacial herpes infection.
- Characterized by the swelling of a finger (usually thumb from sucking) and the apparition of one or several painful, clear, fluid-filled vesicles later becoming opaque.
- Typically side of finger on the distal phalanx. Larger than vesicles seen in HFMD.
- Symptoms last for 1–2 weeks.

Eczema herpeticum

- HSV skin superinfection in patients with underlying eczema.
- In one-third of children, there is a recent history of herpes labialis in one of the parents.
- Vesicles appear in areas of recently healed atopic dermatitis, but rapidly become 'punched out' ulcers and can spread quickly destroying skin.

- Fever develops 2–3 days after the appearance of vesicles and usually last for 4–5 days.
- Toxic symptoms may be severe and viraemia with visceral involvement has been reported.

Herpes gladiatorum—scrum pox
- Lesions present on face, neck or arm of children involved in contact sports such as wrestling or rugby.
- Viral inoculation results from close contact between injured skin and oral secretions.

HSV associated erythema multiforme
- Disease characterized by an autoimmune response to HSV DNA fragments present in the patient's skin with development of distinctive cutaneous target lesions.
- Episodes usually follow an episode of herpes labialis and lasts for 10 days.
- Recurrences are common and direct testing for HSV by culture or PCR is negative.

CNS infection
- HSV is the commonest identified cause of severe encephalitis. HSV-1 is virtually always the agent responsible. The illness is due to a primary infection or most commonly to a reactivation of latent HSV in a nerve or ganglial cell.

Other infections
- A number of other manifestations of HSV have been described in the immunocompetent host, including pneumonitis, exudative tracheo-bronchitis, oesophagitis, hepatitis, recurrent aseptic meningitis, myelitis, and facial nerve (Bell's) palsy.

Diagnosis
- Diagnosis and typing of HSV can be readily performed via immunofluorescence or direct antibody (EIA or ELISA) testing, viral culture or PCR assay of lesions and various body fluids.
- CSF PCR for HSV is the diagnostic method of choice for HSV meningoencephalitis as it has sensitivity and specificity approaching 100%. Timing of CSF sampling is important and the assay is best performed between 3 and 10 days after onset of symptoms. CSF PCR has reduced sensitivity around 24–48 hours after high-dose aciclovir has been commenced.
- Serological testing is available but has limited diagnostic utility.

Management and treatment
A variety of formulations are available for the treatment of HSV including oral, topical and IV aciclovir, oral valaciclovir and famciclovir, and IV foscarnet.
- Gingivostomatitis: pain management is essential. Oral aciclovir decreases the duration of symptoms by around one day and duration of shedding if started early. In adolescents, valaciclovir can be used as it has greater bioavailability. In immunocompromised patients, IV aciclovir

treatment is the preferred option. Foscarnet is the drug of choice in infections caused by aciclovir resistant isolates.

- Skin infections: there are few efficacy data available to recommend treatment in skin infection except eczema herpeticum, which should be treated with IV aciclovir. Treatment of infections in immunocompromised hosts and burn patients should be considered because of the potential severity of symptoms.
- CNS infections: early initiation of treatment with IV aciclovir has shown to significantly reduce morbidity and mortality in patients with encephalitis.

Prevention

- Long-term suppressive therapy in patients with recurrent gingivostomatitis or herpes labialis reduces reactivation but may risk the emergence of aciclovir resistant strains.
- In adults and adolescents with herpes labialis, the administration of a 1-day high-dose regimen with either valaciclovir or famciclovir at the onset of symptoms has been shown to lessen the symptoms and duration of the disease.

Future research

The burden of disease linked to genital HSV infection and neonatal HSV disease has led to research in developing a number of candidate prophylactic herpes vaccines. Early trials have shown some promise in preventing genital disease in seronegative women.

Further reading

Kimberlin D. Herpes simplex virus infection in neonates and early childhood. *Semin Pediatr Infect Dis* 2005;**16**:271–81.

Malm G. Neonatal herpes simplex virus infection. *Semin Fetal Neonatal Med* 2009;**14**:204–8.

Human herpesviruses 6 and 7

📖 see also Chapters 14, 20, 34

Nature and name of organisms

- HHV-6 and 7 are closely related herpesviruses that cause a similar spectrum of disease. This chapter describes HHV-6 in detail, and refers to HHV-7 when there are important differences.
- HHV-6 has a linear, double-stranded DNA of about 160kb. Two major variants A and B have been identified. Variant B is the type associated with the common clinical manifestations in childhood. The virus preferentially infects $CD4^+$ T lymphocytes, but is also found in monocytes, macrophages, brain, and kidney cells.
- HHV-7 has a genome of approximately 145kb, has close homology to HHV-6, and both are more closely related to CMV than to other herpesviruses.

Epidemiology

- Infection is acquired early in life. At birth up to 80% of infants have detectable antibody, which reflects maternal antibody. This declines to a nadir of around 10% at 6 months.
- Neonatal infection has been reported despite high rates of maternal antibody so humoral immunity is not completely protective.
- Rates of seropositivity then steadily climb to a peak of 80–90% by the age of 1–2 years. These rates continue into adult life although the titres decline.
- Epidemiological studies around the world have shown similar rates of acquisition apart from some isolated indigenous communities where rates of seropositivity may be ≤10%.
- HHV-7 tends to be acquired later than HHV-6 but shows a similar pattern of high titres in young children, which decline in adult life.

Transmission

- The fact that infants are infected so early in life suggests that infection within families is the most likely source.
- Congenital infection with HHV-6 has been detected in up to 1% of births, congenital HHV-7 has not been reported.

- HHV-6 and 7 have been isolated from saliva in healthy adults indicating that this may be a major route of transmission.
- HHV-7 has been detected in breast milk.
- HHV-6/7 have been isolated from the cervix so perinatal transmission is possible.

Incubation period
- The mean incubation period for HHV-6 is 9–10 days, The incubation period for HHV-7 is unknown.

Clinical features

Exanthem subitum/roseola infantum
- Exanthem subitum also known as roseola infantum is the classical clinical syndrome associated with HHV-6 and 7.
- Typically this is a disease of infants and young children. There is abrupt onset of a high persistent fever, which may be complicated by seizures. The fever lasts 4–5 days and a rash appears on defervescence. Fever comes down: rash comes out! The rash is comprised of generalized small pink macules.
- The children appear clinically unwell and are often indistinguishable from children with meningitis or severe bacterial sepsis.
- HHV-7 causes an identical clinical syndrome and has been shown to be the cause of a second episode in children with previous HHV-6 infection. Sub clinical infection often occurs, T cell clones against HHV-6 react to HHV-7 and this may protect children from clinical disease with a subsequent HHV-7 infection.

Non-specific febrile illness
- Most young children with acute HHV-6 infection do not present with classical exanthem subitum, but with a high fever (lasting 3–5 days), coryza, and signs of an upper respiratory tract infection.
- Pharyngitis, inflammation of the tympanic membranes, puffy eyes, mild diarrhoea and vomiting, mild lymphadenopathy, and a maculopapular rash are all reported—it is the classic non-specific viral infection.
- In a survey of 1653 children <3 years presenting to an emergency department with acute febrile illness, 160 (9.7%) had serological or culture evidence of HHV-6 infection.
- In the subgroup of children aged 6–12 months this was 20%.
- 17% of those with HHV-6 had a rash, which was only present at initial presentation in a third of patients.

Febrile seizures
- In the same case series 13% with HHV-6 had seizures, compared to 9% of febrile children without HHV-6. This difference was not statistically significant.
- Overall HHV-6 was identified in one-third of children <2 years presenting with a first febrile convulsion.

Encephalitis

- HHV-6 has been associated with severe and fatal encephalitis in otherwise healthy hosts.
- Case series of adult and child patients with encephalitis show a prevalence of HHV-6 in the CSF of 1–3% of patients.
- There are fewer studies reporting HHV-7 but this has also been associated.
- Post-transplant acute limbic encephalitis is discussed below.

Infection of immunocompromised hosts

- HHV-6 was first isolated in lymphocytes from patients with a variety of immune deficiencies.
- It has a particular tropism for T cells and it is not known if it can be a co-factor in reducing immune function in immunocompromised hosts, or if it is simply reactivated in patients with reduced immunity.
- Following bone marrow and solid organ transplantation, HHV-6 is frequently detected by PCR in peripheral blood and is shed in urine.
- It is associated with fever and raised transaminases, but in contrast to CMV infection, neutropenia or other end-organ damage is unusual.
- Co-infection with CMV is common, in which case the risk of disease is greater than with CMV infection alone.
- Post-transplant acute limbic encephalitis (PALE) is seen in patients after solid and bone marrow transplant. Amnesia is the predominant symptom and imaging studies show abnormalities localized to the limbic area. Patients who recover are usually left with some memory impairment.
- There is a strong association with HHV-6 in the CSF and there are anecdotal reports of clinical improvement with ganciclovir and foscarnet.
- The development of amnesia in a transplant recipient should prompt investigations to look for HHV-6 and specific treatment against it.

HIV

HHV-6/7 have not been clearly associated with serious disease in patients with HIV. Some studies have identified HHV-6 DNA in brain lesions in patients with PML but the significance of this is not established. HHV-6 can also be detected in lesions of patients with multiple sclerosis and these findings may just reflect the ubiquity of the virus.

Diagnosis

- In most cases no laboratory diagnosis is made or the child has recovered by the time a diagnosis is made.
- Acute and convalescent serology will show a rising antibody titre
- In the acute phase HHV-6/7 DNA can be detected in peripheral blood mononuclear cells by PCR and culture.

- The viruses can also be detected in throat swabs and in CSF.
- Like other herpesviruses, HHV-6 remains latent and can reactivate, PCR can become positive intermittently in previously infected children without associated symptoms.

Treatment

- In most cases only symptomatic treatment is needed.
- In immunocompromised patients who have co-infection with CMV and HHV-6, treatment of CMV infection with foscarnet and ganciclovir appears to also suppress the HHV-6 viral load.
- Aciclovir has no activity against HHV-6/7.
- There is no trial evidence of benefit from these drugs in generalized or limbic encephalitis but in view of the potential severity of the illness, antiviral treatment should be given when HHV-6/7 encephalitis is suspected.

Prevention

- There is no vaccine against HHV-6/7. As in most cases, the viruses cause mild illness and it is unlikely that mass immunization would be considered even if an effective vaccine were produced.
- Some transplant units routinely monitor patients post transplantation for HHV-6 along with CMV and EBV. Treatment is not given routinely to asymptomatic or mildly symptomatic patients with a detectable HHV-6 viral load but where a rising viral load is associated with a significant clinical problem antiviral treatment might be considered.

Future research

Future research will help to clarify the importance of HHV-6/7 in the immunocompromised host and may identify further clinical syndromes that can be attributed to these pathogens.

Further reading

Hall CB, Long CE, Schnabel KC, *et al.* Human herpes virus in children a prospective study of complications and reactivation. *N Engl J Med* 1994;**331**:432–8.

Levy J. Three new human herpes viruses. *Lancet* 1997;**349**:58–62.

Yamanishi K. Pathogenesis of human herpesvirus 6. *Infect Agents Dis* 1992;**1**:149–55.

Human papillomavirus

📖 see also Chapters 19, 20, 34, 37

Name and nature of organism

- HPV are small, non-enveloped, double-stranded, epitheliotropic DNA viruses. Sequencing of the capsid gene has identified >100 different types.[1]
- HPV are divided into cutaneous and mucosal types depending on the epithelium they infect. Approximately half are mucosal HPVs belonging to the α-papillomaviruses (α-PV) genus. Mucosal HPV are split into high-risk (oncogenic) and low-risk groups (non-oncogenic) types. The remainder are cutaneous HPVs including the β-, γ-, μ-, ν-PV genera and α-PV species 2, 4, and 8.
- The low-risk HPV types 6 and 11 are found in the vast majority (>90%) of anogenital warts. Genital warts are a very common sexually transmitted infection (over 80 000 diagnosed cases/year in all age groups in the UK).
- The high-risk types 16 and 18, are responsible worldwide for about 50% and 20% of cervical cancers, respectively.
- The HPV life cycle is only completed in fully differentiated squamous epithelia with infection of the basal cell layer occurring following minor trauma. Viral gene expression influences the proliferation and maturation of keratinocytes and results in growth of a benign tumour. Virus assembly does not lyse keratinocytes; the infectious virus is shed with desquamating cornified cells.
- Although risk of transmission is considered to be low, HPV can resist desiccation, freezing, and prolonged periods outside host cells.

Epidemiology

Non-genital cutaneous warts

- Cutaneous warts are uncommon in infancy, increase in frequency in childhood and reach a peak in the teenage years, occurring with equal frequency in both sexes. They are seen worldwide and in all age groups with an overall prevalence of approximately 7–12%; most people will have had warts at some time.
- They are most common with a prevalence of up to 20% in school age children.
- Warts usually regress spontaneously; approximately 23% resolve within 2 months and 65–78% within 2 years; in a UK study 90% of children with warts at age 11 had cleared them by age 16 years.[3]

Anogenital warts

- Anogenital HPV prevalence peaks in young women and declines towards middle age. In the UK, seroprevalence data show that 10.7% of 10–29-year-old women are seropositive. Overall, about 25% of women between 14 and 59 years have HPV. Male seroprevalence has been found to be 1.2–73% overall depending on the population with more then half of the studies showing a prevalence ≥20%.
- For the sexually active population the overall lifetime risk of acquiring HPV is about 75%.
- Risk factors for infection with HPV are the numbers of sexual partners, sexual debut at a younger age, oral contraceptive use, and smoking. Risk factors for persistent HPV infection, cytological abnormality and invasive cancer are HPV type, increasing age, smoking, and immune deficiency.
- Only around 10% of all HPV positive individuals have clinically evident lesions
- Most genital HPV infections are transient and are cleared within 2 years with 70% clearance by 12 months and 90% by 2 years.
- For specific HPV types (particularly HPV 16 and 18) there is clear causal evidence of carcinogenicity.

Aerodigestive warts

- Oral warts are rare in children, with an overall prevalence estimated at 0.03%. Warts in the upper airway, predominantly the larynx, are seen in the rare condition recurrent respiratory papillomatosis (RRP) which has a bimodal distribution occurring in children under 5 years or adults.

Transmission

Cutaneous warts

- HPV transmission occurs by direct skin-to-skin contact with individuals with clinical or subclinical HPV-associated lesions, or indirectly via contaminated surfaces and objects, e.g. in swimming pools and bathrooms. Autoinoculation from the lesion to surrounding skin is frequent.
- Productive infection and induction of hyperproliferation are initiated when the virus enters proliferating basal epithelial cells, and this requires abrasion or other minor trauma to the epithelium.
- The incubation period ranges from 1 to 6 months; however, latency periods of ≥3 years may occur.

Anogenital warts

- Transmission usually occurs by direct contact, which can be with clinical lesions, unapparent lesions or genital fluid containing infectious virus and autoinoculation (including digital-genital transmission).
- Perinatal rates of HPV are low with ≤2% in the oropharynx or genitals of infants and 2–3% in children. Perinatally acquired lesions may not become clinically apparent for up to 2 years.

- The exact incubation period is unknown. Estimates are between 1 and 9 months with a median of 3 months, but can be as long as years.
- Persistent HPV infection is a risk factor for neoplasia. Cytological abnormalities can be detected around 7 years after infection, invasive cancer may then follow another decade or two later.
- In prepubertal children, HPV can be acquired through non-sexual contact, however, studies have shown that a significant proportion of children with anogenital warts have been sexually abused.

Aerodigestive warts

- Because the skin of the hand is a common site of infection, most oral warts in children develop from orocutaneous transmission; as in adults, orogenital transmission is also possible.
- Respiratory papillomatosis is probably transmitted during vaginal birth.

Clinical features and sequelae

Clinical manifestations depend on the HPV type involved, the anatomical location, and the immune status of the host.

Cutaneous warts

- Traditionally classified as: common warts (verruca vulgaris); palmoplantar warts (verruca plantaris), including superficial (mosaic) and deep (myrmecia) types; and plane/flat warts (verruca plana).
- In children, the majority (70%) have common warts, one-quarter have plantar warts; plane warts are less common.
- Cutaneous HPV types of α-PV species 2, 4 and 8, μ-, ν-, and γ-PV are those primarily responsible for cutaneous warts.
- Immunosuppressed individuals often have multiple HPV types, notably cutaneous β-PV types. These HPVs were previously thought to occur only in the context of the rare genodermatosis epidermodysplasia verruciformis, but now appear to be widespread in normal skin and hair follicles of the general population from early childhood, and are more prevalent in immunosuppressed individuals.
- Persistent wart infections are common as HPV has evolved mechanisms to evade immune surveillance. However, a successful immune response is eventually generated in most cases; two-thirds of cutaneous warts regress spontaneously within 2 years and multifocal lesions often regress simultaneously. The rate of clearance is influenced by viral type, age of the patient, and extent and duration of the warts and, in particular, host immune status.
- Cell-mediated immune responses appear to be primarily responsible, and impaired cell-mediated immunity is associated with markedly increased incidence and extensive spread of viral warts, e.g. after organ transplantation, HIV infection, chronic lymphatic leukaemia, and lymphoma.

Mucosal HPV-associated disease

- HPV infection in the oral mucosa caused by focal epithelial hyperplasia of 1–5mm size.

- Respiratory papillomatosis is a rare growth of benign papillomas in the respiratory tract, which may be single or multiple, multinodular and exophytic, mainly on the vocal cords and larynx, presenting as a voice change, abnormal cry, and stridor, and may present as an acute respiratory emergency. HPV11-associated disease is more severe than HPV6.
- Anogenital warts (condylomata acuminata) may present as small verrucous papules; discrete, flat, smooth-topped papules or plaques and as large, exophytic/hypertrophic masses. They are often asymptomatic, but may cause pruritus and bleeding, have a cauliflower-type shape and are mostly multiple with size varying from millimetres to several centimetres. They occur in females on the vulva or perianal area, the cervix, or vagina. In males the penis, scrotum, anus and perianal area may be affected.
- Oncogenic HPV is involved in 100% of cervical cancers and 90% of anal cancers (HPV-16, 18). The association is less for other cancers, as around 40% of vulvar, and vaginal cancers (HPV-16, 31, 33), 12% of oropharyngeal, and 3% of oral cancers are due to oncogenic HPV. Cervical dysplasia and invasive cervical cancer may be seen with the high-risk types of HPV-16 and 18.

HPV in the immunocompromised

- Warts occur more frequently in the immunocompromised child and an unusually severe infection with warts should alert the clinician to investigate for immune deficiency, either acquired or congenital.
- HIV-infected adolescents, even those with normal CD4 counts, tend to have a prolonged persistence of HPV.
- A rare HPV associated disease in the immunocompromised is the genodermatosis, epidermodysplasia verruciformis. Skin lesions may be highly polymorphic; red maculaes and plaques; plane wart-like lesions; pityriasis versicolor-like lesions, papillomas and seborrhoeic keratosis-likes lesions. Malignant conversion to squamous cell carcinoma occurs preferentially in sun-exposed sites in the third-fourth decades.

Table 79.1 Clinical, and virological features of warts in childhood.

Name	HPV types	Common sites of infection	Clinical features
Common warts *Verrucae vulgaris*	2, 4 (1, 7, 26, 27, 29, 41, 57)	Usually extremities, especially dorsa of hands/fingers, but may occur anywhere (rarely, oral)	Well-defined papule with irregular, 'cauliflower' surface. Size varies 1mm to >2cm. Skin-coloured to brown to grey. Single or multiple. Clustering and satellite lesions may develop and koebnerization (extension of lesions through trauma) is seen.

Table 79.1 (Contd.)

Name	HPV types	Common sites of infection	Clinical features
Plane or flat warts *Verrucae plana*	3,10 (28, 29)	Dorsa of hands, face (cheek, chin, forehead)	Flat-topped, round/polygonal, smooth or slightly hyperkeratotic. Often multiple, forming confluent plaques. May koebnerize, Facial lesions often flatter and pigmented and hand lesions more elevated and hyperkeratotic.
Deep palmoplantar warts (*Verruca plantaris*; myrmecia)	1 (2, 60, 63, 65)	Usually occur on pressure points of feet	Single, painful, endophytic, deep nodules with hyperkeratotic surface overlying soft keratinous debris and circumscribed by hyperkeratotic ring. Punctate bleeding or 'black dots' when pared (thrombosed dermal capillaries).
Superficial palmoplantar (mosaic) warts	2	Usually plantar	Painless, superficial, often recur, difficult to eradicate, may co-exist with myrmecia.
Epidermo-dysplasia verruciformis	5, 8 (beta types)	Any site	Highly polymorphic; red maculaes and plaques; plane wart-like lesions; pityriasis versicolor-like lesions, papillomas and seborrhoeic keratosis-like lesions. Malignant conversion to squamous cell carcinoma occurs preferentially in sun-exposed sites in the third-fourth decades.
Genital warts (Condyloma acuminata)	6, 11 (16, 18, 2, 27, 57)	On or around the vagina, penis, anus (rarely, oral)	May present as small verrucous papules; discrete, flat, smooth-topped papules or plaques and as large, exophytic/hypertrophic masses. Often asymptomatic, but may cause pruritus and bleeding.
Recurrent respiratory papillo-matosis (juvenile-onset)	6, 11 (16,18)	Approximately 95% involve the larynx, but may occur anywhere in the respiratory tract from the node to the lung	Recurrent growth of benign papillomas in the respiratory tract. Single or multiple. Multinodular and exophytic. Frequently causes hoarseness, poor cry, progressive dyspnoea, or stridor and may present as an acute respiratory emergency.

* most common HPV types involved are presented first followed by other less frequently involved types in brackets.

Diagnosis

- Visual inspection of warts can require internal examination depending on site (speculum, proctoscopy, or urethral meatoscopy).
- Histological and other laboratory tests including HPV DNA detection and serology are usually unnecessary and unhelpful in the diagnosis of most cases.
- Knowledge of the precise infecting HPV type does not necessarily assist in identifying the likely nature of infection. For example, the presence of DNA from high-risk mucosal types in a genital wart is not an unequivocal indication of a sexual mode of transmission and the presence of β-PV types does not occur exclusively in epidermodysplasia verruciformis or other immunosuppressed states.

Management and treatment

- There is no curative treatment for HPV and many warts disappear spontaneously. Recurrence of warts after treatment is common.
- Indications for treatment are pain, interference with function, and psychological morbidity.
- No treatment may be a reasonable option as approximately 23% of warts resolve spontaneously within 2 months and 65–78% within 2 years. A wide range of treatments is currently available; none is 100% effective and treatments may be needed for different types of warts and those at different anatomical sites.
- There is a lack of evidence regarding the efficacy of treatments for non-genital warts. A Cochrane systematic review recommended topical salicylic acid formulations as first-line treatment, since they are effective and safe with clearance rates of 73% in 6–12 weeks.[4] There is less evidence for the efficacy of cryotherapy and some evidence that it is only of equivalent efficacy to salicylic acid. Although other treatments (e.g. topical dinitrochlorobenzene, 5-fluorouracil, intralesional bleomycin and interferons, photodynamic therapy) may have a therapeutic effect, none have significant advantages over simpler, safer topical salicylic acid preparations and their suitability/safety for children has not been clearly determined.
- There is similarly insufficient evidence to direct first- and second-line treatments for genital warts.
- Topical podophyllotoxin, imiquimod, trichloroacetic acid, cryotherapy and electrosurgery/laser are all used. However their suitability/safety for children has not been clearly evaluated.
- Immunomodulators: Imiquimod 5% cream (apply once, three times a week, for up to 16 weeks, wash off with soap and water after 6–10 hours). This immune enhancer stimulates production of interferon and other cytokines, but may cause depigmentation.
- Warts in respiratory papillomatosis may require repeated surgical debulking, usually by microdebridement and laser procedures. Agents such as topical cidofovir may increase the interval between the need for these procedures.

- For detecting cellular abnormalities associated with malignancy in women later in life, screening by a national programme of regular Papanicolaou smears is performed every 3 years.

Prevention

- Patient education: avoid direct contact with warts from other people or other parts of the body; avoid sharing socks, shoes and towels; wear flipflops when using communal showers. Warts should be covered with waterproof tape in wet environments such as showers and swimming pools.
- Exclusion of children with warts from daycare facilities, school, or sports activities is not necessary.
- Condom use reduces the risk of acquiring HPV by 70% if condoms are reportedly used 100% of times. As transmission occurs via skin-to-skin contact, condoms do not completely prevent infection.
- In clinical trials vaccine efficacy for both the bivalent (Cervarix) and quadrivalent (Gardasil) vaccines was very high (≥90%) with the prevention of precancerous lesions associated with HPV-16 or 18 in those without evidence of prior infection. The first head-to-head trial between Cervarix and Gardasil showed similar results regarding virological and precancerous lesion endpoints for HPV-16/18. The immune response (neutralizing antibody titres in blood and cervical-vaginal secretions) appeared better for Cervarix then Gardasil and data suggest that more cross protection also occurred with the bivalent vaccine. However it is not clear whether this translates into differences in clinical outcome. Long-term studies are required to assess the later efficacy of both vaccines; persistence of protection has been shown for 8 years so far (℞ www.immunisation.nhs.uk). Current modelling predicts that a vaccination scheme involving 12-year-old girls is likely to be cost effective should vaccine protection be for >10 years.
- Routine HPV vaccination of teenage girls is therefore now recommended in many European countries.

Future research

- There is a lack of evidence to direct treatment for cutaneous warts.
- No effective antiviral agents have yet been identified for HPV.
- Therapeutic vaccines for conditions such as recurrent respiratory papillomatosis are being investigated.
- Should both genders be vaccinated against HPV?
- The cost-effectiveness of developing a preventive vaccine for non-genital warts has yet to be established.

Key references

1 de Villiers EM, Fauquet C, Broker TR, Bernard HU, Zur HH. Classification of papillomaviruses. *Virology* 2004;**324**:17–27.

2 Gibbs S, Harvey I. Topical treatments for cutaneous warts. *Cochrane Database Syst Rev* 2006;**3**:CD001781.

3 Williams HC, Pottier A, Strachan D. The descriptive epidemiology of warts in British schoolchildren. *Br J Dermatol* 1993;**28**:504–11.

4 World Health Organization Internal Agency for Research on Cancer. *IARC Monographs on the Evaluation of Carcinogenic Risks to Humans*. Volume 90. Human papillomaviruses. Lyon, France, 2007.

Influenza and parainfluenza

📖 see also Chapters 4, 27, 44

Influenza

Name and nature of organism

- Influenza viruses belong to the family *Orthomyxoviridae*, and they have a segmented RNA genome coding for around 10 proteins.
- Influenza viruses are classified into three distinct types: A, B, and C.
- The main surface antigens of the virus are hemagglutinin (16 known subtypes) and neuraminidase (nine known subtypes).
- Birds (waterfowl) are the natural reservoir of influenza A viruses.
- All known subtypes of hemagglutinin and neuraminidase have been found in birds, but few subtypes have been detected in humans.
- Influenza A viruses are divided into subtypes on the basis of their hemagglutinin and neuraminidase content (e.g. H1N1 or H3N2).
- Influenza viruses undergo constant antigenic adaptation because of point mutations in the viral genome ('antigenic drift').
- Major reassortment of gene segments from two different virus subtypes results in 'antigenic shift' with a virus expressing new HA antigens immunologically distinct from the previous strain; this may give rise to a new influenza pandemic.

Epidemiology

- Influenza viruses have a worldwide distribution.
- Epidemics of influenza A occur annually during wintertime in temperate regions of the northern hemisphere.
- Influenza A and B viruses cause large outbreaks. Most seasonal influenza in Europe is due to influenza A, with B causing more major outbreaks every few years; influenza C viruses are responsible for minor respiratory illnesses.
- The severity of the epidemics varies substantially from year to year depending on the antigenic variation of the circulating strains.
- Influenza attack rates are highest in young children.
- During the past 40 years, only A/H1N1, A/H3N2, and B viruses have been circulating among humans in epidemic proportions.
- A/H5N1 ('bird flu') viruses have continued to cause sporadic illnesses since 1997, but there have been no true epidemics.
- Depending on the definition used, four or five influenza pandemics have occurred during the past century (starting year: 1918 H1N1 Spanish flu, 1957 H2N2 Asian flu, 1968 H3N2 Hong Kong flu, 1977 H1N1, and the formal WHO pandemic 2009).

- The latest pandemic caused by a new type of A/H1N1 virus ('swine flu') started in Mexico in the spring of 2009 and has now spread all over the world. Swine-Origin Influenza Virus (S-OIV) A/H1N1 is derived from the original 1918 pandemic strain. Reassortment of virus between humans, bird, and swine influenza viruses continues as humans and animals have close contact.
- The threat of a new influenza pandemic exists all the time.

Transmission and incubation period

- Influenza viruses are spread by virus-laden respiratory secretions from infected subjects.
- Viruses can be transmitted through aerosols, large droplets, or direct contact with secretions.
- Viruses attach to sialic acid-containing receptors on the cell surface of the respiratory mucosa.
- The average incubation period is 2 days (range 1–5 days).
- Virus shedding begins 1 day before the onset of symptoms, peaks at 2–3 days, and continues for 5–7 days after symptom onset.
- Longer periods of shedding are frequently seen in children and immunocompromised patients.

Clinical features and sequelae

- The clinical presentation varies from asymptomatic infection to severe lethal illness.
- The duration of illness is usually between 3 and 8 days.
- Abrupt onset of illness is a classic feature of influenza.
- Typical initial symptoms in adults and older children include fever, chills, malaise, headache, myalgia, cough, and sore throat.
- Most young children with influenza have fever ≥39.0°C, and rhinitis during the early phase of the illness.
- Sepsis-like illness is a common reason for hospitalization of young infants, as well as croup and bronchiolitis.
- Older children have 'flu'-like symptoms, AOM, and pneumonia.
- Other common clinical manifestations include laryngitis, exacerbation of asthma, febrile convulsions, vomiting, and diarrhoea.
- Myositis (very painful leg muscles—especially with influenza B infection—raised creatine kinase—good recovery), myocarditis, encephalitis and encephalopathy are infrequent manifestations of influenza.
- The most frequent complication in children is AOM, which occurs in 40% of children <3 years of age.[1]
- Pneumonia and sinusitis are rarer complications in children. Secondary bacterial pneumonia is the main concern, particularly with *Staphylococcus aureus* or *Streptococcus pneumoniae*. Severe bacterial tracheitis and toxic shock are seen secondary to *S. aureus* disease.
- May cause very severe disease in immunocompromised, and children with pre-existing illness, e.g. cerebral palsy, neurological disease, HIV infection, cardiac disease, etc.

Diagnosis

- Clinical diagnosis of influenza is extremely difficult in young children because of signs and symptoms that overlap with those seen during other respiratory viral infections. A high neutrophil count is often seen in infants.
- Viral culture, antigen detection, and PCR-based assays can be used for laboratory diagnosis of influenza for clinical purposes.

Management and treatment

- Amantadine and rimantadine are active against influenza A viruses.
- Neuraminidase inhibitors oseltamivir and zanamivir are specific antivirals for the treatment of influenza.[2] They reduce symptoms by around 1 day when started within 48 h of symptom onset, but by up to 4 days if started within 24 hours of the onset of symptoms.[3]
- There is only limited evidence that antiviral therapy reduces rates of progression to severe disease in normal children. There are even fewer data on their use in neonates and high-risk children. Guidelines are based on weak evidence, so may therefore vary between countries. In the UK see the NICE website (⅍ www.nice.nhs.uk) for formal guidance.
- Oseltamivir is administered orally (capsules or suspension), and is licensed for children >1 year of age.
- Zanamivir is administered by inhalation with the use of a specific device and can be used in children >5 years.
- In general, antiviral treatment should be started at the latest within 48 hours of the onset of symptoms.
- When started within 48 hours of the onset of symptoms, oseltamivir has been reported to decrease the rate of development of AOM as a complication by approximately 40% in children.
- Antiviral resistance patterns of influenza viruses vary between different drugs, viral subtypes, and geographical areas but the decrease is approximately 80% if the treatment is started within 12 h of symptom onset.[3]
- Acetylsalicylic acid (aspirin) should not be used in children because of increased risk of Reye's syndrome.

Prevention

- Vaccination is the cornerstone of influenza prevention.
- The antigenic composition of influenza vaccine is changed annually in order to accommodate the seasonal changes that have occurred in the hemagglutinin glycoproteins of the circulating viruses.
- The clinical efficacy of influenza vaccine varies between different seasons depending on the degree of match between the strains included in the vaccine and the actual wild-type strains of influenza circulating in the community.
- The currently available inactivated influenza vaccines are administered intramuscularly and they can be given to children >6 months of age.
- Vaccine recommendations vary between different countries, but in developed countries influenza vaccination is generally recommended at least for children with certain chronic medical conditions.[4]
- An intranasally administered live attenuated influenza vaccine has been developed but is not licensed in Europe.

- In certain situations (primarily within households or for high-risk children), postexposure prophylaxis with influenza antivirals could be used to prevent a clinical illness. See ℘ www.nice.nhs.uk.

Future research
- More data on the burden of illness in children are needed to guide vaccine recommendations in this age group.
- Development of vaccines with increased and broader immunogenicity in children is an important goal.

Parainfluenza

Name and nature of organism
- Parainfluenza viruses (PIV) belong to the family *Paramyxoviridae* and have a single-stranded RNA genome.
- The viruses are classified into five types: 1, 2, 3, 4A, and 4B.
- No clinically significant antigenic variants of parainfluenza viruses are known to exist.

Epidemiology
- Parainfluenza viruses have a worldwide distribution.
- Major outbreaks (especially by endemic parainfluenza type 3 viruses—which causes most disease) occur usually in the spring months, but infections may occur at almost any time of the year.
- Type 1 and 2 viruses often cause epidemics in the autumn of every second year.
- Almost all children will be infected by type 3 viruses and most by type 1 and 2 viruses during their first years of life.
- Reinfections by the same virus type are common.

Transmission and incubation period
- Parainfluenza viruses are spread by large droplets or by direct contact with secretions from an infected subject.
- Viruses enter the body via the nose or eyes using sialic acid-containing membrane proteins as receptors.
- Virus replication is mostly limited to the respiratory tract; viraemia is extremely rare.
- The incubation period varies between 2 and 7 days, and it is probably dependent on the size of the inoculum.
- The duration of viral shedding is approximately 1 week, but type 3 viruses in particular may be shed for substantially longer periods.
- Virus shedding may begin several days before the onset of symptoms.

Clinical features and sequelae
- Type 1 and 2 viruses are among the most frequent causes of laryngitis and croup (laryngotracheobronchitis).
- Type 3 viruses are mostly associated with lower respiratory tract infections (bronchiolitis and pneumonia) but may also cause laryngitis and croup.

- Type 3 viruses have been occasionally associated with aseptic meningitis.
- AOM and sinusitis are the most frequent complications of parainfluenza virus infections.
- Immunocompromised children have higher rates of disease and shed virus longer.

Diagnosis

- For clinical purposes, antigen detection and PCR-based assays can be used for laboratory diagnosis of parainfluenza infections.
- The usefulness of serology is limited by substantial cross-reactivity between different types of parainfluenza viruses.
- Except for cases of laryngitis and croup during confirmed parainfluenza activity in the community, distinguishing parainfluenza infections from other viral respiratory infections on clinical grounds alone is very difficult in children.

Management and treatment

Treatment is supportive; no specific antiviral therapy is available.

Prevention

Vaccines against parainfluenza viruses (particularly type 3) are being developed, but currently are not commercially available.

Future research

Because of the substantial impact of parainfluenza virus infections on young children, the availability of both an effective vaccine and an antiviral treatment would be worthwhile goals for research in this area.[5]

Key references

1 Heikkinen T, Silvennoinen H, Peltola V, et al. Burden of influenza in children in the community. *J Infect Dis* 2004;**190**:1369–73.

2 Moscona A. Neuraminidase inhibitors for influenza. *N Engl J Med* 2005;**353**:1363–73.

3 Heinonen S, Silvennoinen H, Lehtinen P, et al. Early oseltamivir treatment of influenza in children 1–3 years of age: a randomized controlled trial. *Clin Infect Dis* 2010;**51**:887–94.

4 Heikkinen T, Booy R, Campins M, et al. Should healthy children be vaccinated against influenza? A consensus report of the Summits of Independent European Vaccination Experts. *Eur J Pediatr* 2006;**165**:223–8.

5 Lee MS, Walker RE, Mendelman PM. Medical burden of respiratory syncytial virus and parainfluenza virus type 3 infection among US children: Implications for design of vaccine trials. *Hum Vaccin* 2005;**1**:6–11.

Legionella

see also Chapters 17, 27

Name and nature of organism

A disease that occurs in three forms:

- A potentially fatal multisystem disease involving pneumonia (legionnaires' disease); a self-limited influenza-like infection (Pontiac fever); and a milder, non-pneumonic form of legionnaire's disease (distinct from Pontiac fever). *Legionella pneunophila*; named following a pneumonia outbreak at the American Legion Convention in 1976.
- Caused by Gram-negative, rod-shaped bacteria with fastidious growth requirements, primarily in aquatic environments as intracellular pathogens of protozoa. The bacteria are also found in biofilms in man-made water systems.

Epidemiology

- *Legionella* causes both sporadic and epidemic community-acquired and nosocomial pneumonia.
- Pontiac fever tends to occur in outbreaks with high attack rates >90% and no mortality.
- *Legionella* infection is rarely diagnosed in children. In the USA, only 1.7% of all cases of legionnaires' disease were reported in the paediatric age group; most paediatric cases are reported in children 15–19 years old.

Transmission and incubation period

- Water systems produce bacteria-containing aerosols that are dispersed into the atmosphere and can be inhaled. In the hospital, the sources of infection are: drinking water, respiratory therapy, and medical equipment (incubators, humidifiers). Nosocomial legionellosis has been reported in a few neonates after water birth.
- The incubation period ranges from 2 to 10 days for legionnaires' disease and from 12 to 48 hours for Pontiac fever.

Clinical features and sequelae

Legionnaires' disease

- Pneumonia is the predominant clinical manifestation of legionnaires' disease. A small proportion of mild, community-acquired pneumonia in older children is due to legionnaire's disease.

- Some clinical signs are associated with severe legionnaire's disease rather than with other causes of pneumonia.
- Abnormal lung: unilateral changes (which may extend to bilateral involvement) with or without pleural effusion, pulmonary infiltrates, and cavitation. Progression of pulmonary infiltrates, despite standard antibiotic therapy for pneumonia.
- Non-specific symptoms: fever, cough (often dry and non-productive), tachypnoea, hypoxia, headache.
- Gastrointestinal manifestations include vomiting, nausea, and diarrhoea.

Pontiac fever

- The symptoms mimic influenza with fever, headache, chills, myalgia, malaise, nausea, non-productive cough, abdominal pain, arthralgia, a dry or sore throat, ear pain, and rash.
- Other symptoms: vomiting, diarrhoea, fatigue, dizziness, dyspnoea, low back pain, thoracic pains, poor concentration.
- The chest radiograph is normal and recovery within 1 week is usual.

Diagnosis

The key to the diagnosis of legionnaire's disease is to perform the appropriate microbiological tests. The following laboratory methods are used to diagnose *Legionella* infection:

- Isolation (culture on buffered charcoal yeast extract (BCYE) agar supplemented with antibiotics) of *Legionella* species from clinical specimens. Culture of *Legionella* spp., with a specificity of 100%, is the gold standard.
- Positive urine ELISA using validated reagents, or seroconversion, or DFA staining of *Legionella* in respiratory secretions
- PCR test
- Non-specific laboratory findings commonly seen in legionnaire's disease in paediatric cases include:
  • Leucocytosis (>15 000 WBCs/ml) or leucopenia (<5000 WBCs/ml)
  • Elevated serum creatinine kinase
  • Elevated LFTs
  • Hyponatraemia.

Management and treatment

- Early initiation of appropriate treatment is crucial for successful treatment reducing the mortality rate. Only symptomatic treatment is recommended for Pontiac fever.
- Antibiotics which have good intracellular penetration into macrophages and achieve high intracellular concentrations should be used (macrolides, fluoroquinolones, tetracyclines, rifamycins, and ketolides).
- Macrolides, usually azithromycin, are an effective and well-tolerated first-line treatment for 5–10 days.

- Fluoroquinolones are very effective in the treatment of legionnaire's disease in immunocompromised children. A 7–10-day course of treatment is usually sufficient.
- Despite advances in the diagnosis and treatment of legionnaire's disease, the reported mortality rate is high.

Prevention

- The disease is not passed from person to person, so isolation is not necessary.
- Legionnaire's disease is the result of inhalation of contaminated aerosol transmitted from the environment. For water births, installation of a filter system into the birthing tub hose is crucial.

Future research

- Improved understanding of the ecology of *Legionella*, i.e. recognition of the factors that effect bacteria survival and growth in the natural environment.
- Improvement of diagnostic methods of identification of all the *Legionella* species and serogroups.
- Further work on the importance of *Legionella* testing in children with undiagnosed pneumonia.

Further reading

DiedeREN BM. *Legionella* spp. and legionnaires' disease. *J Infect* 2008;**56**:1–12.

Greenberg D, Chiou CC, Famigilleti R, Lee CT, Yu LV. Problem pathogens: paediatric legionellosis-implications for improved diagnosis. *Lancet Infect Dis* 2006;**6**:529–35.

Pedro-Botet ML, Yu LV. Treatment strategies for *Legionella* infection. *Expert Opin Pharmacother* 2009;**10**:1109–21.

Leishmaniasis

see also Chapters 2, 3, 22, 34, 42, 45

Name and nature of organism

- *Leishmania* group contains over 20 species of obligate intracellular parasites (Table 82.1).
- Sand flies *Phlebotomus* and *Lutzomyia* are the vectors.

Table 82.1 *Leishmania* species, origin and spectrum of disease

Clinical form	Localization	*Leishmania* species
Visceral leishmaniasis (VL)	Old World	L. donovani, L. infantum
	New World	L. chagasi, L. amazonensis
Cutaneous leishmaniasis (CL)	Old World	L. donovani, L. tropica, L. aethiopica, L. major, L. infantum
	New World	L. mexicana, L. amazonensis, L. venezuelensis, L. braziliensis, L. guyanensis, L. peruviana, L. panamensis, L. chagasi
Mucocutaneous leishmaniasis (ML)	Old World	L. aethiopica
	New World	L. braziliensis, L. guyanensis, L. panamensis

- An estimated 350 million people are at risk worldwide.
- 12 million humans develop the disease (50% are children).
- Incidence of VL is about 0.5 million cases/year. Incidence of the cutaneous form is around 1.5 million cases/year. There are around 70 000 deaths/year globally.
- Leishmaniasis affects countries in tropical and subtropical areas worldwide, particularly Central and South America, southern Europe, North and East Africa, the Middle East, and the Indian subcontinent.
- In Europe, VL has been reported from Greece, Spain and the Balearic Islands, Portugal, Turkey, and many other countries that are popular holiday destinations for sun-deprived northern Europeans.

- VL is predominantly seen in Sudan and India (Bihar).
- CL is more common in Afghanistan, Syria, and Brazil.
- Highest incidence in Europe is in the Iberian peninsula and the Mediterranean Islands, the visceral form being most common.
- Up-to-date information can be obtained from the EU-funded project Leishrisk website (🖰 www.leishrisk.net).

Transmission and incubation period

- Sandflies feeding on infected human beings (anthroponoses) or terrestrial mammals (zoonoses) become infected by the ingestion of macrophage cells containing amastigotes.
- Amastigotes transform into promastigotes and multiply extracellular in the sandfly gut.
- The cycle is completed when infective metacyclic promastigotes are injected at a subsequent blood meal into the skin of the new host (see Fig. 82.1).

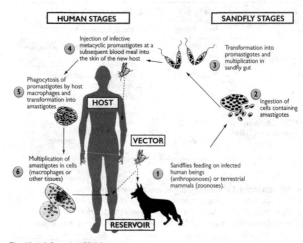

Fig. 82.1 Life cycle of *Leishmania* parasites.

(Adapted from Reithinger et al.,[1] with permission from Elsevier)

- Rarely the parasite can be transmitted without intervention of sandflies. Examples are infections as a result of organ transplantation, transplacental spread, transfusion, and sharing needles.

- Incubation period of the visceral form is 2–6 months after the sandfly bite, but can vary from 2 weeks up to several years.
- Incubation time of the cutaneous forms is shorter, being several days to 2 months.

Clinical features and sequelae

Visceral leishmaniasis (kala-azar)

- *L. infantum* or *L. chagasi* generally affects children <5 years of age in the Mediterranean region and the New World.
- *L. donovani* infects older children and young adults in Africa and Asia.
- Primary lesion at the site of inoculation is the first sign of infection. This is a small papule or ulcer.
- Initial symptoms are non-specific, such as low-grade fever, weakness, malaise, weight loss, and progressive enlargement of liver and spleen. Darkening of the skin, especially on hands, feet, abdomen and forehead, although typical for this disease (kala-azar means 'black fever' in Hindi) is actually infrequent.
- Pancytopenia is common and caused by hypersplenism, bone marrow infiltration, and autoimmune mechanisms. A Coombs positive haemolytic anaemia is seen.
- Children may be misdiagnosed as having leukaemia or lymphoma.
- Without treatment prognosis is poor with mortality rates being >90%. The main causes of death are complications of bacterial infections, haemorrhage, and progressive cachexia.

Cutaneous leishmaniasis

- Affects individuals of any age, but frequently seen in children.
- The lesions typically begin near to the sandfly bite on nocturnally exposed skin such as the face and extremities. It presents as a papule which enlarges to a nodule and ulcerates over weeks to months.
- There are certain differences in the forms of presentation. Generally, in Old World CL, most lesions are papules, nodules or nodule-ulcers—ulcerative lesions are more common in New World CL.
- It looks often like chronic impetigo, i.e. unresponsive to topical or systemic antibiotics.
- In the absence of bacterial superinfection, the lesions usually heal after 3–6 months, leaving a depressed scar.

Mucosal leishmaniasis

- Haematogenous spread from cutaneous lesions to the nasal or oropharyngeal mucosa, with some types of *Leishmania* such as *L. braziliensis*, results in this serious and life-threatening manifestation.
- Generally the patients have had active cutaneous lesions over the past 2 years.
- Nasal mucosa is involved in the majority of cases. Typical symptoms are nasal congestion, epistaxis, and discharge; ulceration and destruction of the oronasal structures.

Diagnosis

Visceral leishmaniasis

- Diagnostic gold standard is by direct visualization of amastigotes in tissue aspiration samples or isolation of the organism by culture.
- Sensitivity for splenic biopsy is >95%, for bone marrow 55–97%, and lymph node aspirate smears 60%.
- Measurement of antileishmanial IgG is diagnostic in high titre. The diagnosis is by serology or Giemsa stain of bone marrow aspirates.
- New methods include freeze-dried antigen (no refrigeration needed), rapid detection of anti-K39 antibody with finger stick blood in an immunochromatographic strip test (sensitivity >90%), and urine testing for leishmanial antigen or antibody.
- Due to increasing numbers of immunocompromised hosts (HIV-infected patients and transplant recipients), testing of peripheral blood and bone marrow by PCR has become increasingly important.

Cutaneous and mucocutaneous leishmaniasis

- Presence of one or more nodular, or ulcerative skin lesion in combination with potential contact with the parasite or travel to endemic regions makes the diagnostic of CL probable.
- Definitive diagnosis is mostly made by direct visualization of amastigotes and culture in biopsies from the ulcer base of the lesion.
- Serological antibody or antigen-searching tests are of less value.

Management and treatment

- Outcome of infection (including spontaneous healing and prevention of reactivation) is determined by the interaction of the host (innate and acquired immune responses) with the pathogen.

Visceral leishmaniasis

- A country's wealth affects the treatment choice (balance between drug efficacy, toxicity, and costs associated with patient care).
- Main treatment options are pentavalent antimony salts and amphotericin B deoxycholate or lipid formulations of amphotericin B.
- Dose and schedule of administration varies according to geographical region and patient profile.
- Currently, various combination therapies are being used and the evidence base is too limited to be able to compare therapies.
- Cure rates are very high, >95% with nearly all standard therapies.
- Aim is to increase treatment efficacy, minimize costs, and risk of parasite resistance development. In Europe, probably the most commonly used regimen is L-amB on day 1, 2, 3, 4, 5, and 10.
- A recent randomized trial in 410 patients in India showed that one single infusion of L-amB was not inferior.[2]

Localized cutaneous and mucocutaneous leishmaniasis

- It is important to distinguish between the different species. Lesions caused by the subgenus *Viannia* should be treated more aggressively because of its high risk of developing mucosal disease.
- Old World lesions self-cure within 2–4 months (*L. major*) or 6–15 months (*L. tropica*).
- New World lesions due to *L. mexicana* resolve spontaneously after 3 month in >75% of cases, but spontaneous resolution of *L. panamensis* and *L. braziliensis* infection is less common.
- Indications for systemic or topical treatment are not clearly defined.

Criteria for systemic treatment

- Lesions in cosmetically or functional critical areas such as the face, hands and feet and/or near joints.
- Lesions with low tendency of self-healing for >6 months.
- More than five lesions or large lesions over 4cm.
- Suspicion of disseminated disease or mucocutaneous disease.

Systemic and local treatment

- Parenteral antimony remains the gold standard for CL. However, in this self-healing disease treatment toxicity must be considered.
- Pentamidine has high efficacy (60–95%; *L. braziliensis* <50%) in a short-course, low-dose regimen particularly in South and Central America.
- Combination of cryotherapy and intralesional antimony has proved to be more effective than either therapy alone.
- Due to the potential for fatal outcome, systemic therapy with parenteral antimony or amphotericin B is indicated in all cases of mucosal disease (ML).[3]

Prevention

Protection against sandfly bites

- Use of insect repellents, appropriate clothes (cover arms and legs).
- In regions where sandflies are endophagic (mainly feeding indoors) bed nets reduces significantly the risk of infection.

Control of zoonotic infection

- In areas such as Latin America, the Mediterranean basin, central and southwest Asia control of dogs, the primary animal reservoir, is of great importance.
- Rapid identification, sensitive and specific diagnostic tests, and effective culling are essential for an effective reservoir control.
- Deltamethrin treated collars are one of the most effective strategies, reducing the number of infected dogs and children.

Insecticide spraying of houses

- House spraying with pyrethroid is the most widely used strategy for controlling endophilic (rest mostly indoors after feeding) sandflies.

Vaccines
- Vaccines based on killed parasites have been shown to be safe and immunogenetic, however long-lasting protection could not be achieved.

Future research

- Standardized protocols of experimental, clinical and epidemiological studies.
- Further understanding into the pathology and immunology of this disease.
- To achieve long-lasting immunity research is focused on the identification of novel antigens, live-attenuated vaccines, recombinant purified proteins, bacteria expressing *Leishmania* antigens and targeting dendritic cells (specialized antigen-presenting cells, which play an important role in the clearance of *Leishmania*-infected cells).

Key references

1 Murray HW, Berman JD, Davies CR, Saravia NG, Advances in leishmaniasis. *Lancet* 2005;**366**(9496):1561–77. Review.
2 Reithinger R, Dujardin JC, Louzir H, Pirmez C, Alexander B, Brooker S. Cutaneous leishmaniasis. *Lancet Infect Dis* 2007;**7**:581–96.
3 Sundar S, Chakravarty J, Agarwal D, Rai M, Murray HW, Single-dose liposomal amphotericin B for visceral leishmaniasis in India. *N Engl J Med* 2010; Feb 11;**362**:504–12.

Further reading

Available at: ℘ www.leishrisk.net (accessed 1 February 2011). Website of an EU-funded project which aims to network the projects working on leishmaniasis under FP5, FP6 and FP7.

Listeriosis

📖 see also Chapters 10, 12, 14, 20, 21, 29, 30

Name and nature of organism

- Listeriosis is a severe but relatively rare infection in the general population and it affects primarily pregnant women, unborn and newly delivered infants, the immunocompromised, and elderly.[1,3,4]
- Genus *Listeria* are non-sporing, aerobic, motile, Gram-positive bacilli, ubiquitous in the environment.
- The genus contains seven species, but almost all cases of human listeriosis are due to *Listeria monocytogenes*.
- Almost all outbreaks of listeriosis have been caused predominantly by serovar 4b strains.
- In clinical specimens, the organisms may be Gram-variable and look like diphtheroids, cocci, or diplococci and therefore can be mistaken for a contaminant. Beware the 'diphtheroid contaminant' in the CSF—could it be *Listeria*—ask the microbiologist again!
- The bacilli exhibit characteristic 'tumbling' motility at 25°C.
- Its ability to survive and multiply under conditions used for food preservation makes *Listeria* problematic to the food industry.

Epidemiology

- *L. monocytogenes* is an important zoonoses in herd animals.
- It has also been recovered from a variety of raw foods, such as uncooked meats and vegetables, or food items that become contaminated during their processing, such as soft cheeses. *L. monocytogenes* is killed by pasteurization and cooking. In ready-to-eat foods contamination may occur after cooking, before packaging.
- The peak incidence of human disease occurs in the summer.
- In 2006, listeriosis was the fifth most common zoonotic infection in Europe, after *Campylobacter*, *Salmonella*, *Yersinia*, and *VTEC*.
- The infection rate in Europe varied between 1 and 10 cases per million of the population, and approximately 20% were neonates.[2]
- There has been a recent increase in pregnancy-related cases in the UK, linked to ethnic minority women.
- Listeriosis is very rare in children >3 months of age (100 cases per million) and pregnant women are 20 times more likely to develop the infection than the general population.

Transmission and incubation period

- Alimentary transmission is the most common route of acquisition.
- Microbiological and epidemiological evidence supports an association with many food types (dairy, meat, vegetable, fish and shellfish, sandwiches) in both sporadic and epidemic listeriosis.
- Maternal infection is associated with abortion, preterm delivery, and fetal death.
- Late-onset neonatal infection can result from acquisition of the organism during birth or from environmental food sources.
- The incubation period is from 1 to 90 days, with an average for intra-uterine infections of around 30 days.

Clinical features and sequelae

Infection in pregnancy

- Most maternal infections occur during the third trimester of pregnancy, when T cell immunity is most impaired.
- Approximately 65% of infected women typically develop a non-specific 'flu-like' syndrome (fever, headache, myalgia), gastrointestinal symptoms or back pain, but may remain asymptomatic.
- 22% of perinatal listeriosis results in stillbirth or neonatal death.[4]

Neonatal infection

- Neonatal listeriosis is classified as early or late infection, depending on timing of the onset of symptoms. Infants are believed to be infected *in utero* because of the maternal bacteraemic phase.
- The mean onset of symptoms is 1.5 days after birth.
- Disease can be early-onset with a sepsis-like picture in the first day or two of life, or late-onset, more commonly presenting with meningitis at around 1–2 weeks of age.
- A sepsis-like picture predominates, but other common manifestations are acute respiratory distress, pneumonia, meconium-staining, fever, rash, jaundice, and more rarely, meningitis or myocarditis.
- In both early- and late-onset neonatal listeriosis, the mortality rate ranges from 10% to 30%.
- Listeriosis in children older than 1 month is very rare, except in those with underlying disease.

Diagnosis

- The organisms can be recovered on blood agar media from cultures of blood, CSF, meconium, amniotic fluid, placenta, gastric washings, placental tissue, and other infected tissue specimens, including joint, pleural, or pericardial fluid.
- When the CNS is infected, polymorphonuclear leucocytes predominate in 70% of cases. Protein levels are usually elevated, and

higher values are correlated with poor prognosis. In 60% of the cases, glucose levels in CSF are normal.
- The Gram stain of CSF is positive in <40% of patients; however, blood cultures are positive in 60–70%.

Management

- No controlled trials have established a drug of choice or duration of therapy for listeriosis.
- *L. monocytogenes* is susceptible to a wide range of antibiotics *in vitro*, including penicillin G, ampicillin, erythromycin, vancomycin, sulfamethoxazole, trimethoprim, chloramphenicol, rifampicin, tetracyclines, and aminoglycosides.[5]
- *Listeria* are always resistant to cephalosporins. This is a problem because ceftriaxone and cefotaxime are the standard first-line drugs for meningitis in many countries. Neonatal sepsis empirical antibiotic regimens without penicillin/ampicillin or gentamicin do not treat listeriosis.
- IV ampicillin and amoxicillin, which are superior to penicillin, are the mainstay of treatment, although high drug concentrations are required for bactericidal effects.
- Gentamicin has had synergistic effects in some studies and should be added initially to the treatment.
- Gentamicin with ampicillin (amoxicillin) is recommended for *Listeria* meningitis to decrease the number of bacteria because most bacteria are extracellular. Almost no resistance has developed to this treatment.
- No systematic study examined the duration of therapy, but the current recommendations are 10–14 days of treatment for invasive infection without meningitis and 14 to 21 days for *L. monocytogenes* meningitis.
- Longer courses are needed for patients who are severely ill or who have endocarditis or thromboencephalitis.
- The prognosis for liveborn children with sepsis is relatively good if they are promptly treated, but long-term neurological deficits are common after meningitis.

Prevention

- Although foodborne outbreaks of listeriosis are uncommon, they remain a major public health problem. Therefore, detecting an outbreak early and identifying its source is a priority.
- There is no vaccine to prevent *Listeria* infection.
- Recommendations for prevention of listeriosis from a foodborne source were developed by the CDC in 1992. They include washing of raw vegetables; avoidance of unpasteurized dairy products; thorough cooking of raw food; washing of hands, knives, cutting boards after exposure to uncooked foods.

- Pregnant women and immunocompromised patients should be advised to avoid unpasteurized soft cheeses, deli meat, and shop bought sandwiches, hot dogs, refrigerated pates, and smoked seafood because they can harbour high levels of contamination.
- Cases of listeriosis should be reported to the local health authorities to facilitate early recognition of outbreaks.

Future research

- *L. monocytogenes* has been used as a model pathogen for >40 years; however, recent studies suggest there are still unidentified immunological aspects of *L. monocytogenes* infection and immunity.
- The epidemiological risk factors for pregnancy acquisition are still not fully understood.
- How *Listeria* precisely interacts with the intestinal barrier is an important issue for understanding later stages of infection. Is there a critical role for other intestinal cells besides enterocytes? How does the interaction with the intestinal barrier shape the immune response?
- Finally, how does *Listeria* precisely cross the placental and the blood–brain barrier? Answering these questions is now a priority.
- At present, there is no satisfactory therapy for the treatment of *Listeria* infection. Thus, new drugs with a better activity against these bacteria need to be discovered.

References

1 Braden CR. Listeriosis. *Pediatr Infect Dis J* 2003;**22**:745–6.
2 Denny J. Human *Listeria monocytogenes* infections in Europe—an opportunity for improved European surveillance. *Eurosurveillance* 2008;**13**:8082.
3 Gillespie IA. Changing pattern of human listeriosis, England and Wales, 2001–2004. *Emerg Infect Dis* 2006;**12**:1361–6.
4 Mylonakis E. Listeriosis during pregnancy. *Medicine (Baltimore)* 2002;**81**:260–9.
5 Hof H. An update on the medical management of listeriosis. *Expert Opin Pharmacother* 2004;**5**:1727–35.

Lyme disease

📖 see also Chapters 14, 34

Name and nature of organism

- A spirochaete, *Borrelia burgdorferi*, causes Lyme disease.
- *B. recurrentis* causes louse-borne relapsing fever, and *B. turicatae*, *B. hermsii*, *B. parkeri*, and *B. duttoni* cause tick-borne relapsing fever.

Epidemiology

- Lyme disease was first recognized in 1975 in Lyme, Connecticut, USA.
- Lyme is the commonest vector-borne human infection in the UK. The infection is endemic in parts of the USA, with around 15 000 cases reported/year. The infection is spread across all age groups. There were 813 laboratory confirmed cases in the UK in 2008 of which 91 were contracted abroad. The incidence is commonest in the summer and early autumn.
- The number of cases may be higher because of the significant seronegative rate in patients tested at the onset of clinical signs.

Transmission and incubation period

- From tick vectors (*Ixodes* species in northern Europe: *Ixodes ricinus* deer or sheep ticks), with a nymph and larval stage. The tick bite needs to be usually longer than 24 hours for human infection to occur.
- Usual vectors are deer in the UK.
- Feeding for several hours on the human being is a prerequisite for transmission
- Person-to-person transmission does not occur.
- Incubation period is 3–20 days with a median of 12 days.

Clinical features and complications

- Clinical disease can be divided into three stages based on the timing after infection. The commonest first feature is the typical rash of erythema migrans, or erythema chronicum migrans, a raised circular lesion (average diameter around 15cm) which spreads out from the site of the tick bite. This usually occurs around 3–30 days after the tick bite, and lasts around 3 weeks.

- Non-specific flu-like symptoms with fever, arthralgia, myalgia, headaches, and neck stiffness may occur at the same time.
- Neurological disease then usually develops between 2 and 10 weeks after the tick bite. Aseptic meningitis, chorea, cerebellar ataxia, and cranial nerve palsies have been reported. Lyme meningitis has been associated with a long duration of headache, cranial neuritis and CSF mononuclear cells.
- Facial palsy is usually unilateral; this occurs usually several weeks or months after infection.
- Arthritis also usually begins around 4 weeks after the tick bite and is most often of a single large joint (knee, shoulder, elbow). This is transient, but may persist or recur for years. It is uncommon in the UK.
- A carditis can also very rarely occur (more in young men).
- The much later neuropsychiatric manifestations (after months or years) and chronic fatigue are extremely rare in children.

Diagnosis

- The skin lesion is pathognomic. With a history of a tick bite, a clinical diagnosis can be made.
- Serological tests may not be positive in the first few weeks of infection.
- In the UK the Lyme Borreliosis Unit of the HPA uses a two stage procedure. The first stage is an EIA screen—positive or indeterminate samples are then tested with an immunoblot or western blot test to confirm the presence of *B. burgdorferi* (Bb) antibodies. There are formal criteria to diagnose a positive western blot, requiring multiple positive bands. Late stage disease should virtually always have a strongly positive IgG. In the UK positive serology is confirmed by the HPA Lyme Borreliosis Unit in Southampton.
- Another test useful for joint aspirates and skin samples is the PCR.

Treatment

- For early, localized Lyme disease and disseminated disease including isolated VIIth nerve palsy and arthritis in a child of ≥12 years use doxycycline or amoxicillin orally for 14–21 days.
- In the younger child amoxicillin in three divided doses is preferred.
- Clarithromycin can be used where there is a definite history of penicillin allergy.
- Use IV ceftriaxone for meningitis and all other neurological disease for between 2 and 4 weeks.
- The great majority of children make a full recovery with no long-term complications.

Prevention

Wearing long trousers and shirts when walking in the woods, using insect repellents, checking children for ticks each day, removing any ticks with tweezers.

Routine prophylactic antibiotics after tick bites are not indicated.

Future research

- Vaccine development is underway for Lyme disease.
- Improved evidence base for different treatment strategies and long-term outcome.

Further reading

Canadian Public Health Laboratory Network. The laboratory diagnosis of Lyme borreliosis: Guidelines from the Canadian Public Health Laboratory Network. *Can J Infect Dis* 2007;**18**:145–8.

Stanek G, Strle F. Lyme borreliosis. *Lancet* 2003;**362**:1639–47.

Wormser GP, Dattwyler RJ, Shapiro ED, *et al.* The clinical assessment, treatment, and prevention of Lyme disease, human granulocytic anaplasmosis and babesiosis: clinical practice guidelines by the Infectious Diseases Society of America. *Clin Infect Dis* 2006;**43**:1089–34.

Chapter 85

Malaria

📖 see also Chapters 3, 41, 42

Name and nature of organism

- Vector-borne infection caused by protozoan parasites of the genus *Plasmodium*.
- Five species known to infect humans.
- *P. falciparum* causes the most severe disease and is responsible for most of the long-term complications and virtually all the deaths related to malaria.
- *P. vivax*, *P. ovale*, and *P. malariae* usually cause milder disease and are not fatal except in individuals with underlying comorbidities.
- *P. knowlesi* usually causes malaria in primates and only infects humans opportunistically, but recent studies have suggested that *P. knowlesi* may contribute to a significant proportion of malaria cases in parts of Southeast Asia, where such infections may be misdiagnosed as *P. malariae*.

Epidemiology

- Malaria is one of the most common infectious diseases globally.
- In 2006, there were ~250 million malaria cases among 3 billion people at risk and 880 000 deaths, mainly in children <5 years; 86% of cases and over 90% of deaths occurred in Africa.
- In Europe, the UK has one of the highest burdens of imported malaria.
- The number of reported cases in all ages peaked in 1995 at 2500 cases and gradually fell to 1370 cases in 2008, when 1087 cases (79%) were due to *P. falciparum* and there were six deaths (0.4%).
- Children account for 15–20% of all cases; the number of childhood malaria cases also peaked in 1996 at 416 cases and has gradually fallen to 226 cases in 2006.
- Children have different risk factors for developing malaria compared with adults and have a higher risk of severe disease as they are more likely to be non-immune to the infection.
- A recent BPSU study estimated the burden of imported malaria in the UK to be 2.8/100 000 children; *P. falciparum* accounted for 85% of childhood cases; 90% of all malaria cases occurred among black African children, who mainly acquired the infection in Africa (particularly Nigeria, 55%).
- Two-thirds of children who developed malaria lived in the UK and had travelled to a malaria endemic country, mainly during school holidays

(July to October and January to February) to visit friends and relatives, and only 8% had taken appropriate antimalarial prophylaxis.
- Families visiting friends and relatives are less likely to seek pre-travel advice, or take antimalarial prophylaxis, or bite prevention measures, and are more likely to travel to rural malaria-endemic areas for longer periods; they are also more likely to delay seeking medical help when returning to their country of residence, often because of cultural and language barriers.
- Imported childhood malaria is generally associated with low mortality of ~1% in Europe; in the UK, 2/1456 children (0.14%) died between 1999 and 2003—but both had been seen by a healthcare professional at least once and malaria had not been suspected.

Transmission

- Malaria in transmitted by the female *Anopheles* mosquito.
- Chronically infected humans are the major reservoir of malaria.
- The *anopheles* mosquito acquires the parasite during a blood meal from an infected person and transfers it to another person during the next blood meal.
- Rare cases have been reported following blood transfusion, or needlestick injury from infected donors.
- Airport malaria occurs in or around international airports when a parasitised mosquito that survived a long-distance air flight from an endemic country infects a person.

Incubation period

- The duration between infection and development of symptoms varies with the species responsible.
- *P. falciparum* infections usually present (85%) within a month, with <1% of cases presenting after 6 months.
- In contrast, 25% of non-falciparum malaria cases present within 1 month, while 60% present within 6 months, and 90% within a year.
- The life cycles of *P. vivax* and *P. ovale* have a hypnozoite form during which the parasite can persist in the liver for months before emerging and causing recurring after the initial infection.

Clinical features

- Symptoms are varied and often mimic other common childhood illnesses particularly gastroenteritis, meningitis/encephalitis, or pneumonia.
- There is increased recognition of the pneumonic and enteric clinical presentation of malaria alone without any secondary bacterial infection.

- Fever is invariably present; but the characteristic regular tertian and quartan patterns are seen in <25% of children; however, children are more likely to have high fever >40°C, which may lead to febrile convulsions.
- Nausea and vomiting are also common and should be taken into consideration if intending to treat the infection with oral anti-malarials.
- Compared with adults, children are less likely to complain of chills, arthralgia/myalgia or headache but are more likely to have hepatomegaly, splenomegaly, and jaundice.
- *P. malariae* infections are also associated with the development of nephrotic syndrome.

Severe malaria

- Severe malaria occurs almost exclusively with *P. falciparum* infections.
- 5–15% of children with imported malaria present with features of severe malaria as defined by the WHO; these criteria, however, were developed for endemic countries and may not necessarily be appropriate for imported malaria.
- In imported cases, severe malaria is associated with young age (<5 years), delayed diagnosis and non-immunity to malaria.
- Immunocompromised children, asplenics, and those with homozygous sickle cell disease are more likely to develop severe malaria.
- Features of severe or complicated malaria include impaired consciousness, coma, seizures, respiratory distress, acidosis (pH <7.3), hypoglycaemia (<2.2mmol/l), severe anaemia (<8g/dl), prostration (the inability to stand or sit), and high parasitaemia (>5% red blood cells).
- Children with severe malaria may also develop focal neurological signs, decerebrate or decorticate posturing, spontaneous bleeding, disseminated intravascular coagulation, hypotension, cardiovascular shock, pulmonary oedema, haemoglobinuria, acute renal failure, and multi-organ failure.
- Concurrent bacterial septicaemia is rare (<5%) but should be considered in children presenting with severe symptoms.
- Children who have taken any antimalarial prophylaxis and those who have been partially treated for malaria may present with minimal symptoms or signs.
- Tropical splenomegaly syndrome, also known as hyperreactive malarial syndrome, usually occurs after repeat exposure to malaria and is characterized by gross splenomegaly, high antibody levels of *Plasmodium* species, hypergammaglobulinaemia (mainly IgM), clinical and immunological response, and regression of splenomegaly over several months after antimalarial therapy.

Diagnosis

- Malaria remains a relatively rare cause of fever in non-endemic areas and requires a high index of suspicion; obtaining a history of foreign travel or of immigration from a malaria-endemic area is vital.
- Delays in diagnosis are associated with an increased risk of severe malaria, requirement for intensive care and death.

- The presence of thrombocytopenia in children with fever following travel to a malaria-endemic area is highly predictive of malaria.
- Diagnosis is usually confirmed by microscopic examination of thick and thin blood films (preferably at the height of fever), which should be requested in any febrile unwell child who has travelled to a malaria-endemic area in the preceding 12 months, irrespective of any chemoprophylaxis taken.
- Thick blood smears are more sensitive in detecting malaria parasites because the blood is more concentrated, allowing for a greater volume of blood to be examined.
- Diagnosis may be missed because of a lack of experienced laboratory support or because the initial blood film may be negative (up to 7% of cases); therefore, three negative blood films should be obtained before malaria can be safely excluded.
- In falciparum malaria, the percentage of parasitized red blood cells, the presence of *P. falciparum* schizonts and pigment deposits in peripheral polymorphonuclear leucocytes may indicate severe malaria.
- Rapid antigen detection tests by means of a 'dipstick' format can distinguish between the four common species and their use in routine diagnosis has increased.
- PCR and serological tests may also be used to confirm the diagnosis, but are usually performed in reference laboratories and reserved for retrospective diagnosis and epidemiological research.

Management and treatment

- Updated guidance on the treatment of malaria in the UK are available on the HPA website (⊗ www.hpa.org.uk) under Malaria—Guidelines.
- Management varies according to the *Plasmodium* species responsible, national guidelines, antimalarial availability, and individual patient factors.
- Treatment does not usually differ between non-immune travellers and immigrants.
- All children with suspected or diagnosed with *P. falciparum* malaria should probably be admitted to hospital for at least 24 hours, because of the possibility of rapid progression in severity of malaria and poor tolerance of oral therapies.
- A thick and thin blood smear, FBCs, electrolytes, blood glucose, and renal and liver function tests should be performed on all patients, as well as testing for glucose-6-phosphate dehydrogenase (G6PD) deficiency.
- Haematological and biochemical parameters are often abnormal.
- Anaemia occurs in 31–100% of cases, although the need for transfusion is rare (<2%).
- Thrombocytopenia (platelet counts <150 × 10^9/l) is characteristic of malaria and occurs in 50–70% but, unlike adults, is not associated with bleeding, even at very low counts.

- Leucocytosis and leucopenia (19–30%) may occur but are usually not associated with severity of malaria or concurrent bacterial infections in imported cases.
- Jaundice (30–50%) and raised liver enzymes (25–40%) are also relatively common but not usually associated with an adverse outcome in imported malaria.
- Children with uncomplicated malaria, low parasitaemia, and no vomiting may be treated with oral antimalarials.
- The combination of oral quinine with a single dose of sulfadoxine-pyrimethamine (Fansidar®) remains highly effective in the UK, with very low relapse rates.
- If sulfadoxine-pyrimethamine is contraindicated (e.g. in children with G6PD deficiency) or is not available, alternatives such as clindamycin and doxycycline may also be given (only in children >8 years because of risk of dental hypoplasia and permanent teeth discoloration).
- Recent data suggest that artemether-based regimens are very safe, well tolerated and clear parasitaemia faster than classical quinine based regimens, but there is limited experience in their use in non-endemic paediatric settings: artemether-lumefantrine is also known as Coartem® and Riamet® (artemether 20mg/lumefantrine 120mg; trade name Riamet®) and is currently licensed for over 12-year olds only
- Atovaquone-proguanil (Malarone®) is expensive but is increasingly gaining popularity for both prophylaxis and treatment of malaria as paediatric tablets are available, but vomiting is a side-effect.
- Mefloquine is also effective but is not recommended for treatment in the UK because of its side effects in adults and high rate of non-completion of treatment courses.
- Halofantrine has also been used in other countries to treat acute, uncomplicated malaria but is associated with potentially fatal cardiac arrhythmias, particularly in individuals receiving drugs that may prolong the QT interval.

Severe malaria

- Guidelines for the management of severe imported childhood malaria in the UK have been proposed recently (☐ see Further reading, p. 623).
- Children with features of severe or complicated malaria should be transferred to PICU and also have a blood gas, blood culture, lactate, clotting profile as well as urine dipstick, and culture on admission.
- Children with respiratory distress should have a chest X-ray.
- Febrile patients with impaired consciousness or repeated seizures should have an LP to exclude meningitis once the patient's condition is stable.
- Aggressive management including consideration of elective ventilation is recommended for those with: depressed conscious level, active seizure activity, irregular breathing, hypoxia, shock, dehydration, hypoglycaemia, metabolic acidosis, and hyperkalaemia.
- Children with anaemia associated with severe malaria may require blood transfusion, although the haemoglobin level at which transfusion should be given remains uncertain.

- Exchange transfusion for hyperparasitaemia >20% (or >10% in the presence of severe symptoms) has been used in children and adults, but there is little evidence that it improves overall outcome.
- Concurrent bacterial infections (meningitis or septicaemia) are rare in children with imported malaria, even in severe cases, but most clinicians would advocate empiric broad-spectrum antibiotics such as a third-generation cephalosporin until bacterial infection can be safely excluded through appropriate blood, urine, and CSF cultures.
- Platelet transfusions for thrombocytopenia, even at platelet levels <20 × 10⁹/l, are generally not recommended because thrombocytopenia is not associated with bleeding problems in children.
- Parenteral quinine is the recommended antimalarial therapy for patients with severe falciparum malaria or non-severe malaria who are unable to tolerate oral medication.
- Current UK guidelines recommend a loading dose of quinine dihydrochloride in 5% dextrose or dextrose saline as a slow infusion over four hours, followed by dosing every 8 hours for the first 48 hours or until the child can swallow.
- The frequency of dosing should subsequently be reduced to 12 hourly if IV quinine continues for more than 48 hours.
- Close monitoring is required for hypoglycaemia, hypoxia, and seizures.
- IV treatment should be changed to oral medication once the patient's condition improves and parasite levels fall.

Non-falciparum malaria

- Uncomplicated non-falciparum malaria does not usually require hospital admission.
- Antimalarial therapy should target both the asexual erythrocytic forms that cause symptoms and, for *P. ovale* and *P. vivax* infections, the liver hypnozoite to prevent relapse.
- Chloroquine remains the treatment of choice for eliminating the erythrocytic forms of non-falciparum malaria.
- In cases of treatment failure (persistent symptoms and/or parasitaemia) or mixed infection with *P. falciparum*, any of the antimalarial combinations recommended for treating *P. falciparum* malaria would be effective in treating the erythrocytic forms of non-falciparum malaria.
- In children without G6PD deficiency, primaquine is recommended routinely in addition for eliminating liver hypnozoites and preventing relapse in *P. ovale* or *P. vivax* malaria, which may occur in up to 25% of cases treated with chloroquine alone.
- In *P. ovale* malaria, a single daily dose should be given for 14 days.
- For *P. vivax* malaria, however, because of increasing resistance to primaquine particularly in Southeast Asia where most UK cases are acquired, a higher single daily dose for 14 days is recommended.
- *P. knowlesi* infections respond adequately to chloroquine and primaquine.
- Children with G6PD deficiency who develop malaria should be referred to specialists in paediatric infectious diseases for further management; treatment options include giving primaquine as a single

weekly dose for 8 weeks in children with mild G6PD deficiency or withholding primaquine and treating any relapse promptly.

Prevention

- Families wishing to travel to a malaria endemic country should be encouraged to visit their general practitioner (GP) or practice nurse, or visit a travel clinic for specific advice, travel vaccinations and antimalarial prophylaxis for the country they are visiting.
- Unfortunately, those at highest risk of developing malaria—the visiting friends and relations group—are the least likely to seek pre-travel advice or take antimalarial prophylaxis.
- The recent BPSU study identified that up to a quarter of children who had travelled to a malaria-endemic country had previously been diagnosed with malaria, reflecting missed opportunities to educate families on malaria prevention when they are admitted to hospital.
- Healthcare professionals providing travel advice should emphasize the ABCD of malaria prevention, which includes Awareness of risk, Bite Prevention, Chemoprophylaxis and prompt Diagnosis and treatment.
- Bite prevention measures include regular use of appropriate insect repellents when outdoors, avoiding areas of stagnant water which may be breeding grounds for mosquitoes, wearing long-sleeved, loose clothing when going outdoors at dawn or dusk, closing doors and windows in sleeping accommodations and using insecticide-containing sprays or mosquito coils, as well as using bed nets (preferably treated with insecticide) and air conditioning where possible.
- Updated guidelines for the prevention of malaria among travellers from the UK are available on the HPA website (𝄞 www.hpa.org.uk) and provide up-to-date guidance on the risk of malaria in different parts of the world, the most appropriate antimalarial prophylaxis as well as indications, contraindications, doses by age/weight, and duration for the different antimalarials.

Future research

- The epidemiology of imported childhood malaria in Europe is now clearly defined: most cases are acquired in children of black African families who are settled in Europe and travel to their country of origin during school holidays without receiving appropriate travel advice or taking antimalarial prophylaxis.
- Future studies should focus on interventions aimed at encouraging antimalarial prophylaxis uptake in this high-risk group.
- With increasing availability of newer antimalarial combinations, there is also a need to standardise recommendations for the treatment of imported childhood malaria in Europe.

Further reading

Chiodini P, Hill D, Lalloo D, *et al.* Guidelines for malaria prevention in travellers from the United Kingdom. London: Health Protection Agency, 2007. Available at: ℘ www.hpa.org.uk; select *Topics A-Z*, followed by *Malaria* and the *Guidelines*.

Ladhani S, Aibara RJ, Riordan FA, Shingadia D. Imported malaria in children: a review of clinical studies. *Lancet Infect Dis* 2007;**7**:349–57.

Lalloo DG, Shingadia D, Pasvol G, *et al.* UK malaria treatment guidelines. *J Infect* 2007;**54**:111–21.
Maitland K, Nadel S, Pollard AJ, Williams TN, Newton CR, Levin M. Management of severe malaria in children: proposed guidelines for the United Kingdom. *BMJ* 2005;**331**:337–43.

World Health Organization. *World Malaria Report 2008.* Geneva: WHO Press, 2008. Available at: ℘ http://apps.who.int/malaria/wmr2008/malaria2008.pdf (accessed 1 February 2011).

Measles

see also Chapters 11, 21, 27, 34, 44

Name and nature of organism

- Measles (also known as rubeola) virus causes an acute illness characterized by rash, fever, and respiratory symptoms.
- Caused by a *Paramyxoviridae* virus of the genus *Morbillivirus*.
- An enveloped single-stranded RNA virus. The genome encodes 8 proteins including haemagglutinin (H) and fusion (F) proteins.
- The complete measles genome has been sequenced allowing differentiation of various wild (23 so far) and vaccine genotypes.

Epidemiology

- Only found in humans.
- Highly infectious. In prevaccination era, >90% of individuals had a symptomatic infection by the age of 10 years.
- In Europe in 2007, the commonest age group affected was 0–4 years, whereas in USA >50% of cases were adults.
- In temperate areas, it is commonest in late winter and early spring, whereas in the tropics it is commonest in the dry season.
- Where infection is common, epidemics occur every 2 years.
- It is estimated that, worldwide, it accounted for over 12.1 million disability-adjusted life years in 2005 and 197 000 deaths in 2007.
- In the EU and EEA/EPTA in 2006 there were 2723 cases and six deaths
- In the UK from a low of around 100 confirmed cases in 2005, this increased to over 1000 cases by 2008 with 1 death in 2006 and 1 in 2008.
- Immunity after natural infection is usually lifelong, due to both neutralizing antibody to the H protein and cell-mediated immunity.

Transmission and incubation period

- Highly infectious, up to 90% of susceptible contacts are infected.
- Spread from person to person via respiratory droplets, which may persist in the air for several hours.
- Can survive on surfaces for up to 2 hours, but its lipid envelope is destroyed by ethanol-based handscrubs.
- Incubation period is from 6 to 19 days (median 13 days). There is a short primary viraemia from the pharynx to local nodes, with a main

secondary viraemia around a week after infection leading to URTI symptoms then rash.
- Virus is shed from 2 days before to 3 days after symptoms appear.
- The period of infectiousness is not known, but is thought to be 1–2 days prior to the appearance of the rash, to 4–5 days after.

Clinical features and sequelae

- Prodrome of high fever, cough, coryza, and conjunctivitis.
- Maculopapular rash appears next around 2–4 days later, first behind the ears—then spreads down the body—generally more rash = more unwell the child—the rash can look almost haemorrhagic.
- Koplik spots (small 1mm bluish white spots on the buccal mucosa) are present about 1–3 days before the onset of the rash and are characteristic of measles though not found in all cases.
- Three days after the rash appears, children improve and are usually fully recovered 7–10 days after onset of illness.
- Complications occur in 6–7% of otherwise healthy individuals in developed countries.
- Complications include otitis media, measles pneumonitis or secondary bacterial pneumonia—difficult to distinguish clinically (38/1000), convulsions (5/1000), encephalitis (1.2/1000), idiopathic thrombocytopenic purpura (1 in 2–3000), and diarrhoea.
- Acute encephalitis occurs around 2–5 days after onset of rash, CSF shows lymphocytosis with elevated protein—may be PCR positive. Most children recover. A severe fulminant encephalitis has been reported.
- Subacute sclerosing panencephalitis occurs in 4/100 000 overall, but 18/100 000 in children infected with measles under a year old. SSPE presents with gradual neurological deterioration around 5–10 years after measles. Proceeds to myoclonic epilepsy, coma, and death. Diagnosis is based on classic EEG pattern of bilateral high amplitude periodic complexes and monoclonal measles antibody titres in the CSF.
- In those malnourished, especially if vitamin A deficient, or immunocompromised, there is a higher morbidity and mortality. There may be *no rash* in the immunocompromised, who present with unexplained pneumonia or encephalitis.
- Mortality is greatest in infants and adults. Overall it is about 1/1000.
- Globally, up to 5% of deaths in the <5s are still due to measles.

Diagnosis

- As the disease has become less common, the accuracy of clinical diagnosis, especially of sporadic cases, has become poor, with as few as 1–2% of suspected cases being confirmed. The differential diagnosis includes adenovirus, rubella, enterovirus or EBV infection, Streptococcal disease, and Kawasaki disease.

- Laboratory diagnosis used to depend on the finding of measles specific IgM or a fourfold rise in IgG in blood.
- Diagnosis is now possible by salivary measles-specific IgM.
- Using RT-PCR, viral RNA can also be found in saliva, allowing genotyping and epidemiological mapping. An oral fluid sample is the best test—ideally using special kits.

Management and treatment

- Treatment of individual cases is symptomatic, with complications being managed individually as they arise. Antibiotics are only needed for secondary bacterial pneumonia.
- WHO recommends that all cases should be treated with vitamin A and that, even in countries where measles is not usually severe, a dose of vitamin A at diagnosis and another a day later, should be given to all severe cases. There is little evidence that this is efficacious in patients not deficient in vitamin A.
- The daily dose of vitamin A is 50 000IU for infants <6 months old, 100 000IU for infants aged 6–11 months and 200 000IU for those ≥12 months. A recent Cochrane analysis reported a fall of over 60% in pneumonia mortality associated with high dose Vitamin A use.
- Patients should be isolated until 5 days after onset of rash.
- Contacts should be traced and consideration given to vaccination or administration of immunoglobulin depending on their age and immunization status and the interval elapsed after contact with the index case. 📖 See Prevention for more details.

Prevention

- Measles vaccines have been available for almost 50 years.
- Initially both live and killed vaccines were used. The latter caused many cases of a severe atypical infection and rapidly gave way to the live attenuated vaccines, which are the only ones now available.
- The measles virus strains in commonest use are derived from the Edmonston strain (named after the boy from whom the measles virus strain was isolated). There is little to choose between them.
- A single dose of a measles-containing vaccine protects 90–95% of recipients, if given to children ≥12 months.
- To attain herd immunity it is necessary to give two doses.
- When given to children <12 months, the efficacy is less, in large part due to the presence of maternal antibodies.
- In countries where measles is a major problem in infants, measles vaccine may be given to individuals as young as 9 months.

- High-titre vaccines were produced in an attempt to protect infants, but they are not in use due to evidence of higher non-measles death rates in recipients.
- Most affluent countries give measles vaccine as part of the combined MMR vaccine. Two doses are given: one at 12–15 months and the other at anything between 2 and 10 years later, with a few countries giving it earlier.
- Side effects of the vaccine usually occur in the second week after vaccination and include a transient rash (2%), fever and other symptoms of measles (5–10%), febrile convulsions (1 in 3000) and idiopathic thrombocytopenia (1 in 30 000). These reactions are much less common after the second dose.
- Anaphylaxis after the vaccine occurs in 1 in 100 000 or less recipients.
- The vaccine is contraindicated in pregnancy and in individuals who are significantly immunocompromised (HIV is an exception).
- In the UK after spurious reports of an association of MMR with autism, immunization rates fell markedly. Following clear evidence of absolutely no link between MMR and autism, national immunization rates are now rising again, but have not returned to pre-scare levels, let alone sufficient to provide herd immunity.
- Cases should be isolated for 4 days from the appearance of the rash. It may be possible to prevent disease in susceptible contacts:
  - Immunosuppressed individuals, whose last contact was within 6 days, should have an urgent assessment of antibody levels and given human normal immunoglobulin if negative or equivocal. If urgent testing is not possible, immunoglobulin as human normal immunoglobulin (HNIG) should be given. The dose recommended is 0.6ml/kg subcutaneously or 0.15g/kg IV. Infants <1 year should be given 0.6ml/kg IM up to maximum of 5ml.
- As the incubation period of the vaccine virus is shorter than that of wild measles virus (7 as opposed to 10 days), if given within 3 days of exposure, MMR or measles vaccination reduces the risk of development of measles.

Future research

- Why does a small proportion of the population not become immune after a single dose of measles vaccine?
- Should the age for vaccination be reduced in countries where maternal immunity is vaccine based?

Further reading

Elliman D, Sengupta N, El Bashir H, Bedford H. Measles, mumps, and rubella: prevention. *Clin Evid (Online)* 2007;**pii**:0316.

Ramsay M, Manikkavasagan G, Brown M, Craig L. Post exposure prophylaxis for measles: revised guidance, May 2009. London: Health Protection Agency.

World Health Organization. Measles vaccine: WHO position paper. *Wkly Epidemiol Rec* 2009;**84**:349–60.

Chapter 87

Meningococcal disease

📖 see also Chapters 29, 34, 36

Meningococcal disease in children is the subject of a National Institute for Health and Clinical Excellence (NICE) guideline.[1]

Name and nature of organism

- Anton Weichselbaum first identified the organism in Vienna in 1887 as an intracellular organism in white blood cells in the CSF of a patient with meningitis and named it *Diplococcus intracellularis*.
- *Neisseria meningitidis* is a Gram-negative diplococcus.
- Meningococci are surrounded by a polysaccharide capsule, the chemical nature of which confers the serogroup of the organism.
- Thirteen serogroups are recognized, but most disease is caused by serogroups A, B, C, Y, and W135.
- Meningococci are also classified by typing of surface proteins found beneath the capsule in the outer membrane (using serology or genetic sequencing).
- The outer membrane contains lipopolysaccharide (endotoxin), which is responsible for the inflammatory response seen.
- Meningococci are commonly isolated from the nasopharynx of healthy individuals; humans are the only natural hosts.

Epidemiology[2]

- The first outbreaks of meningococcal disease were described in Geneva in 1805.
- Globally up to 500 000 cases occur annually, and approximately 1000 of these are in the UK.
- Rates of disease vary over time in any one location and currently range from <0.5/100 000 population in the USA to >1000/100 000 during epidemics in the meningitis belt of sub-Saharan Africa.
- The case fatality rate is approximately 10%.
- Different epidemiological patterns are recognized: epidemics, clusters, hyperendemic disease, and sporadic disease.
- Cycles of *epidemic disease* occur in the sub-Saharan African meningitis belt and most cases are caused by serogroup A, though W135 and X have been recognized in the past decade. Serogroup A epidemics occurred across Europe during the twentieth century conflicts and more recently in Russia, Poland, and parts of Asia.
- *Clusters* of cases occur in closed communities such as schools, colleges and military training camps and have recently been particularly associated with serogroup C meningococci.

- *Hyperendemic disease* occurs in geographically distinct areas most often, due to a single clone of serogroup B (e.g. Normandy in France, New Zealand, and Oregon).
- *Sporadic disease* occurs in most countries and is mostly due to serogroup B, and C in Europe. Serogroup Y causes about one-third of sporadic cases in the USA. Serogroup A causes sporadic cases in Asia and Africa. Distribution of serogroups in any one location varies over time.
- In the UK there are now around 300 laboratory confirmed cases/year of MD in children under 1 year (with 10 confirmed deaths), 400 cases in children aged 1–4 years (10 deaths) and 300 in those 5–19 years (around 5 deaths). These are now nearly all due to group B disease in the UK, but are an underestimate of the total burden of disease.
- Meningococcal disease rates are increased:
  • Among children <2 years of age (especially infants)
  • In adolescents and young adults
  • In household and kissing contacts of an individual with the disease
  • In active and passive smokers
  • During winter (or in the dry season in sub-Saharan Africa)
  • After recent respiratory infection (viral and *Mycoplasma*)
  • Among communities who are exposed to crowded situations (refugee camps, young adults attending bars and nightclubs, the Hajj pilgrimage to Mecca, dormitory accommodation among college freshmen, kissing)
  • In individuals with complement deficiency (especially terminal components, C5–9, properdin or factor D) who have disease caused by rarer serogroups (e.g. Y, 29E, X).

Transmission and incubation period

- *N. meningitidis* colonizes the nasopharynx of up to 25% of adolescents and 10% of adults but is rarely found in the upper respiratory tract of children <10 years of age.
- Transmission is via respiratory secretions and requires close contact with a carrier (hence greatest risk for household and kissing contacts).
- Following acquisition most infections result in harmless colonization which has a duration from days to months before clearance.
- Susceptible individuals develop invasive disease usually within 4 days of acquisition (range 1–10 days but cases developing after many weeks have been documented).

Clinical features and sequelae

The most common clinical syndromes associated with meningococcal infection are:
- Asymptomatic colonization of the nasopharynx
- Meningitis (15% of cases and 5% case fatality rate)

- Septicaemia (25% of cases, also known as meningococcaemia; historically up to 40% mortality)
- A combination of features of meningitis and septicaemia in 60% of cases
- Pneumonia (especially serogroup Y) or occult bacteraemia
- Other syndromes include conjunctivitis, endophthalmitis, pericarditis, osteomyelitis, arthritis, peritonitis, and urethritis
- Chronic meningococcaemia.

Rash

The rash in meningococcal disease is typically a non-blanching petechial or purpuric rash (80% of cases) which evolves from an initial blanching maculopapular rash in 38% of cases. The rash may be absent, especially in early disease. In severe cases large ecchymotic areas develop (*purpura fulminans*) which involve haemorrhage and necrosis in the skin. The great majority of petechial rashes are due to:

- Viral infections (enterovirus, influenza, measles, EBV, CMV, parvovirus)
- Other bacterial infections (Gram-positive and negative infections and especially pneumococcal disease)
- Vomiting or coughing (petechiae on the face and upper chest)
- Accidental and non-accidental injury
- Henoch–Schönlein purpura
- Idiopathic thrombocytopenic purpura
- Leukaemia
- Drug reactions
- Protein C or S deficiency
- Vasculitis.

Meningitis

The presentation of meningococcal meningitis includes:

- Non-specific symptoms (vomiting and irritability, especially in young children)
- Headache. Fever or a history of fever, photophobia
- Neck stiffness, bulging fontanelle in infants
- Decreased level of consciousness
- Seizures or convulsive status epilepticus
- Focal neurological signs
- Petechial or purpuric rash.

Up to 40% also have features of septicaemia.

Signs of raised ICP should be sought, as this is the most common cause of death in pure meningitis cases:

- Reduced level of consciousness
- Relative bradycardia and hypertension
- Focal neurological signs
- Abnormal posturing
- Unequal, dilated or poorly responsive pupils
- Papilloedema.

Laboratory tests are similar to those in other types of bacterial meningitis and include raised WBC and inflammatory markers (CRP, ESR, procalcitonin). Some cases will have normal laboratory values. If a LP is performed, the CSF white cell count and protein are raised and glucose is decreased.

Septicaemia

Features of meningococcal septicaemia (meningococcaemia) include

- Initial influenza-like symptoms (fever, headache, myalgia, vomiting, abdominal pain)
- Maculopapular rash evolving to a petechial/purpuric rash or purpura fulminans—complex coagulation disorder with a combination of intravascular thrombosis and a bleeding diathesis
- Limb pain, cold hands and feet
- Pallor (including a mottled appearance and cyanosis)
- And later confusion, agitation and finally coma.

Evaluation for signs of shock (seen in one third of cases of septicaemia) should be a priority as this is the most common cause of death:

- Tachycardia
- Poor peripheral perfusion (prolonged capillary refill time and cold peripheries)
- Tachypnoea
- Oliguria
- Decreased cerebral perfusion (confusion, agitation, or decreasing consciousness)
- Multiorgan failure
- Hypotension (late sign in children).

Poor outcome is associated with young age, coma, low temperature, and decreased white cell and platelet counts.

Laboratory features in meningococcal septicaemia include raised WBC count and inflammatory markers (CRP, ESR, procalcitonin). Some cases will have normal laboratory values despite severe disease, and those who are most seriously ill and have a rapid onset of disease may have a depressed white cell count. Other common laboratory findings in meningococcal septicaemia are:

- Anaemia, coagulopathy
- Hypoglycaemia, acidosis
- Hypokalaemia, hypocalcaemia, hypomagnesaemia
- Hypophosphataemia
- Raised creatinine.

Chronic meningococcemia

- Recurrent episodes of non-blanching rash with fever, arthralgia, and splenomegaly.
- Untreated cases may develop meningococcal septicaemia.
- Indistinguishable from other causes of petechial rash and fever.
- Check for complement deficiency.

Meningococcal post-infectious inflammatory syndrome

- Relatively common immune complex disease, which causes diagnostic confusion.
- Up to 10% of cases have some features.
- Onset from as early as 4 days after presentation with meningococcal infection but often in second week.
- Features include:
  - Fever

- Maculopapular or vasculitis rash (2%)
- Arthritis (8%), iritis (1%), pericarditis, polyserositis.

Diagnosis

A clinical diagnosis should be made based on the typical features to ensure urgent and appropriate management. In all suspected cases blood should be taken for culture and PCR (whole blood EDTA sample).

A microbiological diagnosis of meningococcal disease is made by identification of the organism in specimens from normally sterile sites, e.g. blood (up to 50% of cases are culture positive but only 5% if obtained after antibiotics), CSF (Gram-stain positive in 65% of cases and >70% are culture positive), joint fluid or the conjunctiva. PCR is highly sensitive in both blood and CSF and increases the diagnostic rate by as much as 40%.

If there are temporary contraindications to LP, the test should be performed as soon as the contraindication has resolved. The following tests are not routinely recommended:
- CSF antigen testing by latex agglutination (insensitive)
- Scrapings or aspiration of skin lesions (no evidence that adds to blood culture and PCR)
- Urinary antigen testing (poor sensitivity)
- Serological testing (not adequately studied)
- Throat swabs (the organism is part of the normal flora).

Management and treatment

Immediate management

The priority in emergency medical care in meningococcal disease is the recognition and management of hypovolaemic shock and raised ICP (see ℘ www.meningitis.org for a paediatric emergency management algorithm). A step-wise approach to initial management is:

1. Involve an experienced clinician and anaesthetist immediately
2. Control the airway, particularly if depressed conscious level (poor cerebral perfusion in shock or raised ICP in meningitis)
3. Give oxygen therapy in case of pulmonary oedema or oligaemia
4. Intubate and ventilate if respiratory failure present as a result of shock or impaired conscious level
5. Give fluid resuscitation (IV or intraosseous) if signs of shock using boluses of 20ml/kg of 0.9% saline over 5–10 minutes
6. If signs of raised ICP present correct the co-existent shock
7. If still shocked after 40ml/kg fluid resuscitation, contact the regional PICU
8. If still shocked after 40ml/kg fluid resuscitation, continue fluids (and inotropes), and electively intubate and ventilate
9. Catheterize to monitor urinary output
10. Correct metabolic derangements (hypoglycaemia, acidosis, hypokalaemia, hypocalcaemia, hypomagnesaemia, hypophosphataemia, anaemia, coagulopathy)

11. Use manoeuvres to improve cerebral perfusion if raised ICP present (mannitol/furosemide, maintain CO_2 in the normal range, use sedation, minimal handling, avoid neck lines, maintain head raised 30 degrees).

If meningococcal disease is suspected antibiotic therapy should be:
- IV ceftriaxone or cefotaxime for 7 days.
- Cefotaxime is preferred in neonates because of hepatic immaturity but ceftriaxone is easier and more cost-effective to administer in other age groups. Importantly, the third-generation cephalosporins provide cover for other organisms, which may present with similar features (e.g. *S. pneumoniae*). Ceftriaxone should not be administered at the same time as calcium containing infusions.
- Adjunctive steroids are beneficial in bacterial meningitis but there is no specific evidence for meningococcal meningitis. However, it is likely that there should be a similar benefit in meningococcal meningitis. Steroids should be given within 4 hours of the first dose of antibiotics when there is a high chance of bacterial meningitis (positive CSF Gram-stain, CSF white cell count >1000 cells/ml, or CSF pleocytosis with a CSF protein >1g/l).
- Treatment doses of steroids should not be used in shock. Some intensivists will use replacement doses of steroids in unresponsive shock with impaired adrenal function.

Management after initial/emergency treatment
- Many children with meningococcal disease can be safely managed on a paediatric ward.
- Because of the risk of deterioration, especially in the first 6 hours after initial management has been instituted, patients with suspected meningococcal disease should be reviewed and reassessed repeatedly after hospital admission.
- Those who do not stabilize after initial intervention should be transferred to a PICU by a specialist paediatric intensive care transfer team.
- After transfer children should be treated in a paediatric intensive care setting and managed according to intensive care protocols.
- Renal failure may complicate meningococcal shock.
- Experimental therapies should not be used in meningococcal disease outside of a clinical trial.
- Skin scarring occurs in about 10% of cases and may be severe enough to require skin grafting.
- Limb ischaemia due to *purpura fulminans* should be managed in conjunction with plastic and orthopaedic surgeons. Severe limb ischaemia may present early, and should be left to demarcate (in the absence of infection) but about 2% of patients will require a delayed amputation.
- Meningococcal post-infectious inflammatory syndrome should be treated with NSAIDs and will usually resolve spontaneously.

Follow up
- Patients who have had meningococcal disease should be reviewed in convalescence (4–6 weeks after discharge).
- All patients should have an audiological assessment (4% hearing loss).

- Neurological developmental and behavioural complications should be considered (occur in 7%) and appropriate referral made.
- Patients who have infection with unusual serogroups of *Meningococcus* should be assessed for complement deficiency.
- If there is a history of recurrent infection, immunological review is advised.
- Chronic renal failure is a rare complication of hypovolaemic shock.
- Orthopaedic and plastic surgical follow-up may be required for some patients.

Prevention

Vaccines

Plain polysaccharide vaccines

- Are available as bivalent meningococcal (Men)A, C or quadrivalent MenA,C,Y,W vaccines.
- Have been used to control outbreaks and for high-risk groups.
- Are generally poorly immunogenic in children <2 years of age (with the exception of serogroup A).
- Provide a relatively short duration of immunity.
- Do not induce immunological memory.
- Do not induce herd immunity.
- May cause a state of immunological hyporesponsiveness of uncertain significance.
- Plain polysaccharide vaccines have been superseded by the conjugate vaccines (see below) and no longer have a place in countries where the conjugate are available.

Protein-polysaccharide conjugate vaccines

- Contain meningococcal polysaccharides conjugated to a carrier protein (tetanus toxoid, diphtheria toxoid or CRM197).
- Are available as monovalent MenC (since 1999) or combination Hib-MenC vaccines (since 2006) in the UK currently.
- Are available in the US as quadrivalent MenA,C,Y,W (since 2005) vaccines and in Europe since 2010.
- Various other combinations are in clinical trials (e.g. Hib-MenCY) and a monvalent MenA vaccine has been developed for Africa.
- MenC has successfully controlled disease caused by serogroup C meningococci in countries where it has been introduced routinely with a catch-up campaign.
- Are generally highly immunogenic from early infancy.
- Induce immunological memory (booster responses are seen with additional doses).
- Appear to induce herd immunity.
- Antibody levels wane if given in early childhood and therefore booster doses are required.

- MenC is recommended for routine childhood immunization in the UK as a two-dose primary schedule (3 and 4 months of age) followed by a booster dose of Hib-MenC vaccine at 12 months of age.
- Booster doses for teenagers may be required and are now recommended in Canada.
- MenC or MenACYW conjugate vaccine should be offered to the household contacts of a case of serogroup A, C, Y or W meningococcal disease as appropriate.

Group B meningococcal vaccines[3]

- The group B polysaccharide is not immunogenic as it shares chemical identity with human antigens and subcapsular antigens have been considered as vaccine candidates.
- Outer membrane vesicle (OMV) vaccines containing surface proteins in a lipid membrane have been developed to control clonal outbreaks (hyperendemic) meningococcal disease in Cuba, Norway, New Zealand, and Normandy.
- Many different clones of meningoccoci cause disease in Europe and a single OMV vaccine is not suitable.
- Vaccines containing multiple OMVs and/or relatively conserved surface proteins are at an advanced stage of development.

Management of contacts

- When a case of meningococcal disease is suspected, the local public health team should be involved as early as possible to plan prevention of secondary cases.
- Household and kissing contacts of a case of meningococcal disease have up to 1000 times the population risk of disease (1–3% of household contacts).
- Healthcare workers are only at risk if directly exposed to secretions in the first 24 hours after antibiotic therapy
- Detailed public health guidance is available from the Health Protection Agency and the local public health team should be notified of the case.[4]
- Those at risk should be offered chemoprophylaxis with:
  - Rifampicin—orally twice daily for 2 days
  - Ciprofloxacin—one oral dose
  - Ceftriaxone—one IM dose.

Future research

The optimal type of fluid (colloid or crystalloid) for resuscitation is not known and the theoretical advantages of colloid warrant investigation.

Vaccines to control serogroup B infection are currently in clinical trials but the huge variation in immunogenic surface structures makes it unlikely that current vaccines will prevent all serogroup B disease. Further research is needed to develop broadly cross-protective vaccines.

Key references

1 National Institute for Health and Clinical Excellence. Bacterial meningitis and meningococcal septicaemia in children: the management of bacterial meningitis and meningococcal septicaemia in children and young people younger than 16 years in primary and secondary care. Clinical guideline 102. London: NICE, 2010. Available at: ℰ www.nice.nhs.uk.

2 Khatami A, Pollard AJ. The epidemiology of meningococcal disease and the impact of vaccines. *Expert Rev Vaccines* 2010;**9**:285–98.

3 Sadarangani M, Pollard AJ, Serogroup B. Meningococcal vaccines—an unfinished story. *Lancet Infect Dis* 2010;**10**:112–24.

4 Health Protection Agency Meningococcus Forum, *Guidance for Public Health Management of Meningococcal Disease in the UK*. Available at: ℰ www.hpa.org.uk/web/HPAwebFile/ HPAweb_C/1194947389261 (accessed 1 February 2011).

Molluscum contagiosum and other poxviruses

📖 see also Chapters 4, 19, 24, 34, 37, 38

Molluscum contagiosum

Name and nature of organism

- Common self-limiting cutaneous wart-like eruption in children and young adults.
- Can cause problems in the immunocompromised host.
- Large, double-stranded DNA virus of the poxvirus group.
- Type 1 is the commonest cause of the condition in children.
- Type 2 is most common in adults (often sexually transmitted).
- Virus replicates in the cytoplasm of epithelial cells.

Epidemiology

- Very common worldwide infection.
- Humans are the only host.
- In a Dutch General Practice Survey there was an incidence of 2.4 per 1000 person-years mainly in children.[1]
- Prevalence may be higher in tropical areas.
- Age distribution is bimodal, most cases occur in preschool children.
- Cumulative incidence of infections in young children is 17%. Infection is rare in children <1 year of age.
- Infection in young adults predominantly sexually transmitted, with a male: female ratio of 3.3:1.
- Infection is more prevalent in individuals with impaired cellular immunity such as HIV infection, in which the prevalence increases with decreasing CD4 count, and in those with skin disease, e.g. eczema.

Transmission

- Mode of transmission is by direct skin to skin contact, involved in contact sports, living in close proximity, sharing of fomites, and sexual contact.
- Incubation period is typically 2–7 weeks (range 1–26 weeks).
- Transmission is increased from disrupted skin lesions following scratching, which may lead to auto-inoculation.
- Period of infectivity unknown but probably whilst lesions present.

Clinical features

- Skin lesions are smooth papular lesions with a pearly appearance and often central umbilication.
- Papules usually are <5mm in diameter but can be as big as 2cm, particularly in the immunocompromised host.
- Typically a patient may have two to three dozen lesions.
- Lesions tend to occur in clusters or sometimes in lines
- The lesions may be anywhere on the body except palms and soles.
- Disrupted lesions can discharge a waxy infectious white material.
- There are no systemic features to the infection.
- Secondary bacterial infection can occur. Lesions on the eyelids can be troublesome particularly in patients with AIDS in whom the lesions become confluent and induce keratoconjunctivitis.

Diagnosis

- The appearance of the lesions is highly characteristic and it is rare that tests need to be performed to confirm the diagnosis—look for the central umbilication.
- Where tests are required a lesion can be punctured and the core material examined either by light microscopy, to show the characteristic intracytoplasmic inclusion bodies, or by electron microscopy.

Management and treatment

- In the immunocompetent host the infection runs a benign, self-limiting course. Individual lesions heal spontaneously in 3 months.
- New lesions will continue to appear and the whole episode of infection may last from 8 to 18 months.
- Scarring is unusual unless there has been a lot of scratching or secondary infection.
- In immunocompromised individuals the lesions may persist for a longer period of time and may enlarge and become disfiguring.
- In the vast majority of cases no treatment is required.
- Treatment is only required in those with immunosuppression. No one treatment has been found to be convincingly effective.[2]
- Surgical treatment involves curettage of individual lesions following topical anaesthesia. This is effective but may result in scarring.
- Cryotherapy has also been used—but is painful.
- Topical treatments include the local immune stimulant imiquimod (produces a local inflammatory response—may cause depigmentation) and the antiviral agent cidofovir.
- In very severe cases associated with underlying immunocompromised states, systemic therapy with antivirals such as cidofovir or with immune modulators such as cimetidine have been used.
- In HIV-positive patients the use of antiretroviral therapy is helpful by correcting the CD4 lymphopenia.

Prevention

- Isolation and exclusion from school are not justified.[3]
- Transmission of infection can be reduced by avoiding the sharing of bath towels, sponges or clothes and minimizing skin-to-skin contact.

- Individuals with molluscum contagiosum should be encouraged not to scratch the lesions, which increases their infectivity.
- In those with lesions confined to a limited area, covering of lesions with bandage or tape prior to participation in contact sports may reduce the likelihood of transmission.

Future research

- Development of an *in vitro* culture system for the virus would help in the development of antiviral agents.
- Where therapy is indicated, controlled clinical trials are required to determine optimal treatment regimens.

Other pox virus infections

Smallpox

- Natural smallpox was eradicated in 1977 after a global immunization campaign. The virus is believed to be held in only two research laboratories in the USA and Russia due to the potential for bioterrorist release. The clinical picture is of a widespread bullous eruption, similar to chicken pox, but with a marked peripheral distribution.

Monkeypox

- Only seen in rural Africa, e.g. Zaire, after animal-to-human contact.
- Severe illness similar to smallpox, with high mortality.

Cowpox and Orf

- Reported in Europe, following animal contact. Causes localized vesicles that ulcerate. In Orf these may be 2–3cm in diameter.

Key references

1 Koning S, Bruijnzeels MA, van Suijlekom-Smit LW, van der Wouden JC. Molluscum contagiosum in Dutch general practice. *Br J Gen Pract* 1994;**44**:417–19.
2 van der Wouden JC, Van der Sande R, Van Suijlekom-Smit LW, *et al.* Interventions for cutaneous molluscum contagiosum. *Cochrane Database Syst Rev* 2009;CD004767.
3 Richardson M, Elliman D, Maguire H, Simpson J, Nicoll A. Evidence base of incubation periods, periods of infectiousness and exclusion policies for the control of communicable diseases in schools and preschools. *Pediatr Infect Dis J* 2001;**20**:380–91.

Chapter 89

Mumps

📖 see also Chapters 14, 15, 29, 44

Name and nature of organism

- An acute illness with swelling of the parotid glands.
- Mumps virus is a paramyxovirus containing negative strand RNA that causes an acute illness with swelling of the parotid glands. Two proteins (haemagglutinin-neuraminidase and fusion) are on the surface and carry neutralizing epitopes.

Epidemiology

- Epidemics of infectious parotitis have been known since ancient times.
- Ubiquitous before the introduction of vaccines, tending to occur in the spring in temperate climates, with outbreaks every few years.
- The peak age before vaccination was in children aged 5–9 years.
- In the USA, the highest yearly incidence of mumps was 250 per 100 000 population. In the UK there have been around 2000 confirmed cases/year, with peak years in 2004 and 2009. The majority of reports are now from university outbreaks.
- Infection is less ubiquitous in the tropics. Serological surveys suggest that eventually 70–90% of individuals are infected, but about one-third are asymptomatic or do not have salivary gland swelling.
- Isolation of cases may have little effect on an outbreak.
- Vaccination has shifted the incidence to higher age groups, and recently in countries that practise vaccination multiple epidemics have occurred in young adults, thought to be the result of waning immunity after vaccination, rather than a change in mumps strains.
- However, even before vaccination the accumulation of susceptibles, as in military populations, resulted in outbreaks.
- Immunity after natural infection is permanent.

Transmission and incubation period

- The virus is excreted in the saliva and urine.
- Transmission is only from human to human, probably in large droplets by the respiratory route as suggested by recent outbreaks in colleges among students not necessarily having intimate contact.
- Less contagious than measles or varicella.

- Incubation period of mumps ranges from 12 to 25 days, with 16–18 days being the most common.
- The virus is often present in the saliva from 2–4 days before symptoms up to 4 to 5 days afterwards
- A case is considered infectious for 5 days after onset of symptoms.
- Virus can also be isolated from urine, blood, and CSF (with or without meningitis) but these are not thought to play a role in transmission, although viruria may persist for two weeks.

Clinical features and sequelae

- Non-specific febrile prodrome of several days, which may include pain in the ears.
- Characteristic symptom is swelling of the parotid glands in about 70% of patients. Parotitis increases for several days and then begins to resolve.
- Involvement may be unilateral.
- The submandibular glands may also be involved.
- Examination of Stensen's duct is likely to show erythema and edema.
- To test for parotitis, give the patient a citrus drink, which causes pain in the gland.
- Inapparent mumps, or mumps presenting with respiratory symptoms is common in young children.
- Mumps involves many different organs, but the principal complications occur in the CNS, cochlea, pancreas, and the testis and ovaries.
- CNS invasion occurs commonly, with lymphocytic pleocytosis seen in about 50% of infections and positive RT-PCR in virtually all patients. Nevertheless, meningismus will be present only in about 10%.
- CNS disease is usually benign in outcome, but symptoms are likely for a week, including signs of general or local neural inflammation.
- True encephalitis occurs only rarely—around a week after clinical infection, is serious but usually has a good outcome.
- Mumps affects hearing in about 4% of cases, and is rarely a cause of permanent acquired deafness.
- Pancreatic glands are involved in about 5% of cases, causing abdominal pain and gastrointestinal symptoms. The serum amylase will be elevated, but is not diagnostic as parotitis can also increase the amylase. Determination of pancreatic lipase can make the distinction. The relationship of mumps pancreatitis to subsequent diabetes mellitus is controversial.
- Orchitis is seen in up to a third of post-pubertal men (rare in younger children), most often unilateral, and usually starting 4–10 days after the appearance of parotitis. Although testicular atrophy is a common result, sterility follows in only 3% of cases.
- Oophoritis also occurs in about 5% of postpubertal females, manifesting as pain.

- Myocardial involvement occurs frequently but is usually asymptomatic. Migratory arthritis, myocarditis, hepatitis and nephritis are other complications that may arise after mumps.
- Mumps virus can pass from pregnant women infected in the first trimester to their fetuses and cause spontaneous abortion. No congenital malformation has been definitely associated with it, although endocardial fibroelastosis is strongly suspected to be a result of intrauterine mumps.

Diagnosis

- During an epidemic the presence of parotitis has a high specificity for the diagnosis of mumps.
- Many other viruses can cause parotitis, notably Coxsackie viruses, and bacterial parotitis must always be suspected if there is pus coming from Stensen's duct.
- HIV, autoimmune disease, cancer, and other non-infectious diseases are considerations if the parotid enlargement is chronic.
- Persistent bilateral parotid enlargement for >3 months is a good sign of paediatric HIV infection.
- Virus isolation in monkey or human cells can be performed using saliva, urine, or spinal fluid.
- However, the best test is RT-PCR to identify mumps RNA directly.
- Serologic diagnosis can be accomplished by a variety of tests; however, mumps-specific IgM, using an ELISA format, is relatively insensitive.
- Although the presence of antibodies in serum is responsible for blocking viraemia, there is no single serological test that definitely correlates with protection. Nevertheless in general, a positive serological test of some sort is evidence for immunity.

Management and treatment

- Ribavirin has been used with possible anecdotal success in very severe disease, but there is no accepted antiviral or immunoglobulin treatment of mumps.
- Symptomatic treatment is important to mitigate the painful swelling of salivary glands and gonads.
- Meningitis and encephalitis are treated conservatively with bed rest and relief of increased CSF pressure.

Prevention

- At least 13 attenuated strains of mumps virus have been produced, but outside Japan generally only three are used: Jeryl Lynn, Urabe, and Leningrad.
- Only one strain, the Jeryl Lynn (and its derivatives), is free of the ability to invade the CNS with aseptic meningitis.

- Mumps vaccine is used almost entirely as a component of the MMR vaccine. The first dose of MMR is routinely recommended to be given between 12 and 15 months of age, with a second dose later in life, often recommended at age 4–6 years. Jeryl Lynn is manufactured in chick embryo cell culture, but allergic reactions have been very rare and allergy to eggs is not a contraindication to vaccinate.
- Vaccinated women should avoid pregnancy for 1 month following vaccination.
- Despite the limitations of the vaccine strains, routine use has had marked effects. In the UK routine vaccination was started in 1988 and by 1994 had profoundly reduced the incidence of mumps. However, the drop in MMR vaccine coverage caused by the autism scare allowed the reappearance of mumps outbreaks.
- In the USA, mumps incidence decreased from the introduction of vaccination in 1967 to reach an all time low in 2003. However, numerous outbreaks have occurred recently throughout the world in adolescents and young adults, many of whom have been previously vaccinated. Although vaccine effectiveness has been moderately high, waning of immunity after one or two doses has been implicated in these outbreaks. Measures to deal with this phenomenon, including third doses, are being evaluated.
- Finland has succeeded in virtual elimination of mumps through a routine two-dose schedule.

Future research

An effective antiviral agent would be a useful treatment option for severe disease due to mumps.

Further reading

Dejucq N, Jegou B. Viruses in the mammalian male genital tract and their effects on the reproductive system. *Microbiol Mol Biol Rev* 2001;**65**:208–21.

LeBaron DW, Foghani B, Beck C, et al. Persistence of mumps antibodies after 2 doses of measles-mumps-rubella vaccine. *J Infect Dis* 2009;**199**:552–60.

Plotkin SA, Rubin SA. Mumps vaccine. In: Plotkin SA, Orenstein WO, Offit PA, eds. *Vaccines*, 5th edn. Philadelphia: Elsevier, 2008:435–66.

Reid F, Hassan J, Irwin F, Waters A, Hall W, Connell J. Epidemiologic and diagnostic evaluation of a recent mumps outbreak using oral fluid samples. *J Clin Virol* 2008;**41**:134–7.

Chapter 90

Mycoplasma

📖 see also Chapters 14, 27, 44

Name and nature of the organism

- Mycoplasmas are prokaryotes that lack a cell wall. They are the smallest free living forms and are ubiquitous pathogens. They can grow in cell-free media and contain both RNA and DNA, clearly separating them from viruses.
- The family *Mycoplasmataceae* is composed of two genera responsible for human infection, *Mycoplasma* and *Ureaplasma*.
- In 1945, Eaton identified an organism which passed through viral filters and could cause focal areas of pneumonia in rodents. This was initially called the Eaton agent and was subsequently classified as *Mycoplasma pneumoniae*.

Mycoplasma pneumoniae

Epidemiology

- Most *M. pneumoniae* respiratory infections occur as a single case or in family outbreaks, but minor epidemics may occur. Infections occur worldwide and show no significant seasonal preponderance.
- The highest attack rate is in people aged 5–20 years, but infection can occur at any age, and neonates can have severe disease. Young children <3 years of age primarily develop upper respiratory tract infections (URTIs), whereas those aged 5–20 years develop bronchitis and pneumonia.
- Outbreaks in the community occur every 3–4 years and very few *M. pneumoniae* infections are seen between outbreaks. Recent outbreaks in the UK have been mild.

Transmission and incubation period

- *M. pneumoniae* infection is spread by respiratory droplets.
- The incubation period is 1–3 weeks.

Clinical features and sequelae

Most *M. pneumoniae* infections are clinically apparent with slow onset of fever, malaise, headache and cough. In about 5–10% infection progresses to tracheobronchitis or pneumonia. The clinical illness continues for 2–3 weeks with a usual subacute course.

On physical examination, the patient usually does not look toxic. The pharynx may be injected and erythematous, usually without significant cervical adenopathy. In children, otitis media can occur. Chest auscultation is usually normal or there may be minimal scattered crackles or wheezes. Infection may be associated with the onset of asthma and bacterial super-infection following *M. pneumoniae* infection is rare. Although pneumonia is usually mild and self-limiting, fulminant and occasionally fatal cases very rarely occur (in normal and immunocompromised children).

The chest X-ray appearance of patients with *M. pneumoniae* infection can vary, but most commonly shows bilateral interstitial pneumonitis. The changes are often more extensive than would be expected from the clinical examination. Hilar adenopathy and lobar consolidation are well described. Pleural effusions can occur, and are usually small but not always small. If thoracentesis is performed, exudative serous fluid with minimal inflammatory cells is found.

Extrapulmonary manifestations
Dermatological involvement

- Many rashes have been reported including macular, morbilliform and papulovesicular eruptions, erythema nodosum, and urticaria.
- Erythema multiforme or even Stevens–Johnson syndrome can occur, causing vesicles, plaques and bullae involving the skin, particularly at mucocutaneous junctions. The conjunctivae, oral and genital mucosa and joints may also be involved. The lesions usually clear within 1–2 weeks without scarring.

Neurological disease

Aseptic meningitis, meningoencephalitis, transverse myelitis, brain stem dysfunction, Guillain–Barré syndrome, and peripheral neuropathy have all been reported. The CSF cellular response is usually minimal, with slightly elevated protein and normal glucose. The diagnosis of *Mycoplasma*-related CNS involvement is made after exclusion of other causes, the presence of an intercurrent febrile and/or respiratory illness and serological evidence of *M. pneumoniae* infection. *M. pneumoniae* has rarely been cultured from the CSF or detected by PCR, and immune-mediated neurological damage has been postulated.

Increased susceptibility to Mycoplasma infections

Persons with sickle cell disease or sickle-related haemoglobinopathies infected with *M. pneumoniae* may develop serious respiratory disease with large pleural effusions and marked respiratory distress. In patients with functional asplenia, with its associated opsonization deficiency, over-whelming pneumonia may occur with *M. pneumoniae* infections.

Other clinical associations

- A Coombs' positive haemolytic anaemia has been reported. Transient reversible vasospasm of the digits on exposure to cold has been described in association with *M. pneumoniae* infections. Cardiac involvement includes pericarditis, arrhythmias.
- Polyarthralgia is common, but arthritis is rare. Renal complications associated with immune complex deposition and high cold agglutinin titres have been reported. There are reports of *M. pneumoniae*-associated aplastic anaemia.

Diagnosis

The laboratory diagnosis of *M. pneumoniae* infections depends on the detection of antibody or the detection of antigen.

Cold agglutinins

Detection of cold agglutinins in plasma is not unique to patients with *M. pneumoniae* infection, but cold agglutinins can be detected before specific antibodies appear. Other diseases that can give rise to cold agglutinins are EBV, CMV, and lymphoma. To rapidly assess for the presence of cold agglutinins put 2–3 millilitres of blood in an EDTA bottle, mix well and then leave in the freezer compartment of a fridge for 5–10 minutes, then look for clumping.

Detection of antibody

Laboratory confirmation is most commonly performed by IgM by ELISA or by complement fixation test (CFT) to show a fourfold rise in complement fixing antibody titres between acute and convalescent serum specimens. The ELISA serology is both insensitive and non-specific with a sensitivity and a specificity of approximately 80% in patients with a syndrome consistent with atypical pneumonia.

Management and treatment

Antimicrobial therapy is not indicated for URTI and this syndrome probably often goes undiagnosed. Pneumonia is self-limiting and usually not life-threatening.

Treatment with effective antimicrobials can shorten the duration of illness and, by reducing cough and the number of organisms, may reduce the spread of infection to contacts. As *Mycoplasma* lack a cell wall, β-lactam antibiotics such as penicillins and cephalosporins are ineffective. Aminoglycosides are effective *in vitro* but the effect *in vivo* is untested.

While antimicrobials shorten the duration of illness, radiographic findings may take much longer to resolve and organisms may be able to be cultured from sputum for several weeks. Erythromycin is often poorly tolerated because of gastrointestinal side affects, including nausea, vomiting, abdominal pain, and diarrhoea. Clarithromycin has probably similar efficacy and fewer side effects. Optimal duration of therapy is unknown and the antimicrobials may work in part through immunomodulation.

Other antimicrobials that have significant *in vitro* and *in vivo* activity against *Mycoplasma* species include quinolones, tetracycline, and the streptogramin antibiotic quinupristin-dalfopristin.

Future research

Future research may involve development of a vaccine or development of more effective antimicrobial agents.

Genital mycoplasmas: *Mycoplasma genitalium, Mycoplasma hominis,* and *Ureaplasma urealyticum*

Epidemiology and clinical significance

- *U. urealyticum* is highly prevalent in the genital tracts of healthy, sexually active women at rates of 60–70%. The prevalence of *U. urealyticum* in the male urethra is lower at 10–20%. Infants can be infected at birth and this organism has been associated with preterm delivery and bronchopulmonary dysplasia in infants. It can rarely cause a diffuse interstitial neonatal pneumonia and neonatal meningitis. The exact role of *U. urealyticum* in chronic lung disease in premature infants remains unclear.
- Genital mycoplasmas are generally commensals in normal flora, although *M. genitalium* is associated with about 20% of non-gonococcal urethritis in males and may have a role in cervicitis or endometriosis. *M. hominis* is less prevalent.
- *M. hominis* has been recovered from a variety of extragenital sites, including kidneys, joints, and surgical wounds. It has been recovered from the blood and CSF of newborns with signs of sepsis and meningoencephalitis and is a rare cause of neonatal meningitis. *M. hominis* has also been isolated from the upper respiratory tract and is thought to be a cause of neonatal pneumonia. It is associated with stillbirths and recovered from fetal lung and liver tissue.
- These organisms can be cultured in the laboratory but with difficulty and are not looked for routinely. PCR has been developed and will become the assay of choice in the future.
- Detection of *U. urealyticum* or *M. hominis* in the genital tract is interpreted as normal flora, but their detection in the blood stream, joints, wound lesions or other sites is significant, and they can cause disease in immunocompromised individuals.

Management and treatment

Susceptibility to antimicrobial agents

- In general, *U. urealyticum* is susceptible to tetracyclines and quinolones, but has limited susceptibility to erythromycin and other macrolides. In vitro, azithromycin and clarithromycin are significantly more active than erythromycin.
- *M. genitalium* is susceptible to the macrolides, erythromycin, azithromycin, and clarithromycin.
- *M. hominis* is intrinsically resistant to erythromycin and other macrolides, but it is susceptible to the lincosamide lincomycin, although lincomycin is not recommended for use in neonates.

Treatment

- Isolation of *U. urealyticum* or *M. hominis* from a normally sterile site, in the absence of other organisms, is justification to consider antimicrobial treatment if there is evidence of inflammation. However, if there is no evidence of inflammation, therapy is probably not warranted, because organisms can be isolated from the blood and CSF of newborns with no adverse outcome and spontaneous clearance without treatment does occur.

- The treatment of choice for *U. urealyticum* neonatal infections (except CNS infections) is erythromycin, although there are no clinical trials and no comparisons with other antimicrobials. Treatment of CNS infections remains difficult. The newer quinolones, moxifloxacin and gatifloxacin, have activity *in vitro*, but *U. urealyticum* is significantly less sensitive to these agents than *M. hominis*.

- Treatment for *M. hominis* neonatal infections is problematic as tetracyclines, the usually recommended agents, are not recommended for use in children <8 years and do not penetrate the blood–brain barrier. There is evidence of *in vitro* sensitivity of *M. hominis* to linezolid, an antibiotic which penetrates the CNS and can be given to neonates and children.

Prevention

There is no mechanism to prevent transmission of genital mycoplasmas either horizontally or vertically. There is no currently effective vaccine.

Future research

Future research may involve development of a vaccine or development of more effective antimicrobial agents. A large randomized study on the role of azithromycin in preventing chronic lung disease in premature infants is underway.

Further reading

Daxboeck F, Blacky A, Seidl R, Krause R, Assadian O. Diagnosis, treatment, and prognosis of *mycoplasma pneumoniae* childhood encephalitis: systematic review of 58 cases. *J Child Neurol* 2004;**19**:865–71.

Gavranich JB, Chang AB. Antibiotics for community acquired lower respiratory tract infections (LRTI) secondary to *Mycoplasma pneumoniae* in children. *Cochrane Database Syst Rev* 2005;**3**:CD004875.

Mabanta CG, Pryhuber GS, Weinberg GA, Phelps D. Erythromycin for the prevention of chronic lung disease in intubated preterm infants at risk for, or colonized or infected with Ureaplasma urealyticum. *Cochrane Database Syst Rev* 2003;**4**:CD003744.

Non-tuberculous mycobacterial infection

📖 see also Chapters 8, 15, 19, 20, 38, 113

Name and nature of organism

- Non-tuberculous mycobacteria are environmental mycobacteria, found throughout the world in soil, dust, water, food, and animals. More than 50 species have been implicated in human disease.
- Acid and alcohol fast, Gram-positive organisms.
- Classification was traditionally based on pigment production and rate of growth. Further differentiation of species by morphology, physiology, biochemistry, and antibiotic sensitivity is routine. PCR and DNA sequencing have increased NTM species identified to >125.
- Rapid identification is by microscopy and staining with fluorochrome. Ziehl–Neelson staining is less sensitive. Culture may take <2 weeks on rapid, broth media for rapid growing NTM or >2 months for slower growing on solid media.
- Can cause invasive, disseminated disease, or local infection.

Epidemiology and aetiology

- Geographical distribution is similar when the environment is sampled, but isolates found in lymphadenopathy vary, with for example, *Mycobacterium avium* complex (MAC) found worldwide, *M. malmoense* in northern areas, *M. haemophilum* in Israel.
- NTM lymphadenopathy typically affects young children between 1 and 5 years, probably reflecting immature mycobacterial immunity—increased incidence has been reported in association with stopping neonatal BCG programmes in Scandinavia.
- Outbreaks of cutaneous NTM infection in older children and adults have been linked to whirlpool footbaths. *Mycobacterium marinarum* is associated with 'fish tank' granulomas on the hands or other water born lesions.
- Respiratory infection is associated with underlying chronic respiratory disease, usually cystic fibrosis. Fast-growing mycobacteria such as *M. abscessus*, *M. chelonae*, and *M. kansasii* are frequently implicated with *M. abscessus* responsible for >80% of pulmonary infection in the USA.
- Disseminated disease occurs with primary or secondary immunocompromise.

Transmission and incubation period

- Infection results from environmental acquisition by inhalation, ingestion or direct contact from a contaminated source. NTM submandibular or cervical lymphadenopathy suggests that the buccal mucosa is a portal of mycobacterial entry
- Unlike tuberculosis, NTM infection is not transmitted from person to person. Hence neither contact tracing nor isolation of an infected child is necessary.

Clinical features and sequelae

NTM lymphadenopathy

- Local lymph node infection in a young child between 1 and 8 years old.
- Any node may be involved but are usually submandibular, cervical or preauricular, with axillary and inguinal nodes occasionally involved.
- Sudden or gradual onset of firm, painless, usually unilateral lymphadenopathy.
- Child remains well, with no systemic upset, no temperature or evidence of dissemination.
- Node gradually increases in size and usually develops a characteristic reddish pink colour over the indurated skin, which deepens to purple blue.
- Often 2–3cm in size but may become very large and disfiguring.
- Eventually nodes soften, rupture and discharge with sinus formation and if not removed or treated can continue to do so for months to years before gradual spontaneous healing.
- Most commonly caused by MAC, rarely now by *M. scrofulaceum*. Classically scrofula was caused by tuberculosis of the neck (King's evil) and was cured by the touch of the monarch of either France or England. No controlled trial supports this intervention.

Other soft tissue infections

- Although not common, sporadic cases and outbreaks of cellulitis, soft tissue abscesses, and rarely extracutaneous disease associated with rapidly growing NTM have been documented in healthy individuals.
- NTM can cause papules and nodules, which may be linear.
- *M. marinatum* follows trauma in water and leads to clusters of nodules that may ulcerate on hands and feet.
- *M. ulcerans* is seen in Australia and Central Africa, causing Buruli ulcer, a single large painless ulcer usually on the extensor surface of the leg, with local necrosis.
- Although some resolve without intervention, infection may result in a severe, protracted, and potentially scarring lesions.

Respiratory infections

- NTM are implicated as occasional pathogens in chronic lung disease in adults. They are isolated regularly in children with cystic fibrosis, though their relevance when found is still not entirely understood.

- The main problem is differentiating colonization from disease.
- Prevalence of NTM in cystic fibrosis appears to be increasing and has variously been quoted at between 6% and 13%, and up to 23% in Israel.
- Risk factors include allergic bronchopulmonary aspergillosis and treatment with steroids, aerosolised medications, and bronchoscopes (contamination).
- Infection is more often associated with markers of severe disease, and disseminated fatal infection has been described post lung transplantation.

CVC-associated NTM infections

- These have been reported in association with leukaemias, lymphomas, and solid tumours.
- Usually these infections are due to rapid growing NTM but *M. avium intracellulare* has also been reported.
- Occasionally NTM in blood cultures may be mistaken for *Corynebacterium* or *Nocardia* species, which leads to a delay in appropriate management or to inappropriate therapy.
- Affected patients are not necessarily neutropenic but are frequently lymphopenic (total lymphocyte count <1000/mm^3) and may also have lung involvement.
- NTM infection should be considered in all persistently febrile children with cancer or leukaemia, particularly those who do not respond to conventional antibiotics or antifungals—do blood cultures in special mycobacterial bottles.

Disseminated disease

- Found in primary and secondary immune deficiency.
- Predisposition for dissemination is seen where the CD4 count is very low, with defects in the IFN-γ, STAT1 signalling, and IL-12 pathways and with significant neutrophil impairment. These include HIV, mendelian susceptibility to mycobacterial diseases (MSMD), SCID, CGD, and malignancy with chemotherapy.
- MSMD describes a newly recognized range of autosomal and X-linked single gene defects in families with an increased predisposition to invasive or recurrent mycobacterial TB (MTB) and NTM disease (e.g. IFN-γ receptor 1 and 2, IL-12β receptor, nuclear factor κB essential modifier (NEMO)). A close relationship between genotype, cellular immune/inflammatory phenotype and the clinical disease manifestations has been observed. NTM and BCG infections appear to predominate but infections with non-typhoidal salmonellae and several herpes viruses have also been problematic.
- Systemic symptoms include fever, weight loss, sweats, diarrhoea, cough, and focal lesions such as bone or joint involvement.
- Infection may be found in blood, bone marrow, lung, bones, joints, gastrointestinal tract, rarely CNS as well as local skin and soft tissue.

Diagnosis

Lymphadenopathy

- Differential diagnosis includes MTB, cat scratch disease, toxoplasmosis, mumps, salivary stone, EBV, malignancy, and CGD.
- Relative risk of NTM and MTB infection depends on the local rate of MTB infection within the population. This will be different in inner London (TB rate >40:100 00) compared with rural Dorset.
- Frequently mistaken for bacterial abscesses, despite lack of systemic or local temperature, no systemic upset, persistent duration, and non-response to oral or IV antibiotics.
- Clinical diagnosis can usually be made based on classic features alone.
- Diagnosis is often made post surgical exploration for incision and drainage when histology subsequently indicates caseating granulomata and/or acid-fast bacilli are seen.
- Initial microscopy of acid-fast bacilli does not distinguish MTB from NTM. Subsequent culture can take from 3 weeks to 2 months. If the clinical situation indicates and there is sufficient acid-fast bacilli-positive material, MTB PCR or commercial DNA probe can distinguish MTB on initial specimens.
- Investigations could include detailed history, including family history of infection, travel and contact with MTB. FBC, CRP, ESR, LFTs, serology—*Bartonella, Toxoplasma*, EBV, ASOT; Mantoux, IFN-γ release assay (IFGRA), CXR.
- Fine needle aspiration may be useful to provide tissue diagnosis.
- Mantoux often weakly positive but less likely to be >15mm.
- IFGRA (QFG in tube and T SPOT TB); some evidence that these are negative in NTM infection in children.

CVC infection

- Although conventional blood cultures will detect rapidly growing NTM, they are unlikely to detect *M. avium intracellulare* or other slow-growing mycobacteria. Specific mycobacterial blood culture bottles are required for this purpose.

Respiratory infection

- Signs and symptoms may be confused with underlying cystic fibrosis or chronic lung disease.
- Deteriorating lung function in face of NTM isolate warrants trial of treatment.
- Consider NTM respiratory disease and drug treatment.

Disseminated disease

- High index of suspicion in immunocompromised. Investigation should include mycobacterial blood cultures, imaging, and guided biopsy for histology and mycobacterial culture.
- Where disseminated infection found in previously well children, the possibility of underlying specific immune deficiency should be explored.

Management and treatment

Lymphadenopathy

The three options are surgical, medical, and observation.
- Parents should be counselled about the chronicity of the condition, the lack of infectivity and eventual resolution. Considerable upset can occur due to the cosmetic appearance and this can lead to social isolation in a child. Both families and doctors often want to 'do something' even if its not very evidence based—a common problem in paediatric infectious diseases.
- Surgical excision, where possible, is curative—although new lesions may appear locally or on the other side.
- The great majority of lesions will also resolve spontaneously over a 1–2-year period. A waxing and waning course is common, with flare-ups associated with minor viral URTIs. In open lesions, secondary infection due to staphylococcal or streptococcal infection may also occur (which is why lesions sometimes seem to partially respond to conventional antibiotics).
- Large lesions, such as those involving significant areas of skin, or deep infection, or close to the facial nerve, may not be possible to safely excise without morbidity or extensive scarring.
- Antimicrobial treatment may be helpful if excision is not possible or incision and drainage has produced an active discharging lesion. Efficacy appears variable and may depend on underlying mycobacterial sensitivities.
- There are limited data on which to base treatment decisions. One randomized trial in 100 children with proven cervical NTM compared surgical excision to 3 months of clarithromycin and rifabutin. Although cure rates were significantly better with surgery (96% vs 66%), substantial rates of complications were also seen with both therapies (28% vs 78%).[1] If the family are in agreement, masterly inactivity (doing nothing) is a perfectly reasonable option.

CVC infection
- Some children have been effectively treated with CVC removal alone. However, standard treatment includes line removal, treatment with at least two anti-mycobacterial drugs for 2–12 weeks for localized disease and 6 months or longer for widespread disease

Drug treatment
- As in all mycobacterial treatment, monotherapy will produce resistance and treatment is required for at least several months. Ideally, a combination of at least two anti-mycobacterial agents is needed to prevent resistance from emerging.
- Tailor to organism, when known, and discuss with laboratory:
  - *M. avium* are generally macrolide sensitive but variably resistant to most other agents
  - *M. malmoense* are variably sensitive to several agents including ethambutol, macrolide, rifampicin, quinolones.
  - *M. chelonae* are often sensitive to tobramycin, clarithromycin, and linezolid, less often amikacin, meropenem, and quinolone.
  - *M. abscessus* may be clarithromycin, amikacin, and cefoxitin sensitive.

- Combinations of a macrolide and rifabutin or rifampicin with or without ethambutol have been used in NTM lymphadenopathy,
- Combinations of at least three, often five, drugs are favoured for disseminated disease in immunodeficiency. These can include a macrolide, rifabutin or rifampicin, ethambutol, quinolones, amikacin, and newer drugs such as moxifloxacin, or linezolid.
- Surveillance for side effects of vision including visual acuity or colour discrimination (ethambutol), the presence of eye pain or uveitis (rifabutin); hepatitis (isoniazid, rifampin, ethionamide, clarithromycin, rifabutin); renal impairment or auditory dysfunction (streptomycin, amikacin); CNS dysfunction (cycloserine, ethionamide); and haematological abnormalities (sulfonamides, cefoxitin, rifabutin) is very important.

Prevention

- Antimycobacterial prophylaxis is unnecessary for localized disease.
- In HIV, low, age-related CD4+ cell counts levels are considered as high risk for MAC warranting consideration of macrolide prophylaxis (℗ www.chiva.org.uk).
- In other immune deficiencies with a specific predisposition to NTM infection, macrolide primary and secondary prophylaxis should be considered.

Future research

- Incidence and prevalence of NTM local and disseminated disease.
- Role of drug treatment in NTM lymphadenopathy.
- Natural history of NTM lymphadenopathy.
- Immune deficiency in disseminated and local disease.
- Stopping secondary prophylaxis in children with immune reconstitution on HAART.

Key reference

1 Lindeboom JA, Kuijper EJ, Bruijnesteijn van Coppenraet ES, Lindeboom R, Prins JM. Surgical excision versus antibiotic treatment for nontuberculous mycobacterial cervicofacial lymphadenitis in children: a multicenter, randomized, controlled trial. *Clin Infect Dis* 2007;**44**:1057–64.

Further reading

Al-Muhsen S, Casanova JL. The genetic heterogeneity of mendelian susceptibility to mycobacterial diseases. *J Allergy Clin Immunol* 2008;**122**:1043–51.

Griffith DE, Aksamit T, Brown-Elliott BA, *et al.* An official ATS/IDSA statement: Diagnosis, treatment, and prevention of nontuberculous mycobacterial diseases. *Am J Respir Crit Care Med* 2007;**175**:367–416.

Heyderman RS, Clark J. Clinical manifestations of nontuberculous mycobacteria. In: Pollard AJ, Finn A, eds. Hot topics in infection and immunity. *Adv Exp Med Biol* 2006;**582**:167–77.

Starke JR. Commentary: The natural history of nontuberculous mycobacterial cervical adenitis. *Pediatr Infect Dis J* 2008;**27**:923–4.

Norovirus

📖 see also Chapters 12, 17

Name and nature of organism

- Noroviruses are a leading cause of mild and severe gastroenteritis worldwide among people of all ages.
- Noroviruses were identified in 1972 as a cause of the illness commonly known as the 'winter vomiting disease', characterized by the sudden onset of self-limiting vomiting and diarrhoea that typically peaked during the colder months. The virus was first identified by immune electron microscopic examination of stools of volunteers challenged with fecal filtrates from students affected by an outbreak of gastroenteritis in 1969 in Norwalk Ohio. The Norwalk virus, the prototype agent of the genus *Norovirus* (previously denoted as 'Norwalk-like viruses'), belongs to the *Caliciviridae* family.
- Three other genera are now described in the *Caliciviridae* family: *Sapovirus* (previously called 'Sapporo-like viruses'), *Lagovirus*, and *Vesivirus*, and a fifth genus (proposed *Nebovirus*) is pending.
- Noroviruses are classified into five genogroups (GI–V) and 32 genotypes, with most human strains clustering within genogroups I and II.
- Noroviruses are positive single-stranded RNA viruses, with no lipid envelope. They are therefore not so easily inactivated by alcohol-based gels, but are inactivated by chlorine-based detergents.

Epidemiology

- Noroviruses are known to infect people of all ages.
- They are the leading cause of epidemic gastroenteritis, causing >90% of non-bacterial and >50% of all-cause epidemic gastroenteritis in many settings worldwide. Disease outbreaks are reported year-round with peaks during months with cold weather in regions with temperate climates. Up to 80% of children may have been infected by school age.
- Noroviruses are also a common cause of severe sporadic gastroenteritis, accounting for up to 30% of gastroenteritis hospitalizations among children and adults.
- Outbreaks occur in hospitals, cruise ships, and other institutions frequently requiring ward closures to terminate the outbreak.
- Children <5 years, immunocompromised persons, and elderly patients are at a greater risk of severe disease from norovirus infection.

Transmission, incubation period, and immunity

- Fecal-oral spread is generally the most important mode of transmission.
- Transmission from infectious vomit, both by mechanical transmission from environmental surfaces (e.g. hand/mouth contact) and aerosolization are likely to propagate spread.
- Foodborne outbreaks occur usually due to infected shellfish and salad.
- Person to person spread among contacts of primary cases further propagates the epidemic. Several characteristics of noroviruses facilitates spread:
  - Low infectious dose (<10 particles)
  - Prolonged shedding (2–4 weeks) even after symptom resolution
  - Viral stability in the environment
  - Repeat infections are common, possibly due to wide strain diversity with incomplete cross-protection and likely short-lived immunity.
- Incubation period is typically 24–48 hours.
- The difficulty in diagnosing norovirus infection and the lack of correlates of protection have made it challenging to assess immunity after norovirus infection. Early volunteer studies suggest that protective immunity after norovirus exposure could be short-lived (i.e. 6–14 weeks). However, decreasing duration of symptoms with increasing age in one community cohort study does suggest the possibility of some protection against severe disease after natural norovirus infection.
- Interestingly, in volunteer studies, approximately 13–40% of exposed persons never became infected and only 50% developed illness. Recent research suggests that host genotype is a prominent factor in development of norovirus infection—it appears that norovirus infection may depend on the presence of specific human histo-blood group antigen receptors in the gut of susceptible hosts.

Clinical features and sequelae

- Disease is characterized by acute onset of nausea, vomiting, abdominal cramps, myalgias, and non-bloody diarrhoea. Fever is reported in nearly half of all patients and typically subsides within 24 hours.
- Sudden onset of continuous severe profuse vomiting is often the first sign of disease. Some studies suggest that vomiting is relatively more common in children >1 year whereas diarrhoea is more common in infants.
- Symptoms typically resolve in 2–3 days but may persist for 4–6 days in some.
- Elderly and the young (in developing countries with limited access to healthcare) may be at greater risk for fatal norovirus disease.
- Norovirus has been associated with necrotizing enterocolitis and postinfectious irritable bowel syndrome, which resolves after 3 months. Prolonged viral shedding with vomiting for over a year has been reported in paediatric oncology patients.

Diagnosis

- Diagnosis rests on finding noroviruses in a fecal or vomitus specimen of patients with suspected gastroenteritis or detecting a rise in significant antibody titres in the sera of an infected patient.
- Because noroviruses have yet to be cultivated, a rapid, sensitive commercial diagnostic assay is not available. RT-PCR and EIAs are two widely used methods of norovirus detection.
  - RT-PCR is more sensitive than EIA because of ability to detect low viral loads and a wider range of strains. PCR has been used in food screening programmes.
  - EIAs are highly specific for some noroviruses, but generally not sensitive enough to detect a wide range of noroviruses.
- Studies have identified and validated four epidemiological features of norovirus disease that can be useful in determining if norovirus is the causative agent in an outbreak, in the absence of access to diagnostic testing:
  - Vomiting in more than half of affected persons
  - Mean (or median) incubation period of 24–48 hours
  - Mean (or median) duration of illness of 12–60 hours
  - Absence of bacterial pathogen in stool culture.

Management and treatment

- First-line therapy for uncomplicated norovirus gastroenteritis should be oral rehydration solutions that provide essential electrolyte replacement plus sugar (glucose or sucrose).
- Significant dehydration or inability to tolerate oral hydration may warrant early parenteral fluid plus electrolyte replacement.
- As tolerated, initiating oral caloric intake early in the illness may enhance patient recovery.
- Antibiotic therapy is not indicated for norovirus gastroenteritis.
- Studies have demonstrated that antimotility agents such as diphenoxylate or loperamide do not reduce intestinal fluid losses. Antimotility agents should be avoided in children <3 years as they are associated with complications (ileus, lethargy, or even death).
- Ward outbreaks in paediatric units need prompt recognition, and action to close the ward and stop transfer of children to other wards.

Prevention

- Prevention of norovirus outbreaks relies on identifying mode of transmission and interrupting it by controlling contamination and reducing spread.
  - Disinfection of environmental surfaces contaminated with vomitus and feces with appropriate solutions is crucial. Depending on the extent of contamination, the facility or institution may have to be closed to interrupt transmission.

- Molecular assays have been developed to detect noroviruses directly from contaminated products and could supplement prevention efforts.
- Strict personal hygiene is critical for prevention of person-to-person transmission, such as through food-handler associated transmission.
- Food-handlers should be excused from work during illness to prevent virus transmission.
- No licensed vaccines are currently available for prevention of norovirus disease.

Future research

- Development of an animal model or cell culture system for cultivating noroviruses will be an important future step towards improving diagnosis and developing a safe and effective norovirus vaccine.
- Studies on immune correlates of protection from natural infection, duration of protection, and cross-protection will improve prospects of vaccine development.
- Better information is needed to identify populations susceptible to infection, for whom the impact of short-term morbidity from gastroenteritis is great (e.g. military troops, travellers), and those at the highest risk of severe disease from norovirus infection (e.g. elderly, infants).
- Systematic surveillance using broadly reactive, state-of-the-art diagnostic assays are needed to fully understand the true burden of noroviruses in the aetiology of severe gastroenteritis, particularly among high-risk populations such as children <5 years and older people. These evaluations are especially necessary in resource-poor countries, where diarrhoea remains a leading cause of childhood death, causing >1.8 million annual deaths.
- Hospital control measures need further investigation, for example duration of ward closure.

Further reading

Green KY. In: Knipe DM, Howley PM, Griffin DE, *et al.* eds. *Caliciviridae: The Noroviruses.* In: *Fields' Virology,* 5th edn, vol. 1. Philadelphia: Wolters Kluwer Health/Lippincott Williams & Wilkins, 2007:949–78.

Lopman B, Vennema H, Kohli E, *et al.* Increase in viral gastroenteritis outbreaks in Europe and epidemic spread of new norovirus variant. *Lancet* 2004;**363**:682–8.

Parashar U, Quiroz ES, Mounts AW, *et al.* 'Norwalk-like viruses'. Public health consequences and outbreak management. *MMWR Recomm Rep* 2001;**50**:1–17.

Patel MM, Widdowson MA, Glass RI, Akazawa K, Vinje J, Parashar UD. Systematic literature review of role of noroviruses in sporadic gastroenteritis. *Emerg Infect Dis* 2008;**14**:1224–31.

Parvovirus

📖 see also Chapters 10, 34

Name and nature of organism

- Parvovirus B19 is a member of the *Erythrovirus* group of parvoviruses—small, non-enveloped single-stranded DNA viruses.
- It binds specifically to P antigen or globoside that is present on erythrocytes, erythroblasts, megakarocytes, endothelial cells, and fetal liver and cardiac cells, explaining clinical specificity.
- Parvovirus B19 tropism for proerythrocytes causes lysis of erythrocyte precursors producing haemolysis and erythroid aplasia.
- Fifth disease gets its name because around 1900 it was the fifth described classical childhood exanthem (the others are: 1. measles, 2. scarlet fever, 3. rubella and 4. Duke's disease—the fourth disease although widely described probably never actually existed).
- Slapped cheek syndrome refers to the characteristic facial rash.
- Humans are the only known hosts of parvovirus B19.

Epidemiology

- Erythema infectiosum or fifth disease is a common disease worldwide.
- Erythema infectiosum is usually a benign infection of early childhood associated with a characteristic facial rash. It is caused by parvovirus B19 and complications may arise in individuals with haemolytic disease, immunocompromised patients, and pregnant women.
- It affects children of all ages. In Europe up to 10% of children are seropositive by the age of 5, up to 50% by 10, and 75% by age 30.[1]
- It is highly infectious, and a child with erythema infectiosum may infect up to 50% of susceptible household contacts.
- Outbreaks are common in childcare facilities and schools, with 10–60% of children being infected during an outbreak.
- Outbreaks occur most commonly in late winter and spring and have a 3–4-year cycle.
- Infection with parvovirus confers lifelong immunity.

Transmission and incubation period

- The incubation period of erythema infectiosum is 4–14 days, but can be as long as 21 days.
- Children are infectious before the facial rash develops (Table 93.1). Parvovirus B19 can be detected in respiratory secretions and saliva during the prodromal period, which is usually 3–6 days before the rash. This partially explains why outbreaks occur as it is hard to diagnose the disease in the most infectious period.
- The appearance of parvovirus B19 IgG and IgM coincides with the onset of the rash, so once the rash is present, they are less infectious.

Table 93.1 Duration of infectivity by manifestations of parvovirus B19

Clinical condition	Duration of infectivity
Slapped cheek syndrome	Until rash appears
Polyarthropathy syndrome	Until joint symptoms occur
Papular purpuric gloves and socks syndrome	While symptoms are present
Transient aplastic crisis	For at least 7 days after symptoms start
Chronic persistent anaemia	Indefinitely in the immunocompromised host

- It is generally spread via respiratory droplets.
- Vertical transmission from mother to fetus can occur.
- It can also be transmitted via blood and blood products including packed cells, platelets, and clotting factors.
- Those with haemolytic disease or immunocompromised have high viral titres in respiratory secretions and blood and are infectious.

Clinical features and sequelae

See Table 93.2.

Table 93.2 Clinical manifestations of parvovirus B19 infection

Clinical condition	Typical host
Slapped cheek syndrome	Healthy child
Asymptomatic infection	Healthy child or adult
Respiratory illness with no rash	Healthy child or adult
Papular purpuric gloves and socks syndrome	Healthy child or adult

Table 93.2 *(Contd.)*

Clinical condition	Typical host
Polyarthropathy syndrome	Healthy adult female
Chronic persistent anaemia	Immunocompromised child or adult
Transient aplastic crisis	Individual with haemolytic disease
Foetal hydrops/congenital anemia	Fetus (first 20 weeks' gestation)

- In previously healthy children erythema infectiosum is a benign, self-limiting illness with no long-term sequelae.
- In 20–50% of children, infection is asymptomatic.
- There is a prodromal period of mild flu-like symptoms: fever (30% of children), headache (20%), sore throat (15%), and myalgia. There may also be abdominal pain, nausea, fatigue, and rhinorrhoea. This usually lasts 3–6 days before the onset of the rash.
- Adults are more likely to develop arthralgias in the prodromal period than children.
- The characteristic rash of erythema infectiosum is an erythematous rash on both cheeks, with sparing of the nose, nasolabial folds, and circumoral and periorbital regions, giving the appearance that the cheeks have been slapped. This rash is most common in younger children. It usually lasts 1–4 days.
- A rash subsequently develop on the trunk, spreading to the arms and legs. This is an erythematous rash that clears from the centre outwards, giving a characteristic reticular or 'lacy' morphology. The rash may be itchy. It usually fades after a couple of weeks, but may recur for months after recovery with stimuli including exercise or sunlight.
- There is occasionally an associated oral enanthem with erythema of the tongue and pharynx and red macules on the palate and buccal mucosa.
- Associated symptoms are rare in childhood, although about 10% of children develop arthralgia or occasionally arthritis. This predominantly affects large joints such as the knee. Adults, especially females, with parvovirus B19 infection are more prone to a polyarthropathy affecting the knees and small joints such as the digits. The arthritis may exist without a rash.
- A separate exanthem caused by parvovirus B19 is **papular purpuric gloves and socks syndrome**. This starts as erythema and oedema of the hands and feet associated with mild fever. Purpuric papules develop on the palms and soles extending as far as the wrists and ankles. The rash is itchy and treatment is symptomatic with antihistamines. It usually resolves in 1–2 weeks without sequelae. Other viruses including HHV-6, HHV-7, CMV, and measles have been associated with the syndrome.
- **Unilateral laterothoracic exanthem (ULE)** is marked by unilateral coalescing erythematous papules on one side of the chest. It is most often seen in children, and is benign but lasts around a month.

It has been associated with various viral infections—most commonly parvovirus B19.

- In healthy children, complications of parvovirus B19 infection are rare and include transient bone marrow suppression (anaemia, leukopenia and thrombocytopenia), vasculitis, myocarditis, encephalitis, and glomerulonephritis.
  - In haemolytic disease: patients with high red cell turnover such as sickle cell disease and haemolytic anaemia are at risk of aplastic crisis if infected with parvovirus B19. This is usually transient but may be profound and longlasting.
  - In immunocompromised: in patients with either primary immunodeficiency or those who are immunocompromised secondary to chemotherapy or bone marrow transplantation, or in individuals with HIV, infection with parvovirus B19 may persist and lead to severe relapsing-remitting anaemia.
  - In pregnant women: parvovirus B19 infection in non-immune pregnant women (around 50% in Europe) can cause intrauterine growth retardation, pleural and pericardial effusions, hydrops fetalis and fetal death. It is the most frequent cause of non-immune fetal hydrops. The transmission risk is around 30%; the risk of fetal loss is 2–6% and is greatest in the first 20 weeks of pregnancy.

Diagnosis

- Diagnosis in healthy children is usually made clinically because the rash is so characteristic. The differential diagnosis includes rubella in which a maculopapular rash also starts on the face.
- PCR is the mainstay of laboratory diagnosis of parvovirus B19 infection as it is rapid and accurate. PCR can be done on blood, respiratory secretions or CSF.
- Diagnosis can be made serologically with IgM and paired IgG titres in serum from the onset of the rash. This is not a useful test in an aplastic crisis or in immunocompromised patients.

Management and treatment

- As the infection is usually benign and self-limiting, treatment is generally supportive, with antipyretics and analgesia as necessary.
- There is no effective antiviral therapy but antibody is key to viral clearance.
- Patients with aplastic crisis or immunodeficiency require admission, intensive monitoring and packed red cell transfusions to treat the severe anaemia.
- Patients who are immunocompromised with chronic severe anaemia due to parvovirus B19 infection may be treated with IVIG. Regimens of 0.5g/kg for 3–5 days have been used.
- Pregnant women with suspected infection or contact with erythema infectiosum should have serology checked. If parvovirus infection is confirmed, this may have implications for the fetus, so the mother

should be counselled and referred for a specialist opinion. Serial ultrasounds to monitor for hydrops fetalis may be indicated. If hydrops is diagnosed early, intrauterine transfusions can prevent the most severe outcomes.

Prevention

- Primary prevention of parvovirus B19 infection is currently not possible as there is no commercially-available vaccine. However, a recombinant vaccine has shown promise in a phase I trial.[2]
- Prevention of secondary cases of parvovirus B19 infection is difficult because cases are infectious before the disease is usually diagnosed with the appearance of the rash. By the time the characteristic facial rash appears, the patient is no longer infectious and therefore exclusion from childcare facilities, school or work is usually unnecessary. As transmission is by respiratory droplets, hand-washing precautions are likely to have an effect on spread of infection.
- Pregnant parents of children at risk should be warned of this infection so appropriate action can be taken if there is a contact.
- Pregnant healthcare workers should be advised about the risk to their unborn child of caring for a child with parvovirus B19.
- In hospitals, prevention of secondary cases usually focuses on those at risk of severe complications: patients with haemolysis, immunocompromised patients, and pregnant women.
- In patients with transient aplastic crisis, respiratory droplet precautions should be continued for 7 days.

Future research

- Although there has been a successful phase 1 trial, there is as yet no vaccine available.
- There are no anti-viral drugs to treat parvovirus infection. An effective drug would be an important advance for high risk patients or those who develop complications from parvovirus B19 infection.
- IVIG has been used to treat severe parvovirus B19 infection, but reports are limited to case reports and no controlled trial has been undertaken.
- There is no effective prophylaxis in high-risk patients when they have contact with parvovirus B19 infection. It is possible that IVIG could be used, but this needs study.

Key references

1 Mossong J, Hens N, Friederichs V, *et al.* Parvovirus B19 infection in five European countries: seroepidemiology, force of infection and maternal risk of infection. *Epidemiol Infect* 2008;**136**:1059–68.

2 Ballou WR, Reed JL, Noble W, Young NS, Koenig S. Safety and immunogenicity of a recombinant parvovirus B19 vaccine formulated with MF59C. *J Infect Dis* 2003;**187**:675–8.

Pertussis

📖 see also Chapters 27, 44

Name and nature of organism

- Pertussis is an infectious disease of the respiratory tract caused by *Bordetella pertussis* or, less commonly, *B. parapertussis*.
- *B. pertussis* produces the large complex pertussis toxin as well as other toxins that cause most of the clinical disease.
- *Bordetella* spp. are aerobic, Gram-negative coccobacilli that express tropism for ciliated epithelial cells.

Epidemiology

- Before the introduction of pertussis vaccines, pertussis was an endemic disease with epidemic peaks occurring around every 3 years. Most cases occurred in young children and mortality was high.
- Worldwide, whole cell pertussis vaccines have led to a significant reduction in the incidence and severity of pertussis in infants. However, pertussis remains one of the main causes of vaccine-preventable deaths; there are 20–40 million cases per year worldwide and an estimated 200 000–400 000 deaths.
- As part of routine immunization (diphtheria/tetanus/pertussis combination vaccine), it is estimated that more than 80% of infants worldwide routinely receive three doses of the pertussis vaccine in the first year of life. The impact of vaccination is demonstrated by comparisons between neighbouring countries with and without vaccination programmes, and within countries when vaccination programmes are interrupted (e.g. the UK in the 1970s and 1980s; Fig. 94.1).
- More recently the proportion of cases occurring in younger, unvaccinated children appears to be increasing. In some countries this is accompanied by an increase in the absolute numbers of cases in this age group and suggests a persisting reservoir of infection.
- Vaccine-induced immunity wanes 6–10 years after primary immunization and pertussis in these older individuals is likely to be under-diagnosed and untreated. The major source of infection for young children therefore comprises older children, adolescents and adults. As a consequence, pertussis booster doses in adolescents and adults have been introduced in several countries.

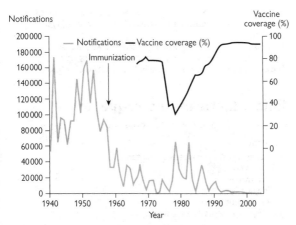

Fig. 94.1 Pertussis notifications and vaccine coverage of children by their second birthday, England and Wales (1940–2003).

(Reproduced from *Immunisation against Infectious Disease*, 3ʳᵈ edition. Department of Health, 2006. Reproduced under the terms of the Click-Use Licence.)

Pathogenesis

The disease process in pertussis is multifactorial and dependent on several *B. pertussis* virulence factors. These factors, alone or in combination, enable the organism to:
- Attach to and damage the respiratory epithelium
- Avoid local immune mechanisms
- Elaborate toxins that cause the systemic effects of pertussis.

The principal factors include those that have been included in the new acellular pertussis vaccines:
- Pertussis toxin
- Filamentous haemagglutinin
- Pertactin
- Agglutinogens.

Other factors may also include:
- Tracheal cytotoxin
- Tracheal colonization factor
- Adenylate cyclase factor.

Transmission

- Transmission of the infection is by aerosol droplet from infected cases to susceptible hosts.
- Infected cases are most infectious during the early catarrhal phase.

- The incubation period is usually 1–3 weeks and cases are infectious from 6 days after exposure to 3 weeks after the onset of typical paroxysms.
- There is no evidence for a prolonged carrier state, though asymptomatic individuals have been identified during epidemics.
- The secondary attack rate in household contacts is 80–100%.

Clinical features and sequelae

There are typically three stages of pertussis disease.

Catarrhal

- This stage includes non-specific symptoms:
  - Rhinorrhoea
  - Sore throat
  - Conjunctivitis
  - Non-productive cough.
- This stage typically lasts for 2 weeks.

Spasmodic

- During this stage the cough becomes paroxysmal, i.e. bouts of continuous coughing.
- This causes venous congestion and may result in cyanosis or facial discoloration.
- In typical cases, the paroxysms of cough may end with a deep inspiration (whoop) and very commonly vomiting.
- Paroxysms of cough may occur more than 30 times per 24 hours and are common at night.
- There is commonly production of profuse secretions with the coughing.
- Paroxysms can occur spontaneously or are precipitated by external stimuli such as noise and cold air.
- Between coughing episodes, there are few clinical signs—chest examination is usually normal and the child is afebrile.
- Very rarely the spasms are so severe that ventilatory support may be required.
- This stage also typically lasts 2 weeks.

Convalescent

- The coughing gradually subsides in this phase.
- If another viral upper respiratory infection is acquired, relapse of the disease may occur.
- This stage can last from 2 weeks to several months.

Atypical features
- In infants may include:
  - Apnoea
  - Cough (with no whoop)
  - Cyanotic episodes
  - Vomiting

- Poor feeding
- Fever
- Seizures
- Sudden infant death syndrome.
- In the partially immunized:
  - Duration of catarrhal phase may be reduced
  - Whoop may not occur.
- In adolescents and adults:
  - Prolonged cough—persistent cough for over a month and vomiting are key signs suggestive of pertussis
  - Paroxysmal cough
  - Whoop—rare
  - Phlegm
  - Post-tussive vomiting.

Major complications and deaths occur most commonly in infants <6 months of age. These include:
- Bronchopneumonia—clues for secondary pneumonia are high fever and chest signs; do a CXR looking for focal consolidation (infiltrates and atelectasis seen in pertussis)
- Vomiting—leading to severe weight loss; weekly weights are very important
- Cerebral hypoxia and haemorrhage—along with apnoea and bradycardia, and seizures.

Minor complications include:
- Subconjunctival haemorrhages
- Epistaxis
- Facial oedema
- Ulceration of the tongue or surrounding area
- Suppurative otitis media.

Diagnosis

Pertussis is largely diagnosed clinically. Confirmation of the diagnosis or corroborative evidence may be obtained from a history of contact with a case and/or laboratory investigations. Advances in diagnostic techniques such as PCR assays have improved laboratory diagnosis of pertussis in addition to the traditional culture and serology testing.

Culture of secretions

- Currently the gold-standard investigation; high specificity, but only 80% sensitivity.
- A specimen is collected via a pernasal swab or by nasopharyngeal aspiration. Direct inoculation of the sample onto culture medium at the bedside increases sensitivity, but transport to the laboratory in an appropriate medium is more practical. Yield is very low after any antibiotics have been given.
- *B. pertussis* is fastidious, requiring a special culture medium.
- Growth occurs over 3–7 days.

PCR analysis
- More sensitive than culture and is highly specific.
- PCR enables rapid diagnosis of pertussis, particularly in infants, but the validity of the results must be assured by careful controls.
- PCR-based tests are recognized as a reliable diagnostic tool, even in the later stages of the illness and after the commencement of antibiotic treatment.

Serology
The diagnostic sensitivity of serology depends on the timing of sample collection relative to disease, and on the choice of antigen and class of antibody. The most widely used antigens are pertussis toxin and filamentous haemagglutinin using IgA or IgG antibodies.

Responses can be measured by ELISA. Specimens should be obtained in the acute and convalescent phases of the disease. Age-adjusted normal ranges have also been formulated for certain antibodies that may aid in the interpretation of single sample results.

Lymphocytosis
This finding is non-specific but a lymphocytosis of over 15 000cells/mm^3 is suggestive of pertussis. There is some evidence that severity of lymphocytosis and disease may be linked, possibly through pertussis toxin levels.

Management and treatment

Supportive
Oxygen therapy and suction of pharyngeal secretions may be required during paroxysms of cough. Previously used specific treatments for the cough include:
- Corticosteroids
- Salbutamol
- Pertussis-specific immunoglobulin.

However, there is currently insufficient evidence to draw any conclusions about the benefits of these interventions and the treatment is generally supportive.

Medication
- Erythromycin given for 7 days reduces transmission by eradicating *B. pertussis* from the respiratory tract.
- Azithromycin and clarithromycin have been shown to be as effective in eliminating *B. pertussis* but, as with erythromycin, have little effect on the clinical course of the illness.
- Treatment should be started within 21 days of the onset of symptoms.
- An association of hypertrophic pyloric stenosis with erythromycin has led to the preferred use of clarithromycin in younger infants.

Prevention

- Routine infant vaccination with whole cell or acellular pertussis vaccines is the mainstay of pertussis prevention.
- Postexposure prophylaxis with clarithromycin for cases and for families/close contacts of infants at high risk of complications (unimmunized or partially immunized) is recommended.
- In view of the increasing burden of disease in older individuals, booster vaccination of adults and adolescents has been considered, and in some countries employed, as an additional strategy.
- To protect the infant until they reach the age of active immunisation, vaccination of new parents is also recommended in some countries. Both vaccination in pregnancy and neonatal vaccination are possible theoretical strategies.

Future research

- Further studies are required to assess the potential use of maternal and neonatal vaccination which may prove valuable in protecting infants against pertussis from birth.
- Continuing research into new PCR methods including real-time PCR may assist in the detection of pertussis even in later stages.

Further reading

Altunaiji SM, Kukuruzovic RH, Curtis NC, Massie J. Antibiotics for whooping cough (pertussis). *Cochrane Database Syst Rev* 2007;**3**.

Dodhia H, Crowcroft NS, Bramley JC, Miller E. UK guidelines for use of erythromycin chemoprophylaxis in persons exposed to pertussis. *J Public Health Med* 2002;**24**:200–6.

Gangarosa E, Galazka A, Wolfe C, *et al.* Impact of anti-vaccine movements on pertussis control: the untold story. *Lancet* 1998;**351**:356–61.

Plague

📖 see also Chapters 42, 45

Introduction

First documented in the Old Testament, plague has caused three large pandemics, the Black Death, multiple epidemics, and still has widespread outbreaks, mainly in resource-poor countries. It also has the potential for use as a bioterrorist agent (class A pathogen).

Name and nature of organism

- Gram-negative coccobacillus, *Yersinia pestis* (family Enterobacteriaceae).
- Originally *Pasteurella pestis*, it was renamed in 1967 after Alexander Yersin who first isolated the bacterium in 1894 and developed an antiserum for treatment.
- Pleomorphic facultative anaerobe. V and W antigens determine virulence.
- Stains with characteristic bipolar appearance (closed safety pin).
- Combination of endotoxin, lipopolysaccharide, coagulase and fibrinolysin allow evasion of the host immune response.

Epidemiology

- Naturally zoonotic disease cycle, primarily affecting wild rodents.
- Humans are accidental hosts.
- Over 23 000 human cases were reported to WHO between 1998 and 2008, affecting 11 countries (mortality rate approximately 10%).
- Over 90% cases occur in Africa, including Madagascar.
- Other endemic regions include China, India, Peru, and Vietnam.
- Disease foci in Europe lie around the Caspian Sea and Caucasus.
- >50% of cases are in people <20 years.

Factors that favour hosts and vectors of the bacteria increase disease prevalence, including global warming and the expanding world population (with poorer sanitation/hygiene and increased risks of animal contact).

Transmission and incubation period

Transmission

- Three main routes:
  - Host to human via bite from vector (e.g. rat to person via rodent flea)
  - Direct inhalation or ingestion of bacterium

- Close contact with infected tissue or body fluids (e.g. through broken skin).
- Most important vector is the Oriental rat flea (*Xenopsylla cheopis*).
- Main vector reservoir hosts are rats, then squirrels and cats.
- Highly infectious nature so only small number of organisms needed to cause disease (inhaled infectious dose is 100–500 organisms).

Incubation period
- Varies depending on the transmission method and form of plague
  - Via flea bite: 2–8 days.
  - Via airborne/aerosol: 1–3 days.

Clinical features and sequelae

- Toxic appearance with fever, chills, myalgia, general malaise, weakness, and headaches.
- Pathognomonic feature = bubo—classic large lymph nodes (also seen in syphilis, TB, gonorrhoea).
  - Necrotic and haemorrhagic lymph node draining area of skin containing vector bite
  - Very tender with overlying erythema and pitting oedema
  - 2–10cm, oval in shape
  - Over 70% affect inguinal nodes
  - Intra-abdominal buboes can mimic a surgical abdomen.
- Often rapid progression to systemic shock with diffuse infection leading to DIC.
- Commonly spread via lymphatic channels, then haematogenous route with vascular seeding to multiple organs.

Complications include
- ARDS or lung abscess.
- Superinfection of buboes (commonly staphylococcal or *Pseudomonas*).
- Gangrene of extremities.
- Lymphoedema.
- Polyarthritis.

Diagnosis
The initial symptoms are very similar to many, more common, infections. Suspicions should be raised if
- History of flea bite (only remembered in 10% people).
- Travel to endemic plague area, with close contact with potential animal reservoir.
- Sudden increase in severe pneumonia cases in a previously healthy population.

Take three sets of blood cultures during the first hour (before starting antibiotics), CSF (if relevant), sputum, and bubo fluid.

Label all specimens as high risk so laboratory staff take appropriate handling precautions.
- Direct microscopy reveals bacilli with bipolar staining. Appropriate stains include Gram, Wayson, and Giemsa.

- Rapid diagnosis using:
  - Biochemical test strips (*Y. pestis* is catalase positive and oxidase negative)
  - Dipstick assay (using immunochromatography) to detect F1 antigen
  - Direct immunofluorescence of fluid or other cultures for anti-F1 antigen antibody.
- ELISA to detect IgM and IgG antibodies:
  - Acute and convalescent serum is useful in culture-negative cases (positive if fourfold or higher rise in titre).
  - Immediately inform: local and national authorities.

Management and treatment

- Plague is a notifiable disease and a public health emergency.

General

Population

- Eradicate fleas, rats, other vectors, and reservoirs associated with infected case.
- Available vaccines not recommended for immediate protection in outbreaks (takes 4 weeks to develop protective immune response).
- Strict infection control precautions when dealing with suspected or confirmed cases (human or animal).

Individual

- Keep isolated until effective antibiotics given for 2–3 days or until sputum culture negative (if ever positive).
- Must be in strict respiratory isolation if any signs of pneumonia.
- Gangrenous areas may require amputation.
- Incision and drainage of buboes if large or fluctuant.

Antibiotics

- Antibiotics are most effective if given within the first 24 hours of symptoms.
- Aminoglycosides and ciprofloxacin are first line, unless meningeal plague.
- Use chloramphenicol in plague meningitis (better blood–brain barrier penetration).
- Resistance to antibiotics has been reported.
- Length of treatment:
  - Minimum of 14 days, and for at least 3 days after the last fever
  - If suspected meningeal involvement then 21 days minimum
- Can convert to oral antibiotics (e.g. doxycycline) after 48 hours if symptoms are improving.
- Although fever and symptoms can settle in <1 week with appropriate treatment, a primary bubo may take months to resolve.

Postexposure prophylaxis
- Give to humans in close contact with an infected animal or body fluids or a case of pneumonic plague within the last 6 days.
- Complete a 7-day course.

Prevention

The main aim is to prevent contact with zoonotic foci.

Individual led
- Insect sprays on exposed body areas and bedding.
- Avoid contact with known animal reservoirs, especially if dead or sick.
- Avoid visiting endemic plague regions.

Vaccines
- Live attenuated and killed whole cell vaccines have existed for over a century but both are reactogenic.
- Newer candidates, in ongoing trials, include rationally attenuated mutants and subunit vaccines (using F1 and V antigens).

Future research

Keys areas for vaccine development involve anticipating an imminent bio-terrorist attack, including having a vaccine effective against the pneumonic plague, which gives more immediate protection.

Further reading

ECDC factsheet. Available at: ℜ http://ecdc.europa.eu/en/healthtopics/Plague/basic_facts/Pages/basic_facts.aspx (accessed 1 February 2011)

HPA Centre for Infections. *Plague: Information includes Guidelines for Action in the Event of a Deliberate Release* (section 2.7 contains briefing note for the public). www.hpa.org.uk/Topics/InfectionsDiseases/InfectionsAZ/PlagueDR/Guidance/. (accessed 1 February 2011).

Chapter 96

Pneumocystis pneumonia (PcP)

📖 see also Chapters 19, 20, 24, 27

Name and nature of organism

- The organism was identified in guinea pig and rat lung tissue by Chagas and Carini in the early twentieth century; initially classified as a protozoon and named as *Pneumocystis carinii* by Delanoes in 1912, it was reclassified as a fungus (phylum Ascomycetes) in 1988.
- *Pneumocystis jiroveci*, named after Otto Jirovec, a Czech parasitologist who demonstrated *Pneumocystis* as the aetiological agent of interstitial 'plasma cell' pneumonia in premature infants in early 1950s, is the species infecting humans (versus *Pneumocystis carinii*, the species that infects rats).

Epidemiology

- The organism is ubiquitous in mammals worldwide, with unique tropism for the lungs and stringent host specificity (i.e. no cross-infection from species to species).
- Children are exposed to the organism early in life, as more than 85% of healthy children have detectable antibodies by the age of 20 months; colonization (by detection in nasopharyngeal aspirates), particularly in infants, occurs in ~10% of healthy and ~15% of those with respiratory symptoms, so infants may represent the human reservoir.
- The disease was initially identified after outbreaks of pneumonia in orphanages in Central and Eastern Europe.
- The incubation period is unknown, but work based on animal models suggests 4–8 weeks from exposure to clinical disease is usual.
- Clinically significant disease occurs in children with primary (genetic), as well as in those with secondary immunodeficiency, such as premature or severely malnourished children, children on immunosuppressive treatment (following solid organ and haemopoietic stem cell transplantation, for malignancy and autoimmune/rheumatic disorders) and especially children with AIDS due to infection with HIV.

Transmission

- The organism's source in nature has not been identified, and so the issue of transmission has been difficult to examine.
- Person-to-person transmission is the most likely mode of acquiring new infections, although acquisition from environmental sources may also occur.

Clinical features and sequelae

- *Pneumocystis* infections are virtually always limited to the lung, but the host characteristics that allow infection are not completely understood.
- Classically, PcP presents with subtle onset of progressive tachypnoea, dyspnoea, low-grade fever and non-productive cough; however, a more abrupt onset of respiratory insufficiency can occasionally be the initial presentation. Hypoxia out of proportion to the apparent clinical disease is a good clue.
- Physical examination is often surprisingly normal, even in the presence of significant disease and hypoxaemia: tachypnoea, tachycardia, and normal findings on lung auscultation or crackles may be heard.
- Typical radiographic features are bilateral perihilar interstitial infiltrates, which may become increasingly homogeneous and diffuse as the disease progresses. Pneumatoceles and or pneumothorax can be seen less commonly but with a white out CXR are strongly predictive of PcP; HRCT may reveal extensive ground glass attenuations or cystic lesions.
- The mortality rate ranges from 5% to 20% if treated, to close to 100% if untreated.

Diagnosis

- No combination of symptoms, signs, and chest radiographic findings is diagnostic of PcP.
- The diagnosis requires microscopic examination of respiratory specimens (induced sputum, bronchoalveolar fluid, or lung tissue). The organism is not usually present in nasopharyngeal secretions specimens and cannot be cultured, thus invasive procedures are often required to isolate organisms.
- Bronchoscopy with BAL is the preferred diagnostic test (reported sensitivity 89% to >98%); sputum induction procedure with hypertonic saline (reported sensitivity 74–83%) is less invasive, but often not possible in children <10 years old; bronchoscopic or open lung biopsy is sometimes needed to identify organisms.
- Specimens are stained in the laboratory using Giemsa, Grocott– Gomori silver stain or fluorescent antibody stains.
- PCR assays are still not in routine use, but in particular those assays using primers for the gene for *Pneumocystis* mitochondrial large subunit ribosomal RNA are more sensitive, though less specific compared with traditional microscopic methods. Most of the PCR assays are based on amplifying *Pneumocystis* DNA. This may persist for an indeterminate amount of time after cell death, thus providing no information concerning the organism's viability or infectivity. These tests appear to result in many 'positive' diagnosis of disease.
- The usefulness of elevated serum levels of LDH and lower plasma levels of S-adenosylmethionine are still not confirmed as valued diagnostic tests.

Management and treatment

- Co-trimoxazole (trimethoprim-sulfamethoxazole) (divided in 2, 3, or 4 doses) given IV remains the first-line treatment option; oral therapy can be given in less severe disease.
- Pentamidine isetionate once daily given IV (beware—risk of severe hypotension) is an alternative for children who cannot tolerate co-trimoxazole or who have not responded to it after 5–7 days of treatment.
- Second-line and/or treatment for mild to moderate disease (NB unlicensed indications; associated with considerable toxicity; experience in children limited).
  - Combination of clindamycin orally given four times/day and primaquine orally once daily (need testing for G6PD activity).
  - Combination of dapsone orally once daily with trimethoprim orally given every 6–8 hours.
- Duration of therapy is 21 days.

Because of the ongoing and sometimes exuberant lung inflammation, adding corticosteroids is considered of benefit in patients being treated for PcP.

- Guidelines/standard recommendation is prednisolone at 2mg/kg per day (maximum 80mg):
  - Adolescents—prednisolone 40mg given twice daily for the first 5 days, followed by 40mg once daily for 5 days and 20mg once daily until day 21
  - Smaller children—methylprednisolone or prednisolone 1–2mg/ kg per day divided in 2–4 doses for the first week, followed by a tapering dose until day 21.

Prevention

Primary prophylaxis is to prevent a first case of PcP. Secondary prophylaxis is to prevent a relapse in a child who has already had PcP.

- Primary prophylaxis should be given to children with significant primary or secondary immunodeficiency. The precise risks are complicated and not well quantified for many diseases. This includes children with SCID and other primary immunodeficiency (PID), leukaemia and other malignancies, HIV, and those receiving immunosuppressive drugs, e.g. high-dose prolonged methotrexate.
- Secondary prophylaxis should be given to all children with a history of the infection who are severely immunocompromised until their immunity recovers sufficiently.
- Prophylaxis should not be discontinued if the child is still receiving cytotoxic therapy or long-term immunosuppressive therapy. For children with HIV, primary prophylaxis can be stopped when their CD4 count has been over 200/µl for >6 months.
- Primary prophylaxis regimens vary between underlying disease, reflecting the poor evidence base. Co-trimoxazole is the drug of choice.

- A simple regimen of co-trimoxazole once daily three times a week usually on Monday, Wednesday, and Friday is:
  - Infants <1 year: 120mg
  - Average-sized children aged 1–3 years: 240mg given once daily
  - Children aged 4–9 years: 480mg once daily
  - Children ≥10 years: 960mg once daily.
- Pentamidine isetionate, intermittent inhalation once daily every 4 weeks or 150mg every 2 weeks.
- Other less effective regimens for primary prophylaxis in those allergic or intolerant of the above, include dapsone orally or atovaquone orally once a day.

Future research

- Determining whether one single simple prophylaxis regimen is adequate for all children with immunocompromise at risk of PcP.
- The dose and duration of therapy is poorly evidence based.

Further reading

Huang L, Morris A, Limper AH, Beck JM, on behalf of the ATS Pneumocystis Workshop Participants. An official ATS Workshop Summary: recent advances and future directions in *Pneumocystis* pneumonia (PCP). *Proc Am Thorac Soc* 2006;**3**:655–64.

Thomas CF, Limper AH. *Pneumocystis* pneumonia. *N Engl J Med* 2004;**350**:2487–98.

Chapter 97

Polio

📖 see also Chapters 14, 29

Name and nature of organism

- Poliovirus is a single-stranded RNA virus belonging to the family *Picornaviridae*, genus *Enterovirus*.
- The virus particle consists of an icosahedral non-enveloped protein capsid with RNA core.
- The capsid consists of four structural proteins: VP1, VP2, VP3, and VP4.
- There are three serotypes: these are antigenically distinct with little heterologous protection. Infection gives immunity to the serotype.

Epidemiology

- Humans are the only known natural host.
- Poliovirus infection occurs predominantly in summer and autumn in temperate climates, but year round in tropical regions.
- Prior to the twentieth century, most children were exposed to poliovirus in early infancy while still protected by maternal antibodies, hence clinical infections were sporadic and largely confined to younger children. However, following the industrial revolution and improvements in hygiene and sanitation, children increasingly encountered poliovirus at older ages without the benefit of passively conferred immunity, leading to epidemics of poliomyelitis.
- Attempts to control poliomyelitis through vaccination programmes have led to a dramatic fall in the incidence of poliomyelitis, with WHO declaring transmission interrupted in the Americas, Western Pacific, and Europe. Furthermore, wild poliovirus type 2 was last identified in India in 1999. However, by the end of 2009, wild poliovirus types 1 and 3 remained endemic in Nigeria, Afghanistan, India, and Pakistan, and, following importation, poliovirus transmission had been re-established in a number of other countries.

Transmission and incubation period

- Transmission is primarily by the faecal-oral route.
- The virus enters through the gastrointestinal mucosa and, after initial replication in the pharynx and gastrointestinal tract, spreads to local lymph nodes. After a further period of local replication, a minor viraemia ensues with viral replication in blood, muscle, fat, liver, spleen, and bone marrow. In the majority of patients, the virus will be contained at this stage, but in 4–8% of individuals experiencing a

minor viraemia, a secondary major viraemia ensues. During a major viraemia patients may experience mild non-specific illness ('abortive poliomyelitis') or, in a minority of patients, the virus may invade the CNS leading to non-paralytic aseptic meningitis or paralytic poliomyelitis.

- The incubation period is generally between 7 and 14 days but can range from 3 to 35 days.
- Patients are most infectious immediately before and 1–2 weeks after onset of paralytic disease.

Clinical features and sequelae

- 90–95% of infections are asymptomatic.
- 4–8% of individuals with a primary viraemia will develop a secondary major viraemia which may be associated with a minor non-specific illness ('abortive poliomyelitis'). The signs and symptoms may include fever, sore throat, myalgia, anorexia, malaise, nausea, vomiting, abdominal pain, and constipation or diarrhoea.
- A small proportion of patients experiencing a major viraemia will manifest signs and symptoms of CNS invasion. These include:
  - Non-paralytic polio (1–2% of poliovirus infections) with specific features of aseptic meningitis. Patients experience the non-specific features of abortive poliomyelitis, but in addition may complain of severe headache and neck, back, and lower limb pain. They may display nuchal rigidity and CSF lymphocytosis.
  - Spinal poliomyelitis—characterized by acute flaccid paralysis secondary to selective destruction of spinal motor neurons and subsequent denervation of the associated skeletal musculature. Children exhibit a biphasic illness with 2–3 days of minor non-specific illness, followed by up to 5 days without symptoms. Abrupt onset of headache, fever, vomiting, neck stiffness, and intense muscle pain is followed after 24–48 hours by flaccid weakness and paralysis, which are usually asymmetrical. Multiple muscle groups and limbs may be involved, with proximal involvement usually more severe than distal. The lower limbs are involved more frequently than the upper limbs. Deep tendon reflexes may initially be hyperactive, but are rapidly lost. Sensory loss has been described but is rare. Bladder paralysis and bowel ileus commonly occur but tend to improve over a few days.
  - Bulbar poliomyelitis—characterized by paralysis of muscle groups innervated by cranial nerves. Patients present with dysphagia, nasal speech, and respiratory compromise secondary to involvement of medullary respiratory centres.
  - Bulbospinal poliomyelitis—where both the brainstem and spinal cord are affected resulting in a mixed clinical picture.
  - Paralytic poliomyelitis—occurs in 0.1–1% of all cases of poliovirus infections. Cranial nerve dysfunction is reported in 5–35% of paralytic polio cases. Respiratory compromise is an important complication, resulting from involvement of both the diaphragm

and intercostal muscles, the medullary respiratory centre and the IX, X, and XII cranial nerves affecting pharyngeal, palatal, and vocal cord function. In the pre-vaccination era, mortality rates of up to 60% were reported, mainly due to respiratory compromise. With modern intensive care, mortality rates of 2–5% in children have been described.

- Most cases of paralytic disease will show clinical improvement but approximately 60% of affected individuals will experience a residual deficit. Complete recovery is rare if the paralysis is severe or ventilatory support is required. Patients who survive bulbar involvement often recover quickly to normal function.
- Certain risk factors for paralysis have been identified. These include pregnancy, B cell immunodeficiencies, strenuous exercise during the first days of the illness and IM injections which seem to predispose to paralysis in the limb injected (provocation paralysis).
- Complications of infection include respiratory compromise, myocarditis, gastrointestinal haemorrhage, and ileus.
- Up to 30% of patients who have recovered from paralytic polio may experience new-onset weakness, pain, and atrophy in the previously affected muscle groups some 25–35 years after the primary illness, referred to as the post-polio syndrome.

Diagnosis

- The virus may be cultured from throat and stool swabs.
- Isolation of virus from CSF is diagnostic but seldom achieved. CSF may show raised cell count (10–200 leucocytes/ml) and mildly raised protein (40–50mg/dl).
- The virus is shed from the throat for between 1 and 3 weeks and excreted in stool for 4–8 weeks following infection.
- The virus produces cytopathogenic effects in monkey kidney cell and human cell monolayers within 1 week.
- Neutralizing antibody can be detected in serum as early as 1 week post infection. A fourfold rise in acute and convalescent IgG titres demonstrates acute infection but cannot distinguish between vaccine and wild-type virus.
- RT-PCR for poliovirus can be performed for stool, throat swabs, and CSF specimens.

Management

- There is no specific antiviral therapy.
- Management is supportive:
  - Analgesia and bed rest in the acute phase to reduce extension of paralysis
  - Decompression of bladder where indicated
  - Ventilatory assistance/tracheal intubation where indicated

- Avoid IM injections—risk of 'provocation paralysis' (see clinical features)
- Physiotherapy during recovery phase.

Prevention

- Vaccination against poliovirus, first introduced in the 1950s, has had a dramatic effect on the incidence of polio.
- The first vaccine to be introduced was Salk's inactivated poliovirus vaccine (IPV) in 1955. This immunized against all three strains of poliovirus and reduced the incidence of paralytic poliomyelitis in the USA from 13.9 cases per 100 000 in 1954 to 0.5 cases per 100 000 in 1961.
- In 1961, Sabin developed monovalent live oral polio vaccines (OPVs) which were replaced by a trivalent OPV in 1963. These were seen to offer the advantage of superior immunogenicity, ease of oral administration, induction of local mucosal immunity, and the potential public health benefit of the spread of live vaccine (attenuated) viruses from immunized to unimmunized contacts. However, the genetic instability of the Sabin vaccine strains, combined with the potential for recombination with other viruses allows reversion of attenuated strains to neurovirulence, leading to rare cases of vaccine-associated paralytic poliomyelitis (VAPP).
- VAPP is defined by the WHO as poliomyelitis that occurs in a vaccinee between 7 and 30 days after a dose or in a close contact of a vaccinee between 7 and 60 days after receipt of the dose. VAPP is most common after the first vaccine dose. Hypogammaglobulinaemic individuals have a 3000-fold higher risk of developing VAPP than healthy vaccinees. OPV is contraindicated in patients with immunodeficiency or household contacts of immunodeficient individuals.
- In addition to VAPP, a further consequence of OPV is the development of vaccine-derived polioviruses (VDPV). A VDPV is defined as a Sabin poliovirus with ≥1% genetic variation compared to prototype sequence (reflecting sustained viral replication over at least 1 year in one or more persons). These viruses can be further sub-divided into circulating VDPV (cVDPV), associated with person-to-person transmission in the community with reversion to neurovirulence, and immunodeficiency related VDPV (iVDPV), arising from prolonged virus replication in an immunodeficient individual. Individuals with deficient B cell immunity may fail to clear the virus after OPV vaccination and may continue to excrete the virus for prolonged periods (months to decades).
- Outbreaks of cVDPV, with sustained transmission in affected communities, have occurred primarily in areas where poor vaccine coverage has led to diminished herd immunity and have involved all three serotypes (including serotype 2 which has been eradicated in its wild form). These outbreaks have been interrupted with widespread targeted vaccination programmes using OPV.

- In 1988, the WHO announced the Global Polio Eradication Initiative, setting the goal of global eradication of poliomyelitis by 2000. By this target year, the global incidence of poliomyelitis cases had declined from approx 350 000 in 1988 to 719, with the last isolation of wild-type poliovirus 2 in 1999. But in 2008 and 2009, >1600 cases of polio were reported worldwide each year.
- The reasons for failure to date of the global initiative to achieve its goal are multiple. Interruption of vaccination programmes due to military conflicts, local cultural or political misconceptions regarding the vaccine, and fears of VAPP impact on herd immunity all predispose to local outbreaks. Reintroduction of virus into previously polio-free countries has occurred through travel. Low OPV vaccine efficacy has been reported in certain states in India, with children requiring multiple doses to achieve levels of population immunity to stop poliovirus transmission.
- Current approaches to eradication of polio:
  - As wild-type poliovirus was eliminated from circulation in Western countries with effective immunization programmes, the risks of VAPP inherent in OPV became unacceptable. Many developed countries have now switched their immunization programmes from live OPV to 'enhanced potency' IPV which induces comparable or superior serum neutralizing antibody responses compared with OPV. The UK changed to IPV in 2004 and the schedule of immunization now advises a three-dose primary course of IPV at 2, 3, and 4 months, with boosters at preschool and school-age visits.
  - IPV remains unaffordable for many developing countries. The suboptimal efficacy of trivalent OPV against serotypes 1 and 3 has led the WHO to recommend the use of monovalent and bivalent OPV for targeted supplementary immunization activities in addition to trivalent OPV immunization programmes.

Further reading

De Jesus NH. Epidemics to eradication: the modern history of poliomyelitis. *Virol J* 2007;**4**:70.

Ehrenfeld E, Modlin J, Chumakov K. Future of polio vaccines. *Expert Rev Vaccines* 2009;**8**:899–905.

Kew OM, Wright PF, Agol VI, *et al.* Circulating vaccine-derived polioviruses: current state of knowledge. *Bull World Health Organ* 2004;**82**:16–23.

Minor P. Vaccine-derived poliovirus (VDPV): Impact on poliomyelitis eradication. *Vaccine* 2009;**27**:2649–52.

World Health Organization. Conclusions and recommendations of the advisory committee on polioyelitis eradication, November 2009. *Wkly Epidemiol Rec* 2010;**85**:1–12.

World Health Organization. *Global Polio Eradication Initiative.* Available at:
ℜ www.polioeradication.org (accessed December 2010).

Rabies

📖 see also Chapters 14, 42, 45

Name and nature of organism

- Rabies is a zoonosis caused by a rhabdovirus that can affect the nervous system of all mammals, including humans, causing an acute encephalomyelitis and leading to painful death in almost all cases.
- Caused by the RNA rhabdovirus, genus *Lyssavirus* (*Lyssa*—Greek God of raging fury/madness) (this genus has seven genotypes, type 1 of which represents the classic rabies virus). The virus causing clinical rabies in bats is distinct from that causing rabies in dogs.
- Less frequently, rabies may result from infection with rabies-related *Lyssavirus*, including European bat lyssaviruses (EBLVs).
- A strain of rabies called European bat lyssavirus (EBLV-2) has been found in UK Daubenton bats.

Epidemiology

- WHO estimates that over 50 000 people die from rabies each year (95% in Asia and Africa).
- The epidemiology of human rabies mirrors the disease prevalence in the local animal population.
- Rabies in animals is found in all continents except Antarctica.
- Individual countries report being rabies-free in terrestrial animals.
- Animal rabies is predominantly found in dogs but may affect all mammals. It has been found in cats, foxes, skunks, and bats.
- In Europe, the main indigenous animal reservoirs are:
  - Eastern Europe/borders with Middle East: Dogs
  - Central/Eastern Europe: Fox
  - North-Eastern Europe: Racoon
  - Pan-Europe: Insectivorous Bat.
- Most human deaths result from a bite from an infected dog; 30–60% of those bitten by dogs are children <15 years.
- Children, especially from poorer backgrounds, are more likely to play outdoors with dogs. As they are shorter than adults, they are more likely to be bitten and scratched around the head and face, and will therefore have a worse clinical outcome.

- The European incidence is <5 cases per year. From 2008 to 2009 there were four reported cases of human rabies: two in the Ukraine, one in the Russian Federation and one in the UK. The former two countries reported 960 and 632 cases of rabies in domestic animals, respectively, while the UK case was imported.
- In the UK the last case of human rabies from an indigenously affected terrestrial animal occurred in 1902.
- There was a fatal case of human rabies from an indigenous bat in Scotland in 2002, and imported cases occurred following a dog bite in Goa in 2005 and South Africa in 2008.[1]
- Wound cleansing and immunization performed as soon as possible after potential exposure prevents clinical onset of rabies in nearly all cases but once symptoms appear the disease is usually fatal.

Transmission and incubation period

- Rabies is spread by the saliva of an infected animal.
- Transmitted to humans through bites, scratches, licks on broken skin, or mucous membranes.
- Incubation period is generally between 3 and 12 weeks but may range from 4 days to 19 years depending on salivary viral load, inoculation site (quicker if closer to brain), and viral strain.
- There is a shorter incubation period for inhalational, face, and upper body exposure.
- Experimental studies indicate dogs may shed virus (and hence be infectious) for 13 days before onset of symptoms. Bats may be infected without symptoms.
- Virus enters the body through transdermal inoculation (infectious virus in saliva from rabid animal) penetrating skin through bite or scratch or direct contact with mucous membranes, or broken skin.
- The rhabdovirus binds to cell receptors. It may directly infect nervous cells or replicate within striated muscle cells.
- Virus moves via retrograde axoplasmic transport at 1–40cm/day to the CNS where rapid viral replication occurs. The virus then travels via anterograde axoplasmic flow within peripheral nerves with infection of neighbouring tissue (such as salivary glands) en route.
- There is salivary viral shedding from the new victim when symptoms are manifest, thus completing the infectious cycle.

Clinical features

- Initially there is a prodromal phase from 2 to 10 days of non-specific symptoms of fever, malaise, headache, and anxiety. There may be pain or paraesthesia at site of exposure.
- Then there are two distinct presentations:
  - *Encephalitic ('furious')*—presents with agitation, delirium, hydrophobia. May also demonstrate hyperventilation, hypersalivation, and priapism. Progresses to fluctuant conscious

level and generalized convulsions. This leads to coma and death usually within a week of onset of symptoms.
- *Paralytic ('dumb' rabies)* is more commonly seen after bat exposure and looks clinically similar to Guillain–Barré syndrome, with an ascending flaccid paralysis and extreme weakness at site of exposure.

Diagnosis

- The early diagnosis is difficult if no classic history of exposure is obtained.
- Specialist laboratories may be able to detect the virus in CSF or saliva by culture or PCR.
- Brain biopsy in an animal may show virus in brain tissue.
- In England, the Virus Reference Division of the HPA has expertise with diagnosis of rabies in humans. Colindale also issues post-exposure prophylaxis immunoglobulin.
- Laboratory diagnosis supported by DFA of hair follicles, virus PCR, brain biopsy for histology (cytoplasmic inclusion bodies consistent with Negri bodies), and PCR.

Treatment

- There is no specific antiviral therapy for rabies.
- Until 2003, there have been only five survivors reported, all of whom received some form of immunization after exposure but before onset of symptoms. Four patients had severe neurological sequelae.
  - A case was reported from Milwaukee, USA, in 2005 of a 15-year-old girl bitten on her hand by a bat, who cleaned her wound immediately but did not seek medical advice, and then developed fatigue, diplopia, ataxia, and paraesthesia 1 month later. She was treated by induced coma to buy time for the innate immune response to develop and was given amantadine and ribavirin. Rabies vaccine was not administered and an LP 8 days into the illness showed rabies antibody. She was discharged home at 76 days and at 5-month follow up was alert and communicative but with unsteady gait and choreoathetosis.[2]
- Given the high mortality of rabies, treatment is often palliative. Sedatives, neuromuscular blockade, narcotic analgesics, and antiepileptics may offer symptomatic relief. The 'Milwaukee protocol', as the induced coma therapeutic option is now known, has never been successfully replicated.
- Patients with rabies should be barrier nursed to avoid potential healthcare worker and family contacts to infectious material.
- All suspected human rabies cases should be notified to the appropriate local public health team.

Prevention

Pre-exposure

- Avoid exposure by being careful around dogs and bats.
- Pre-exposure vaccination are recommended for travellers to high-risk countries, laboratory workers handling the virus, and those who frequently handle imported animals.
- Pre-exposure immunization involves three immunizations by the deep IM or subcutaneous route with the inactivated vaccine at 0, 7, and 21–28 day intervals.
- Animal vaccination helps with environmental control (easier in domestic animals).

Post-exposure

- Washing the site of exposure aggressively with repeated irrigation and soap can reduce the risk of developing clinical rabies by 50–90%.
- Avoid suturing wounds and occlusive dressings.
- The slow time-course of rabies with slow axoplasmic viral transport to the CNS allows time for successful intervention with post-exposure prophylaxis.
- Post-exposure prophylaxis includes both the vaccine and rabies immune globulin (RIG) (human or equine).
- In previously unimmunized individuals, vaccine should be given on days 0, 3, 7, 14, 30, and 90, and RIG 20IU/kg (most infiltrated into exposure site and the residual given by parenteral injection).
- Two vaccine booster doses at 0 and then 3–7 days rather than RIG are indicated for patients completely vaccinated pre-exposure.
- The vaccine does not contain live organism and cannot cause rabies disease.
- RIG is obtained from pooled immunized and screened donors.
- There have only been seven reported failures of post-exposure prophylaxis before onset of symptoms when both the vaccine and RIG has been used according to the WHO protocol.
- WHO guidelines state if the biting animal remains well under quarantined observation after 10 days, there is no risk of rabies transmission and the vaccine course can be stopped.[3]
- The modern cell-culture vaccine is safer than nerve-tissue based vaccines.

Future research

- Monoclonal antibodies as vaccines/therapy.
- Intradermal vaccine as pre-exposure prophylaxis.

Key references

1 Willoughby RE, Tireves KS, Hoffman GM. Survival after treatment of rabies with induction of coma. *N Engl J Med* 2005;**352**:2508–14.
2 Available at: ✍ www.hpa.org.uk/ (accessed 1 February 2011). Follow links to updated country risk tables.
3 Available at: ✍ www.who.int/rabies/en/ (accessed 1 February 2011).

Respiratory syncytial virus

📖 see also Chapters 17, 27, 44

Name and nature of organism

- RSV is a negative-sense, single-stranded RNA paramyxovirus of the genus *Pneumovirus*.
- There are two main immunodominant surface glycoproteins—the F fusion protein and the G attachment protein, which divide RSV into two antigenic subtypes A and B.
- The incubation period is 2–8 days with 4–6 days being most commonly observed.

Epidemiology

- RSV is the commonest viral cause of bronchiolitis and severe respiratory illness in infants and young children. It has very predictable yearly epidemics worldwide, identifiable in virtually every country—from November to March in temperate climates and during the rainy season in tropical climates.
- The sharp winter peaks demonstrate limited variability in respect of timing or size—most notably Christmas/New Year period in temperate climates. The sharpness of the disease peak appears to be latitude related, flattening closer to the equator. Severe RSV disease is most common in younger infants in the first 6 months of life in Europe and the second 6 months of life in Africa.
- Approximately 20% of paediatric admissions for lower respiratory tract infection in the UK are due to RSV. The annual UK incidence of RSV-related hospital admissions is 28.3/1000 for infants, and 1.3/1000 for children between 1 and 4 years. Mortality is estimated at 0.1%. All children will have been infected by 2–3 years of age. Length of hospital stay for RSV bronchiolitis varies markedly across Europe.
- Primary infection induces an immune response with the production of specific antibodies but it does not prevent repeated infections each year, although these are usually much milder. Antigenic variation both between the main subgroups and within each subgroup may be one of the factors in enabling RSV to cause reinfections. RSV A and B may co-circulate during an epidemic, but the specific proportions of the two groups will vary each year and also by location. Despite both RSV and influenza A outbreaks being prevalent in the winter months, their peaks seldom overlap.

- Risk factors for severe lower respiratory disease include congenital heart disease, prematurity, immunodeficiency, and respiratory or neuromuscular conditions. Passive smoking is also a risk factor. Elderly patients and immunosuppressed patients can also suffer severe disease.

Transmission

- Spread is by large droplets of secretion from an RSV-infected person, by direct hand-to hand contact or via contaminated surfaces and objects. Studies suggest that aerosol spread via small particles is less important outside families as infection does not occur at distances greater than 1.8m (6ft) from an infected person. The virus can remain viable on surfaces for about 4–7 hours.
- Clinical severity dictates the duration and degree of viral shedding. RSV can be shed for prolonged periods, up to 4 weeks in young infants and 6 weeks in immunocompromised patients. Older children and adults shed the virus for 3–4 days.
- Transmission between infants and staff may be more important than between infants, in hospitals, childcare centres, and institutions. At home, infants are usually infected via an older sibling with few symptoms. Studies demonstrate that increasing family size correlates with increasing incidence of disease.

Pathophysiology

- Inoculation is via the upper respiratory tract. The nose and eye are more effective routes compared with the mouth. After inoculation RSV is confined to the respiratory mucosa, spreading down the lower respiratory tract by fusion of the infected cells with uninfected cells. This results in giant masses of cells with multiple nuclei known as syncytia—hence the name respiratory syncytial virus.
- A marked peribronchiolar cellular infiltrate occurs in RSV bronchiolitis. In the early stages this consists of monocytes, lymphocytes, eosinophils, and neutrophils. In the later stages of the infection T lymphocytes predominate with monocytes. An inflammatory cascade is triggered involving a wide range of immunoregulatory and inflammatory molecules including toll-like receptors, chemokines, cytokines, and surfactant proteins. Extensive research continues in this area to try to delineate the fine balance between protective effects of the immune process and disease severity.
- Subsequent necrosis of the epithelium and submucosal oedema of small airways occurs. Mucous plugging is also present. All of which contribute to hyperinflation and/or collapse of lung tissue. Ventilation perfusion mismatches occur. Full recovery may take several weeks. In RSV pneumonia studies have demonstrated an interstitial infiltration of mononuclear cells, with more generalized involvement of bronchioles, bronchi and alveoli.

Clinical features

- RSV accounts for over 50% of all cases of bronchiolitis. In Europe this typically is seen in an infant around 1–5 months of age. It begins as an URTI quickly followed by signs of respiratory distress with tachypnoea, a typical bronchiolitic cough, occasional wheeze, but more commonly end-expiratory crackles, recession and hyperinflation. Older children present with a RSV viral pneumonia, or a viral induced wheeze picture.
- Antibiotics are not required in the great majority of infants. Bacterial secondary infection is very rare.
- Acute illness gets worse, stabilises, then usually resolves within 7 days, but infants may cough and wheeze post recovery. High risk infants may quickly progress to respiratory failure. Preterm infants may present with apnoea or non-specific signs of sepsis. Older children and adults will have symptoms similar to a cold (cough, runny nose, low grade fever). Less commonly, RSV can also cause croup, ear infections, conjunctivitis, and laryngitis.

Diagnosis

- The availability of a rapid RSV test is useful for infection control measures and facilitating cohorting of patients for bed management. Nasopharyngeal aspirate immunofluorescence testing is the routine test available in hospitals. It has estimated 60–90% sensitivity in the acute illness. The diagnosis of bronchiolitis is a clinical one.
- CXR findings include hyperinflation, and focal areas of collapse, which may rotate between different areas of the lungs during the course of the disease.

Management and treatment

- Most children can be managed at home. Hospitalization should occur in children needing fluids/oxygen or ventilatory support. Generally a respiratory rate in an infant of over 60 breaths/min, and/or taking less than two-thirds of normal feeds is a good marker for needing admission. Oxygen saturation <90% also mandates admission.
- Where possible milk feeds should be continued via a nasogastric tube but when these are not tolerated IV fluids may be required. Oxygen should be delivered by nasal cannula or head box to ensure saturations are >93%. Supportive treatment is the only management option available. Studies have shown that adrenaline, bronchodilators, and oral, inhaled, and IV steroids offer no benefit and may even be harmful in the acute phase. There is little evidence of benefit for chest physiotherapy.
- Around 2% of admitted infants with RSV bronchiolitis require short-term ventilation due to apnoea or respiratory failure. Underlying prematurity, chronic lung disease, cardiac disease or neurological problems are associated with longer intensive care stays. Medical management is supportive. Many treatments have been tried in PICU. None are of proven benefit.

- Ribavirin should only be considered as IV therapy in immunocompromised children with severe RSV disease in the intensive care setting, where it may have a very small effect on reducing length of ventilation and hospital stay.

Complications

- Studies have shown that RSV infections in infancy may result in long-term respiratory problems, with recurrent wheezing, reactive airways disease and 'asthma', which may persist into adolescence. This risk is increased if parents smoke, so clear advice and support for stopping smoking should be given to all parents of a child diagnosed with RSV bronchiolitis.
- Children who have been hospitalized with RSV disease require more frequent hospital outpatient attendances for respiratory complaints. Recent studies have shown that regular inhaled corticosteroids do not reduce these late respiratory complications, so smoking advice is the only possible therapeutic intervention to prevent subsequent respiratory disease.

Prevention

- Infants with RSV should be isolated or cohorted. Particular attention should be paid to standard infection control measures such as hand-washing with alcohol-based gels, aprons, and cohort nursing.
- Currently, passive immunization with palivizumab, an IM monoclonal antibody, is the only licensed option available for certain high-risk groups. This is given monthly, usually for 5 months over the winter RSV season. The original studies demonstrated a 55% reduction in RSV hospitalization in those deemed high risk. Its cost-effectiveness remains debatable. Systematic reviews are in agreement that the potential costs of palivizumab nearly always outweigh any potential savings generated by reduced hospital admissions. Mortality from RSV bronchiolitis is now extremely low, even in high risk groups.
- National guidance varies based on local epidemiology and hospital costs.
- In the UK the Joint Committee on Vaccination and Immunisation advise it to be considered for the prevention of RSV only in:
- Infants with chronic lung disease (oxygen dependency for at least 28 days from birth) who have the following specific risk factors:
  - Infants born up to 30 weeks premature who are <3 months old at the start of the RSV season.
  - Infants born up to 26 weeks premature who are <6 months old at the start of the RSV season.
- Infants with chronic lung disease with a sibling at school or in daycare including:
  - Infants born at ≤35 weeks' gestation, and <3 months at the start of the RSV season

- Infants born at ≤30 weeks' gestation, who are <6 months at the start of the RSV season
- Infants born at ≤26 weeks' gestation, who are 9 months at the start of the season
- Infants with haemodynamically significant acyanotic congenital heart disease <6 months old.
- Children with SCID until they achieve immune-reconstitution.
- Prophylaxis of RSV using palivizumab is not in the UK considered a cost-effective strategy for other preterm infants and children with congenital heart disease except for the groups mentioned above.

Future research

- The development of a safe, effective RSV vaccine is a worldwide priority. Vaccine development has been slow, following deaths due to an apparently enhanced immunological response to wild RSV after vaccination with an early formal inactivated RSV vaccine.
- An active vaccine will need to be deliverable within the routine primary immunization schedule if it is to have any practical effect, as the average age of hospital admission with RSV bronchiolitis is <3 months. Live attenuated strains, vector-based, and viral protein subunit/DNA-based candidates are currently in development. A live attenuated RSV/parainfluenza vaccine delivered intranasally is in clinical trials. An oral small molecule RSV fusion inhibitor is also in early trials.

Further reading

Abarca K, Jung E, Fernandez P, *et al.* Safety, tolerability, pharmacokinetics and immunogenicity of motavizumab, a humanised, enhanced-potency monoclonal antibody for the prevention of respiratory syncytial virus infection in at-risk children. *Pediatr Infect Dis J* 2009;**28**:267–72.

Gill MA, Welliver RC. Motavizumab for the prevention of respiratory syncytial virus infection in infants. *Expert Opin Biol Ther* 2009;**9**:1335–45.

Olszewska W, Openshaw P. Emerging drugs for respiratory syncytial virus infection. *Expert Opin Emerg Drugs* 2009;**14**:207–17.

Nokes JD, Cane PA. New strategies for control of respiratory syncytial virus infection. *Curr Opin Inf Dis* 2009;**21**:639–43.

Schickli JH, Dubovsky F, Tang RS. Challenges in developing a pediatric RSV vaccine. *Hum Vaccines* 2009;**5**:582–91.

Chapter 100

Rotavirus

📖 see also Chapters 12,17

Name and nature of organism

- Rotavirus is a double-stranded, non-enveloped RNA virus.
- It belongs to the *Reoviridae* family of viruses. On electron microscopy the appearance is of a wheel (Latin *rota*) with spokes.
- Group A rotaviruses are the major cause of infection worldwide.
- Seven serotypes, G1–4, 9 and P1 are thought to cause the majority of disease in the US and Europe, although in sub-Saharan Africa these account for less than 70% of infection and G8, as well as other P serotypes appear to be important causes of disease in those regions.

Epidemiology

- Rotavirus is the commonest cause of severe gastroenteritis in children worldwide.
- Recent data from the WHO European region identified that rotavirus infection causes an estimated 6550 deaths and 150 000 hospital admissions each year in children aged <5 years. Hospital admission rates were similar across income groups.
- Seven countries, mostly in the low- and lower-middle-income groups, accounted for 93% of estimated deaths. Disease burden varied dramatically by income level in the European region. Rotavirus vaccination in Azerbaijan, Kazakhstan, Kyrgyzstan, Tajikistan, Turkmenistan, Uzbekistan, and Turkey could potentially prevent 80% of all regional rotavirus deaths.
- It is an important cause of mortality in children in the resource-poor world, where approximately 300 000 children <5 years die from rotavirus infection yearly. The number of deaths from rotavirus in the UK is now low, and may be <5 per year.
- Rotavirus infection is ubiquitous worldwide, and by the age of 5 years, almost every child will have been exposed to and become infected with rotavirus, fewer than half of which will have clinically apparent infection.
- Although the mortality rate in the developed world is low, rotavirus is an important cause of morbidity. It is estimated that rotavirus is responsible for 2.5% of all hospital admissions annually; 20% of adult household contacts develop disease, causing lost workdays, with the knock-on economic impact, as well as the direct cost to the health service. In the UK it has been estimated that there are around 15 000 admissions due to rotavirus in children each year. Severe rotavirus

disease appears to be less common than previously in children in the UK.
- Rotavirus infections show marked seasonality. In temperate climates, the disease occurs in the late winter months.
- This seasonality is less pronounced in tropical climates, but tends to occur during the drier, cooler months of the year.

Transmission and incubation period

- Transmission is faecal-oral in nature, and so breaking the transmission cycle is heavily dependent on meticulous hand hygiene. Humans are the only reservoir for infection and the virus is excreted solely in faeces.
- As it is an unenveloped virus, it can survive for long periods on fomites, such as toys, hard surfaces, and door handles. This increases the risk of transmission and needs to be remembered when instituting infection control programmes in the hospital setting and breaking the cycle of infection in nurseries and daycare centres.
- Although animals can be infected with rotavirus, spread is species specific and animal to human spread of disease has not been documented.
- Rotavirus is shed in high concentrations in the stool of infected patients, and shedding begins just prior to the development of diarrhoea.
- Virus can be shed in stool for up to 2 weeks after infection in the immunocompetent patient and in immunocompromised hosts has been isolated from stool more than a month after the onset of symptomatic disease.
- Asymptomatic shedding of virus, both in adults and children has been described and can be a cause of ongoing transmission. This explains the rapid spread of infection in the family setting and in daycare centres.
- Water and contaminated foods are other possible routes of transmission, but this is not well documented.
- Incubation period is usually around 2 days.

Clinical features

- The clinical picture ranges from a short-lived mild gastrointestinal illness to severe dehydration, lactic acidosis, electrolyte abnormalities and death. A low serum bicarbonate is often seen.
- The disease typically starts abruptly, with high fever and watery non-bloody diarrhoea. Profuse vomiting often precedes the development of the diarrhoea and fever.
- Complications such as seizures and encephalitis have been described, although it is not clear whether the CNS signs are a result of direct infection of the CNS with rotavirus. A mild hepatitis is not uncommon.

- The typical duration of illness is 3–8 days.
- Immunocompromised children develop more severe and prolonged infections.
- There is an association between wild-type rotavirus and intussusception.

Sequelae

Long-term sequelae are few, the most important of which is ongoing chronic diarrhoea as a result of damage to the intestinal mucosa during the infection. Cow's milk protein and lactose intolerance may be seen which can last 3–6 months.

Diagnosis

- A number of tests exist for the diagnosis of rotavirus infection.
- The most commonly used ones are antigen detection assays, PCR, and cell culture isolation.
- Antigen detection assays are very specific but false-positives do occur in neonates and patients with underlying chronic intestinal diseases.
- Electron microscopy is useful in the direct identification of the virus.
- Cell culture is the gold standard for detecting rotavirus. It has the advantage of identifying the infective strain, but is time consuming and requires specific expertise. It is used mainly as a research tool.

Management and treatment

- This is supportive only.
- There is no effective antiviral agent for the treatment of rotavirus infection.
- Rehydration and the correction of electrolyte imbalances are key to management.
- ORS has revolutionized treatment of diarrhoea worldwide, and has had a marked impact on the reduction of mortality from rotavirus in the developing world.
- Persistent diarrhoea and poor weight gain may represent post rotavirus enteropathy. The differentiation between a mild recovering post rotavirus enteritis and true cow's milk protein and lactose intolerance may be difficult. The key is growth rather than persistent diarrhoea. Failure to grow post rotavirus should be investigated and may require a temporary change to a diet free from cow's milk protein and lactose.
- There are two vaccines currently available.
- A monovalent rhesus reassortant vaccine (RotaRix) is licensed in around 30 countries, and has been introduced into the routine vaccination schedule in some South American countries. This has an 84% efficacy in the prevention of severe rotavirus gastroenteritis.

- An oral quintavalent bovine vaccine (RotaTeq) was licensed in the USA in 2006 and has a 98% efficacy in prevention of severe rotavirus induced gastroenteritis.
- A rhesus reassortant vaccine (Rotashield) was withdrawn from the USA market after post-licensure surveillance identified a small increase in intussusception rates in the vaccinated population. The relationship between intussusception, rotavirus disease, and the vaccine is complex. Post-licensing surveillance has not identified any increase risk associated with the two currently licensed vaccines.
- Rotavirus vaccination is recommended as part of the routine schedule in the USA, but has yet to be introduced into the UK. However, although the two vaccines currently licensed provide protection against the four serotypes that cause 90% of disease in the USA and Europe, these strains are estimated to cause <70% of the disease in sub-Saharan Africa.
- In June 2009, the WHO recommended the introduction of rotavirus into all national immunization programmes worldwide. This has the potential to prevent over half a million deaths from severe gastroenteritis, in the <5-year age group yearly.
- In the clinical, childcare centre, and home setting, meticulous hand-washing and disinfection of fomites such as door handles and taps is vital to contain infection and prevent spread among patients or family members. The use of soap and water should be used, followed by a 70% ethanol solution to inactivate the virus and break the transmission cycle.

Future research

- Post-licensure surveillance mechanisms to detect rare events.
- Monitoring of changes in the prevalent circulating pathogenic rotavirus strains worldwide.
- Safety and efficacy of vaccination of immunocompromised children.

Further reading

Dennehy PH. Rotavirus vaccines: an overview. *Clin Microbiol Rev* 2008;**21**:198–208.

Tharpar N, Sanderson I. Diarrhoea in children: an interface between developing and developed countries. *Lancet* 2004;**363**:641–53.

Williams CJ, Lobanov A, Pebody RG. Estimated morbidity and hospital admission due to rotavirus in the WHO European Region. *Epidemiol Infect* 2009;**137**:607–16.

Chapter 101

Rubella

see also Chapters 10, 30, 34

Name and nature of organism

- Rubella is caused by the rubella virus, an RNA enveloped virus in the togavirus family.
- It is usually a mild disease in children, but infection in early pregnancy can be transmitted to the developing fetus with serious outcomes including fetal death or congenital rubella syndrome (CRS), characterized by multiple defects affecting the heart, eye and ear.

Epidemiology

- Humans are the only host for rubella.
- In the absence of comprehensive rubella immunization programmes, rubella was a common childhood infection and endemic worldwide; epidemics occurred about every 4–9 years.
- Worldwide it is estimated that more than 100 000 infants are born with CRS each year, mostly in developing countries.
- Circulation of infection can be interrupted with effective rubella immunization programmes, and several WHO regions have set targets for the elimination of CRS (<1 case of CRS/100 000 births).
- Since the introduction in 1988 of the combined MMR vaccine for young children of both sexes in the UK, the incidence of rubella infection has declined substantially. Fewer than 20 infants with congenital rubella were reported in the UK during the 10 years 1999–2008.

Transmission and incubation period

- Transmission is by direct contact or droplet spread.
- The infectious period is from about a week before to up to a week after the onset of the rash.
- The incubation period is about 14–21 days.
- Infants with congenital rubella may continue to excrete virus for ≥6 months after birth.

Clinical features and sequelae

- Up to half of all cases of rubella infection are asymptomatic and in the remainder the disease is rarely serious.
- In children there is usually little if any prodrome, but in adolescents and adults low-grade fever, malaise, headache, conjunctivitis, sore throat and cough may precede the rash, if it occurs, by up to 5 days.

- At all ages there may be a generalized lymphadenopathy, usually the suboccipital, postauricular, and cervical nodes.
- The pink-red maculopapular rash appears first on the face, and spreads rapidly to the rest of the body. The rash then disappears from the face, coalesces on the trunk, and is gone by day 4.
- The lymphadenopathy may take longer to resolve. The rash may appear similar to measles, scarlet fever or parvovirus B19.
- Transient arthritis or arthralgia is sometimes associated with rubella infection in adults and adolescents, particularly in women.
- Other rare complications include purpura (with normal or low platelet counts) that is usually self-limiting. Rubella encephalitis is extremely rare.

Congenital rubella

- The risks associated with rubella are highest in non-immune women who acquire infection in the first 10 weeks of pregnancy, at which stage transmission to the fetus is extremely likely, and the probability of damage, frequently severe and multiple, is about 90%.[1]
- The likelihood of transmission diminishes as pregnancy progresses, and after about 13 weeks' gestation damage is usually confined to sensorineural hearing loss; maternal infection after the sixteenth week of pregnancy is not normally associated with any adverse effects.
- Clinical manifestations of congenital rubella include fetal death and stillbirth, growth retardation, cardiac anomalies (septal defects, patent ductus, pulmonary artery stenosis), eye involvement (cataract, microphthalmia, retinopathy), sensorineural deafness, thrombocytopenia, and jaundice.

Diagnosis

- Clinical diagnosis of rubella infection is uncertain and should not be relied on, particularly if a pregnant woman is, or has been in contact with, the suspected case.
- The virus can be recovered from the nasopharynx and the urine in the acute phase, and a clinician notifying a case of rubella will normally be asked to take an oral fluid sample for PCR.
- In recent years in the UK over 1000 cases of rubella in children and adults have been reported annually but <3% are confirmed rubella.
- Routine antenatal testing for rubella susceptibility does not distinguish between recent and past infection, and is not diagnostic—its sole purpose is to indicate whether or not a woman requires post-partum vaccination with MMR to protect future pregnancies. The screening test is on one sample only; women with rubella IgG antibodies detectable at 10IU/ml or more are reported to have detectable antibody, and those with antibody levels <10IU/ml are reported not to have detectable antibody, and advised to have rubella immunization after delivery.
- Any pregnant woman with a rubella-like rash, or contact with suspected rubella, should be investigated as soon as possible and managed in accordance with current guidelines.[2] Normally oral fluid for

PCR testing and a serum sample for rubella specific IgM and IgG testing would be requested, with a subsequent serum sample taken 10 days later.
- Confirmation of maternal infection is on the basis of detection of rubella virus or RNA in a clinical sample, the detection of rubella IgM with low avidity IgG in serum, and/or a significant increase in rubella IgG in serum samples taken 10 days apart. Close consultation between the clinician managing the woman and the virologist is essential to ensure proper timing of samples and correct interpretation of results. Confirmed infection in early pregnancy is an indication for offering a termination of pregnancy.
- Congenital rubella can be confirmed in an infant by virus isolation or PCR on clinical specimens.

Management and treatment
- There is no specific treatment for rubella; treatment should be based on alleviating any symptoms.
- Individuals with congenital rubella should have regular clinical review so that any late onset problems, for example deterioration in sight or hearing, or development of autoimmune conditions such as diabetes or thyroid disorders, are identified and managed appropriately.

Prevention
- A child with confirmed rubella should be kept away from school or nursery for 6 days after the first symptoms, and contact with pregnant women should be avoided if possible.
- The main prevention strategy relies on:
  - Ensuring high uptake of the combined MMR vaccine among children, to maintain herd immunity in the community and prevent circulation of rubella infection.
  - Ensuring women are not susceptible to rubella when they become pregnant.

Vaccination strategy
📖 see the NHS immunization information website (🖱 www.immunisation.nhs.uk).
- A live attenuated vaccine has been available for over 40 years. The original approach in the UK was to ensure individual protection by allowing the virus to circulate amongst children, with vaccination offered to all schoolgirls at around age 11–14, to protect those who had not acquired infection naturally. Rubella vaccine was also promoted for health professionals and susceptible women of child-bearing age. In 1988 the strategy changed when MMR vaccine was

introduced for all children at 13 months of age, with the aim of preventing circulation of all three diseases. A second MMR dose was subsequently introduced for children aged 3–5 years.

- Both the vaccine and the disease are thought to provide lifelong protection for most individuals, but reinfection does sometimes occur; there have been a few cases of congenital rubella in infants born to women known to have been immune in the past, though this is rare.
- Rubella vaccine should not be administered during pregnancy, but there is now substantial evidence to suggest that though vaccine virus can cross the placenta, it does no harm. Inadvertent vaccination in pregnancy is therefore no longer considered to pose a risk, and termination of pregnancy is not recommended under these circumstances. Women who are rubella-susceptible at antenatal screening should not be immunised during pregnancy, but offered MMR vaccine as soon as practical after delivery, preferably before discharge from the maternity unit. If anti-D immunoglobulin is required, the two may be given at the same time, but different sites.

Migrants

People migrating to the UK from countries where rubella vaccination is not routine, or has not been longstanding, are at particular risk of being susceptible to rubella, and should be tested for rubella antibodies, and/or offered MMR vaccine.

Healthcare staff

All healthcare staff, male and female, should be screened for rubella, and immunized if susceptible.

Surveillance of congenital rubella

- Surveillance of congenital rubella was established in 1971 to monitor the impact of the newly implemented vaccination programme. Prior to that there was no routine monitoring, but studies suggested that about 200–300 children were born with congenital rubella damage in the UK every year, and many more in epidemic years. During the 1970s >50 children a year were reported to the National Congenital Rubella Surveillance Programme (NCRSP), but there was probably substantial underreporting. Several hundred terminations associated with rubella disease or contact were also reported every year. The number of affected pregnancies declined slowly during the late 1970s and 1980s, but much more rapidly after the introduction of MMR.[3]
- In the 10 years 1999 to 2008 <20 UK-born infants were diagnosed and reported altogether. About half of these infants were born to women who acquired infection abroad, usually in their country of origin in early pregnancy, and more than half of the remainder had mothers who, though they acquired infection in the UK, were themselves born abroad.

Notification of cases of rubella and congenital rubella

Rubella in children and adults is a notifiable disease in the UK and should be reported through the normal channels. In addition, infants born with congenital rubella should be notified to the NCRSP by paediatricians on the BPSU's monthly surveillance card.

Future research

- Long-term immunity of MMR as maternal age at pregnancy increases.
- Impact of drop in MMR uptake rates in the UK.

Key references

1 Miller E, Cradock-Watson JE, Pollock TM. Consequences of confirmed maternal rubella at successive stages of pregnancy. *Lancet* 1982;**2**:781–4.
2 Morgan-Capner P, Crowcroft NS, on behalf of the PHLS Joint Working Party of the Advisory Committees of Virology and Vaccines and Immunisation. Guidelines on the management of, and exposure to, rash illness in pregnancy (including consideration of relevant antibody screening programmes in pregnancy). *Commun Dis Public Health* 2002;**5**:59–71.
3 Tookey PA, Peckham CS. Surveillance of congenital rubella in Great Britain, 1971–96. *BMJ* 1999;**318**:769–70.

Further reading

Best JM. Rubella. *Semin Fetal Neonatal Med* 2007;**12**:182–92.

Scabies

📖 see also Chapters 34, 38, 41

Name and nature of organism

- A mite, *Sarcoptes Scabiei* var. *hominis*, belonging to the class Arachnida (Scabere—Latin—to scratch!).
- The adult female mite is approximately 0.4mm by 0.3mm, the male being smaller at 0.2mm by 0.15mm, with four pairs of legs. The body is white with bristles and spines on the dorsal surface.
- The mite is an obligate human parasite, living burrowed into skin.
- After mating, the male mite dies. The female lays two or three eggs each day in the burrows in the epidermis. A total of 40–50 eggs are laid during the remainder of the female mite's life, which lasts 4–6 weeks in total.
- A larva emerges after 3–4 days. After a number of moults it becomes a nymph and after further moults, an adult mite. Development from egg to adult takes about 10–15 days.
- <10% of eggs become mature mites.
- The average infestation is with 12 mites. Individuals who are immunocompromised may be heavily infested, with thousands or even millions of mites—crusted or Norwegian scabies.

Epidemiology

- Scabies affects all ethnic and socioeconomic groups globally.
- In many tropical and subtropical areas, scabies is endemic.
- In industrialized countries, scabies occurs as sporadic cases and institutional outbreaks, particularly in elderly people.
- There are about 300 million cases of scabies worldwide each year.
- Poverty, overcrowding (especially bed sharing), malnutrition, and poor hygiene are all predisposing factors.
- It has been claimed there are cyclical rises in incidence approximately every 20 years, but this is disputed.
- Infestation is commonest in young children and becomes less frequent, with increasing age.
- In UK it seems to be commoner in winter.
- In some countries it is commoner in rural populations, whereas in others it is commoner in urban areas. This may be related to the frequency of predisposing factors.
- In one area of Poland, the reported prevalence ranged from 7.9–80 per 100 000 people.

Transmission and incubation period

- On warm skin, mites crawl at about 2.5cm a minute. They are unable to jump or fly.
- Away from a human host, in bedding, clothing etc., they can survive for 24–36 hours under average conditions. However, transmission is most likely if contact of the materials with the human host was very recent.
- Spread is mainly by direct skin to skin contact, such as prolonged hand-holding, sharing a bed, sexual intercourse, etc. Therefore, it occurs mainly within households.
- Casual contact is rarely important, however, carers of those with scabies, may become infected.
- A large study in Sheffield (UK), about 40 years ago found that infested school children and teenagers, especially girls, were the most common route of introduction into households.
- 38% of family contacts within a household became infested. The secondary attack rate was highest for preschool children (49%) and lowest for men (30%). This may be related to closeness and duration of contact.
- In the case of a first infection, once infestation has occurred, symptoms usually occur 7–27 days later, but the incubation period may be longer.

Clinical features and sequelae

- The probable cause of the symptoms is an immune response, immediate and delayed type hypersensitivity, to the mites and their products (saliva, eggs and faeces).
- The main symptom is itching which does not necessarily occur at the site of the burrows. It tends to be worse at night.
- Erythematous papules, excoriation and sometimes vesicles are most likely to occur at the interdigital spaces, flexor surfaces of the wrists, axillae, waist, periumbilical skin, scrotum, feet, and ankles.
- In young children, the palms, soles, face, neck, and scalp are often affected.
- Very young children often have widespread eczema-like lesions, particularly on the trunk, and there may be multiple crusted nodules on the trunk and limbs.
- In infants, the commonest lesions are papules and vesicopustules, which are particularly common on the palms and soles.
- Pinkish brown nodules are particularly seen with scabies in babies.
- The distribution of lesions tends to be symmetrical.
- Using a magnifying glass, linear burrows can be seen in the interdigital spaces, and on wrists and ankles.
- Skin may develop bacterial infection due to damage caused by scratching.

Crusted or Norwegian scabies

- These are heavy infestations, found particularly in immunocompromised individuals.
- The skin lesions most commonly seen are hyperkeratotic crusted nodules and plaques.
- The nails are frequently thickened, with subungual debris.
- Secondary bacterial infection with *Staphylococcus aureus*, GAS, or peptostreptococci can occur.
- Glomerulonephritis, septicaemia, and death may follow infection.
- In some communities, the secondary infection is an important cause of rheumatic fever and rheumatic heart disease.

Diagnosis

- Usually based on the clinical presentation, including itching worse at night, the distribution of the skin lesions and contact with other cases. Burrows may be seen.
- Differential diagnosis includes bites from insects such as midges, fleas, and bedbugs; and infections such as folliculitis, impetigo, tinea, and some viral exanthemata.
- Diagnosis is more difficult with secondary bacterial infection.
- Confirmation of the diagnosis can be made by gently scraping the skin off a burrow with a blunt scalpel blade or needle. The mite may stick to the scalpel or needle point, and may be seen with the naked eye. If not seen, the sample can be examined under a microscope or sent to a laboratory. This method is only about 50% sensitive. As yet, there are no reliable laboratory tests in routine use.

Management and treatment

- For classic scabies, topical permethrin is the treatment of choice and is very effective.
- A 5% preparation should be applied to the whole body. Even though the manufacturers recommend exclusion of the head and neck, these areas should be included. Particular attention should be paid to the webs of the fingers and toes and it should be brushed under the edges of the nails. It should be washed off after 8–12 hours. If the hands are washed during this time, it should be applied again. It can sting. The treatment should be repeated 7 days later.
- Topical lindane (gammabenzene hexachloride) is equally effective, but is no longer used in many affluent countries because of concerns about potential neurotoxicity.
- Benzyl benzoate is less effective and should be avoided in children as it is irritant.
- Topical malathion may be as effective as permethrin.
- Oral ivermectin (as a single dose) appears to be as effective as topical malathion, however it is licensed for use in children in few countries and has no clear benefit over permethrin.

- Crusted scabies should be treated with topical permethrin and oral ivermectin.
- There is evidence of *in vitro* resistance to ivermectin, when used frequently in scabies-endemic communities.
- Secondary bacterial infection should be treated with an appropriate antibiotic.
- Even in the presence of effective treatment, itching may persist for up to 6 weeks. If it continues beyond this, re-treatment is indicated, as it is likely to indicate continuing infestation.
- Treatment for pruritus with oral histamines has not been shown to be effective, but given at night may help sleep.

Prevention

- As classic scabies is not highly infectious, it is unnecessary to exclude infested children from school.
- Asymptomatic household contacts, sexual partners, people that share a bed and close contacts (those that have had >5 minutes direct, continuous skin-to-skin contact with the affected person) should receive a single treatment of topical permethrin.
- Clothes and bedding that have had contact with an infested individual within the previous 72 hours should be machine washed at 50–60°C. and machine dried. If this is not possible, they may be kept in a sealed plastic bag for 72 hours. Either method should kill the mites.

Future research

There has been no recent systematic survey of the prevalence and management of scabies in the community.

Further reading

Chosidow O. Clinical practices. Scabies. *N Engl J Med* 2006;**354**:1718–27.

Mounsey KE, Holt DC, McCarthy JS, Currie BJ, Walton SF. Longitudinal evidence of increasing in vitro tolerance of scabies mites to ivermectin in scabies-endemic communities. *Arch Dermatol* 2009;**145**:840–1.

Strong M, Johnstone P. Interventions for treating scabies. *Cochrane Database Syst Rev* 2007;**3**:CD000320.

Schistosomiasis

📖 see also Chapters 3, 41, 42

Organism

- Schistosomes are flat worms of the trematode family.
- The adult schistosome is an unsegmented leaf-like organism, 1–2cm in length and is either male or female. They have an average lifespan of 3–7 years, although they can live for as long as 30 years.
- They have an amazingly complex life cycle with both parasitic (snail and humans) and free living forms (cercariae).
- Cercariae are shed by the snail into water and penetrate human skin to transform into schistosomulae, which travel through veins via the lungs to the liver where they become a sexual form. They pass down the portal system to the bowel or bladder to mate and deposit eggs (ova). These are passed in stool or urine into freshwater and hatch into miracidia that invade snails.
- The ova released by the female worm are distinctive, oval in shape with a hook, the placement of which varies depending on species.
- Schistosomiasis causes a number of different clinical syndromes, dependent on the infecting species, the infective load, the distribution of ova, and the host response to them.
- Disease can be both acute and short lived or chronic, with long-term sequelae.
- There are five main species which cause disease in humans: *S. mansoni*, *S. haematobium*, *S. japonicum*, *S. mekongi*, and *S. intercalatum*.

Epidemiology

- Schistosomiasis is found almost worldwide and is an important cause of chronic ill-health in the resource-poor, affecting over 200 million people.
- Around 200 000 people die from schistosomiasis annually.
- Although more common in people who live in endemic areas, particularly rural areas, brief exposure to infected water can result in infection.
- Infection in endemic areas amongst local communities occurs in childhood, but the peak prevalence and severity of disease occurs between the ages of 15 and 20.
- Generally, only one adult worm pair persists in a host. Severity of disease is related to the egg load produced.

- Although schistosomiasis infection is widespread, different species are responsible for disease in different regions.
- Each species of schistosome has a predilection for a specific snail species as its intermediate host. It is the presence and location of these snail species which determines the geographical distribution and species of schistosome.
- *S. mansoni* (intestinal/hepatic) and *S. haematobium* (bladder/renal) account for 95% of all infections.
- *S. mansoni* is widespread through Africa, parts of the Caribbean, the Middle East and South America (Brazil, Venezuela).
- *S. haematobium* is endemic throughout Africa, Mauritius, the Middle East, a few parts of India and is also found in the eastern Mediterranean region.
- *S. japonicum* (gastrointestinal and hepatic disease) is widespread throughout East Asia and the Pacific region.
- *S. mekongi* is confined to a small area in the Mekong river delta, in South East Asia.
- *S. intercalatum* is limited to West and Central Africa.
- In the UK there are around 50–100 cases reported each year, with Malawi and Zimbabwe the commonest country of origin.

Transmission and incubation period

- Humans (particularly young children) are the principal hosts in the life cycle, with water snails being the intermediate hosts.
- Fresh water becomes infected from human faeces and urine in which schistosomal ova are excreted.
- Miracidia are hatched from these eggs into the water where they infect snails, the intermediate hosts.
- The asexual lifecycle takes place in the snail, where the miracidia multiply as sporocysts. These mature into cercaria, which are released into the water.
- Cercaria have bifurcated tails, which allow them to propel through the water and seek the definitive host, humans. They enter the host through the skin, shedding their tails at this point, and are now known as schistosomulae. The lifecycle continues with the migration of these organisms into the blood and lymph vessels.
- The adult worms develop in the arterial blood vessels, primarily of the lungs and liver. This process takes 4–6 weeks and both male and female worms develop. Adult worms live in a state of permanent copulation, and produce ova, but do not replicate themselves, in the human host.
- The female worm sits within the groove of the adult male worm and 1–3 months after the development of the adult worms, the female begins to release ova into the circulation which are then excreted either in the faeces or the urine. The lifecycle begins again.
- The incubation period is thus 4–8 weeks. However, symptoms related to the entry of the cercaria through the skin can cause a more acute syndrome.

Clinical features

- Different species of *Schistosoma* cause different clinical syndromes, the reason for its variable clinical presentation.
- Many infections are asymptomatic and go undetected.
- Symptomatic disease is more common in travellers who are non-immune, than people who live in endemic areas, who are more likely to suffer from chronic schistosomiasis and the sequelae.
- Severity of disease is related to infective burden.
- The majority of the clinical features and underlying pathology of schistosomiasis are related to the *Schistosoma* eggs, and the host response to them.
- In the initial stages of infection, when the cercariae penetrate the skin, the first presentation can be one of dermatitis (swimmers itch). In endemic areas where exposure and infection with cercariae is repeated, this can be severe. It is caused by a delayed hypersensitivity reaction, which is immune mediated, in addition to the immediate allergic reaction more commonly associated with this phenomenon.
- Katayama fever is an immune-mediated syndrome occurring about 2–8 weeks after infection with *S. mansoni* or *S. japonicum*. It presents with non-specific symptoms of fever, chills, myalgias, arthralgias, headaches, and dry cough, which can resemble many other infections which present non-specifically, such as malaria (endemic in similar geographic regions), viral infections or serum sickness. Lymphadenopathy and hepatosplenomegaly can also be part of the syndrome. The presence of eosinophilia helps in the diagnosis, but is not consistent. Pulmonary infiltrates can be seen on CXR. Ova are infrequently found, as this clinical presentation coincides with the early production of ova, making diagnosis more difficult.
- Dysuria associated with terminal haematuria is a common presentation of *S. haematobium*.
- Intestinal symptoms and signs, bloody diarrhoea, abdominal pain and cramping, and poor appetite are common presentations of all species of *Schistosoma*, although much rarer in *S. haematobium* infection, which generally presents with urinary symptoms.
- Hepatic symptoms and signs are the predominant clinical features of *S. mekongi*, and can occur with other species of *Schistosoma* as well. Marked hepatosplenomegaly is a hallmark of infection. Ascites and varices can occur, and are important causes of morbidity and mortality.
- Occasionally, neurological disease occurs, presenting as transverse myelitis, seizures, limb pain, increased intracranial pressure, or focal impairment.
- Pulmonary involvement, manifesting most commonly as dyspnoea can occur.
- Weight loss, poor appetite, fatigue, and iron deficiency anaemia are commonly associated with all types of infection.

Sequelae

- Anaemia, fatigue, malnutrition and growth restriction are important and common sequelae of chronic infection in endemic areas.
- Depression of cognitive function has been noted in children.
- Ongoing bladder inflammation is a risk factor for bladder cancer, more prevalent in areas where *S. haematobium* is endemic, and is related to chronic inflammation caused by deposition of ova in the bladder wall.
- Deposition of ova in the genitourinary tract is also a risk factor for acquisition of HIV in young adults, particularly young women.
- Hepatic infection can be a prelude to hepatic fibrosis and portal hypertension, with an increased risk of oesophageal varices.
- In patients with ongoing intestinal disease, polyps, ulcers and intestinal strictures can develop.
- With heavy infestations affecting the lungs, pulmonary hypertension and cor pulmonale can occur.
- Infertility, both male and female, is a rare sequelae of chronic *S. haematobium* infection.
- Secondary bacterial infection is a common complication of schistosomiasis.
- Co-infection with the hepatitides is common, and can cause more severe morbidity related to liver damage.
- Malaria and schistosomiasis have similar geographical distributions and can occur concurrently. The two diseases have variable effects on each other, with some suggestion that in younger children schistosomiasis has a protective effect against severe malarial disease.

Diagnosis

- Non-specific findings on blood film include eosinophilia in up to 70% of patients, usually early in the disease process.
- Iron deficiency anaemia occurs in patients with chronic infection.
- Abnormal liver transaminases can be found in patients with hepatic sequestration of ova.
- Haematuria, either macroscopic or microscopically detected on dipstick is almost pathognomonic of *S. haematobium* infection in children who live in endemic areas.
- Isolation and identification of ova is a simple and definitive method of diagnosis, although this is not sensitive early in the disease process or in light infections.
- *S. haematobium* eggs can be seen in urine specimens as well as faecal samples, and, although similar in size to those of *S. mansoni*, have a large terminal rather than lateral spine. *S. intercalatum* is similar to *S. haematobium*, but much larger. *S. japonicum* and *S. mekongi* are similar but smaller.
- Rectal snips have a better sensitivity for the detection of ova than faecal samples, even in *S. haematobium* infection.

- The use of concentration techniques for both urine and faeces increases the sensitivity of detection of ova in these samples. Yield is greater in samples taken in the middle of the day, or after exercise.
- Serology is a useful means of diagnosis, though more expensive, and becomes positive later in the disease process. Antibodies are produced to the schistosomal ova, so tests are seldom positive before 4–6 weeks after infection and sometimes are absent for much longer. Serology does not differentiate between present and past infection, so is most useful when positive in travellers to confirm diagnosis, and when negative in residents of endemic areas, to rule out infection.

Treatment

Praziquantel is the only drug available for treatment of all types of schistosomiasis. It has very few side effects and is usually effective as a single oral dose in one or two divided doses. It has no effect on ova and immature worms, and so a repeat dose 6–12 weeks later is sometimes necessary, if the first dose is given early in the infection. Ova can continue to be shed for 4–6 weeks after successful treatment.

Prevention

There is no vaccine for prevention, so public health programmes are based on:
- Advice to travellers about avoidance of wading or swimming in fresh water lakes or rivers in endemic countries—especially Lake Malawi!
- Eradication programmes: elimination of snail species, the intermediate hosts, is an important strategy for breaking the life cycle of *Schistosoma* species and decreasing transmission of disease and is effective when used in conjunction with mass treatment of communities with praziquantel.

Future research

- Antigen detection assays are currently being developed.
- PCR tests are in development phase and look promising, with good sensitivity and specificity.
- New therapeutic strategies and drugs are required and an important focus for future research.

Further reading

Gryseels B, Palman K, Clerinx J, Kestens L. Human schistosomiasis. *Lancet* 2006;**368**:1106–18.

National Travel Health Network and Centre (NaTHNaC). Available at: ℘ www.nathnac.org/travel/factsheet/schistosomiasis (accessed 1 February 2011).

World Health Organization. Schistosomiasis. Available at: ℘ www.who.int/schistosomiasis (accessed 1 February 2011).

Chapter 104

Shigellosis

📖 see also Chapters 12, 69

Name and nature of organism

- Shigellae are non-motile Gram-negative bacilli within the family Enterobacteriaceae. The organism invades intestinal macrophages triggering localised inflammation and necrosis.
- The genus *Shigella* comprises four serogroups and many serotypes:
  - Serogroup A: *S. dysenteriae* (12 serotypes—produces Shiga toxin)
  - Serogroup B: *S. flexneri* (6 serotypes)
  - Serogroup C: *S. boydii* (23 serotypes)
  - Serogroup D: *S. sonnei* (1 serotype).

Epidemiology

- It is estimated that *Shigella* serogroups infect over 200 million people and cause more than one million deaths each year worldwide.
- Shigellosis is endemic in conditions of overcrowding, poor sanitation, and inadequate water supply (especially in confined populations such as refugee camps).
- In tropical areas there is a seasonal peak of shigellosis, usually before the rainy season starts, when water supplies are low.
- *S. flexneri* is the most frequently isolated serogroup worldwide, accounting for 60% of cases in resource-poor countries. However *S. sonnei* is the most common serogroup in developed countries.
- *S. sonnei* is endemic in the UK, causing around two-thirds of the 1000 cases reported each year of shigellosis. *S. boydii*, *S. dysenteriae*, and most *S. flexneri* infections originate outside the UK.
- The major burden of disease in resource-poor countries is in children aged 1–4 years, who account for 70% of cases and 60% of deaths. Illness in infants <6 months is uncommon.
- Epidemics of *S. dysenteriae* occur particularly in confined populations, and affect all age groups. *S. dysenteriae* type 1 causes the most severe form of disease, including toxic megacolon and HUS, with a case fatality rate up to 20%.

Transmission

- Shigellae are resistant to gastric acid, and the infective dose is very low: ingestion of 10–100 bacteria is sufficient to produce disease.
- Transmission is mainly faecal-oral from people with diarrhoea, especially in households, schools, and nurseries.

- The secondary attack rate in households may be as high as 40%.
- Outbreaks occur in crowded conditions with poor sanitation.
- Occasionally spread via food or water that has been contaminated by people with shigellosis.
- Incubation period: 1–7 days.
- Period of communicability: during the acute illness and for up to 4 weeks afterwards. Rarely, the carrier state persists for months.
- Appropriate antimicrobial treatment usually reduces duration of carriage to a few days.

Clinical features and sequelae

- The spectrum of shigellosis ranges from mild watery diarrhoea to full-blown dysentery with fever, abdominal pain and severe diarrhoea with blood, mucus, or pus. The infection primarily affects the colon, and less frequently the terminal ileum.
- The bacteria invade the intestinal mucosa resulting in mucosal ulcerations and confluent colonic crypt abscesses. Despite the intense superficial destructive process in the colonic epithelium, bacteraemia and disseminated infection are relatively rare.
- Nausea, vomiting, headache (± meningism), lethargy, confusion, and convulsions (mainly in small children) may occur and have been attributed to a neurotoxin.
- Less common presentations include a morbilliform rash and conjunctivitis (which may be confused with measles) and pneumonia.
- Dehydration and electrolyte imbalance is the main cause of death. There is a high mortality rate in neonates and infants.
- *S. sonnei* usually causes mild illness that is self-limiting within a few days, except in immunocompromised patients.
- The other *Shigella* serogroups cause more severe disease: *S. dysenteriae* type 1 causes the most serious illness.
- HUS is a complication of *S. dysenteriae* type 1, caused by the production of Shiga toxin.
- Reactive arthritis occurs in up to 5–10% of patients 2–5 weeks after the dysenteric illness, especially in patients with HLA-B27.

Diagnosis

- *Shigella* serogroups can be cultured from faeces or rectal swabs.
- Culture media that are selective for *Shigella* (and *Salmonella*) are used to enhance sensitivity.
- Faeces samples should be cultured as soon as possible after collection to obtain the best diagnostic yield.

Management and treatment

- Most cases of non-bloody diarrhoea can be managed supportively with rehydration and correction of electrolyte imbalance.

- Antibiotic therapy is usually recommended for shigellosis as it:
  - Shortens the duration of illness.
  - Lessens the severity of illness in patients with underlying conditions (e.g. malnutrition, immunosuppression).
  - Terminates excretion of bacteria in faeces, and therefore antibiotic therapy reduces person-to-person spread of shigellosis.
- The choice of antibiotic therapy should be based on knowledge of local susceptibility patterns (multidrug resistance is increasingly common) and adjusted if resistant. There are high rates of plasmid-mediated antibiotic resistance globally.
- Empirical treatment options include ciprofloxacin, azithromycin, and ceftriaxone. There are no controlled trials suggesting superiority of any specific antibiotic.
- Amoxicillin or trimethoprim is effective if the organism is sensitive.
- Antimotility drugs, such as loperamide or diphenoxylate, are contra-indicated.
- Avoid analgesics such as codeine that have an antimotility effect.

Prevention

- Good hygiene and sanitation. Hospitalized patients should be isolated using enteric precautions.
- Children with *S. sonnei* should be excluded from school until 48 hours after first normal stool.
- Children with other *Shigella* serogroups may require confirmation of microbiological clearance before returning to school.
- Exclusion is particularly important for young children and others who may find adherence to hygiene practices difficult.
- Children should be excluded from swimming pools for 2 weeks following the last episode of diarrhoea.
- In the UK shigellosis is a notifiable disease.

Future research

- Vaccination probably offers the best prospect for controlling shigellosis: several candidate vaccines are currently in development.
- In the absence of an effective vaccine, more research into the control and treatment of antibiotic-resistant shigellosis is required.

Further reading

Clinical Knowledge Summaries. *Gastroenteritis*. 2009 Available at: ℞ www.cks.nhs.uk/gastroenteritis (accessed 1 February 2011).

World Health Organization. *Guidelines for the Control of Shigellosis Including Epidemics Due to Shigella dysenteriae 1*. 2005. Available at: ℞ www.who.int/vaccine_research/documents/Guidelines_Shigellosis.pdf (accessed 1 February 2011).

Staphylococcal infections including MRSA

📖 see also Chapters 5, 6, 8, 11, 15, 17, 27, 28, 30, 31, 34, 36, 38, 39, 40

Name and nature of organism

- Staphylococci are amongst the most frequently encountered causes of localized and systemic bacterial infections, as well as being ubiquitous commensals of skin and mucosa. Staphylococci are Gram-positive cocci, which characteristically appear in clusters (Greek *staphyle*— bunch of grapes).
- Staphylococci are subdivided by the coagulase test into *Staphylococcus aureus* (coagulase-positive) and other species that are coagulase-negative. These are less virulent acting as opportunistic pathogens.
- *S. aureus* is a major human pathogen. Most strains remain sensitive to commonly used antibiotics (including flucloxacillin) and are referred to as MSSA. Meticillin (or methicillin) is an old narrow-spectrum β-lactam antibiotic, now no longer used clinically; resistance to meticillin denotes staphylococci that are flucloxacillin resistant. Strains that are resistant to flucloxacillin are also called meticillin-resistant (MRSA).
- *S. aureus* produces multiple exotoxins that are either membrane active or superantigens.

Meticillin-sensitive *S. aureus*

Epidemiology

- Carried by around 30% of the population at any one time.
- Nose is the commonest carriage site.
- Other carriage sites include: throat, axillae, perineum, gastrointestinal tract.
- Can also be carried by pets and other animals.
- Acts an opportunistic pathogen when body's defences are breached.

There has been a steady rise in reported bacteraemia in children due to *S. aureus*. It is now the commonest identified cause of bacteraemia in the UK after CONS. Recent data suggest increased hospital admissions due to abscesses, osteomyelitis and other *S. aureus* clinical disease syndromes. Whether this is reporting bias or a true rise and if so, the underlying cause, is not clear.

Risk factors for infection with S. aureus
- Primary immunodeficiencies, especially those with neutrophil dysfunction e.g. hyper IgE syndrome, chronic granulomatous disease
- Acquired immunodeficiencies, especially neutropenia
- Healthcare workers
- Skin or mucosal damage: recent surgery
- Presence of a foreign body, e.g. intravascular catheters
- Cystic fibrosis.

Infections are common in all age groups: serious infections are most common in infancy and as healthcare-associated infections.

Different strains of S. aureus produce different virulence factors some of which are associated with characteristic syndromes.

Transmission

Infections may be endogenous or exogenous.
- Endogenous infections occur when commensal bacteria become invasive.
- Exogenous infections are acquired from other people (occasionally animals).

Transmission may be via direct contact with a colonized or infected individual or indirect contact with a contaminated environment: S. aureus can survive on surfaces for at least 24 hours.

Staphylococcal food poisoning is caused by pre-formed exotoxin (enterotoxins) in food. Source is nearly always a colonized foodhandler: contaminated food is then stored under inappropriate conditions allowing S. aureus to multiply and produce enterotoxin.

Clinical features and sequelae

Less serious infections
Superficial skin infections:
- Folliculitis, furuncles (boils) and carbuncles (confluent boils with sinus formation), cervical adenitis.
- Neonatal septic spots, breast abscesses, omphalitis.
- Impetigo: S. aureus is the main pathogen in both types of impetigo.
  - Non-bullous (70% of cases). Mainly affects face and limbs, often commencing in an area of traumatised skin
  - Bullous. More commonly affects the trunk: more rapidly progressive with larger and multiple bullae. Commonest in infants.
- Infected atopic dermatitis: S. aureus common in exacerbations, but clinical significance in the absence of overt infection is not certain.
- Surgical site infections:
  - Urinary tract infections (especially catheter-associated)
  - Ocular infections: conjunctivitis, dacryocystitis, endophthalmitis.

Serious infections
- Primary bacteraemia—bacteraemia (contamination from skin colonisation possible) and septicaemia.
- Pneumonia
  - Primary (📖 see Panton-valentine leucocidin producing S. aureus, p. xxx)

- Secondary to viral infections, especially chickenpox, influenza
- Ventilator-associated.
- Device-related infections (e.g. central venous catheters).
- Endocarditis (native valve and prosthetic valve).
- Osteomyelitis, septic arthritis, discitis, pyomyositis, psoas abscess.
- Meningitis
  - Shunt-associated, or post-trauma
  - Uncommon cause of primary meningitis, mainly in neonates.

Specific virulence factor-related conditions

Staphylococcal food poisoning

- Abrupt onset 2–6 hours after ingestion of food of vomiting, followed by abdominal pain and watery diarrhoea. Usually self-limiting with resolution of symptoms within 8 hours.

Toxic shock syndrome

- Rapid onset multisystem superantigen-mediated disease:
  - Menstrual: strongly associated with strains that produce toxic shock syndrome toxin 1 (TSST-1)
  - Non-menstrual: usually associated with enterotoxins.

Staphylococcal scalded skin syndrome

- Caused by strains of S. aureus that produce exfoliatin toxins A and B, which cleave desmosomal junctions in epidermis.
- Initial infection (which may be trivial) followed by:
  - Acute fever
  - Diffuse tender erythroderma: redness accentuated around the eyes and mouth and in flexures
  - Clear bullae form and rupture leading to separation of sheets of skin
  - Nikolsky's sign: intact-appearing skin is easily rubbed off.

Panton-valentine leucocidin (PVL) producing S. aureus

PVL production is strongly associated with virulence and transmissibility. Features of CA-MRSA (see later), but most PVL-producing strains are not MRSA. Infections characteristically cause:

- Skin and soft tissue infections:
  - Infections may be recurrent and/or unusually severe
  - Pain and erythema are prominent
  - May progress to necrosis and intravascular thrombosis
- Necrotizing pneumonia.

Suspect where:
  - Airway bleeding/haemoptysis
  - Hypotension
  - Flu-like illness (temp>39°C, tachycardia, myalgias)
  - Leucopenia, high CRP (>200mg/l)
  - Gram-positive cocci on Gram stain of sputum
  - CXR multilobular infiltrates
  - Raised serum creatine kinase
- Osteomyelitis, septic arthritis, pyomyositis.

Diagnosis

- May not be necessary to collect samples in infections of superficial sites where *S. aureus* is the likely pathogen, unless unusually severe, recurrent or unresponsive to empiric therapy.
- Not all cases of *S. aureus* in blood cultures will be clinically significant. The proportion of significant bacteraemia is unknown and depends on the clinical setting.
- Gram stain of clinical material (especially from sites that are normally sterile) may be useful in making a presumptive diagnosis.
- Culture of *S. aureus* from the site of infection is main diagnosis.
- Blood cultures are often positive in deep-seated infections: always look for a focus of infection when *S. aureus* is isolated from blood.
- Once *S. aureus* has been cultured:
  - Antibiotic sensitivities are required, especially to distinguish between MSSA and MRSA
  - Further tests may be required to identify specific virulence factors or to investigate possible outbreaks.

Management and treatment

Less serious infections

- Superficial pyodermas and eye infections: generally respond to topical antimicrobials.
- Impetigo: topical fusidic acid is widely used, although there are increasing reports of resistance. Resistance may be due to selection of resistant mutants during treatment, or mediated by a transmissible gene. The risks in primary care are probably overstated, because swabs are only collected from selected patients. However, use of topical fusidic acid in hospitals is not recommended.
- Other established topical antibiotics (neomycin, mupirocin) are used for MRSA decolonization, and their widespread use for other indications is not recommended.
- Retapamulin is a novel topical pleuromutilin antibacterial. It appears to be effective with a low risk of resistance, but is expensive.
- Concern about antibiotic resistance has led to renewed interest in antiseptics: limited data indicate that 1% hydrogen peroxide in stabilized cream has comparable efficacy with topical antibiotics, is well tolerated, and carries no risk of antibiotic resistance.
- Widespread or severe impetigo may require treatment with oral antibiotics, usually flucloxacillin or a macrolide.
- Exacerbations of atopic dermatitis: topical corticosteroids are the mainstay of treatment. Although *S. aureus* is frequently isolated from such patients, there is little evidence that addition of an antibiotic hastens recovery, unless there is clear evidence of infection.

Serious infections

- Flucloxacillin remains the main treatment of invasive infections with MSSA in the UK. Sometimes combined with another agent, although there is little evidence to support this approach:
  - Fusidic acid or rifampicin penetrate well into difficult sites, e.g. bone. Never used as monotherapy because of the high rate of emergence of resistant mutants.

- Aminoglycosides (e.g. gentamicin) sometimes recommended, especially for endocarditis. Recent work suggests that even at low dose, the risks of nephrotoxicity may outweigh benefits.
- A macrolide, clindamycin or a glycopeptide are alternatives to flucloxacillin for patients who are allergic to penicillin.

PVL-producing *S. aureus* infections

Mild-moderate infections—flucloxacillin or clindamycin
Serious skin and soft tissue infections—aggressive surgery where indicated: clindamycin and/or a glycopeptide
Pneumonia—clindamycin + linezolid + rifampicin; consider IVIG
Bone and joint infections—clindamycin + linezolid or rifampicin

Prevention

- The ubiquity of *S. aureus* means that it is not realistic to avoid it. Nevertheless, general good hygiene should be encouraged.
- Families with recurrent boils and abscesses due to MSSA disease may require whole family decolonization with mupirocin nasal cream daily for a week with chlorhexidine baths (one capful and a good wash in the groins and axillae ± systemic antibiotics for active disease). There is no point treating one family member!
- Specific measures for higher risk people may be considered:
  - Screening and decolonization treatment for patients at increased risk of infection
  - Surgical antibiotic prophylaxis
  - Long-term antibiotic prophylaxis for high-risk patients
  - Screening and/or decolonization treatment of close contacts of PVL cases.

Meticillin-resistant *S. aureus* (MRSA)

Epidemiology

There are two types of MRSA:

- Healthcare-associated: The most common in the UK. In the UK dominated by two epidemic hospital strains: EMRSA 15 and 16.
- Community-associated: Currently much less common in the UK, but prevalent in the USA, especially USA300 clone. These strains also produce PVL and are therefore more virulent—usually clindamycin sensitive (used as a marker for community-acquired MRSA—but now less clear).

Hospital-associated MRSA versus community-associated-MRSA (Table 105.1)

Table 105.1

	Healthcare-associated	**Community-associated**
Typical patients	Elderly; neonates; chronically ill patients who are frequent healthcare attendees	Young healthy people
Transmission	Within healthcare settings; little spread among household contacts	Community acquired; spreads within families and institutions where close contact
Infection sites	Sites of nosocomial intervention	Often spontaneous: skin commonest
Antibiotics	Usually resistant to several antibiotic classes	Usually resistant mainly to β-lactam antibiotics

Diagnosis
- As with MSSA, culture together with antibiotic sensitivity testing.
- Use of chromogenic culture media allows a presumptive diagnosis to be made in 18–24 hours.
- PCR is increasingly being used as a screening, and sometimes diagnostic, test for MRSA in high-risk patient groups. However, these tests are expensive and their accuracy and cost-effectiveness in children (a low prevalence population) is currently uncertain.
- MRSA bacteraemia rates in children in the UK are low (<100 cases/year). Most cases can be linked to either NICU or PICU admission and indwelling CVCs.

Treatment
- Glycopeptides (e.g. vancomycin, teicoplanin) are main treatment.
- Linezolid may have more favourable pharmacodynamics and could offer better outcomes in some type of infection. It is also available for oral administration.
- For strains that are macrolide-sensitive clindamycin is sometimes suitable (preferred to other macrolides because emergence of resistance requires two mutations).
- Routine use of more than one agent is not recommended. Adding a second agent, e.g. rifampicin or fusidic acid, is indicated for bone and joint infections or meningitis or for severe infections with PVL-producing community-acquired MRSA (see earlier).
- Newer agents, e.g. daptomycin, should be used after specialist advice only.
- Decolonization treatment: The most commonly used regimen is mupirocin + a daily antibacterial bodywash and shampoo (usually chlorhexidine gluconate) for 5 days.

Prevention

In contrast to MSSA, MRSA is not ubiquitous and is more preventable. Hospital-acquired MRSA is controlled by isolation, decolonization, and appropriate prophylaxis of MRSA-positive patients. MRSA bacteraemia rates are now falling dramatically in the UK. Most adult patients admitted to hospitals in the UK are now screened for MRSA. This allows early detection of colonized patients, but the cost-effectiveness and clinical effectiveness of this approach in a low-prevalence paediatric population is uncertain.

In the UK only high-risk children (multiple previous admissions/chronic underlying condition) or high-risk surgery (cardiac/transplantation, etc.) are being routinely screened on admission. All PICU and NICU admissions should be screened.

Community-acquired MRSA is currently rarely seen in the UK. However the US approach has been around preventing and managing the five Cs: Contaminated items, Close contact, Crowding, Cleanliness, Cuts and other compromises to skin integrity.

Coagulase-negative staphylococci (CONS)

Epidemiology

- Ubiquitous skin commensals. Do not produce enzyme coagulase (clots rabbit plasma!). Around 30 species. Act as opportunistic pathogens in immunocompromised and/or with indwelling devices.
- Most frequent cause of late onset (2–28 days) bacteraemia in neonates; majority in VLBW babies and clinical significance often uncertain. *S. epidermidis* is the commonest species, but there are many others. Slime production is an important virulence factor: interferes with opsonophagocytosis and impedes antibiotic penetration.

Many infections are endogenous. Direct or indirect person-to-person spread in hospitals is also possible.

Clinical features and sequelae

- Almost exclusively HCAIs. Traditionally regarded as low-virulence pathogens, but growing evidence in neonates that they may be associated with a poorer long-term neurodevelopmental outcome than was originally thought.
- Late-onset neonatal infections: Bacteraemia, pneumonia, meningitis. Meningitis rare, usually in VLBW babies with recurrent or persistent CONS bacteraemias.
- Bacteraemia in neutropenic patients.
- Device-related infections: Intravascular devices, CSF shunts, prosthetic joints, peritoneal dialysis catheter-related peritonitis.
- UTI: Especially catheter associated. *S. saprophyticus* is a cause of UTI in older girls.
- Endocarditis (usually post operative or prosthetic valve).

Diagnosis

Isolation of the bacterium from a site that is normally sterile. Challenge is to distinguish true infection from contamination. Isolation of the same bacterium (e.g. based on antibiogram) on more than one occasion and/or in association with other laboratory and clinical markers of infection increase certainty that CONS are pathogenic. In the neonatal setting approximately 50% of CONS bacteraemias are probably clinically significant.

Management and treatment

- Strains causing infections are often multipe antibiotic-resistant. Glycopeptides (e.g. vancomycin, teicoplanin) are main treatment.
- Occasionally addition of a second agent (e.g. rifampicin in meningitis) is indicated. Newer anti-Gram-positive antibiotics (e.g. linezolid, daptomycin) should only be used on specialist advice.

Prevention

- No specific measures can protect against acquiring CONS, although good hygiene practices in hospitals can help prevent spread of nosocomial strains.
- The most important preventative measure is good care and early removal of indwelling medical devices, the main foci of infection.

Future research

- Use of screening and decolonization treatment to prevent hospital acquired infections with MSSA: this may be effective.
- Improved understanding of the apparent rise of MSSA disease
- More data on the prevalence and screening of MRSA in children.
- Better data on distinguishing true infection due to CONS from contamination, especially in the neonatal setting.
- Use of anti-staphylococcal polyclonal and monoclonal antibodies to prevent neonatal staphylococcal infections.

Further reading

Coia JE, Duckworth GJ, Edwards DI, *et al.* Guidelines for the control and prevention of meticillin-resistant *Staphylococcus aureus* (MRSA) in healthcare facilities. *J Hosp Infect* 2006;**63** Suppl 1:S1–S44.

Gould FK, Brindle R, Chadwick PR, *et al.* Guidelines (2008) for the prophylaxis and treatment of methicillin-resistant *Staphylococcus aureus* (MRSA) infections in the United Kingdom. *J Antimicrob Chemother* 2009;**63**:849–61.

PVL Sub-group of the Steering Group on Healthcare Associated Infection. *Guidance on the Diagnosis and Management of PVL-associated Staphylococcus Aureus Infections (PVL-SA) in England*, 2nd edn. London: Health Protection Agency, 2008.

Streptococcal infections

📖 see also Chapters 5, 6, 8, 15, 16, 25, 27, 28, 29, 30, 34, 36, 38, 39, 40, 44

Name and nature of organism

Streptococci are Gram-positive cocci, appearing either in chains as with β-haemolytic streptococci or viridans streptococci, or as diplococci as with *Streptococcus pneumoniae*. According to the type of haemolysis produced around colonies growing on blood agar, streptococci are classified into two main groups:

- β-haemolytic streptococci = pyogenic streptococci: Colonies are surrounded by a zone of complete haemolysis on blood agar. The cell wall contains Lancefield group-specific antigen which defines the following medically important groups:
  - Group A: *Streptococcus pyogenes*
  - Group B: *Streptococcus agalactiae*
  - Group C and group G: *S. dysgalactiae* and *S. equisimilis* (now classified as one species *S. dysgalactiae* subsp. *equisimilis*)
- α-haemolytic or viridans streptococci: Colonies on blood agar are surrounded by a zone of greenish colour due to altered haemoglobin (partial or incomplete haemolysis). Of medical importance in this group are:
  - *Streptococcus pneumoniae*
  - *Streptococcus anginosus* (previous *S. milleri*) group
  - Other viridans streptococci colonize the oral cavity and may be associated with dental or other oral infections, endocarditis and disease in immunocompromised patients.

β-haemolytic streptococci

Streptococcus pyogenes (GAS)

Epidemiology

- GAS is one of the most important bacterial pathogens of humans.
- It is the most common cause of bacterial tonsillopharyngitis in children between 5 and 15 years of age, accounting for 15–30% of cases.
- About 10% of children carry GAS asymptomatically.
- In temperate climates the incidence of GAS infection peaks during the winter and early spring, coinciding with the influenza season.

Transmission

- Pharyngitis and scarlet fever arise following transmission of GAS via respiratory droplets, usually from a contact with GAS pharyngitis. Occasionally spread via contaminated food.
- Impetigo is acquired from another person with impetigo by direct contact. GAS does not penetrate intact skin. Colonization of healthy

skin usually precedes infection. Any minor (even unrecognized) skin break may result in infection.

Incubation period

- 1–5 days for streptococcal pharyngitis and 7–10 days for impetigo. May be shorter (12–24 hours) in cases with subcutaneous inoculation of organisms (e.g. childbirth or penetrating trauma).

Period of communicability

- When untreated, infectivity lasts for 7–21 days.
- Treatment with antibiotics reduces infectivity to 24 hours.
- Some children carry GAS in the pharynx for weeks or months and may be contagious for this time, although the risk of transmission is low in the absence of acute infection.

Clinical features

- Purulent pharyngotonsillitis is the most common GAS infection. It may be complicated by otitis media, sinusitis, suppurative cervical lymphadenopathy, or tonsillar, retropharyngeal or peritonsillar abscess (quinsy). Meningitis or brain abscess may occur as a rare complication resulting from direct extension of an ear or sinus infection or from bacteraemic spread.
- The Centor criteria are used to predict GAS pharyngitis. The four criteria are fever, anterior cervical lymphadenopathy, tonsillar exudate and absence of cough.
- Scarlet fever usually occurs in association with pharyngitis. It has a characteristic confluent erythematous 'sandpaper-like' rash which is caused by one or more of several erythrogenic exotoxins produced by GAS strains. The rash usually starts on the head and neck and is accompanied by circumoral pallor and a strawberry tongue. Subsequently the rash expands rapidly to cover the trunk followed by the extremities and ultimately desquamates; the palms and soles are usually spared.
- The skin is the second most common site of GAS infections, i.e. impetigo, erysipelas and cellulitis. Eczema, minor trauma, burns, and VZV infection are predisposing conditions.
- Invasive infections are defined as bacteremia, pneumonia ± empyema, or any other infection associated with the isolation of GAS from a normally sterile body site. Invasive infections also include necrotizing fasciitis (characterized by severe pain which is often disproportionate to cutaneous findings especially in the early stage, fever, tachycardia, malaise, myalgias, diarrhoea, anorexia, and hypotension) and spontaneous gangrenous myositis.
- Streptococcal TSS is associated with shock and multiorgan involvement including rapidly progressive renal failure. The most common portals of entry are skin, vagina, pharynx, and mucosa. However, the focus cannot be ascertained in about 50% of cases.
- Neonatal GAS infection results from vertical transmission from the mother (puerperal fever) or from nosocomial acquisition from medical personnel. Early onset disease causes severe sepsis and pneumonia, while late onset neonatal disease can cause severe soft tissue infections.
- Perianal and vulval infection may be seen in young children with marked erythema, itching, and bleeding.

Sequelae

- Acute rheumatic fever (ARF) occurs 2–3 weeks following initial pharyngitis. Manifestations include arthritis, carditis, chorea, subcutaneous nodules and erythema marginatum. ARF remains an important public health problem in resource-poor countries.
- Post-streptococcal glomerulonephritis (PSGN) more commonly follows streptococcal skin infection than pharyngitis. The clinical spectrum varies from asymptomatic microscopic haematuria to acute nephrotic syndrome with frank haematuria, oedema, hypertension, and acute renal failure.
- PANDAS (Paediatric Autoimmune Neuropsychiatric Disorder associated with group A Streptococci) is a term that describes the onset (usually rapid) or an exacerbation of obsessive compulsive disorder or tic disorders following GAS infection. This association remains controversial.

Diagnosis

- *Culture* of GAS from normally sterile sites is diagnostic. Throat culture is the gold standard for the diagnosis of acute pharyngitis due to GAS with a sensitivity of 90–95%.
- *Rapid antigen detection tests (RADT)* are available as 'near patient tests'. RADT have a specificity of ≥95%; sensitivity varies between 65% and 90%. It is recommended that throat culture be performed in children with a negative RADT.
- Neither throat culture nor RADT can differentiate patients with acute GAS pharyngitis from GAS carriers with intercurrent viral illness.
- *Serology*: Antistreptococcal antibody tests including measurement of ASO and anti-deoxyribonuclease B (DNAse B) are useful in the diagnosis of sequelae of streptococcal infection such as ARF. As the antibody response does not occur until 2–3 weeks after the onset of infection, serology is not helpful in the diagnosis of acute GAS infection. The antibody response is frequently aborted by early and appropriate antibiotic therapy.

Management and treatment

Invasive GAS infection

- Supportive (often intensive) care is essential. Established GAS infection is treated with a combination of IV benzylpenicillin and clindamycin. Clindamycin acts by inhibiting protein synthesis; in GAS it suppresses synthesis of bacterial toxins and of the antiphagocytic M-protein.
- In necrotizing fasciitis, debridement of affected tissue is essential. Antibiotic treatment should be started with a broad-spectrum β-lactam (e.g. meropenem) in combination with clindamycin as organisms other than GAS may be involved.
- The use of IVIG may be considered as adjunctive treatment in streptococcal TSS or necrotizing fasciitis in severely ill patients.

Non-invasive GAS infection

- Is treated with penicillin or amoxicillin unless contraindicated.
- GAS remains uniformly susceptible to penicillin. Resistance to erythromycin is currently around 5% in the UK (>25% resistance rates

have been reported from Scandinavia and other European countries). Clindamycin may be effective in erythromycin-resistant strains.

- The great majority of children with pharyngitis do not need an antibiotic or a throat swab. The aims of antimicrobial treatment of GAS proven upper respiratory tract disease are:
  - To reduce duration and severity of illness (by around 1 day)
  - To reduce incidence of acute rheumatic fever and of acute suppurative complications (such as quinsy) (the number of sore throats needed to be treated to prevent one such case is many thousands)
  - To reduce infectivity and transmission to contacts.
- Oral antibiotic therapy has to be continued for 10 days in order to achieve pharyngeal eradication. Treatment failure is more common with penicillin than with other agents, mainly due to problems with compliance.
- In penicillin allergy, a 10-day-course of erythromycin or clarithromycin may be given, or a 5-day-course of azithromycin.
- A 10-day-course of a narrow-spectrum cephalosporin is an alternative in patients with recurrent GAS infection.

Prevention
- Handwashing is the single most important measure to reduce cross-infection.
- If GAS is diagnosed in a newborn baby or its mother, both baby and mother must be treated.
- In case of invasive GAS infection prophylaxis may be offered to close contacts with underlying risk factors. For this purpose, as well as for surveillance purposes, invasive GAS infections have to be notified to public health authorities.
- Secondary prophylaxis for patients who have had rheumatic fever (without residual heart disease) should be continued for 5 years or until the twenty-first birthday, whichever is later, and may have to be lifelong for patients with persistent valvular disease.

Streptococcus agalactiae (GBS)
Organism
- Grows easily on a variety of media; detection from genital/gastrointestinal tract specimens is optimized using selective media
- Serotypes: 9 type-specific capsular polysaccharides (Ia, Ib, II-VIII; 5 serotypes account for 95% of invasive disease); can be further classified according to surface localized protein antigens.

Epidemiology
- Group B streptococcal infection is the leading cause of neonatal sepsis in Europe. Rare cause of invasive disease in children but increasingly reported in pregnant women, immunocompromised, and elderly adults.
- GBS colonizes the genitourinary or gastrointestinal tract of approximately 25% of pregnant women.
- Around 1% of infants born to colonized women may develop early-onset GBS disease (<7 days of age) in the absence of intrapartum antimicrobial prophylaxis.

- Infection usually occurs within the first 3 months of life, two-thirds occur <7 days of age and 90% of these occur on day 1 of life.
- GBS infection occurring later in infancy (after the first 90 days of life) is commonly associated with a history of extreme prematurity or immunodeficiency.

Transmission

- Transmission from mother to baby may occur *in utero* or during passage through the birth canal. Approximately 50% of babies born to colonized mothers will be colonized.
- Exposure to GBS in hospital, home or community may result in late onset disease.

Incubation period

- By definition, less than 7 days in early-onset disease but in majority will be 1–2 days; otherwise unknown.

Clinical features and sequelae

- GBS infection is classified by age of onset into:
  - **Early-onset infection**—defined as <7 days of age but majority present within 24 hours of birth.
  - **Late-onset infection**—usually occurs at 4–5 weeks of age (range 7 to 89 days).
- Sepsis without a focus of infection occurs in 80–85% of cases of early-onset GBS disease. Signs of sepsis are non-specific and include irritability, lethargy, respiratory distress, hypoxia, temperature instability, poor perfusion and hypotension.
- Pneumonia occurs in approximately 10% of cases of early-onset disease. It may be accompanied by septicaemia. In the pre-term baby, clinical findings may be very similar to those of respiratory distress syndrome due to surfactant deficiency. Pleural effusions are more common in GBS pneumonia than in hyaline membrane disease.
- Meningitis may be associated with early-onset GBS infection (7%) or with late-onset infection (25–30%). In late infection, the onset is more insidious and septicaemia is less common. Clinically apparent seizures are more likely to occur in late onset disease.
- Late-onset disease may present as pneumonia, meningitis, osteomyelitis (classically of the upper humerus in a baby—beware late-onset 'Erb's palsy'—think GBS!), cellulitis, neck adenitis, and abscesses. Rare presentations of late-onset infection include endocarditis, myocarditis, pericarditis, pyelonephritis, endophthalmitis, and brain abscess, among others.

Diagnosis

- Identification of Gram-positive cocci in chains on Gram stain of specimens from normally sterile sites in a neonate is an indication for GBS infection, but a positive culture result is necessary for definitive diagnosis. Intrapartum antibiotic prophylaxis may inhibit growth of GBS from blood or CSF cultures.
- RADTs for GBS in body fluids other than CSF are not recommended due to lack of specificity.

- Molecular tests exist but have not yet been established in clinical practice.

Management and treatment

- Supportive care and antimicrobial therapy combined with drainage of abscesses/collections are essential in treatment of GBS disease in neonates and small infants.
- Benzylpenicillin or amoxicillin plus an aminoglycoside should be commenced in cases of suspected GBS infection. Cephalosporins are also effective, but carry an increased risk of resistance development. When GBS infection has been confirmed and a clinical response documented, benzylpenicillin can be given as single therapy.
- Treatment duration for GBS bacteraemia is 10 days and for meningitis at least 14 days, although complicated infections have to be treated for longer.

Prevention

- Intrapartum antibiotics reduce the risk of neonatal GBS infection by interrupting transmission to newborn infants during delivery.
- In the UK a 'risk-based strategy' is in place (in contrast to an antenatal maternal swab-based 'screening strategy' in the USA where the incidence of neonatal GBS infection was much higher). Intrapartum prophylaxis should be given to mothers who have:
  - Previous delivery of an infant with GBS disease
  - GBS isolated in urine or vagina during pregnancy
  - Chorioamnionitis
  - Pre-term delivery
  - Prolonged rupture of membranes
  - Pyrexia during labour.
- GBS vaccines are in development.

Lancefield group C or G streptococci

These are primarily pathogens of horses, cattle, and pigs, which have adapted to the human host. *S. dysgalactiae* subsp. *equisimilis* (Lancefield group C or G) may cause epidemic sore throat in schools, nurseries and other institutions, often associated with unpasteurized milk. Skin infections are less common; endocarditis, septicaemia, or meningitis are very rare.

α-haemolytic streptococci

Streptococcus pneumoniae

Organism

- *S. pneumoniae*, also known as the pneumococcus, is distinguished from other viridans streptococci by its appearance on Gram stain as lancet-shaped diplococci and its sensitivity to optochin and solubility in bile salts.
- Colonies classically have a 'draughtsmen' appearance (sunken centre due to spontaneous autolysis of older organisms).
- The carbohydrate capsule protects the organism against phagocytosis.

- The capsule contains the polysaccharide carbohydrate antigen which is type-specific. 84 capsular types are recognized (91 serotypes).

Epidemiology

- *S. pneumoniae* is a major cause of pneumonia, meningitis, otitis media and sinusitis.
- It is a common commensal of the upper respiratory tract (approximately 50% of preschool children). Carriage rates are highest in children during the winter months.
- Disease occurs in association with a viral URTI or in the presence of a particularly virulent strain. The majority of infections are associated with the lower numbered serotypes.
- Risk factors for severe infection include congenital and acquired immunodeficiency (especially HIV), asplenia, nephrotic syndrome, and sickle cell anaemia.

Transmission

- Transmission is via respiratory droplets. Infectivity is low in most cases, and patient isolation is not required.

Incubation period

- Uncertain, may be as short as 1–3 days.

Clinical features and sequelae

- Pneumococcal pneumonia is usually lobar. Infection in the right upper lobe may be associated with meningism and of the lower lobe with abdominal pain. Pneumonia may be associated with pleural effusion/ empyema.
- Pneumococcal meningitis cannot be distinguished on clinical grounds from that caused by *N. meningitidis* or *H. influenzae*, although the onset may be more gradual compared with the other two agents. Long-term complications (sensorineural deafness and disability) occur more commonly following pneumococcal meningitis.
- Recurrent episodes of meningitis suggest immunodeficiency or a defect in the structures surrounding the CNS, which may or may not be associated with chronic leakage of CSF.
- Septicaemia may occur in young children and in older children post splenectomy or with functional asplenia (e.g. sickle cell disease).
- Pneumococci also cause otitis media, mastoiditis, sinusitis, conjunctivitis, periorbital cellulitis, osteomyelitis, and septic arthritis.
- Complicated invasive pneumococcal infection is associated with HUS.

Laboratory diagnosis

- Gram stain and culture is the mainstay of laboratory diagnosis. However, culture may fail as pneumococci lyse readily.
- Molecular tests are increasingly important in diagnosis of pneumococcal infection.
- Antigen detection tests are often not more sensitive than culture.

Treatment

- In the UK almost all strains (96–98%) remain sensitive to penicillin, whereas in some countries penicillin resistance is a significant problem. Macrolide resistance in the UK was 5% in 2009 (HPA data). Resistance to third-generation cephalosporins is negligible. Treatment is with penicillin or amoxicillin unless contraindicated. Uncomplicated infections other than meningitis due to pneumococci with reduced susceptibility to penicillin usually respond to penicillin or amoxicillin at appropriate dose.

- Cefotaxime or ceftriaxone should be given initially for pneumococcal meningitis.

Prevention

- A 7-valent conjugate pneumococcal vaccination was introduced in September 2006 as part of the UK infant vaccination schedule, given at 2, 4, and 13 months of age, containing serotypes 4, 6B, 9V, 14, 18C,19F, and 23F. There has been rapid serotype replacement with rates of invasive pneumococcal disease almost as high in 2010 as they were prior to the introduction of the conjugate vaccine. This also appeared to happen in some countries of Europe, especially the 19A (although not perhaps as fast as in the UK). From 1 April 2010 the 7-valent conjugate pneumococcal vaccine (Prevenar™) has been replaced with a new vaccine, Prevenar 13x™, which protects against the seven strains contained in the previous vaccine as well as six further common pneumococcal strains—1, 3, 5, 6A, 7F,19A. It remains to be seen how quickly serotype replacement will occur with the new vaccine—there are over 90 serotypes!

Viridans (α-haemolytic) streptococci other than S. pneumoniae

- The *S. anginosus* (previously called *milleri*) group and *S. bovis* are the most important members of this very heterogeneous group. Other viridans streptococci are often not identified further by clinical laboratories but simply reported as 'α-haemolytic' or 'viridans' streptococci.
- Most 'viridans' streptococci are part of the normal oral flora e.g. *S. mitior*, *S. sanguis*, *S. mutans*, *S. salivarius*.
- The *S. anginosus* (previously *milleri*) group which comprises *S. anginosus*, *S. constellatus*, and *S. intermedius* may inhabit the oropharynx, gastrointestinal tract, or vagina.
- *S. bovis* is primarily an animal organism but may be found in the human intestinal tract. It may be α-haemolytic or non-haemolytic and reacts with Lancefield group antigen D.

Epidemiology and clinical features

- The *mutans* group of streptococci has a role in development of dental caries.
- Viridans streptococci are associated with subacute endocarditis in patients with pre-existing valvular damage (congenital heart disease or rheumatic fever). Dental or other surgical procedures in the mouth cause transient bacteraemia; the viridans streptococci have a particular ability to adhere to platelets, fibronectin, fibrinogen and laminin which are present on damaged heart valves.
- Viridans streptococci may cause sepsis in immunocompromised patients, particularly septicaemia secondary to translocation of organisms in patients with mucositis or central line infections.

- *S. bovis* is particularly associated with endocarditis and, in a different association, with underlying malignancy.
- The *S. anginosus* (previously *milleri*) group may cause dental, brain, liver, abdominal, and pelvic abscesses when organisms move from the sites which they colonize to deeper tissues.

Transmission
- Derived from the patient's own flora.

Treatment
- Resistance to penicillin is increasing among viridans streptococci (20–30% in the UK from 2004–2008, HPA data). Treatment of endocarditis may include penicillin or vancomycin ± gentamicin according to results of susceptibility testing.
- *S. bovis* is susceptible to penicillin in >90% of isolates in the UK. As for other viridans streptococci, treatment of endocarditis needs to be planned with a microbiologist.
- The *S. anginosus* (*milleri*) group remains sensitive to penicillin (<5% of isolates in the UK are penicillin-resistant). Macrolide resistance is currently around 10%. Treatment of choice is penicillin or amoxicillin. Macrolides or cephalosporins may be used alternatively where indicated. For initial empirical therapy metronidazole should be added as mixed infections with anaerobes are not uncommon. Abscesses must be drained.
- Infections of the oral cavity may respond to penicillin or amoxicillin, however, due to increasing penicillin resistance among anaerobic organisms, co-amoxiclav is frequently used as first-line agent with clindamycin as alternative in patients allergic to penicillin.

Prevention
- According to NICE guidelines (Clinical Guideline 64, March 2008) routine antibiotic prophylaxis for endocarditis is no longer recommended.
- Oral hygiene is essential in preventing infections due to viridans streptococci and particularly important in patients with valvular heart disease and in immunocompromised patients.

Future research

- The rapid serotype replacement following the introduction of conjugate pneumococcal vaccination requires further study.
- Maternal GBS vaccine development.

Further reading

Centers for Disease Control and Prevention (CDC). Invasive pneumococcal disease before licensure of 13 valent pneumococcal conjugate vaccine—United States 2007. *MMWR Morb Mortal Wkly Rep* 2010;**12**:253–7.

Health Protection Agency. Sensitivity data from Health Protection Report. Weekly report Vol **3** No 46, 20 November 2009.

Ohlsson A, Shah VS. Intrapartum antibiotics for known maternal Group B Streptococcal colonisation. *Cochrane Database Syst Rev* 2009;**8**:CD007467.

Syphilis

📖 see also Chapters 10, 30, 37

Name and nature of organism

- Syphilis is caused by the spirochaete bacterium *Treponema pallidum* subspecies *pallidum*.
- It is worth noting that three other diseases are associated with *T. pallidum*. Yaws (subsp. *pertenue*), Bejel (subsp. *endemicum*) Pinta (subsp. *carateum*) and syphilis all probably diverged from a single disease.
- These clinical diseases cannot be distinguished using current serological tests.

Epidemiology

- Syphilis is now an uncommon infection in developed countries, but remains endemic in many resource-poor countries.
- Although numbers remain small, there has been a resurgence of syphilis in the UK and USA in recent years. Diagnoses of primary and secondary infectious syphilis in UK genitourinary medicine clinics increased from 342 in 2000 to 2524 in 2008. However, congenital syphilis remains rare, with 37 reported cases in 2005 and 9 in 2008.

Transmission

- Syphilis is primarily an STI.
- The incubation period for primary syphilis after sexual transmission is usually between 14 and 28 days (range 10–90 days).
- Infection via transfusion of blood from unscreened donors is another mode of transmission in resource-poor countries.
- Congenital syphilis is usually due to transplacental transmission. This occurs most often where the mother has untreated or inadequately treated early syphilis (i.e. within the first four years after infection). The likelihood of mother-to-baby transmission approaches 100% where the mother has symptomatic early syphilis; overall it is around 70% in early syphilis and 10–20% where the mother has late latent syphilis.
- Mother-to-baby transmission may also occur during delivery by contact of the newborn with infectious genital lesions.
- Congenital disease usually commences *in utero*. Spirochaetes have been detected in the fetus as early as 9–10 weeks of pregnancy.

Clinical features and sequelae

Congenital syphilis

- Congenital infection can be manifest as spontaneous abortion, stillbirth, premature birth, neonatal death, intrauterine growth retardation, hydrops fetalis, neonatal disease, or latent infection.
- At least one-third of cases of transplacental transmission will result in spontaneous abortion or intrauterine death.
- About two thirds of liveborn infected infants do not have any abnormal physical findings at birth but present later.
- Congenital syphilis is usually classified as early congenital syphilis, presenting in children <2 years of age, and late congenital syphilis, where stigmata of congenital infection develop later in childhood or in adult life.

Early congenital syphilis

- The earliest classic sign is usually rhinitis with nasal discharge ('snuffles') that turns bloody later, soon followed by a diffuse, maculopapular, desquamative rash with extensive sloughing of the epithelium, particularly of the palms, soles, and around the mouth and anus. A vesicular rash and bullae may also develop containing large numbers of spirochaetes and are highly infectious.
- Some infants present with nonspecific signs, including rash, generalized lymphadenopathy, anaemia, hepatosplenomegaly, thrombocytopenia and jaundice, with hepatomegaly and hepatitis.
- Osteochondritis/periostitis is common, and may present as pseudo-paralysis of one or more limbs. X-ray abnormalities include metaphyseal lesions, periostitis and ostial lesions which are usually symmetrical and more commonly seen in the long bones. Wimberger's sign (the cat bite) is a classical destruction of the medial part of the proximal tibial metaphysis.
- CNS involvement occurs in at least one-fifth of neonates. The CSF is abnormal in around half of affected babies.
- Necrotizing funisitis is an uncommon sign, seen almost exclusively in preterm infants, caused by inflammation of the umbilical cord.

Late congenital syphilis

- Manifestations include:
  - Hutchinson's triad: interstitial keratitis, Hutchinson's incisors (centrally notched, widely spread, peg-shaped upper central incisors) and VIIIth nerve deafness.
  - Characteristic deformities resulting from osteochondritis, perichondritis and periostitis, including depression of the nasal bridge (saddle nose) and anterior tibial bowing (sabre shin).
  - Recurrent arthropathy and bilateral knee effusions (Clutton's joints), prominent frontal bones and reduced maxillary bones.

- Neurosyphilis is a common late presentation, but the late
  development of cardiovascular syphilis is rare.
- The patient is non-infectious during this stage.

Acquired syphilis

Untreated sexually acquired syphilis progresses through four stages:
primary, secondary, latent, and tertiary. Primary, secondary, and early
latent phase are the infectious stages of syphilis.

Primary syphilis

The primary lesion is a painless indurated ulcer or chancre at the site of
entry of the infection. Untreated, the chancre heals in 2–6 weeks. The
inguinal lymph nodes are moderately enlarged, mobile, discrete and painless. This stage is often unnoticed, especially in females.

Secondary syphilis

Without treatment, spirochaetes later migrate into the bloodstream and
the disease progresses to the secondary stage 6–12 weeks after exposure.
Clinical manifestations include fever, malaise, sore throat, headache, a
generalized maculopapular rash, and condylomata lata in the genital area.
Patients are highly infectious at this stage. Because syphilis is uncommon,
the diagnosis may not be considered when patients present to medical
services with these symptoms.

Latent syphilis

Untreated, the manifestations of secondary syphilis resolve, and the infection becomes asymptomatic and latent. During this stage the number of
spirochaetes in the blood declines, so that after 2–4 years only dormant
bacteria remain in deeper organs and tissues.

Tertiary syphilis

Around one-third of untreated patients subsequently develop tertiary
syphilis, at least 10–20 years later. Gummas may affect any organ in the
body. Other late manifestations include cardiovascular syphilis (especially
aortitis) and neurosyphilis.

Diagnosis

General principles

- In primary, secondary, and early congenital syphilis, examination
  by dark-ground microscopy or immunofluorescent staining of
  mucocutaneous lesions is the quickest and most direct laboratory
  method of establishing the diagnosis.
- *T. pallidum* cannot be cultured *in vitro*.
- Molecular methods such as PCR can be used to detect *T. pallidum*
  DNA in clinical material.
- Serological tests are the mainstay of screening and diagnosis. There
  are two types of serological test: treponemal and non-treponemal.
  Neither test is specific for *T. pallidum* subspecies *pallidum*. This is rarely
  a problem in Europe where other treponemal infections do not occur,

but needs to be considered when interpreting serological results from patients from abroad.

- Non-treponemal antibody tests use non-specific antigens. The commonest are the Rapid-Plasma-Reagin (RPR) and Venereal Disease Research Laboratory (VDRL) tests. These tests have a high rate of biological false positives. They become reactive 4–7 days after development of the primary lesion and are always reactive in secondary syphilis. Non-treponemal tests are mainly used to monitor the response to treatment, because titres decrease after effective treatment. They can be regarded as a sort of 'syphilis ESR' and should not be used to diagnose syphilis without confirmation of seropositivity with a treponemal test.

- Treponemal tests use specific treponemal antigens. These include EIAs for detection of IgG and/or IgM, the *T. pallidum* haemagglutination assay (TPHA) or *T. pallidum* particle agglutination assay (TPPA), and the fluorescent treponemal antibody-absorbed test (FTA-ABS). With the exception of EIAs for IgM, these tests remain positive indefinitely.

- EIAs are now the most commonly used screening tests for syphilis. EIAs that detect specific anti-treponemal IgM antibodies are useful in diagnosing congenital and early acquired syphilis.

Diagnosis of congenital syphilis

- *T. pallidum* can be demonstrated directly by dark-ground microscopy and/or PCR of exudates from suspicious mucocutaneous lesions or nasal discharge or placenta if suspected at delivery.

- Serological testing should be performed on the infant's blood (not cord blood).
  - Where screening tests are negative and there are no signs of congenital infection, no further testing is necessary.
  - Infants with a positive screening test must be investigated further to determine whether the infant has been infected or the seropositivity relates to passive transfer of maternal antibodies.
  - A positive IgM test and/or a sustained fourfold or greater difference of VDRL/RPR titre or TPPA titre above that of the mother is diagnostic of congenital syphilis.
  - Where the IgM is negative and other tests are reactive with titres below those diagnostic of congenital syphilis, previously reactive tests should be repeated at 3, 6, and 12 months of age, or until all tests become negative. The IgM should be repeated at the age of 3 months in case the infant's response is delayed.

- Further investigations to assess infants with congenital syphilis include: FBC, LFTs, U&Es, CSF examination for cells, protein and serological tests, X-rays of long bones and ophthalmic assessment.

Management and treatment

General principles

- Manage with a genitourinary medicine physician.
- Penicillin remains the drug of choice for treatment of syphilis during pregnancy.

- Recommendations for penicillin G dosage and duration of therapy vary according to the stage of disease and clinical manifestations.
- Alternative antimicrobial treatment options include azithromycin and ceftriaxone, but these agents have not been proven to be as effective as penicillin in preventing transplacental transmission.
- Consider other STIs.
- Adequate early treatment of a pregnant woman with syphilis usually, but not always, ensures that the fetus will be unaffected.

Management of infants with congenital syphilis
Groups of infants who need full treatment for congenital syphilis
- Infants with proven or probable congenital syphilis
- Infants born to mothers with syphilis who have had:
  - Treatment only within 4 weeks' of delivery
  - Treatment with drugs other than penicillin
  - No treatment or inadequate treatment
  - No documentation of treatment.
- If mothers have been treated adequately with a documented history or a full treatment course of a penicillin-based regimen more than 4 weeks prior to delivery, and there is no evidence of reinfection or relapse, serological monitoring of the infant alone is recommended.

Treatment regimens
- Benzylpenicillin sodium 12 hourly in the first 7 days of life and 8 hourly thereafter for 3 days (10 days in total) is the preferred treatment regimen.
- Alternatively, procaine penicillin daily IM for 10 days.
- If >1 day of treatment is missed, the entire course should be restarted.

Prevention

- All pregnant women are screened for syphilis at the initial antenatal visit. Additionally, for patients at high risk, serological testing should be repeated at 28–32 weeks of gestation and at delivery.
- Acquired syphilis may be prevented by sexual education and by identification and treatment of infected individuals.

Further reading

British Association for Sexual Health and HIV (BASHH). UK National Guidelines on the Management of Syphilis 2008. *Int J STD AIDS* 2008;**19**:729–40.

Chakraborty R, Luck S. Syphilis is on the increase: the implications for child health. *Arch Dis Child* 2008;**93**:105–9.

French P, Gomberg M, Jonier M et al. IUSTI: 2008 European Guidelines for the management of Syphilis. *Int J STD AIDS* 2009;**20**:300–9.

Tetanus

see also Chapters 30, 40

Name and nature of organism

- *Clostridium tetani* is an obligate anaerobic spore-forming Gram-positive bacillus.
- Spores are found in soil, house dust, animal intestines, and human faeces and remain viable for years.
- Wounds become contaminated with *C. tetani* spores. Spore germination is favoured by anaerobic and acidic conditions, resulting in release of exotoxin (a neurotoxin—tetanospasmin).

Epidemiology

- Tetanus is rare in Western Europe. In the UK, <20 cases of tetanus are reported each year. The main risk groups are the elderly (who may not be fully vaccinated) and injecting drug users. In resource-poor countries neonates are another important risk group, but neonatal tetanus has been eliminated in Western Europe.
- Worldwide, tetanus remains a major public health problem, causing 200 000 to 300 000 deaths each year.
- The mortality rate for untreated tetanus is up to 90%, but with high quality intensive care it is less than 10%. The mortality rate of those who have received 1 or 2 doses of vaccine, but not a previous complete course, is around half that of the unvaccinated.

Transmission and incubation period

- Tetanus is transmitted by direct inoculation of *C. tetani* spores in soil and animal manure: it is not transmitted from person to person.
- Traumatic wounds (most commonly), burns, ulcers, gangrene, frostbite, and the neonatal umbilical stump are portals of entry.
- Incubation period: 4–21 days (around 10 days) after injury.

Clinical features and sequelae

- Tetanus may be generalized (the most common form) or localized. Complications may be due to direct toxin effect or secondary to spasms.

Generalized tetanus
- Usually commences with muscles spasms, especially of the jaw muscles (trismus or lock jaw).
- As the disease progresses muscle stiffness and spasms become more generalized.
- Mild stimuli such as noise, light and touch may trigger reflex spasms. Other symptoms and signs include facial grimacing (risus sardonicus), dysphagia, restlessness.
- Without supportive care the disease usually progresses to death.
- Tetanus neonatorum is generalized tetanus in neonates born to unimmunized mothers caused by unhygienic delivery and/or application of local treatments to the umbilical stump. The baby first presents with generalized weakness, apnoea, and poor feeding. This progresses to classic tetanic spasms and opisthotonus. Mortality is very high, as is residual neurological damage in survivors.

Localized tetanus
- This presentation is less common, and usually occurs in people who are partially immune.
- Symptoms and signs remain localized to the region of the infection, with weakness of the involved extremity, and intense painful spasms in severe cases.
- Cephalic tetanus is a rare form of localized tetanus secondary to craniofacial injuries or infections. The incubation period is usually very short (1–2 days), presenting with cranial nerves palsies.
- Cephalic tetanus is more likely to progress to generalized tetanus.

Diagnosis
- Because tetanus is a rare disease the first challenge is to suspect the diagnosis, based on the clinical history. It is important to remember that the wound site may not be obvious.
- Obtain advice from a microbiology laboratory.
- Bacterial cultures from the wound site are only positive in a few cases.
- Detection of *C. tetani* neurotoxin in serum: blood must be collected early before anti-toxin is administered.

Management and treatment
- Early recognition and treatment can be life-saving.
- Human tetanus immunoglobulin should be given immediately IV (preferably), or IM in multiple sites. In the UK this is available from the HPA.
- Toxin production at the site of infection is reduced by thorough wound toilet and antimicrobial therapy, usually IV metronidazole or benzylpenicillin.
- Muscle spasm can be reduced by isolating the patient from noise and bright light stimuli. Sedation with benzodiazepines can decrease rigidity, and control spasms. Diazepam alone or anticonvulsants such as phenobarbital and chlorpromazine can be used.

- Respiratory failure is managed in a specialist unit by tracheostomy and assisted ventilation after neuromuscular blockade. Paralysing agents such as pancuronium can worsen sympathetic overdrive: magnesium sulphate infusions are used to reduce this.

Prevention

Tetanus vaccine

- Primary prevention is with tetanus vaccine. This is made from a cell-free purified *C. tetani* toxin that is treated with formaldehyde to turn into toxoid, and adsorbed onto an adjuvant.
- In the UK, it is only available as a component of Diphtheria, Tetanus, Polio (DTP) with or without Hib.
- Individuals who have received five doses at appropriate intervals are considered fully immunized. Routine boosters every 10 years are no longer considered necessary.
  - Primary immunization consists of three doses of tetanus-containing vaccine with an interval of 1 month between each dose, given at any stage from 2 months up to 10 years of age.
  - A first booster dose is given around 3 years after the primary course, and a second booster after another 10 years.

Management of wounds

- Thorough cleaning of all wounds is essential.
- The opportunity to check that the injured individual is fully immunized against tetanus should always be taken.
- Tetanus-prone wounds are:
  - Wounds or burns that require surgical intervention that is delayed more than 6 hours.
  - Wounds or burns that show a significant degree of devitalized tissue or a puncture-type injury.
  - Wounds containing foreign bodies, soil or manure, or compound fractures.
  - Wounds or burns in patients who have systemic sepsis.
  - Injecting drug users with skin abscesses and poor hygiene.
- Human tetanus immunoglobulin may be indicated for patients who have sustained tetanus-prone wounds.

Future research

Long-term follow-up to determine if early childhood immunization will provide lifelong protection to the elderly.

Further reading

Rushdy AA, White JM, Ramsay ME, Crowcroft NS. Tetanus in England and Wales 1984–2000. *Epidemiol Infect* 2003;**130**:71–7.

Chapter 109

Threadworm

📖 see also Chapter 22

Name and nature of organism

- *Enterobius vermicularis* is a small white roundworm with a threadlike appearance, hence it is commonly referred to as the threadworm or pinworm.
- The adult female worm measures about 9–12mm in length and is much larger than the male worm, which is approximately 2.5mm long.
- Humans are the only reservoir. Ingested threadworm eggs hatch in the duodenum. Within 5–6 weeks the larvae develop into adult worms and live in the terminal ileum, appendix, caecum, and ascending colon. The female worm can live for 4–6 weeks and the male worm for only 2 weeks. Threadworms do not multiply within the body. At the end of the life cycle the gravid female worms migrate to the perianal region, where they deposit up to 10 000 eggs and die. This occurs usually during the night, as inactivity of the host causes the worms to migrate. The sticky eggs adhere to the anal skin and embryonate to become infective within 4–6 hours.

Epidemiology

- Threadworm infection is the most common helminth infection throughout the world, and the most common parasitic infection of children in Europe.
- It is most frequent among preschool and school-aged children up to the age of 10 years. Western European studies indicate that up to 20% of children are affected at any one time.
- Children living in overcrowded conditions or in institutions are most affected. However, higher social economic status and good sanitation do not prevent from infection.
- Within a household other family members, most often the mother and other children, are commonly infected.

Transmission and incubation period

- The most common mode of transmission of eggs is via hands, particularly underneath fingernails, from scratching the anal/perianal region.
- From contaminated hands, eggs may be passed directly into the mouth or indirectly via toys, food, etc.

- Transmission may occur by exposure to viable eggs in soiled bed linen, house dust, or clothing. Eggs can remain infectious for up to 2 weeks.
- Reinfection is common, and occurs either by autoinfection or by infection following ingestion of eggs from another person.
- Another possible means of transmission is retro-infection, in which eggs hatch on the anal mucosa and larvae migrate into the large intestine.
- The incubation period is 2–6 weeks.

Clinical features and sequelae

- Most threadworm infections are asymptomatic.
- The most common symptom is pruritus ani—itchy bottom—(mainly at night), which varies from mild itching to acute pain. Scratching of the perianal region may lead to excoriation of the skin and secondary bacterial infection.
- Some children present because worms have been seen on the perianal skin or, less commonly, in stools.
- General symptoms may include anorexia, weight loss, restlessness, irritability, and insomnia.
- It has been suggested that threadworms can cause symptoms resembling appendicitis (without mucosal invasion) and threadworms have been found in the lumen of the appendix, but the relationship between threadworm infection and appendicitis is not clear.
- Uncommonly, vulvovaginitis with pruritus vulvae and mucoid vaginal discharge may occur in young girls.
- Rarely, abnormal migration of the worms leads to ectopic disease, such as pelvic, cervical, vulvar, and peritoneal granulomas, which may be mistaken for other disease processes. Threadworms have also been found in the inguinal area, the prostate, the liver, and even the lungs. Tissue invasion does not occur.

Diagnosis

- Occasionally, adult worms may be seen in the perianal region, typically 2–3 hours after the child is asleep.
- Detection of eggs by microscopic examination of material collected using a moistened perianal swab is the preferred diagnostic method. This is more sensitive than, and has largely superseded, the use of transparent adhesive tape applied to the perianal skin.
- Microscopy of stool specimens is not recommended, because very few eggs are present in stool. The detection rate from faecal samples is only 5–15%.

Management and treatment

- Treatment is indicated if threadworms have been seen or their eggs detected.
- Treatment should also be given if the test result is negative, but symptoms are highly suggestive.
- The drug of choice is mebendazole, which can be given in children >2 years of age. A second dose may be given 2 weeks later because of the frequency of reinfection. Mebendazole acts by inhibiting the uptake of glucose by the worm. It is poorly absorbed from the gastrointestinal tract, and side effects are rare. It should not be used in pregnancy.
- Piperazine may be given to children >3 months of age at a schedule of two doses 2 weeks apart. It acts by blocking the neurotransmitter acetylcholine in the worm, leading to paralysis. Piperazine preparations often contain senna or another laxative, to aid the expulsion of the paralysed worm. As piperazine is systemically absorbed, its side effect profile is less favourable than mebendazole.
- As anthelmintics have no effect on threadworm eggs, treatment needs to be combined with strict hygiene measures to prevent reinfection. These measure include:
  • Good hand hygiene before each meal and after using the toilet
  • Having a bath or shower every morning to remove large amounts of eggs laid during the night
  • Frequent changes of underwear, night clothes and bed sheets
  • Fingernails kept short
  • Avoidance of nail biting and finger sucking
  • Wearing of close fitting night clothes to discourage night time scratching
  • Avoidance of sharing towels/flannels
  • Cleaning and vacuuming of the home daily for several days after treatment of cases
  • Elimination of overcrowded living accommodation.
- It is recommended that all family members are treated simultaneously in order to minimize reinfection. Hygiene measures should continue for 6 weeks.
- It is not necessary to exclude children from school and other day care facilities, as asymptomatic infection is often involved in transmission, and threadworm is generally a mild illness in childhood.

Prevention

- Maintenance of high standards of personal hygiene can reduce the risk of threadworm infection.
- Children should be taught to wash their hands with soap and water regularly, particularly after using the toilet and before eating or preparing food.

Further reading

Clinical knowledge summaries. Threadworm. Available at ℰ www.cks.nhs.uk/threadworm. (Accessed 1 February 2011)

Tinea

📖 see also Chapter 38

Introduction

- Dermatophytic infestations are common in childhood.
- Caused by a group of spore-forming fungi.
- Of 40 species identified, a third are important causes of disease.
- Anthropophilic and zoophilic species primarily infect humans and animals, respectively, while geophilic species reside in the soil.
- Infections tend to become chronic if not treated.
- Asymptomatic carriage is relatively common.

The clinical picture and management depends on the site involved. The organism responsible changes from time to time and place to place. All four clinical conditions are found worldwide.

Tinea capitis (scalp ringworm)

Name and nature of organism

- *Trichophyton tonsurans* and *Trichophyton violaceum* are the most prevalent anthropophilic species, which tend to be restricted to particular geographic areas.
- *Microsporum canis* is the most prevalent zoophilic species and is found worldwide.
- The main reservoirs for *M. canis* are cats, dogs, and a number of other mammals.
- *Trichophyton schoenleinii*, an anthrophilic species, causes favus, a clinically distinct form of tinea capitis.

Epidemiology

- The prevalence varies between and within countries.
- In many areas, it is the most common dermatophytosis of childhood.
- Of physician visits for tinea capitis in USA, 85.6% were in those <15 years old.
- Reported in 2.5% of south-east London school children.
- Disease is commonest in 3–7 year olds.
- The prevalence has increased in the past 2–3 decades.
- In North America and the UK, *T. tonsurans* is responsible for more than 90% of cases of tinea capitis, whereas previously *Microsporum* species predominated.
- *M. canis* is still the most important organism in Europe.
- Anthropophilic species may be linked to immigration from Africa.

Transmission and incubation period

- Transmission is by passage of spores (arthroconidia) or infected hairs by close contact, often head to head.
- Children who are household contacts of symptomatic cases are frequently (50% or more) carriers. This is much less so for adults.
- After about four human-to-human transmissions, *M. canis* lose virulence and returns to an animal host to survive.
- Indirect spread from combs, brushes, hats, etc. is unclear.
- The incubation period is unknown.

Clinical features and sequelae

- There is usually hair loss (alopecia) with hairs breaking at the scalp surface.
- There may be patchy areas of dandruff-like scaling, erythema and oedema.
- Lymphadenopathy often occurs.
- **Kerion** is an inflamed fungal abscess. It presents as a boggy mass covered with pustules.
- **Favus** (Latin for honeycomb), a particular presentation, is characterized by yellowish, circular, cup-shaped crusts (scutula) grouped together to give the appearance of a piece of honeycomb, each a few millimetres across, with a hair projecting through the centre. These increase in size and become crusted over, so that the characteristic appearance can only be seen round the edge of the scab. Growth continues to take place for several months, when scab and scutulum come away, leaving a shining bald area.

Diagnosis

- Alopecia areata usually has no local inflammation or scaling. Hairs in tinea are said to look like commas, whereas those in alopecia areata are like exclamation marks. Seborrheic dermatitis usually has no hair loss.
- Diagnosis based on clinical presentation may be inaccurate, and so should ideally be confirmed by microscopy of hairs and hair fragments, pre-treated with potassium hydroxide, which may reveal fungal spores. To get a suitable sample, scrape the affected areas with a blunt scalpel, to collect affected hairs and scalp scales.
- Fungal cultures can be performed for precise identification of the species but is not always reliable and it can take 6 weeks to get results. It is not routinely of value.
- Under Wood's light (UV light) hairs infected with *Microsporum audouinii* and *M. canis* produce a brilliant yellow-green fluorescence, while *Trichophyton schoenleinii* causes a dull green fluorescence. However, *T. tonsurans,* is not detectable.
- A PCR diagnostic test has been developed specifically for *T. tonsurans*.

Management and treatment

- Topical treatment is unlikely to eradicate symptomatic infection.
- Griseofulvin, a fungistatic, given daily for a period of 6–8 weeks is usually successful in treating the condition and has been the treatment

of choice for decades. Give with fatty meal—continue for 1–2 weeks after clinical resolution.

- Terbinafine (an allylamine) and fluconazole (azoles), are as efficacious as griseofulvin in infections caused by *Trichophyton* spp. Even though more expensive than griseofulvin, terbinafine, a fungicidal, is preferable for *Trichophyton* infestations as treatment for 2–4 weeks is sufficient.
- Terbinafine may not be as effective as griseofulvin in treatment for *Microsporum* species.
- For the first two weeks of therapy, twice weekly, topical treatment, with a shampoo, such as either selenium sulphide or ketoconazole, may be given in addition to oral therapy.
- Carriers should also be given a 2-week course of topical therapy.

Prevention

- As symptomatic children are likely to have been infested for some while, isolation is not necessary, but treatment should be prompt.
- Hats, combs, hairbrushes, etc. should not be shared.
- If the infecting agent is *M. canis*, an animal source should be sought and treated.
- Further cases within a household should be treated.
- When an outbreak occurs in a school, it is advised that children should have a scalp inspection, using scalp brushes.

Tinea corporis (body ringworm)

Name and nature of organism

- *T. rubrum* is the commonest cause.

Epidemiology

- Commonest in children, before they reach puberty.
- Of physician visits for tinea corporis in USA, 46.0% were in those <15 years old.

Transmission and incubation period

- Direct contact with an infected person or animal, for example dogs, cats, guinea pigs, and cattle.
- **Tinea corporis gladiatorum** refers to infestation as a result of contact sports, such as wrestling and judo.
- Indirect contact with contaminated items such as clothing, towels, bedclothes, and chairs handled by infected people.
- Incubation period of 2–4 weeks.

Clinical features and sequelae

- Round or oval red scaly patches, often less red and scaly, or even healed, in the middle, giving rise to an **annular** appearance. One ring may be superimposed on another. Usually pruritic.
- In tinea corporis gladiatorum, the disease is often on the head, neck and arms, the areas likely to come into contact with the infected skin of participants in close contact sports.

Diagnosis

- Usually clinical. If any doubt or unresponsive to treatment, take skin scrapings for microscopy and culture.

Management and treatment

- Except for chronic or widespread disease, topical therapy is the first line treatment.
- Topical terbinafine applied as a 1% cream, gel or solution, once or twice daily for 7–14 days results in clinical cure rates ranging from 75% to 84%.
- Treatment with a combination topical antifungal/corticosteroid cream can prolong the course of therapy for months as inflammation may be suppressed but disease not cured. Best not used.
- If unresponsive or widespread disease is present, use an oral antifungal agent, such as griseofulvin or terbinafine.

Prevention

- Clothing, towels, bedding, etc. should be carefully washed and not shared with infected individuals. No exclusion from school.

Tinea pedis (athletes' foot)

Name and nature of organism

- *T. rubrum*, followed by *T. interdigitale,* both anthropophilic species, are the commonest cause.

Epidemiology

- A study in Australian schoolchildren found a prevalence of 2.1% in 4–6 year olds, rising to 9.7% in 16–18 year olds. It was about 50% commoner in males. Less than 40% of those with a confirmed diagnosis said they had disease when asked on questionnaire.

Transmission and incubation period

- Disease is spread by sharing infected towels, socks, etc. as well as walking barefoot on an infected surface
- Incubation period is 2–3 weeks.

Clinical features and sequelae

- Typically cracking and fissuring of the skin in the webbing between the toes, with pruritus.
- Less commonly, there may be a more diffuse, scaling pattern involving the sole and side of the foot (moccasin type). May also have vesicles and blisters.

Diagnosis

- Usually clinical, with microscopy if unresponsive to treatment.

Management and treatment

- Topical treatment is usually adequate, the most effective being terbinafine. Other topical agents such as azoles, ciclopiroxolamine, butenafine, tolnaftate, and undecanoate are also effective. Relapse is common.

- Of oral treatments, griseofulvin has been the mainstay, but newer, treatments such as terbinafine and the azoles have a higher cure rate. On the basis of limited comparative data, terbinafine appears most efficacious.

Prevention

- Footwear should keep feet cool and dry. Cotton socks are best.
- Feet should be dried well, after washing, especially between toes.
- Towels should be washed well and not shared.
- Infected feet should be covered when walking in public places
- Avoid scratching affected skin as this may spread the infection.

Tinea unguium (onychomycosis, infestation of the nails)

Name and nature of organism

- *T. rubrum* is the commonest cause of toe onychomycosis (about 80%), whereas it accounts for <20% of finger onychomycosis, most being due to *Candida* species. Rare in children.

Clinical features and sequelae

- Onychomycosis, in general, is classified clinically as distal and lateral subungual onychomycosis (DLSO), superficial white onychomycosis (SWO), proximal subungual onychomycosis (PSO), candidal onychomycosis, and total dystrophic onychomycosis.
- In DLSO, infection starts at the distal end of the nail bed, often laterally, and spreads proximally, causing hyperkeratosis and onycholysis. The nail is pitted. It is due to *T. rubrum* in the majority of cases. There is nearly always tinea pedis.
- SWO is less common and affects the nail plate rather than the nail bed. The surface of the nail is flaky and the colour white rather than cream. Tine pedis is not usually present. It is usually due to *T. mentagrophyes*.
- *Candida* infection of the nail plate generally results from paronychia and starts near the nail fold (the cuticle). The nail fold is swollen, tender and red. White, yellow, green, or black marks appear on the nearby nail and spread.

Diagnosis

- Differential diagnosis includes other fungal infections such as *Candida albicans*, *Scopulariopsis brevicaulis*, and *Fusariоum* species (more likely with finger nail infections), eczema of the nails, and congenital or acquired chronic nail dystrophies.
- The diagnosis should be confirmed microbiologically by taking nail clippings, examining them microscopically and attempting culture.

Management and treatment

- There is little evidence that topical treatments are effective. There is some evidence that ciclopiroxolamine and butenafine are effective but they need to be applied daily for prolonged periods (at least a year). Oral treatment is therefore essential.
- Oral therapy with terbinafine is probably superior to that with griseofulvin, but there are few good comparative trials.
- Any treatment should continue until, at least, all signs of infection have gone.
- Terbinafine should be given for at least 6–8 weeks (fingernails) or 3–4 months (toenails).
- The addition of topical therapy may improve cure rates.
- Removal of the nails is not indicated.

Prevention

- Exclusion from school is not necessary.
- Tight footwear and trauma to the nails predispose to tinea.

Future research

There is a strong need for large randomized controlled trials of the optimal management of tinea infections.

Further reading

Bell-Syer SEM, Hart R, Crawford F, Torgerson DJ, Tyrrell W, Russell I. Oral treatments for fungal infections of the skin of the foot. *Cochrane Database Syst Rev* 2002;(**2**):CD003584.

Borman AM, Campbell CK, Fraser M, Johnson EM. Analysis of the dermatophyte species isolated in the British Isles between 1980 and 2005 and review of worldwide dermatophyte trends over the last three decades. *Med Mycol* 2007;**45**:131–41.

Crawford F, Hollis S. Topical treatments for fungal infections of the skin and nails of the foot. *Cochrane Database Syst Rev* 2007;**3**:CD001434.

Ginter-Hanselmayer G, Weger W, Ilkit M, Smolle J. Epidemiology of tinea capitis in Europe: current state and changing patterns. *Mycoses* 2007;**50** Suppl 2:6–13.

González U, Seaton T, Bergus G, Jacobson J, Martínez-Monzón C. Systemic antifungal therapy for tinea capitis in children. *Evid Based Child Health* 2009;**4**:132–221.

Toxocariasis

📖 see also Chapters 3, 31, 45

Name and nature of organism

- Toxocariasis is human infection caused by the dog roundworm *Toxocara canis* or (less commonly) cat roundworm *Toxocara cati*.
- 50% of puppies are infected and produce the highest number of eggs (up to 10 000 eggs/g of faeces). Around 20% of adult dogs are infected, and they produce eggs at lower levels.
- Eggs passed in dog and cat faeces are initially unembryonated and non-infectious: they become infective in the environment 10–21 days after shedding, and thereafter can remain viable for years.
- The human is an accidental host; development stops at the larval stage, causing toxocariasis, visceral larva migrans, or ocular toxocariasis.

Epidemiology

- Toxocariasis occurs worldwide.
- Around 2–10% of the population in western world is seropositive with higher rates in children.
- The incidence of symptomatic toxocariasis is difficult to ascertain. Only around 10 cases are reported each year in the UK, but this is likely to be an underestimate of the true incidence: the incidence of ocular toxocariasis alone may be up to 6–10 per 100 000 children.
- Severe disease occurs sporadically and affects mainly children between 2 and 4 years of age: this is the age group that is most prone to exposure and ingestion of eggs.

Transmission and incubation period

- Direct or indirect transmission of infective Toxocara eggs from contaminated soil or surfaces contaminated with animal faeces.
- Toxocariasis may also be transmitted via handling or ingestion of undercooked meat.
- After ingestion, embryonated eggs hatch in the intestine, larvae penetrate intestinal wall and migrate to the liver and other tissues via lymphatic and circulatory system.
- From the liver, larvae spread to other tissues, particularly lungs, abdominal organs and brain (visceral larvae migrans) or the eyes (ocular larva migrans), and induce granulomatous lesions. Humans tend to get *either* visceral *or* ocular larva migrans.
- Incubation period: weeks or months, ocular manifestation may take 4–10 years to develop.

Clinical features and sequelae

Most cases are asymptomatic: when symptoms do occur they are caused by migration of second stage larvae. There are two major forms of symptomatic toxocariasis:

- Visceral larva migrans
  - Clinical presentation depends on the organs affected. It is classically an infection of younger children.
  - Symptoms include coughing, fever, nausea and vomiting, abdominal pain, headaches, and changes in behaviour and sleep.
  - Signs include lymphadenopathy, hepatosplenomegaly, fever and pallor. Occasionally there may be signs of pneumonia, cardiac dysfunction, nephrosis, and neurological lesions (fits, epilepsy, pareses, and transverse myelitis). An asthma-like syndrome can occur.
  - Most children will have a marked eosinophilia and hypergammaglobulinaemia.
  - The term covert toxocariasis is sometimes used to refer to less serious cases of visceral larva migrans.
- Ocular toxocariasis
  - Usually affects only one eye, and presents in older children.
  - Loss of visual acuity over days or weeks is commonest symptom.
  - Other clinical features may include red eye, white pupil, fixed pupil, retinal fibrosis, retinal detachment.
  - Presentations may be confused with retinoblastoma.

Diagnosis

- Demonstration of larvae is difficult and biopsy of the lesions is seldom justified. Serological diagnosis by ELISA is now the test of choice. The sensitivity depends on the worm burden in the patient.
- In ocular toxocariasis, serology is less reliable. It may be possible to demonstrate larvae in vitreous and/or aqueous humour, but often the diagnosis is based on clinical findings alone.

Management, treatment, and prevention

- Treatment is indicated for symptomatic cases only.
- Albendazole orally for 5 days is the standard treatment
- Mebendazole, thiabendazole, and diethylcarbamazine are also effective. Diethylcarbamazine may be the most effective treatment, but is less well tolerated: often reserved as a second line agent.
- Systemic corticosteroid therapy is indicated in ocular toxocariasis and serious visceral larva migrans.
- Eosinophilia may persist for months after clinical cure. Regular treatment of dogs and bitches as well as newborn puppies with anthelmintics is essential, with prompt disposal of animal faeces.

Toxoplasmosis

📖 see also Chapters 3, 10, 15, 19, 20, 31, 45

Name and nature of causative organism

- *Toxoplasma gondii*—an obligate intracellular protozoan parasite.
- It exists in three forms (stages)—tachyzoites are seen in acute infection, bradyzoites in cysts are seen in chronic latent infection, and sporozoites are the sexual form in oocysts that occur only in intestines of the cat family.

Transmission and incubation period

- Worldwide—many species of mammal are infected.
- Cats are definitive hosts and become infected by feeding on mice containing bradyzoites.
- The parasite replicates in the cat small intestine and oocysts are then shed 3–30 days after primary infection.
- The oocysts mature and sporulate outside the cat and may be ingested by intermediate hosts including cattle, pigs, and sheep. Tissue cysts develop in the organs of these animals.
- Infection of the human results from ingestion of inadequately cooked meat or from infected cat faeces.
- Most infection in early childhood has been thought to result from congenital infection: transmission occurs at any stage in pregnancy.
- Infection can occur postnatally and may be important.
- The incubation period is approximately 7 days (may be 21 days).

Epidemiology

- The incidence of congenital toxoplasmosis in northern Europe and the USA is thought to about ≤1 per 10–100 000 births.
- Congenital infection is associated with maternal primary infection in pregnancy. Around 50% of women in western Europe are seropositive by childbearing age.
- About one third of infected women produce an infected fetus; first trimester infection tends to produce more severe disease.
- By adolescence 10–30% of infected infants will have developed retino-choroiditis.
- In a UK surveillance study performed from 2002 to 2004 involving paediatricians, ophthalmologists and the Toxoplasma laboratory service 38 children with *Toxoplasma* infection were identified—22 (58%) were classified as congenital infection (3.4/100 000 livebirths); 2 (9%) were

stillborn; 7 (32%) had intracranial abnormalities and/or developmental delay, five of whom also had retino-choroiditis; 10 (45%) had retino-choroiditis alone. A further 16 children (42%) had been infected after birth and had retino-choroiditis.
- There appears to be considerable regional variation in the disability produced by infection; eye lesions in Brazil for instance are more frequent and severe than those in northern Europe.

Clinical features

Acquired toxoplasmosis
- This may be asymptomatic or a mild infection with low-grade fever, headache, myalgia, sore throat, and lymphadenopathy.
- Generalized cervical lymphadenopathy may last several weeks.
- In those with immunodeficiency including HIV infection, encephalitis or pneumonitis may develop.
- In children with AIDS the commonest presentation is with focal neurological signs, including hemiparesis, speech abnormalities, and convulsions. The CT scan classically shows multiple bilateral ring enhancing lesions, often at the cortico-medullary junction.

Congenital toxoplasmosis
- Characterized by the classic triad of choroido-retinito-choroiditis, hydrocephalus from aqueduct stenosis, and intracranial calcification.
- CT scan may show classic parenchymal and periventricular calcification.
- Other features include rashes, lymphadenopathy, hepatomegaly, splenomegaly, jaundice and thrombocytopenia.
- There is a high mortality and morbidity in the small number of infants with the classic triad and systemic illness.
- Survivors may develop epilepsy and learning difficulties.
- In those with retino-choroiditis the macula is often involved. Relapsing disease produces a combination of old scars and active disease. Visual problems (usually unilateral) tend not to present until later childhood.

Diagnosis

- This is complex and advice should be obtained from the Toxoplasmosis Reference Laboratory.
- In normal children a fourfold rise of IgG, or the presence of specific IgM or IgA can be diagnostic. In the immunocompromised child the presence of specific *T. gondii* IgG demonstrates the possibility of reactivation causing disease.

In pregnancy
- Some countries such as France have screening programmes in pregnancy but their value and benefits are not entirely clear. Cost efficacy of screening programmes depends on the varying prevalence of infection.

- All pregnant women should be counselled to avoid handling cat litter and eating under-cooked meat.
- The investigation of possible infection during pregnancy has to establish whether this occurred before or after conception.
- IgG assays are used in combination with the IgM EIA. The Sabin Feldman Dye test is also used to detect previous infection. An IgG avidity test can also be used to identify when infection developed. The tests are complex and further advice is provided by a Toxoplasma reference unit.

Fetal testing

- With serological evidence of maternal infection there may be an indication for cordocentesis to obtain specimens for both serology and detection of the parasite using PCR.
- Even with fetal infection IgM antibodies are undetectable in most.
- Amniocentesis, which provides a lower risk to the fetus, is as sensitive in detecting the presence of *Toxoplasma*.

In the newborn

- By collection of cord blood or preferably a neonatal blood sample (to reduce the risk of contamination) and maternal specimen.
- Comparison of neonatal and maternal IgG by immunoblot. In an infant born to a mother with acute toxoplasmosis, the diagnosis can be made by high levels of specific IgG, which continues to persist at high levels in the first year of life. Passive transfer of maternal IgG leads to a rapid decline in these levels.
- Detection of neonatal IgM and IgA by EIA and/or immunosorbent agglutination assay (ISAGA) are diagnostic for neonatal infection.
- IgM /IgA may be present in under 60% of children with congenital infection in the first month of life, so continued testing is required.
- Disappearance of IgG in infancy excludes *Toxoplasma* infection.

Treatment

- There are no adequate treatment trials in the literature.
- The treatment currently available is at best of marginal benefit. Recent cohort data have questioned the efficacy of both antenatal and postnatal therapy.
- Consequently in the UK, toxoplasmosis does not fulfil the criteria to be included in the national screening programmes during pregnancy. The low prevalence leads to concern about over diagnosis, over treatment, and perhaps unnecessary terminations of pregnancy.
- If there is maternal infection consider spiramycin, a macrolide, that only reduces the risk of maternal transmission to the fetus.
- If fetal infection is confirmed, use pyrimethamine and sulfadiazine in the mother from 30 weeks' gestation until delivery.
- When there is clear evidence of congenital infection in the newborn then pyrimethamine and sulfadiazine are recommended until the age of a year. This may be alternated with spiramycin if there are toxicity problems. Steroids may be used in the presence of ocular infection.

- Pyrimethamine may produce severe neutropenia and folinic acid can be used to prevent this.
- For acquired infection resulting in choroido-retinitis treat with pyrimethamine, sulfadiazine, and steroids. Because of the toxicity of this regimen newer options being used in small case series, include co-trimoxazole combined with azithromycin.

Prognosis

- No treatment is usually required in healthy children with acute toxoplasmosis, although lymphadenopathy and some symptoms may persist for up to a year.
- In immunocompromised children treatment usually leads to resolution of clinical and radiological abnormalities, but permanent neurological damage sometime occurs. Only correction of the underlying immune deficit prevents further relapses.
- The outcome of children with congenital infection depends on the severity of *in utero* cerebral damage along with prompt diagnosis and treatment. Severe hydrocephalus is a poor prognostic sign. In children with less severe disease prompt treatment can be associated with good neurological and cognitive outcomes. This is a rare disease and large prospective cohort studies are limited.
- Retinal scars can progress and long-term ophthalmological review into adult life is very important. Relapses can occur when treatment is stopped at 1 year.

Further research

- There is a need for better understanding of how to improve the effectiveness of education programmes during pregnancy.
- Randomized controlled trials of both antenatal and post natal treatment are required—with safer and more effective therapy.

Further reading

Montoya JG, Liesenfeld O. Toxoplasmosis. *Lancet* 2004;**364**:579.

SYROCOT. Effectiveness of prenatal treatment for congenital toxoplasmosis; a meta-analysis of individual patient data. *Lancet* 2007;**369**:823–4.

Tuberculosis

📖 see also Chapters 15, 19, 20, 27, 29, 42, 91

Name and nature of organism

- TB is an infectious disease caused by bacteria belonging to the *Mycobacterium tuberculosis* complex (includes *M. tuberculosis*, *M. bovis*, and *M. africanum*).
- The genus *Mycobacterium* consists of a diverse group of bacilli that retain specific dyes strongly despite treatment with acid-alcohol (hence called acid- and alcohol-fast).

Epidemiology

- About nine million new cases of TB disease, and nearly two million deaths from TB, are estimated to occur around the world every year.
- It is estimated that there are 1.3 million cases annually in children <14 years leading to 450 000 deaths per annum.
- Most of the estimated cases are in Asia (55%) and Africa (31%), with small proportions of cases in the Eastern Mediterranean Region (6%), the European Region (5%) and the Region of the Americas (3%).
- The increasing burden of TB in many parts of the world has been attributed to poor TB control, development of drug resistance, and increasing HIV infection in the population.
- Accurate figures for the burden of childhood TB in the world are not readily available because of the difficulty in accurately diagnosing TB in children and the reliance of national reporting systems on sputum smear positivity which effectively excludes most children.
- In the WHO European Region, 422 830 cases of TB were notified in 2006 with an overall notification rate of 48 cases per 100 000, with large variability between countries and an incremental west-to-east gradient.
- Paediatric cases represent approximately 4% of notifications, in both national and foreign-born children in Europe.
- In a BPSU study of TB in children in the UK, pulmonary disease (including hilar adenopathy) occurred in >70% of children and CNS disease in <10% of children. Of those children that had samples sent for culture, only 43% were positive (58% in sputum samples and 28% in gastric aspirates). Drug resistance was reported in <1% of cases.

Transmission and incubation period

- Transmission of *M. tuberculosis* is usually from person to person, through inhalation of aerosolized drops produced by someone with pulmonary TB who is coughing or sneezing.
- The most important factor for contagiousness is the presence of bacilli in the sputum of individuals with pulmonary TB—smear-positive individuals. Most children are usually less infectious, unless they have extensive or cavitating disease. Most non-pulmonary forms of TB are usually non-infectious.
- Following exposure, initial infection in the lung is characterized by the primary complex (Ghon focus with regional adenitis). In most individuals, the primary complex resolves spontaneously with residual scarring or calcification.
- In some individuals, especially infants and children, progressive primary disease may occur causing mediastinal lymphadenopathy, invasion and compression of surrounding structures (such as bronchi, pleural and pericardial spaces) or haematogenous extra-thoracic spread (CNS disease, bone and joint disease).
- Post-primary or reactivation disease may occur following resolution of initial primary complex, usually in adolescent and adults.
- The incubation period from infection to development of a delayed-type hypersensitivity reaction (skin test conversion) is 2–12 weeks. Clinical manifestations of disease after infection usually occur in the first 6 months, although disease can occur many years after infection (post-primary or reactivation disease).
- Due to the nature of most TB disease in children (progressive primary and extrapulmonary disease), children with TB who are <10 years are usually not infectious.

Clinical features and sequelae

- Most children with latent TB infection (LTBI) caused by *M. tuberculosis* are asymptomatic and will have normal chest radiography.
- TB disease is characterized by the development of clinical symptoms, signs or radiographic changes.
- A clear decision has to be made whether a child has TB infection or disease.
- The commonest clinical features include fever, growth delay, weight loss or poor weight gain, chronic cough >3 weeks and night sweats.
- Clinical examination is often normal, but cachexia, focal chest signs, lymphadenopathy, pleural effusion, and hepatosplenomegaly may occur.
- Radiographic findings include lymphadenopathy (hilar, subcarinal, paratracheal or mediastinal), atelectasis or infiltrate, pleural effusion, cavitary lesions or miliary disease. Marked hilar adenopathy with less parenchymal disease may be seen.
- Pleural effusions are mostly seen in older children >6 years old. Pleural tap shows a high protein, low sugar, white cells and usually no

organisms as it represents reactive disease. Pericarditis and an effusion can lead on to a constrictive pericarditis.

- Lymph node disease is common in children, usually supraclavicular or cervical nodes, with slow enlargement of a firm fixed node. Low grade symptoms of chronic inflammation are common. Neck node disease is secondary spread from a pulmonary focus, seen on CXR in around a quarter of children.
- TB meningitis is secondary to lympho-haematogenous spread. It occurs in young children from 6 months up to school age. Presentation may be slow or more fulminant. Clinical presentation can be staged into:
  - Stage I: with slow non-specific headache, drowsiness, and no focal signs
  - Stage II: more rapid disease with meningism, neck stiffness, and focal neurological and cranial nerve signs
  - Stage III: with coma, hemiplegia and signs of raised ICP.
- Outcome is related to stage. CSF sugar is low, protein high, with increased lymphocyte count and TB stains only positive in a minority of cases. CT signs include basal meningeal thickening, hydrocephalus, or in children with focal disease a tuberculoma may be seen mimicking malignancy.
- Miliary disease is seen in infants and young children with high fevers, cachexia, respiratory distress, widespread nodular changes on CXR, and hepato-splenomegaly.
- Abdominal TB presents most frequently with weight loss, gastrointestinal symptoms, lymphadenopathy, and ascites.
- Bone disease includes dactylitis, focal knee, hip, elbow or ankle chronic osteomyelitis. Vertebral disease leads to bone destruction and collapse with spinal malformation. Local spread is common into soft tissue, causing paraspinal (Pott's disease) or psoas abscess.
- Renal disease is very rare in children due to the long incubation period but may occur in adolescents.
- Severe forms of TB, such as miliary disease or meningitis, are associated with higher mortality and morbidity, often with long-term neurological sequelae.
- Congenital TB is relatively rare and occurs following *in utero* transmission of TB across the placenta.
- Clinical findings in patients with drug-resistant TB disease are indistinguishable from those with drug-susceptible disease.

Diagnosis

- Isolation of *M. tuberculosis* by culture from specimens of gastric aspirates, sputum, bronchial washings, pleural fluid, CSF fluid, urine, or other body fluids or biopsy specimens establishes the diagnosis.
- Microscopic examination of samples using Ziehl–Neelsen or fluorochrome stains may also be used to identify acid-fast bacilli although yields are lower than with culture.
- Sputum samples are usually obtained from older children and adolescents who are able to produce a sputum sample or by induction with nebulized hypertonic saline.

- In younger children and infants who cannot produce sputum, three consecutive early morning gastric aspirates are collected. This involves leaving a nasogastric tube in overnight then aspirate 10–20ml of saline in the morning before feeds.
- The diagnostic yield from three early morning aspirates remains <50% on culture.
- Radiological studies will depend on the site of disease, most commonly a CXR or chest CT scan for pulmonary disease. CT imaging may also be useful for diagnosing CNS disease (TB meningitis or tuberculoma).
- PCR on sputum and other samples appears to have lower sensitivity and specificity in children, primarily because of the type of disease seen in children (primary disease as opposed to post-primary/reactivation disease seen in adults—paucibacillary).
- TST: Intradermal injection of two tuberculin units (0.1ml) of purified protein derivative (PPD) followed by measurement of induration (not erythema) 48–72 hours later.
- Positive TST: induration of 5–14mm (no previous BCG) or induration >15mm (previous BCG)
- TST suffers from false-positives (previous BCG vaccination, non-tuberculous mycobacterial infection) and false negatives (severe disease, malnutrition, immunosuppression).
- Interferon gamma release assays (IGRAs) rely on the measurement of IFNγ production by lymphocytes following stimulation with antigens specific to *M. tuberculosis* (ESAT-6, CFP-10). Two IGRAs are commercially available, 'QuantiFERON-TB Gold' and 'T-Spot-TB', and have been introduced in several countries on the basis of limited evidence to either replace TST or performed to exclude false-positive TST due to BCG or non-tuberculous mycobacteria.
- IGRAs do not differentiate LTBI and active TB disease.
- While IGRAs have been found to have a high sensitivity and specificity in diagnosing LTBI in immunocompetent adults, they may have limited sensitivity in diagnosing active TB in children.
- Further long-term follow-up studies are being conducted to determine the predictive role of these assays in the diagnosis of LTBI and TB disease in children.

Management and treatment

- Treatment of LTBI: preferred regimen—3 months of isoniazid and rifampicin (or 6 months of isoniazid).
- Treatment of pulmonary disease (including hilar lymphadenopathy): 2 months of isoniazid + rifampicin + pyrazinamide (+ ethambutol if resistance suspected or at increased risk) for 2 months followed by isoniazid + rifampicin for 4 months (Table 113.1).
- Treatment of extrapulmonary non-CNS disease (including bone and joint disease, cervical lymphadenitis, gastrointestinal disease): 2 months of isoniazid + rifampicin + pyrazinamide (+ ethambutol if resistance suspected or at increased risk) for 2 months followed by isoniazid + rifampicin for 4 months.

- Some experts recommend longer duration of therapy (12 months) for osteoarticular disease, especially spinal TB, and miliary TB.
- Treatment of CNS TB (including meningitis and tuberculoma): isoniazid + rifampicin + pyrazinamide (+ ethambutol if resistance suspected or at increased risk) for 2 months followed by isoniazid + rifampicin for 10 months.
- Corticosteroids are indicated for children with tuberculous meningitis, because they decrease rates of mortality and long-term neurological impairment.
- Corticosteroids may be considered for children with bronchial obstruction due to enlarged intrathoracic lymph nodes, pericardial effusion and pleural effusion, severe miliary disease and endobronchial disease. A dose of prednisolone at 1–2mg/kg/day (maximum 60 mg/day) for 4–6 weeks followed by weaning doses is usually recommended.
- Most cases of pulmonary TB in children caused by isoniazid-resistant *M. tuberculosis* can be treated with rifampicin, pyrazinamide and ethambutol.
- Treatment of multidrug resistant TB should include at least 4 effective agents for at least 12–18 months.
- The treatment of children with drug-resistant TB should only be carried out by or in conjunction with specialists with appropriate experience in the management of such cases.

Table 113.1 Management and treatment

Hilar adenopathy	2 months of RHZ(^{a}E) then 4 months of RH
Pulmonary TB	2 months of RHZ(^{a}E) then 4 months of RH
Extrapulmonary TB	2 months of RHZ(^{a}E) then 4 months of RH
TB meningitis/tuberculoma	2 months of RHZ(^{a}E) then 10 months of RH

R, rifampicin; H, isoniazid; Z, pyrazinamide; E, ethambutol.

[a]Where resistance suspected or at increased risk.

Prevention

- Prompt treatment of infectious cases of TB and contact tracing of household and close contacts of such cases are important preventive measures.
- BCG vaccine is a live attenuated vaccine prepared from a strain of *M. bovis*. It is used in more than 100 countries globally as part of routine vaccination programmes of infants to prevent disseminated and severe forms of TB.

- Two meta-analyses of published clinical trials and case–control studies suggest a protective efficacy of 80% against miliary and meningeal TB and 50% for pulmonary TB.
- BCG vaccination continues to be used in many countries in the world, primarily given to neonates and infants to prevent severe forms of TB, particularly miliary TB and TB meningitis.

Future research

- New diagnostics methods (including IGRAs) for TB disease and LTBI in children.
- Development of vaccines that are more protective than BCG.
- Development of new drugs, particularly for drug-resistant TB.

Further reading

National Collaborating Centre for Chronic Conditions. *Tuberculosis: Clinical Diagnosis and Management of Tuberculosis, and Measures for its Prevention and Control.* London: Royal College of Physicians, 2006.

Shingadia D, Novelli V. Diagnosis and management of childhood tuberculosis. *Lancet Infect Dis* 2003;**3**:624–33.

WHO. *Global Tuberculosis Control: Epidemiology, Strategy, Financing.* WHO Report, 2009.

Typhoid and paratyphoid—enteric fever

📖 see also Chapters 5, 12, 15, 21, 22, 33, 35, 42, 45

Name and nature of organism

- *Salmonella enterica* Typhi and *Salmonella enterica* serovar Paratyphi A (rarely Paratyphi B and C) are Gram-negative bacilli causing typhoid and paratyphoid fevers, respectively, collectively known as the enteric fevers.
- Serotypes of *Salmonella enterica* (about 2500) are based on three main surface antigens O (somatic), H (flagellar) and Vi (capsular). Virulence genes determine invasion and pathogenicity.
- The organisms cause infection exclusively in humans. Human faecal or urinary carriers are the sources of infection. The organisms can persist in food and water contaminated by sewage.

Epidemiology

- Enteric fever is prevalent in low- or middle-income countries in areas where there is inadequate sanitation, poor hygiene.
- More than 27 million new cases are estimated to occur worldwide, with approximately 200 000 deaths.
- It is most common in children and young adults (ages 2–35 years).
- The majority of UK infections occur in patients who have travelled to the tropics on holiday or visiting friends and relatives. Occasional cases result from chronic carriers where there is a breakdown in food hygiene. Increasing numbers of reports are being seen—in the UK now about 500 confirmed cases/year in all ages.
- Compared with non-typhoidal salmonellas (mainly *S. enteriditis* and *S. typhimurium*) which cause 2500 cases in children/year in the UK.
- Typhoid fever cases are estimated to outnumber paratyphoid cases worldwide by 10:1 although in some areas of Asia paratyphoid has recently become more common.
- Although paratyphoid fever is usually less severe than typhoid fever, it can sometimes cause life-threatening disease.

Transmission and incubation period

- The disease is spread by the faeco-oral route usually by ingestion of food or water contaminated with faeces and/or urine from an infected person excreting the bacteria. Uncooked or undercooked foods are common routes of infection.

- Average incubation period of 1–3 weeks, but may be longer depending on size of infecting inoculum. Severity of disease is related to high ingested dose, reduced gastric acid, young infants and immunocompromise—especially HIV and sickle cell disease. The evidence that typhoid is more severe in HIV infection is scanty (as opposed to nontyphoidal salmonellosis).
- Chronic carriers (e.g. the cook Typhoid Mary) continue to excrete for months or years. When you admit a child with typhoid—check the parent's occupation!

Clinical features and complications

Enteric fever is a systemic bacterial disease with a wide range of clinical presentations. Classic symptoms include in the first 2 weeks a gradually more severe illness including:

- Continued high spiking fever
- Malaise; headache; dry cough
- Diarrhoea ± blood and/or mucus—later constipation.

Physical findings can include:

- High fever that can go on for weeks—spiking once or twice a day
- Apathetic facies
- Splenomegaly; hepatomegaly
- Relative bradycardia—not usually seen in children
- Rose-coloured spots (2–4mm pink blanching papules) on trunk.

The most important acute complications usually occur after 2–3 weeks of illness and are:

- Septicaemia—especially in children aged <2 years or the immunocompromised
- Intestinal perforation
- Gastrointestinal haemorrhage
- Encephalopathy and shock
- Myocarditis.

Many other focal complications have been described but are relatively rare including

- Cholecystitis; hepatitis
- Osteomyelitis; septic arthritis (especially in children with sickle cell disease)
- Pneumonia
- Meningitis (rare and usually in infants); brain abscesses
- Psychotic states
- Glomerulonephritis.

Some patients initially present with the disease complication (e.g. acute abdomen due to typhoid perforation, or encephalopathy/confusion).

The disease may also be complicated by relapse (recurrence of the illness 1–2 weeks after recovery from the first episode) and by chronic faecal or urinary carriage (defined by persistent excretion of the organism in faeces or urine for >1 year).

Diagnosis

Confirmation of the diagnosis requires isolation of the organisms from a normally sterile site. This is much more difficult if the child has already received oral antibiotics, which is often the case.

The diagnosis may have to be on clinical probability alone in a child with a prolonged swinging fever, who has recently returned from a typhoid endemic area, and does not have either malaria or any other common focal infection (e.g. UTI, otitis media, etc).

Blood culture

Blood culture is the usual site of isolation:
- Only positive in 40–60% of cases, often early in the disease.
- Sensitivity affected by prior antibiotic use, stage of illness, level of bacteraemia, and volume of blood taken.

Bone marrow culture

Bone marrow culture is more sensitive than blood culture and remains positive later in the disease process.
- Positive in 80–90% of cases.
- May remain positive for several days after antibiotics started.
- Of less use practically in children.

Stool and urine cultures

- Worth doing, although may reflect chronic bacterial carriage, not acute infection.
- Important in follow up to exclude faecal and urinary carriage.

Serology

- The Widal Test detects agglutinating antibodies to *Salmonella* Typhi O and H antigens. Used extensively in resource poor countries but is an unreliable diagnostic test.
- HPA Centre for Infections, UK offer an immunoblot test in place of the Widal test. This new test has high sensitivity and specificity but is technically demanding.
- Rapid diagnostic tests detecting IgM antibodies are being developed and evaluated in endemic areas. Examples include Typhidot-M and TUBEX. May be more sensitive than blood culture, but inadequate specificity remains a problem.

NAATs

- Nested and real-time PCRs have been used in research studies.

Other laboratory findings in typhoid

- A mild normochromic anaemia, mild thrombocytopenia, and an increased ESR are common.
- Most patients have a total WBC within the normal range or mild leucocytosis. Very high leucocytosis may suggest either perforation or other diagnosis (e.g. appendicitis, ulcerative colitis).
- Laboratory evidence of mild DIC is common but rarely of clinical significance.

Management and treatment

- Prompt treatment with appropriate antibiotics as well as full supportive care reduces the mortality to <1%. Widespread use of antibiotics has led to an increase in multidrug resistance, especially in South East Asia and the Indian subcontinent.
- Fluoroquinolones, such as ciprofloxacin, have been the first-line treatment for many years. However, isolates with decreased susceptibility to ciprofloxacin are now common in Asia. The laboratory may report these as ciprofloxacin susceptible, but patients infected with these isolates with decreased susceptibility frequently do not respond to ciprofloxacin. Resistance to nalidixic acid is a surrogate laboratory marker of decreased susceptibility. Alternatively, the laboratory can measure the ciprofloxacin MIC.
- In an ill child with suspected enteric fever, start with IV ceftriaxone, while awaiting culture and sensitivity results. Treatment courses can be completed with high-dose oral azithromycin (or ciprofloxacin if susceptible) once resolution of fever has occurred.
- Delay in resolution of fever for 2–3 days after starting IV antibiotics is common in typhoid fever, even if the infection is fully susceptible. There is often a period of concern where the antibiotics have been started and the fever persists for a few days before slowly settling. It is reasonable to wait this out if the child remains clinically stable.
- Prolonged treatment courses are required to prevent relapse. Bacteraemia or severe clinical enteric fever should be treated for 10–14 days, focal disease, including osteomyelitis and meningitis 4–6 weeks.

Severe typhoid

Typhoid gastrointestinal perforation

- Nasogastric suction, administration of fluids to correct hypotension, and prompt surgery.
- Simple closure of perforations is adequate but experienced surgeons use procedures to bypass the worst-affected sections of the ileum in order to reduce postoperative morbidity. Closure of perforations should be accompanied by vigorous peritoneal toilet.
- Metronidazole or clindamycin should be added to the therapy of ceftriaxone or fluoroquinolone-treated patients.
- Altered conscious level and shock—dexamethasone may be used.
- In one study in Indonesia, dexamethasone, 3mg/kg infused IV over half an hour, followed by eight doses of 1mg/kg 6 hourly, resulted in a 10% case fatality compared to 55.6% in controls.

Prevention

- Improvements to public health and sanitation in endemic areas are crucial.
- Eradication of carriage in long-term carriers may be necessary, especially if they are food handlers. Eradication requires prolonged, high-dose antibiotics to which the bacteria are susceptible.

- Notification to the public health authorities is mandatory.
- Vaccination is important in endemic areas and for travellers.

Vi polysaccharide vaccine

- IM injection.
- Provides cover for 3 years.
- Not considered suitable or effective for children <2 years.

Live attenuated vaccine (Ty21)

- Oral vaccine.
- Three doses of a single capsule every alternate day.
- Provides 12 months protection.
- Not considered suitable or effective for children <6 years.

Future research

- Diagnostics are a major challenge. It is difficult to distinguish typhoid and paratyphoid fever from other tropical febrile illnesses. Development and evaluation of cheap and simple rapid diagnostic tests that are usable in resource-limited settings must remain a priority.
- Antimicrobial resistance, especially to fluoroquinolones is a major issue. Continually changing patterns of resistance demand regular microbiological surveillance of *Salmonella* infections.
- The failure to use vaccination as a programmatic tool in endemic areas means that typhoid remains a major public health problem. The International Vaccine Institute (IVI) is conducting research on the efficacy of the programmatic use of typhoid vaccines in Asia.
- The lack of a paratyphoid vaccine is also a gap as paratyphoid fever is of increasing in importance in Asia. A bivalent Typhi and Paratyphi A vaccine is in development.

Further reading

Bhutta ZA. Current concepts in the diagnosis and treatment of typhoid fever. *BMJ* 2006;**333**:78–82.

Health Protection Agency. *Pilot of Enhanced Surveillance of Enteric Fever in England, Wales, and Northern Ireland, 2007.* London: HPA, 2008.

World Health Organisation. *Background Document: the Diagnosis, Treatment, and Prevention of Typhoid Fever.* Geneva: WHO/V&B/03.07, 2002.

Chapter 115

Typhus

see also Chapters 15, 33, 34, 41, 42

Introduction

- 'Typhus', which is derived from the Greek word '*typos*', represents 'fever with stupor'.
- Typhus is a group of infectious bacterial diseases of the *Rickettsia* genus. It comprises two main Gram-negative obligate intracellular bacteria: *Rickettsia typhi* (causes murine or endemic typhus) and *Rickettsia prowazekii* (causes epidemic typhus).

Endemic or murine typhus (fleaborne typhus, *Rickettsia typhi*)

Name and nature of organism
- A rickettsial disease caused by the organism *R. typhi* and less commonly by *Rickettsia felis*.

Epidemiology
- Fleaborne rickettsioses are widely distributed, especially throughout the tropics and subtropics and in port cities and coastal regions. In Europe, it is prevalent in Portugal, Spain (included the Canary Islands) and Greece.
- Most of cases occur in summer and autum. It is also reported among travellers returning from Asia, Africa, and southern Europe, and has also been reported from Hawaii, California and Texas.

Transmission and incubation period
- Reservoirs: wild rats, mice, and other rodents. It is maintained in nature by the rodent-flea cycle.
- *R. typhi* infects the gut epithelial cells of the flea and is excreted in its faeces as it feeds on the reservoir (the rodent). The rodent is infected and carries *R. typhi* without ill effect.
- Rat fleas (*Xenopsylla cheopis*) and probably cat fleas transmit the agents to humans. Distribution is sporadic but worldwide; incubation period ranges from 6 to 18 days (mean 10 days).

Clinical features and sequelae
- Endemic is milder than epidemic typhus, causing shaking chills, headache, fever and rash.

- The patient's temperature increases steadily over the first few days and may become intermittent when the rash appears, with the morning temperature tending to be normal.
- Children may have fever as high as 41°C (106°F). Fever usually lasts approximately 12 days, then gradually returns to normal.
- The rash and other manifestations are similar to those of epidemic typhus but less severe. The early rash is sparse and discrete.
- Mortality is low but is higher in elderly patients.

Diagnosis

- Consider this diagnosis in patients with fever and/or rash and a history of cat contact or flea bite.
- The gold standard of diagnosis of murine typhus is IFA; a fourfold increase in titre between the acute- and convalescent-phase serums is considered to be diagnostic.
- Murine typhus can be identified by immunohistology of a skin biopsy, PCR with use of peripheral blood, buffy coat, and plasma specimens, or serum ELISA.

Management and treatment

- Primary treatment is doxycycline until the patient improves and has been afebrile for 24–48 hours but is continued for at least 7 days, or 2–4 days after defervescence to preclude relapses. The risk of dental staining by doxycycline is very low when a short course of therapy is given (5–10 days).
- Patients can also be treated with IV or IM doxycycline. In pregnant women and children <8 years of age, whose disease course is mild, macrolides may be used.
- Chloramphenicol is second-line treatment.

Prevention

- Incidence has been decreased by reducing rat and rat fleas.
- No effective vaccine exists.

Epidemic typhus (louseborne typhus, *Rickettsia prowazekii*)

Name and nature of organism

- A rickettsial disease caused by the organism *R. prowazekii*, a small Gram-negative intracellular bacterium.

Epidemiology

- In Europe, this rickettsiosis is a long-known infectious disease and remains important in some communities.
- The Plague of Athens is the oldest recorded epidemic which occurred around 429BC. Outbreaks have often been tied to periods of war, poverty, and natural disasters, especially during the colder months when louse infested clothing is not laundered.

- It reappeared in Europe during the Napoleonic Wars and more recently during the world wars. Following improvements in hygiene, outbreaks have largely been controlled.

Transmission and incubation period

- Transmitted by body lice (*Pediculus humanus corporis*) when louse faeces are scratched or rubbed into bite or other wounds.
- Humans may occasionally contract epidemic typhus after contact with flying squirrels in the USA (flying squirrel disease).
- *R. prowazekii* is a potential category B bioterrorism agent, because it is stable in dried louse faeces and can be transmitted by aerosols.
- The natural reservoirs are humans, wild rodents.
- Incubation period ranges from 7 to 14 days.

Clinical features and sequelae

- Patients usually have 1–3 days of malaise before abrupt onset of severe headache and fever. Prolonged high fever up to 40°C persists, with slight morning remission, for about 2 weeks.
- Intractable headache accompanied by CNS manifestations (e.g. delirium, coma, and seizures) in 80% of cases.
- Maculopapular rash, which appears on the fourth to sixth day, rapidly covers the body, usually involving the axillae and the upper trunk but not the palms, soles or face. Eschars are absent. In severe cases, the rash becomes petechial or haemorrhagic.
- Splenomegaly is sometimes present. Hypotension occurs in most seriously ill patients.
- **Brill–Zinsser disease** is a mild form of relapsing epidemic typhus that occurs in convalescent patients with a subclinical infection.
- Fatal outcome is observed in up to 40% of untreated cases.
- Fatalities are rare in children <10 years, but mortality increases with age and may reach 60% in untreated patients >50 years old. However, it is approximately 4% if effective antibiotics are given.
- Poor prognostic signs are vascular collapse, renal insufficiency, encephalitic signs, ecchymosis with gangrene, and pneumonia.

Diagnosis

- Diagnosis of epidemic typhus is based on detection of specific antibodies in sera. Plate microagglutination is a sensitive test.
- Indirect immunofluorescence test is the current reference method, an IgG titre of 1:128 or an IgM titre of 1:32 confirms the diagnosis.
- Louse infestation is usually obvious and strongly suggests typhus if history (e.g. living in or visiting an endemic area) suggests possible exposure.
- Culture (shell vial assay) is now used to isolate from clinical samples (blood or skin biopsy) using L929 fibroblast cell monolayers, and identification of rickettsial isolates may be done by microscopic examination after Gimenez staining or by immunofluorescence.

Management and treatment

- Primary treatment is doxycycline until the patient improves and has been afebrile for 24–48 hours but is continued for at least 7 days, or 2–4 days after defervescence to preclude relapses. Patients can also be

treated with IV or IM doxycycline. In pregnant women and children <8 years of age, whose disease course is mild, macrolides clarithromycin or azithromycin may be administered.
- Chloramphenicol for 7 days is second-line treatment.

Prevention
- Louse control is highly effective for prevention. Delousing methods consist of removing and destroying all lice by bathing the patient, and changing and boiling infested clothes.
- Lice may be eliminated by an insecticide (10% DDT, 1% malathion, or 1% permethrin)—also an effective method.

Future research
- Mouse models may be useful for studying and assessing new therapeutic molecules and vaccine candidates.

Scrub typhus (tsutsugamushi disease, *Orientia tsutsugamushi* (formerly called *Rickettsia tsutsugamushi*))

Name and nature of organism
- An acute febrile, potential fatal zoonotic disease caused by intracellular Gram-negative bacterium *O. tsutsugamushi* (formerly called *R. tsutsugamushi*).
- *O. tsutsugamushi* is a very tiny (0.5 × 1.2–3µm in size) organism without peptidoglycan and lipopolysaccharide in its cell wall.
- More than 30 antigenically distinct serotypes are present in the endemic area.

Epidemiology
- First described in China in AD313. The '*tsutsugamushi*' is derived from two Japanese words '*tsutsuga*' (something tiny and dangerous) and '*mushi*' (a live organism, bug).
- Approximately one billion people are at risk of this disease and one million cases are reported annually. (Between 25% and 50% of cases are children in endemic areas.)
- Distributed widely in the western Pacific area and Asia (know as the 'Tsutsugamushi triangle'), covering from northern Japan and South Korea, as far south as northern Australia and to the west as far as Afghanistan and Pakistan.
- Significantly more common in men than women and similarly, boys are more often infected than girls among school-age children.
- Children (incidental hosts) are infected mainly in summer.

Transmission and incubation period
- *O. tsutsugamushi* is transmitted by the bite of trombiculid mite larvae (chiggers) to vertebrate animals.

- Rodents are the main recipients of transmission by infected chiggers bites, however, humans (local residents, farmers, outdoor workers, soldiers, and travellers) are opportunistic hosts.
- About 20 species of the trombiculid mite (*Leptotrombidium* spp.) are the primary vectors and reservoirs of *O. tsutsugamushi*. It is tiny (0.2–0.4mm).
- The incubation period is about 5–21 days (with a mean around 10–12 days) after the initial chigger bite.

Clinical features and sequelae

- The most common symptom is abrupt fever of unknown origin.
- The other characteristic feature is one or more typical eschars, which can be accompanied by regional lymphadenopathy that may be tender, seen in 60–70% of patients.
- An eschar is a non-painful ulcer covered by a centrally depressed dark scab and surrounded by a red areola. The dark scab may be absent when scratched off. Eschars are more commonly found in scrub typhus than murine typhus.
- Major clinical manifestations of paediatric scrub typhus are fever and chills, cough, anorexia, eschar, and lymphadenopathy.
- Other symptoms and signs include headache, maculopapular rash, diffuse abdominal pain, vomiting, neck stiffness, hepatosplenomegaly, pitting oedema, jaundice and seizures.
- Children with mild cough may have evidence of interstitial pneumonitis on CXR.
- Typical eschar location varies between adults and children: mainly within 30cm below the umbilicus on the anterior trunk and on the lower extremities in adults, and mainly in the axillary and genital regions (moist and warm areas of the body) in children.
- Maculopapular skin rash appears after the onset of fever, lasts for 5–8 days and is transient, pale, and easy to miss.
- Seizure with mental change or delirium is reported, particularly in children with CNS involvement, including meningomyelitis and encephalitis (reported in about 13% patients).
- Serious complications of scrub typhus may involve liver, lungs, heart, brain, or kidneys. The most common complications are hepatic dysfunction (over 90%) and pneumonitis (over 50%). Typical pathology is a focal or diffuse vasculitis with destruction of endothelial cells and perivascular infiltration of leucocytes.
- Multiorgan dysfunction, such as fulminant hepatic failure, pericardial effusion, myocarditis, severe pneumonitis with progressive acute respiratory distress syndrome, thrombocytopenia, DIC, cardiogenic and septic shock are the most serious complications of scrub typhus.
- Most children respond well to adequate antibiotic treatment and recover completely. However, relapses may occur and are associated with short duration of therapy.
- Mortality rates vary widely, ranging from 3% to 60% in adults and 5% only in Taiwanese children. Factors determining outcome include appropriate timely antibiotic treatment, prior status of the patient and the strain of *O. tsutsugamushi*.

Diagnosis

- Clinical and laboratory features are non-specific; the diagnosis of scrub typhus is difficult to make. Physicians should maintain a high index of suspicion, especially in children with a fever of obscure cause, with hepatic dysfunction or pneumonitis in endemic areas.
- The key to diagnosing scrub typhus is finding a typical eschar. Although not present in all cases, can be found in about 50–67% of children with scrub typhus after careful examination.
- Patients respond promptly to antibiotic treatment with rapid improvement, becoming afebrile within an average of 1.5 days. Serological tests, based on a fourfold antibody rise for *O. tsutsugamushi* measured in acute and convalescent paired sera, are the most reliable tool for diagnosis. Tests include IFAs and immunoperoxidase assays.
- Non-specific laboratory values; raised CRP (>96% of children), elevation of liver enzyme levels (90–100% children) with or without hypoalbuminaemia, may also help in diagnosis.
- CXR abnormalities seen in scrub typhus include diffuse, bilateral, reticulonodular opacities.
- Abdominal ultrasound may show pictures of acute cholecystitis (double wall of gallbladder, hydrops of gallbladder) and hyperechogenicity of the liver parenchyma.

Management and treatment

- β-lactam antibiotics are ineffective treatment for scrub typhus since *O. tsutsugamushi* does not have peptidoglycan in its cell wall and is an intracellular obligate infection. A few studies report that aminoglycosides, such as gentamicin, are ineffective in human and in mice scrub typhus infection.
- Doxycycline (age >8 years) and chloramphenicol are the drugs of choice for childhood scrub typhus. However, doxycycline-resistant *O. tsutsugamushi* has been reported in northern Thailand. Rifampin may be effective in drug-resistant areas.
- 1 week of oral doxycycline or newer macrolide antibiotics (roxithromycin, azithromycin) are recommended for mild and uncomplicated paediatric scrub typhus.
- Most severely ill children respond well to doxycycline for 7–10 days or until afebrile for 2–3 days with supportive therapy during hospitalization.

Prevention

- Application of insect repellents (dibutyl phthalate, benzyl benzoate, and diethyltoluamide) to skin and clothes to prevent chigger bites.
- Avoid sitting in overgrown grass and brush in endemic areas. Wearing long pants, sleeves, socks or other suitable covering garments.
- Rodent control and public health education (via media to local residents and travellers).
- No effective vaccine is available. High antigenic variation makes this difficult.

Boutonneuse fever—Mediterranean spotted fever

This tick-borne disease is caused by *R. conorii* and is seen across the Mediterranean basin, including Portugal and into Africa and Asia. The disease is transmitted by the dog tick. The illness causes a high fever around a week after the tick bite, with the classic spotted rash being seen a few days after the fever starts. Boutonneuse fever is generally a milder disease, though severe complications can occur. The management is similar to scrub typhus.

Further reading

Bechah Y, Capo C, Grau GE, Raoult D, Mege JL. A murine model of infection with *Rickettsia prowazekii*: implications for pathogenesis of epidemic typhus. *Microbes Infect* 2007;**9**:898–906.

Bechan Y, Capo C, Mege JL, Raoult D. Epidemic typhus. *Lancet Infect Dis* 2009;**8**:471–26.

Blanco JR, Oteo JA. Rickettsiosis in Europe. *Ann N Y Acad Sci* 2006;**1078**:26–33.

Civen T, Ngo V. Murine typhus: an unrecognized suburban vector borne disease. *Clin Infect Dis* 2008;**46**:913–18.

WT Jim, NC Chiu, WT Chan, et al. Clinical manifestations, laboratory findings and complications of pediatric scrub typhus in eastern Taiwan. *Pediatr Neonatol* 2009;**50**:96–101.

Watt G, Parola P. Scrub typhus and tropical rickettsioses. *Curr Opin Infect Dis* 2003;**16**:429–36.

World Health Organization. *Frequently Asked Questions: Scrub Typhus*. 2009. Available at: Ⓝ www.searo.who.int/LinkFiles/CDS_faq_Scrub_Typhus.pdf (accessed 1 February 2011).

Viral haemorrhagic fevers

📖 see also Chapters 13, 14, 34, 42

Name and nature of organisms

- Viral haemorrhagic fevers (VHFs) comprise a diverse group of infections characterized by febrile illnesses and in some, high case fatality rates. Many are transmitted from person to person.
- The diseases include: Lassa fever, Ebola haemorrhagic fever, Marburg haemorrhagic fever, Crimean-Congo haemorrhagic fever (CCHF), the South American haemorrhagic fevers (Argentinian, Bolivian, Venezuelan and Brazilian), Kyasanur forest disease and Omsk haemorrhagic fever, and haemorrhagic fever with renal syndrome (HFRS). Some forms of dengue virus infection can lead to serious haemorrhagic disease, known as dengue haemorrhagic fever (DHF).
- The VHFs are caused by distinct RNA viruses that are members of four viral families: *Arenaviridae*, *Bunyaviridae*, *Filoviridae*, and *Flaviviridae*.
- Arenaviruses: six viruses are currently known to cause haemorrhagic disease in humans. The family is divided in Old World (Lassa and Lujo viruses), and New World (Junin, Machupo, Chapare, Guanarito and Sabiá viruses). All arenaviruses are enveloped, pleomorphic, bisegmented, single-stranded, 60 to >200nm.
- *Bunyaviridae*: The family includes CCHF virus (genus *Nairovirus*), and hantaviruses including Seoul, Puumala, Dobrava. The viruses are enveloped, segmented, and single-stranded, 90–120nm.
- *Filoviridae*: This family contains only Marburg and Ebola viruses. There are five subtypes of Ebola, four of which cause disease in humans; Sudan, Zaire, Cote d'Ivoire, and Bundibugyo. The fifth ebolavirus type, Reston, has been found in primates and pigs, and while inducing an antibody response in humans, has not thus far caused symptomatic infection. The viruses are enveloped, filamentous and non-segmented, 80 × 800–1000nm.
- *Flaviviridae*: This large family of viruses includes dengue and yellow fever viruses as well as the agents responsible for Kyasanur forest disease and Omsk haemorrhagic fever. There are four distinct serotypes of dengue virus (DEN 1, DEN 2, DEN 3, and DEN 4). They are enveloped, non-segmented, single-stranded, 50nm.
- The arenaviruses, filoviruses, and CCHF virus are classified as hazard group 4 as they present a serious hazard to laboratory workers.

Epidemiology

- **Lassa fever:** Reservoir is the multimammate rat (*Mastomys* species). Disease is endemic in West Africa, particularly Guinea, Liberia, Sierra Leone, and Nigeria. Many thousand cases are thought to occur each year in these endemic countries. Imported cases are rare, but have occurred in Europe, North America and elsewhere, almost exclusively in persons with high-risk occupations such as medical or other aid workers.

- **Lujo virus:** This has been recently described following a small outbreak in South Africa in 2008. The index case acquired infection in Zambia, and three secondary and one tertiary transmissions followed after the patient was repatriated to a hospital in South Africa. Four infections were fatal. Little is yet known of the epidemiology of this virus, but a rodent reservoir is likely.

- **South American Arenaviruses:** All are rodent borne (field voles, cane rats, cotton rats), and each virus occurs in a different country; Junin virus in Argentina, Machupo and Chapare viruses in Bolivia, Guanarito virus in Venezuela, and Sabiá virus in Brazil. Argentine HF (Junin virus) is the commonest of these, although its incidence has declined since use of an effective vaccine. A resurgence of Bolivian HF was noted in 2007–8. Imported cases are very rare outside the Americas. Laboratory-acquired infections have occurred.

- **Ebola:** The reservoir is probably in bats; non-human primates and other mammals also susceptible. The four pathogenic subtypes are found in Central and West Africa: Republic of Congo, Democratic Republic of Congo, Gabon, Sudan, and Uganda. Ebola Reston has only been found in the Western Pacific and has not to date caused illness in humans. Sporadic outbreaks occur which may be extensive with hundreds of cases. Imported cases are very rare. Laboratory-acquired infections have occurred.

- **Marburg:** The reservoir is almost certainly fruit bats, and certain monkey species are susceptible to infection. Found in Central and West Africa: Kenya, Uganda, Democratic Republic of Congo, Angola. Sporadic cases and outbreaks occur, the largest of which was in Angola in 2004–5. Imported cases are very rare. Two cases occurred in 2008, one in Holland and one in the USA, and both followed a visit to a bat infested cave in the Maramagambo Forest, Uganda.

- **CCHF:** Reservoir in livestock, small mammals and birds; tick-borne. CCHF virus is the most widely distributed agent of severe haemorrhagic fever known and is enzootic from western China across to eastern Europe, the Middle East, and down to southern Africa. This range reflects the distribution of the *Hyalomma* ticks which are the main vector. Several hundred cases occur per year in Turkey, the Balkans, and southern parts of the Russian Federation. Epidemic years can occur. Imported cases appear to be rare.

- **Hantaviruses:** Rodent borne (various species including voles, mice, rats) and each virus has a specific rodent host. There is variable distribution in Europe, Asia, and the Americas depending on both viral and rodent species. Seoul virus is found worldwide, particularly in Asia, while Puumala and Dobrava virus occur in Europe. Puumala virus is responsible for a mild form of HFRS known as nephropathia endemica. About 150 000 cases of HFRS are thought to occur worldwide each year, and many thousand of those are in Europe.

- *Dengue:* A mosquito-borne infection transmitted by *Aedes* species, principally *Aedes aegypti* and *Aedes albopictus*. Dengue is endemic in over 100 countries in tropical and subtropical regions of the world. WHO estimates there are ~50 million cases of dengue fever per year, of which up to 500 000 are DHF. Imported cases of dengue fever are relatively common in Europe, and cases of DHF are also seen.
- *Omsk haemorrhagic fever/Kyasanur forest disease.* These tick-borne infections are geographically limited to the western Siberia regions of Omsk, Novosibirsk, Kurgan, and Tyumen, and the Kyasanur Forest in southern India, respectively, and so are not considered further.

Transmission and incubation period

- *Lassa fever:* Virus is shed in the urine and droppings of infected multimammate rats, and most human infections arise through contact with materials contaminated by these. Person-to-person transmission also occurs via direct contact with body fluids (blood, semen, respiratory secretions, urine) of an infected person. Symptomatic patients are considered infectious, and urine may be intermittently positive for up to 2 months. Sexual transmission is possible as virus remains detectable in semen for up to 3 months post-symptom onset. The incubation period is 7–10 days, with a range of 3–21 days.
- *South American arenaviruses:* Transmission to humans occurs via direct contact with infected rodents, or through inhalation of infectious rodent fluids and excreta. Argentine haemorrhagic fever is particularly seen in agricultural workers harvesting maize fields where rodents are plentiful. Person-to-person transmission has been documented with Junin and Machupo viruses. The incubation period is from 7 to 14 days, with a range of 5–21 days.
- *Ebola and Marburg:* The index case in an outbreak usually follows contact with an infected animal (a non-human primate or other mammal, or a bat). Virus is then transmitted to others through direct contact with the blood, secretions, organs or other body fluids of infected persons, or with fomites contaminated by body fluids. Symptomatic patients are considered infectious, and are most infectious as disease becomes severe. Infection in healthcare workers and caregivers has been a notable feature in outbreaks. Sexual transmission has been reported 3 months post onset of symptoms. The incubation period for Ebola is 2–21 days, and for Marburg is 3–10 days.

- **CCHF:** Infection is acquired through the bite or crushing of an infected tick, or through contact with blood of an infected animal. Person-to-person transmission occurs via direct contact with the blood, secretions, organs or other body fluids of infected persons; symptomatic patients are considered infectious. Nosocomial transmission remains a problem in endemic areas. The incubation period appears to vary with route of transmission. Following a tick bite, it is usually 1–3 days, and up to 9 days; but following contact with infected blood or tissues it is usually 5–6 days, up to 13 days.
- **Hantaviruses:** Virus is shed in urine, faeces, and saliva of the rodent host, and most human infections are thought to arise via inhalation of infected aerosols from these excreta. Person-to-person transmission is rare. The incubation period is 2–4 weeks for the viruses causing HFRS.
- **Dengue.** Infection follows the bite of an infective *Aedes* mosquito. Person-to-person transmission does not occur, although during the viraemic phase blood is infective for biting mosquitoes. The incubation period is 4–7 days, with a range of 3–14 days.

Clinical features and sequelae

- **Lassa fever:** Clinically infection ranges from mild to asymptomatic (80% of cases) to a severe fulminating infection. Onset is gradual with fever, chills, malaise, headache, myalgia, and sore throat. Nausea, vomiting, diarrhoea or cough may be present, and exudative pharyngeal inflammation is common. In severe cases, shock, encephalopathy, renal and circulatory failure may develop progressing to severe haemorrhage. Overall the mortality rate is 1–3%, but is around 15% in hospitalized cases. Mortality rates are high (~30%) in the third trimester of pregnancy, and fetal death approaches 100%. The most notable complication is acute hearing loss and sensorineural hearing deficit occurs in 25–30% of patients and may persist for life. It does not appear to be associated with disease severity.
- **South American haemorrhagic fevers:** The clinical picture is consistent for all these viruses: onset is gradual with fever, malaise, myalgia, back pain, and headache. Petechiae and haemorrhage develop after a few days, and neurological manifestations may follow with tremor of hands and tongue, seizures, and coma. Blood loss is usually minor, but the haematocrit rises as capillary leak syndrome becomes more severe. Renal impairment is very common in Argentine haemorrhagic fever. Overall mortality rates vary from 5% to 30%, and are highest in the third trimester of pregnancy. Fetal mortality is high.
- **Ebola and Marburg:** Onset is sudden with headache, high fever, and back pain. Prostration follows rapidly with pharyngitis, vomiting, severe watery diarrhoea, conjunctivitis, and a measles-like rash. Neurological manifestations include severe lethargy, irritability, and confusion. Haemorrhagic manifestations develop after ~5 days, and may progress to severe blood loss and death. Overall the mortality rates are very high; between 50% and 90%. Fetal loss is common when infection

occurs during pregnancy. Convalescence is slow and debilitating, and survivors may have prolonged amnesia.

- *CCHF:* Onset is sudden with fever, myalgia, dizziness, neck pain and stiffness, backache, headache, sore eyes, and photophobia. Nausea, vomiting, diarrhoea, and sore throat may also occur. Haemorrhagic manifestations develop after ~5 days and may be extensive with petechial rash, bruising, ecchymoses and generalized bleeding of the gums and orifices. In severe cases multiorgan failure develops. Up to 50% of cases are fatal, but mortality rates vary considerably.

- *HFRS:* These are a group of clinically similar illnesses characterized by fever, headache, malaise, gastrointestinal symptoms, and renal impairment. Onset is sudden. Petechial and conjunctival haemorrhage may precede periods of hypotension followed by hypovolaemic shock. Most infections do not exhibit overt signs of bleeding or internal haemorrhage. The mortality rate is up to 15%, but in Europe, Puumala virus infection is generally a mild disease (nephropathia endemica) that is rarely haemorrhagic and has a case fatality rate <1%.

- *Dengue fever/DHF.* Most dengue infections are either asymptomatic, or a febrile influenza-like illness. However, DHF is a potentially fatal complication of classical dengue fever, the pathogenesis of which is still unclear. Strain variability may have a role, but the main hypothesis surrounds the immune response to sequential infections with different viral serotypes. Dengue fever starts with fever, nausea, severe headache, and back pain. Acute illness is relatively short-lived although incapacitating. DHF is typically seen in children <15 years old and is characterized by rapid deterioration and prostration, with haemorrhage and shock secondary to circulatory collapse. Petechiae and ecchymoses appear. Mortality rates of DHF can exceed 20% in the absence of circulatory support, but are <2% with appropriate management.

Diagnosis

- For all the hazard group 4 haemorrhagic fever viruses, diagnostic testing must be carried out in a designated laboratory with containment level 4 facilities.
- The diagnosis of a VHF should be considered in all patients returning from an endemic area and presenting with compatible symptoms.
- In the first few days of illness, diagnosis is achieved by virus detection in blood or tissue samples—virus isolation; detection of viral antigens in tissue by immunofluorescence or EIA; detection of viral nucleic acid by PCR.
- Serological testing by detection of IgM and IgG antibodies in serum by ELISA or fluorescent antibody test (FAT). IgM may be detectable very soon after symptom onset. For dengue diagnosis, serological cross-reactions with other flaviviruses must be rigorously excluded.
- There may be a number of possible differential diagnoses depending on the country of exposure, including malaria, typhoid, leptospirosis, rickettsial infections.
- Dual pathology is possible.

Management and treatment

- Seek advice as soon as possible, and transfer patient to a specialist unit if appropriate
- For Lassa, CCHF, Ebola, Marburg, and South American arenaviruses, patients must be managed in strict isolation (in a negative pressure room if available), with full infection control precautions. Contacts should be restricted to essential personnel only, and invasive procedures including venepuncture should be minimized.
- Symptomatic and supportive treatment is essential, particularly fluid and electrolyte balance, replacement of plasma loss during period of capillary leakage, volume replacement, and replacement of coagulation factors and platelets.
- The supportive care of patients critically ill with a VHF should be the same as the conventional care provided to patients with other causes of multisystem failure.
- Renal failure with oliguria is a prominent feature of HFRS and may be seen in other VHFs as intravascular volume depletion becomes more pronounced. In HFRS, the management of oliguria may require haemodialysis or peritoneal dialysis.
- Monitor platelets and haematocrit, and virological indices (i.e. PCR positivity and viral load) in blood and urine.
- In severe cases, therapy will be required for shock and blood loss.
- Antiviral therapy with ribavirin is recommended for Lassa fever, Argentine HF (and is probably effective for other arenaviruses), and CCHF.
- IV ribavirin should be given early in the course of disease. There is some evidence that ribavirin treatment reduces renal complications in HFRS.
- Convalescent immune plasma has been used with beneficial effect against Argentine haemorrhagic fever, but is only available in Argentina.
- No antiviral therapeutic options currently exist for other haemorrhagic fevers.

Prevention

Lassa and other arenaviruses, CCHF, Ebola, Marburg

- Strict barrier precautions when managing patients are essential to minimize exposure of healthcare workers, other hospital staff, and family members, and thus prevent nosocomial transmission. Non-essential staff and visitors should be restricted.
- All persons entering the room must be gloved and gowned, with face shields and eye protection for those coming within 1m (3ft).
- Prevention of percutaneous injuries associated with the use and disposal of sharps is vital.
- Keep laboratory tests to the minimum necessary for clinical management in order to reduce potential exposures to laboratory staff. Samples must be appropriately labelled and the laboratory alerted as to their high-risk status.

- Standard protocols for laundry, cleaning, and disinfection may be followed where there is no contamination by blood/body fluids.
- Safe and effective disinfection and decontamination procedures are required for materials contaminated with blood/body fluids (including personal protective equipment, linens, fomites, equipment, and patient samples sent for diagnostic investigations). Persons carrying out decontamination must be appropriately protected. Contaminated environmental surfaces should be cleaned with hypochlorite solution (5000ppm available chlorine), unless the contamination is heavy, in which case hypochlorite solutions containing 10 000ppm available chlorine should be used. Where possible, contaminated materials and samples should be double-bagged then autoclaved or incinerated.
- Contact tracing: All persons having contact with the case since they became symptomatic must be identified and risk assessed. Those with close contact must be monitored by daily temperature checks for 21 days following their last contact.
- There is no evidence to suggest that postexposure prophylaxis with ribavirin is effective.
- No vaccines are currently available, except for Argentine haemorrhagic fever. This vaccine is only available in Argentina, where it has been used since the 1990s, and been responsible a decrease in incidence of this disease.
- Prevention of naturally acquired cases in endemic areas—control of rodent and insect vectors, rodent-proof storage containers, and avoidance of insect bites or exposure to body fluids of infected animals.

Dengue and hantavirus
- Normal control of infection procedures apply when managing patients.
- Contact tracing not required.
- No vaccines currently available.
- Prevention of naturally acquired cases in endemic areas—control of rodent and insect vectors, rodent-proof storage containers, and avoidance of insect bites.

Further reading

Howard CR. *Viral Haemorrhagic Fevers, Perspectives in Medical Virology*, Volume **11**. 2003, Elsevier.

Yellow fever

📖 see also Chapter 18, 41

Name and nature of organism

- A systemic viral (haemorrhagic) arthropod borne disease with sudden onset and a broad clinical spectrum.
- Yellow fever virus is a member of the family *Flaviviridae*, genus *Flavivirus*.
- The prototype member of the genus *Flavivirus*, yellow fever virus is a small, single-stranded, positive sense, RNA virus with a lipid envelope.
- At least seven genotypes have been distinguished in specific geographical regions; there is a single serotype.

Epidemiology

- Yellow fever probably originated in Africa 3000 years ago. It was transported to the Americas during the seventeenth century on slave ships and to Europe via the maritime trade route.
- Widespread epidemics occurred in North America and Europe up to the late nineteenth century.
- Yellow fever now is a risk only in the tropical regions of sub-Saharan Africa, South America, and Trinidad in the Caribbean and Panama.
- In 2007, the WHO received reports of 11 laboratory confirmed cases in Africa and 48 cases in South America. In endemic countries, the number of cases and deaths is likely to be grossly underreported. It has been estimated that for every symptomatic case, there are seven sub-clinical infections. In the 1980s and early 1990s there were several thousands of cases reported annually.
- The majority of cases and deaths occur in sub-Saharan Africa, where there are 33 countries with a risk of yellow fever transmission.
- The epidemiology of yellow fever is dynamic and the virus may emerge in areas previously considered free of the disease.
- Since 1996, there have been six fatal cases of yellow fever in unvaccinated travellers returning to their country of origin.

Transmission and incubation period

- Yellow fever is a zoonotic infection. Non-human primates are the main reservoir.
- Yellow fever virus is transmitted by mosquitoes most active during the daytime.

- In Africa, *Aedes* spp. mosquitoes transmit infection. In jungle areas of South America, *Haemagogus* spp. transmit infection, with *Aedes aegypti*, the predominate species in urban outbreaks.
- Transmission occurs year round. In Africa, the risk of transmission is highest during the rainy season in areas of habitation which border the rainforest (intermediate cycle). In the South American rainforest, transmission in the monkey population increases intermittently, resulting in waves of disease activity. Humans living or visiting in these areas are at risk of infection (sylvatic cycle).
- Transmission occurs in urban environments (urban cycle), where breeding conditions are favourable for *A. aegypti* (water storage containers and collections of rainwater).
- The incubation period after an infective bite is 3–6 days.

Clinical features and sequelae

- Infection can be subclinical, a mild febrile infection, or a severe illness with jaundice, haemorrhage, multiorgan failure and death.
- Onset of symptoms is abrupt.
- During the first 3–4 days (viraemic stage) symptoms include fever, headache, prostration, myalgia, photophobia, anorexia, irritability, epigastric tenderness, and hepatomegaly.
- Bradycardia relative to fever (Faget's sign) can be present. Fever can be as high as 40°C (105°F).
- There is leucopenia with relative neutropenia.
- Jaundice occurs 48–72 hours after onset of symptoms, with elevation of liver enzymes.
- After a period of remission (48 hours), around 15% progress to more serious disease. Symptoms include return of fever, jaundice, nausea, vomiting, and oliguria.
- Complications are haemorrhage (e.g. DIC, melaena, petechiae, epistaxis), myocardial damage and arrhythmias, profound hypotension and shock, encephalopathy, coma, and renal and liver failure.
- Five to 10 days after onset of symptoms, the patient recovers, or death occurs as a result of multiorgan failure (case fatality rate: 20–50%).

Diagnosis

- Clinical symptoms (differential diagnoses include leptospirosis, louse-borne relapsing fever, other VHFs, viral hepatitis, Q fever, Rift Valley fever, typhoid, and malaria).
- Specific laboratory diagnosis by detection of virus or viral antigen in blood or body tissue:
  - Viral culture, RT-PCR
  - Post-mortem diagnosis by immunocytochemical staining for yellow fever antigen in liver, heart or kidney.

- Detection of yellow fever antibody in sera: IgM-capture ELISA (presumptive diagnosis on a single sample, confirmed by rise in titres in acute and convalescent samples).
- Yellow fever is a notifiable infectious disease in the UK and globally under International Health Regulations (2005).

Management and treatment

- There is no specific antiviral treatment.
- Intensive supportive care with management of complications is necessary for severe cases. In high-income countries, all cases or suspected cases of yellow fever should be managed in a specialist unit for infectious or tropical disease.

Prevention

- Prevention is by vaccination, mosquito bite avoidance, and vector control.
- Vector control (using insecticides and larvicides) in the urban environment can interrupt the mosquito breeding cycle and transmission of the virus.
- Vaccination is included in the expanded programme of immunization in some countries where there is a risk of yellow fever transmission.
- Vaccination should be given to:
  - Children aged ≥9 months and adults who plan to visit yellow fever risk areas.
  - Laboratory workers handling infected material.
- Vaccination should be given at least 10 days before travel to allow protective immunity to develop. Protective levels of neutralizing antibody are seen in about 90% of vaccinees within 10 days of vaccination and in up to 99% of vaccinees within 30 days.
- The administration of yellow fever vaccine is regulated under the WHO International Health Regulations (2005) which stipulate that 'State parties shall designate specific yellow fever vaccination centres within their territories in order to assure the quality and safety of the procedures and materials employed.'
- Vaccination is a requirement for entry into some countries under International Health Regulations (see National Travel Health Network and Centre, Country Information Pages, ℘ www.nathnac. org). Vaccination must be recorded in an International Certificate of Vaccination or Prophylaxis (ICVP).
- The ICVP becomes valid 10 days after administration of vaccination in first time vaccinees and immediately after if reimmunized.
- Vaccination should be repeated at 10-yearly intervals if a person remains at risk.
- In the UK, vaccination is with yellow fever 17D (204 strain), live, attenuated vaccine which contains no antibiotics or preservatives (alternative but similar vaccines are in production globally). It is

supplied in a lyophilized preparation with a diluent and must be reconstituted immediately before use.

- 17D vaccine is manufactured in chick embryo cell culture; the vaccine contains very small amounts of egg protein.
  - There are specific contraindications and precautions associated with yellow fever vaccine. A careful risk assessment should be made before administration and specialist advice sought as appropriate.
- 17D vaccine has been used for >60 years and has a well-documented history of tolerability and safety. However, rare severe and fatal adverse reactions to the vaccine have been reported:
  - Anaphylaxis is rare (one case per 156 000–250 000 doses)
  - Yellow fever vaccine-associated neurologic disease (VAND) (approximately four to eight cases per 1 000 000 doses):
    — First time recipients of vaccine only
    — Onset 3–28 days after vaccination (median 14 days)
    — Fever, focal neurological dysfunction, convulsions, paresis
    — Nearly all patients recover.
  - Yellow fever vaccine-associated viscerotropic disease (VAVD) (approximately five cases per 1 000 000 doses):
    — First time recipients of vaccine only
    — Onset 1–8 days post vaccination (median 3 days)
    — Fever, malaise, headache *progressing to*
    — Hepatitis, hypotension, respiratory failure, renal failure, coagulopathy
    — Case fatality rate is approximately 60%.
- Risk of either VAND or VAVD increases for first time vaccinees aged ≥60 years (around 20 cases per 1 000 000 doses).
- Risk of severe adverse neurological events is increased for infants aged <9 months with the risk being inversely proportional to age. The vaccine should never be given to infants aged <5 months because of the risk of post-vaccination encephalitis. Infants aged 6–9 months should only be immunized if the risk of yellow fever during travel is unavoidable.
- Mosquitoes can be repelled by N, N-diethylmetatoluamide (DEET). DEET preparations are safe to use in concentrations of up to 50%, in adults (including those pregnant or breastfeeding) and infants and children aged >2 months. Infants who are too young to receive yellow fever vaccination and where travel to risk areas is unavoidable, should ideally be nursed under an insecticide impregnated mosquito net, day and night.

Future research

- Clinical trials underway or planned:
  - Further evaluation of the safety and immunogenicity of 17D vaccine
  - Evaluation of the safety, tolerability, and immunogenicity of inactivated yellow fever vaccine, as well as other vaccine types.
  - Study of immune memory generated against yellow fever vaccine.

- Mechanism of severe adverse events following yellow fever vaccination.
- Comparative assessment of viraemia, immunogenicity and safety of live attenuated yellow fever vaccine given alone or in combination with human immunoglobulin.
- WHO Yellow Fever Working Group (representatives from the WHO, CDC, Pan-American Health Organization, NaTHNaC, and others) to review best evidence for yellow fever geographical distribution and agree risk maps to be used for travellers.

Further reading

Advisory Committee on Dangerous Pathogens. *Management and Control of Viral Haemorrhagic Fevers*, December 1996. London: The Stationary Office, 1996. Available at: ℘ www.hpa.org.uk/web/HPAwebFile/HPAweb_C/1194947382005 (accessed 23 September 2010).

Barnett ED. Yellow fever: epidemiology and prevention. *Clin Infect Dis* 2007;**15**:850–6.

Centers for Disease Control and Prevention. Yellow Fever Vaccine. Recommendations of the Advisory Committee on Immunization Practices (ACIP). *MMWR* 2010;**59**(RR-7):1–26.

Monath TP, Cetron MS, Teuwen DE. Yellow fever vaccine. Chapter 36. In: Plotkin S, Orenstein W, Offit P, eds. *Vaccines*. 5th edn. Philadelphia, PA: WB Saunders/ Elsevier, 2008.

National Travel Health Centre and Network. Health Information Sheet. Yellow Fever. March 2010. Available at: ℘ www.nathnac.org/pro/factsheets/yellow.htm (accessed 1 February 2011).

World Health Organization. International travel and health. Geneva 2010. Available at: ℘ www.who.int/ith/en/ (accessed 1 February 2011).

World Health Organization. *International Health Regulations*, 2005. Geneva: World Health Organization, 2005:1–60. Available at: ℘ www.who.int/csr/ihr/en/ (accessed 23 September 2010).

Yersiniosis

📖 see also Chapter 12, 15, 22, 69

Name and nature of organism

- *Yersinia enterocolitica* and *Yersinia pseudotuberculosis* are short pleomorphic Gram-negative rods or cocco-bacilli, which often exhibit bipolar staining.
- Grow on simple laboratory media, including those containing bile salts (e.g. MacConkey agar).

Epidemiology

- *Y. enterocolitica* and *Y. pseudotuberculosis* are zoonotic infections.
- Main reservoir is the gastrointestinal tract of a wide range of animals, including pigs, cattle, cats, dogs, rodents, and birds.
- Infections are more common in children than in adults.
- *Y. pseudotuberculosis* infections is more common in males.
- Most cases occur in autumn or winter.
- More common in Scandinavia and northern Europe, though cases have been reported worldwide.
- Infections are more common and more severe in patients with iron overload, e.g. haemochromatosis, thalassaemia.

Transmission and incubation period

- Infection follows ingestion of inadequately cooked meat (especially pork) or other food contaminated with *Yersinia spp.* (e.g. milk).
- Infection may also occur after contact with infected pet.
- Ability of *Y. enterocolitica* to grow at +4°C means refrigerated meat can be source of infection.
- In northern Europe most cases are sporadic.
- In USA foodborne outbreaks associated with contaminated chocolate, dairy products, tofu, lettuce, and carrots have been described.
- Incubation period: *Y .enterocolitica* 3–10 days, *Y. pseudotuberculosis* 7–21 days.

Clinical features and sequelae

Although both organisms cause a similar spectrum of infections, the majority of *Y. enterocolitica* infections present as acute enteritis or acute terminal ileitis whereas *Y. pseudotuberculosis* is more commonly associated with mesenteric adenitis or acute pseudo-appendicitis.

- Acute enteritis or acute enterocolitis is characterized by thin, watery diarrhoea, abdominal pain, lower right quadrant tenderness, and low grade fever, especially in infants.
- There may be blood and mucus in the stool, mimicking shigellosis.
- Mesenteric adenitis, acute pseudo-appendicitis or terminal ileitis are characterized by abdominal pain in the right lower quadrant and low-grade fever. In some cases the pain may be so severe, acute appendicitis is suspected. Intussusception may occur.
- The majority of cases of enteritis and mesenteric adenitis are self-limiting with recovery after 1–3 weeks.
- Post-infectious complications include a reactive arthritis (especially in HLA-B27 +ve individuals) and erythema nodosum.
- Bacteraemia may occur in otherwise healthy children as well as in those with underlying comorbidities. Children with conditions associated with iron overload, including haemolytic anaemias, thalassaemia, sickle cell anaemia, diabetes mellitus and immunosuppression (including HIV), are at risk. Infants <3 months of age are also at increased risk of developing a bacteraemia.
- A range of extra-intestinal complications of *Y. enterocolitica* bacteraemia have been reported. These include hepatic and splenic abscess, pneumonia, empyema, septic arthritis, meningitis, endocarditis, and mycotic aneurysms.
- *Y. pseudotuberculosis* infection has been associated with a clinical syndrome resembling Izumi fever, an illness that occurs epidemically in Japan, or Kawasaki disease. Symptoms and clinical findings include fever, rash, diarrhoea, vomiting, desquamation, strawberry tongue, abdominal pain resembling acute appendicitis, arthralgia, lymphadenopathy, hepatosplenomegaly, and conjunctivitis. Coronary artery aneurysms have been reported.

Diagnosis

- *Y. enterocolitica* can be isolated from stool cultures on a selective medium. A cold-enrichment technique of incubation at +4°C for up to 3 weeks may be necessary to recover the organisms. Clinicians should inform the laboratory if they suspect a yersinial infection.
- *Y. pseudotuberculosis* is rarely isolated from stool culture but may be recovered from mesenteric lymph node culture.
- Blood cultures should be taken.
- Serological tests, including agglutination tests and ELISA may be used. False-positive results from cross-reacting antibodies to salmonellae, *Escherichia coli* and *Brucella* spp. occur.

Management and treatment

- The majority of cases of *Yersinia* enteritis and mesenteric adenitis are generally self-limiting and do not require antimicrobial therapy. However, antimicrobials should be administered to ill children and immunocompromised patients.
- Septicaemia, extraintestinal foci of infection, and enteritis in immunocompromised patients should be treated with antimicrobials.
- *Y. enterocolitica* is generally resistant to penicillin, ampicillin, and first-generation cephalosporins.
- Ciprofloxacin, co-trimoxazole, and aminoglycosides have all been used successfully to treat *Y. enterocolitica* infections.
- *Y. pseudotuberculosis* is usually susceptible to penicillin and ampicillin.

Prevention

- Good hygienic practices should be observed at all stages of the production and preparation of food.
- All meat, especially pork, must be thoroughly cooked before consumption.
- Vegetables and salads should be washed before consumption.
- Children visiting farms and handling animals should wash their hands thoroughly before eating.

Future research

- Further studies of the natural history and epidemiology of *Y. enterocolitica* and *Y. pseudotuberculosis*.

Further reading

Abdel-Haq NM, Asmar BI, Abuhammour WM, Brown WJ. *Yersinia enterocolitica* infection in children. *Pediatr Infect Dis J* 2000;**19**:954–8.

Hoogkamp-Korstanje JAA, Stolk-Engelaar VMM. *Yersinia enterocolitica* infection in children. *Pediatr Infect Dis J* 1995;**14**:771–5.

Tauxe RV. Salad and pseudoappendicitis: *Yersinia pseudotuberculosis* as a foodborne pathogen. *J Infect Dis* 2004;**189**:761–3.

Vento S, Cainelli F, Cesario F. Infections and thalassaemia. *Lancet Infect Dis* 2006;**6**:226–33.

Appendix 1

The contribution of infectious diseases to neonatal and childhood deaths in England and Wales

Introduction

- The UK has one of the highest mortality rates in children <5 years (6.5/1000 livebirths) among Western European countries and the second highest among industrialized countries worldwide after the USA (8/1000 livebirths).[1, 2]
- Infections are a significant and potentially preventable cause of death, particularly in young children.
- In England and Wales, there are around 650 000 births annually, with ~3000 stillbirths, ~2000 neonatal deaths (<28 days), ~3000 infant deaths (<1 year) and ~4500 childhood (0–15 years) deaths a year (Fig. A1.1).
- In the UK, the recent Confidential Enquiry into Maternal and Child Health (CEMACH, ℘ www.cemach.org.uk) reported infection to be the 'largest single cause of death in children dying of an acute physical illness … despite comprehensive and expanding immunization programmes, antibiotic availability, training in resuscitation and life support.'

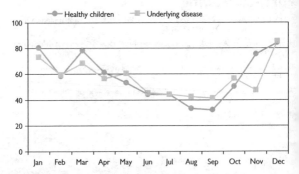

Fig. A1.1 Number of infection-related deaths by month of death among previously healthy children and those with underlying disease, England and Wales 2003–05.

Childhood deaths

- The CEMACH report estimated that infection was relevant in at least 20% of the childhood deaths it reviewed, and this was supported by a recent analysis of childhood death certificates.[3]
- Among infection-related deaths, the median age was 1 year; and, half of all children who died had an underlying medical condition recorded on their death certificate.
- The contribution of infection to childhood deaths was highest in the 1–4 year age group (27% of all deaths), followed by <1 year olds (21%) and 5–14 year olds (12%).
- The proportion of children who died of an infection and had an underlying medical condition recorded on their death certificate increased with age.
- Underlying medical conditions varied with age—prematurity and associated problems were most common in infants (<1 year olds), cerebral palsy and its complications in 1–4 year olds and malignancy in 5–14 year olds.
- Girls who died were more likely to have an underlying medical condition than boys.
- Septicaemia was recorded in half of all infection-related deaths, followed by respiratory tract infections (30%), and infections of the CNS (15%).
- Previously healthy children were more likely to present with meningitis or encephalitis, while those with underlying medical conditions were more likely to have septicaemia.
- Among previously healthy children, respiratory tract infections were most prevalent in infant deaths, septicaemia in 1–4 year olds and meningitis or encephalitis in 5–14 year olds.
- Where a pathogen was specified on the death certificate, 60% were bacterial, 30% viral, 8% fungal, and 2% other infections (Table A1.1).
- In previously healthy children, meningococci were the most commonly reported organisms (28%), followed by pneumococci (18%) and other streptococci (13%).
- In children with underlying medical conditions, Gram-negative enteric bacilli accounted for over half of all bacterial infections, while enterococcal and staphylococcal infections contributed a further 20% of deaths.
- Viral infections contributed equally to deaths among previously healthy children and those with underlying medical conditions (20%)—over half the deaths attributed to viral infections were caused by four viruses: RSV (16%), adenovirus (12%), influenza virus (12%), and CMV (10%).

Table A1.1 Pathogens noted on death certificated in previously healthy children and those with an underlying medical condition (excluding deaths in the neonatal period, <28 days after birth) in England and Wales between 2003 and 2005

	Previously healthy (n = 681)		Underlying conditions (n = 676)		All cases (n = 1357)	
Bacterial (total)	339	%	155	%	494	%
Meningococcal	133	39.2	5	3.2	138	27.9
Pneumococcal	72	21.2	17	11	89	18
Other streptococci	51	15	11	7.1	62	12.6
Unspecified Gram-negative	6	1.8	36	23.2	42	8.5
Staphylococcal	15	4.4	23	14.8	38	7.7
Klebsiella	1	0.3	16	10.3	17	3.4
E. coli	4	1.2	12	7.7	16	3.2
Pseudomonas	5	1.5	9	5.8	14	2.8
Unspecified Gram-positive	2	0.6	1	0.6	3	0.6
Other/not specified	50	14.7	25	16.2	75	15.2
Viral (total)	122		134		256	
RSV	8	6.6	34	25.4	42	16.4
Adenovirus	11	9	21	15.7	32	12.5
Influenza	18	14.8	12	9	30	11.7
CMV	17	13.9	10	7.5	27	10.5
Varicella	8	6.6	11	8.2	19	7.4
Other/not specified	60	49.2	46	34.3	106	41.4
Fungal (total)	5		64		69	
Candida	3	60	23	35.9	26	37.7
Aspergillus	0	0	22	34.4	22	31.9
Pneumocystis	0	0	6	9.4	6	8.7
Other/not specified	2	40	13	20.3	15	21.7
Tuberculosis	12		4		16	
Other	3		2		5	
Not specified	203		317		520	

Neonatal deaths

- The neonatal death rate (defined as deaths among infants <28 days of age) in England and Wales has remained constant at 3.4–3.9 per 1000 livebirths over the past decade, which is significantly lower than the global neonatal mortality rate of 30 per 1000 livebirths.
- Worldwide, the largest cause of neonatal mortality is infection, accounting for 36% of deaths, but in England and Wales, as in the rest of the developed world, the most significant cause of neonatal mortality is prematurity and its complications, with infection playing a smaller role.[4]
- In England and Wales, analysis of death certificate data estimated that at least 11% of neonatal deaths were infection-related, which is similar to the 10% estimated by the 2007 CEMACH report.
- Overall, 36% of the neonatal infection-related deaths occurred in term neonates, 17% in preterm neonates (28–36 weeks) and 47% in extremely pre-terms (<28 weeks' gestation).
- 57% of all and 49% of term neonatal infection-related deaths had an underlying medical condition recorded on their death certificate, mainly respiratory in premature and extremely premature neonates and cardiac, respiratory, and birth asphyxia in previously healthy term neonates.
- Septicaemia was the most common clinical presentation (50%) followed by pneumonia (15%) and meningitis (5%).
- A pathogen was recorded on the death certificate of only 44% of neonatal deaths—of these, 80% were bacterial, 10% were fungal, and 9% were viral (Table A1.2).
- GBS was recorded in a third of neonatal deaths where a bacterial infection was specified and in 11% of all infection-related neonatal deaths.
- Among preterm and extremely preterm deaths, Gram-negative pathogens (particularly *Escherichia coli*), staphylococci (mainly CONS) and fungi (mostly *Candida* species) predominated.
- Deaths caused by viral infections were rare, except for HSV infections, which almost exclusively affected healthy term neonates.

Table A1.2 Pathogens reported on the death certificates of neonates who died in England and Wales between 2003 and 2005

	Healthy term neonates (>36 weeks' gestation)		Preterm neonates (28–36 weeks' gestation)		Extremely preterm neonates (<28 weeks' gestation)	
Bacterial (total)	111		42		120	
Gram-positive	81	73.0%	18	42.9%	58	48.3%
Streptococci:	75	67.6%	11	26.2%	23	19.2%
• GBS	58	52.3%	10	23.8%	19	15.8%
• Pneumococcus	4	3.6%	1	2.4%	0	0%
• Other streptococci	13	11.7%	0	0%	4	1.6%
Staphylococci:	6	5.4%	6	14.3%	29	24.2%
• CONS	0	0.0%	2	4.8%	11	9.2%
• S. aureus	1	0.9%	1	2.4%	3	2.5%
• MRSA	2	1.8%	1	2.4%	1	0.8%
• Unspecified Staphylococcus sp.	3	2.7%	2	4.8%	14	11.7%
Other/unspecified Gram-positive	0	0.0%	1	2.4%	6	10.3%
Gram-negative	27	24.3%	24	57.1%	60	50.0%
E. coli	10	9.0%	9	37.5%	18	30.0%
Pseudomonas sp.	6	5.4%	3	12.5%	10	16.7%
Klebsiella sp.	2	1.8%	1	4.2%	5	8.3%
Other/unspecified Gram-negative	9	8.1%	11	45.8%	27	45.0%
Unspecified bacteria	3	2.7%	0	0%	2	1.7%
Viral (total)	**23**		**3**		**3**	
Herpes simplex	13	56.5%	1	33.3%	0	0%
Coxsackie	3	13.0%	0	0%	0	0%
RSV	1	4.3%	0	0%	1	33.3%
Other/unspecified viral	6	26.1%	2	66.6%	2	66.6%
Fungal (total)	**2**		**4**		**31**	
Candida sp.	2	100.0%	2	50%	19	61.3%
Aspergillus sp.	0	0.0%	0	0%	1	3.2%
Other/unspecified fungal	0	0.0%	2	50%	11	35.5%

Conclusions

- Infections contribute to at least 11% of neonatal and 20% of childhood deaths in England and Wales.[5, 6]
- Around half the neonates and children who die have other comorbidities.
- GBS contribute significantly to neonatal deaths, while meningococci and pneumococci are important causes of death among previously healthy infants and young children—these infection-related deaths may be preventable through routine infant immunization in the near future.[7]
- Among children with underlying medical conditions as well as preterm and extremely preterm neonates, Gram-negative enteric pathogens and fungi contribute significantly to death—this group of children share similar risk factors, such as recurrent and prolonged hospitalizations, exposure to multiple antibiotics and immunosuppressive medications, and insertion of in-dwelling vascular catheters.

Key references

1 Collison D, Dey C, Hannah G, Stevenson L. Income inequality and child mortality in wealthy nations. *J Public Health (Oxf)* 2007;**29**:114–17.

2 Roush SW, Murphy TV. Historical comparisons of morbidity and mortality for vaccine-preventable diseases in the United States. *JAMA* 2007;**298**:2155–63.

3 Pearson GA, ed. *Why Children Die: A Pilot Study 2006, England (South West, North East and West Midlands), Wales and Northern Ireland.* London: Confidential Enquiry into Maternal and Child Healty (CEMACH), 2008. Available at: ℅ www.cemach.org.uk/Publications-Press-Releases/Report-Publications/Child-Health.aspx (accessed 1 January 2010).

4 Lawn JE, Cousens S, Zupan J. 4 million neonatal deaths: when? Where? Why? *Lancet* 2005;**365**:891–900.

5 Ladhani S, Pebody RG, Ramsay ME, Lamagni TL, Johnson AP, Sharland M. Continuing impact of infectious diseases on childhood deaths in England and Wales, 2003–2005. *Pediatr Infect Dis J* 2010;**29**:310–13.

6 Confidential Enquiry into Maternal and Child Health. *Confidential Enquiry into Maternal and Child Health (CEMACH) Perinatal Mortality 2007: United Kingdom.* London: CEMACH, 2009. Available at: ℅ www.cemach.org.uk/Publications-Press-Releases/Report-Publications/Perinatal-Mortality.aspx (accessed 1 January 2010).

7 Vergnano S, Embleton ND, Collinson A, *et al.* Missed opportunities for preventing GBS infections. *Arch Dis Child Fetal Neonatal Ed* 2010;**95**:F72–F3.

Appendix 2

Guidance on infection control in school and other childcare settings

Prevention of the spread of infections is best ensured by: routine immunization, high standards of personal hygiene and practice, particularly handwashing, and maintaining a clean environment. Once infection has occurred, it may be necessary to exclude children from contact with others so as to prevent further cases. Advice on exclusion periods often varies across Europe. Table A2.1 is based on unpublished work carried out for the European Centre for Disease Prevention and Control.

In England it is advised to discuss community infection control with the local Health Protection Unit (HPU).

Table A2.1 Guidance on infection control in school and other childcare settings

Illness	Recommended period to be kept away from school, nursery, or childminders	Comments
Diarrhoea and vomiting		
Diarrhoea and/or vomiting	48 hours from last episode of diarrhoea or vomiting	Exclusion from swimming should be for 2 weeks following last episode of diarrhoea
E. coli 0157 VTEC	Symptomatic cases should be excluded, until they have had normal stools for 48 hours. Children <5 years may need to be excluded until they have had two consecutive negative faecal samples	Exclusion from swimming should be for 2 weeks following last episode of diarrhoea
Shigella (dysentery)	Symptomatic cases should be excluded. Children <5 years should be excluded for a further 48 hours. Always consult with your health protection unit (HPU)	Exclusion from swimming should be for 2 weeks following last episode of diarrhoea
Typhoid[a] (and paratyphoid[a]) (enteric fever)	Symptomatic cases should be excluded. Children <5 years should be excluded until three negative stools have been collected. Always consult with HPU	Exclusion from swimming should be for 2 weeks following last episode of diarrhoea
Respiratory infections		
Influenza	Until recovered	
Tuberculosis[a]	Always inform HPU if smear positive for at least 2 weeks after starting treatment	Not usually spread from children. Requires prolonged close contact
Whooping cough[a] (pertussis)	5 days from commencing appropriate antibiotic treatment or 21 days from onset of illness if no antibiotic treatment	Preventable by vaccination. After treatment non-infectious coughing may continue for many weeks

(Continued)

Table A2.1 (Contd.)

Illness	Recommended period to be kept away from school, nursery, or childminders	Comments
Rashes/skin		
Athletes foot	None	Athletes foot is not a serious condition. Treatment is recommended
Chicken pox	5 days from onset of rash	Contacts who are immunosuppressed or pregnant should seek urgent advice
Cold sores (herpes simplex)	None	Avoid kissing and contact with the sores. Cold sores are generally a mild self-limiting disease
German measles (rubella)[a]	6 days from onset of rash	Preventable by immunization (MMR ×2 doses). Pregnant female staff in contact with rubella in the period 7 days before to 6 days after the development of the rash should consult their GP or obstetrician
Hand, foot, and mouth disease	None	Contact HPU if a large number of children are affected. Exclusion may be considered in some circumstances
Impetigo	Children should be excluded from school until all the sores have crusted over or for 48 hours after starting antibiotic treatment	Antibiotic treatment by mouth may speed healing and reduce infectious period
Measles[a]	4 days from onset of rash	Preventable by vaccination (MMR × 2 doses.) Contacts who are immunosuppressed or pregnant should seek advice
Molluscum contagiosum	None	A self-limiting condition
Ringworm	Exclusion is not necessary, but treatment should be commenced as soon as possible	Different treatments are required for the different forms of the disease; not all are available from a pharmacist. Also check/treat symptomatic pets
Roseola (infantum)	None	None

Table A2.1 (Contd.)

Illness	Recommended period to be kept away from school, nursery, or childminders	Comments
Scabies	Child can return after treatment	Two treatments 1 week apart for cases. Contacts should have one treatment; include the entire household and any other very close contacts. If further information is required contact your local HPU
Scarlet fever[a]	24 hours after commencing antibiotics	Antibiotic treatment recommended for the affected child
Slapped cheek/ fifth disease. Parvovirus B19	None	Pregnant contacts and carers of children with sickle cell disease should seek advice from their GP or obstetrician
Warts and verrucae	None	Verrucae should be covered in swimming pools, gymnasiums, and changing rooms
Other infections		
Conjunctivitis	None	If an outbreak/cluster occurs consult HPU
Diphtheria[a]	Exclusion is important	Preventable by vaccination. HPU will organize any contact tracing
Glandular fever	None	About 50% of children get the disease before they are five and many adults also acquire the disease without being aware of it
Head lice	None	Treatment is recommended only in cases where live lice have definitely been seen. Close contacts should be checked and treated if live lice are found. Regular detection (combing) should be carried out by parents
Hepatitis A[a]	Exclusion may be necessary. Always consult with HPU	Good personal and environmental hygiene will minimize any possible danger of spread of hepatitis A
Hepatitis B[a] and C[a]	None	
HIV/AIDS	None	HIV is not infectious through casual contact. There have been no recorded cases of spread within a school or nursery.

(Continued)

Table A2.1 (Contd.)

Illness	Recommended period to be kept away from school, nursery, or childminders	Comments
Meningococcal meningitis[a]/septicaemia	Until recovered	Meningococcal C meningitis is preventable by vaccination. There is no reason to exclude siblings and other close contacts of a case. The HPU will give advice on any action needed and identify contacts requiring antibiotics
Meningitis[a] due to other bacteria	Until recovered	Hib meningitis and pneumococcal meningitis are preventable by vaccination. There is no reason to exclude siblings and other close contacts of a case. Always contact the HPU who will give advice on any action needed and identify contacts requiring antibiotics
Meningitis viral[a]	None	Milder illness than bacterial meningitis. There is reason to exclude siblings and other close contacts of a case. Contact tracing is not required
MRSA	None	Good hygiene, in particular handwashing and environmental cleaning, are important to minimize any danger of spread. If further information is required contact your local HPU
Mumps[a]	5 days from onset of swollen glands	Preventable by vaccination. (MMR × 2 doses)
Threadworms	None	Treatment is recommended for the child and household contacts
Tonsillitis	None	There are many causes, but most cases are due to viruses and do not need an antibiotic

[a]**Denotes a notifiable disease in England.** It is a statutory requirement that doctors report a notifiable disease to the proper office of their local authority. In addition, organizations may be required via locally agreed arrangements to inform their local HPU.

Outbreaks: If a school, nursery, or childminder suspects an outbreak of infectious disease they should inform their HPU. Advice can also be sought from the school health service.

This table is based on HPA guidance. (Guidance on infection control in schools and other childcare settings). ✍ www.hpa.org.uk/web/HPAwebfile/HPAweb_C/1194947358374 (accessed October 2010), and unpublished work from the European Centre for Disease Control and Prevention.

Immunization of the normal and immunocompromised child

Immunization of the normal child

Immunization schedules vary considerably around Europe. There is little evidence base of regional variation in disease to explain this variation. Resources for immunization programmes also vary considerably between EU countries. Different countries perceive different priorities in vaccine preventable diseases. Some differences are due to historical variation in vaccine delivery programmes and funding arrangements. It is likely that there will be increased harmonization of schedules for newer vaccines due to regulatory approval for specific schedules by the European Medicines Agency.

The European Centre for Disease Prevention and Control (ECDC) is working towards defining the core requirements for an immunization programme, with a number of very useful summary guidance documents by the Scientific Panel on Childhood Immunisation Schedule (see, for example, the report on DTP ℘ www.ecdc.europa.eu).

The WHO also has an important role in promoting immunization (e.g. the European Immunization Week highlights the continuing role of vaccines in preventing disease across the EU (℘ www.euro.who.int/eiw)).

The WHO Vaccine Preventable Diseases Monitoring System maintains a very useful website containing each country's different immunization schedules by antigen and selection centre (℘ www.who.int/immunization_monitoring/resources/en/)

In the UK, independent expert advice is provided to the ministers of the Department of Health by the Joint Committee on Vaccination and Immunisation. The minutes are available at ℘ www.dh.gov.uk/ab/JCVI and are well worth reading.

The HPA's Immunisation Division monitors the uptake of immunization and the epidemiology of vaccine preventable diseases. Full details of the current UK immunization schedule can be found at ℘ http://www.dh.gov.uk/en/Publichealth/Information/index.htm.

The 2011 UK immunization schedule

2 months
- Diptheria, acellular pertussis (whooping cough), tetanus (DTaP), polio and *Haemophilus influenzae* type b (Hib) given as a 5-in-1 single combination vaccine known as DTaP/IPV/Hib
- 13 valent Pneumococcal conjugate vaccine (PCV-13)

3 months
- 5-in-1, second dose (DTaP/IPV/Hib)
- Meningococcal serogroup C (Men C)

4 months
- 5-in-1, third dose (DTaP/IPV/Hib)
- PCV-13, second dose
- Men C, second dose

12–13 months
- Men C, third dose
- Hib, booster dose (Hib/Men C given as a single combination vaccine)
- MMR given as a single dose
- PCV-13, booster dose

3 years and 4 months, or soon after
- MMR second dose
- DTaP/IPV, given as a 4-in-1 pre-school booster

12–13 years
- Human papilloma virus (HPV) vaccine, which protects against cervical cancer (girls only): three doses given within 6 months

13–18 years
- Diphtheria, tetanus and polio booster (Td/IPV), given as a single dose.

Immunization of the immunocompromised child

The number of children considered to be immunocompromised is increasing as more and varied treatment regimens are used to treat malignant disease and inflammatory disorders, whilst the numbers of children undergoing organ and haematopoietic stem cell transplantation also continue to increase. With a few notable exceptions there is a paucity of published evidence on which to base firm recommendations for immunization and general principles need to be applied. The key questions when deciding about immunization in these circumstances are (see Table A3.1):

- Risk of the infection?
- Risk of the vaccine?
- Likelihood of efficacy.

General principles—non-live vaccines
- Safe in all groups.
- Increasing evidence for efficacy in those with secondary immunosuppression.
- Few data on primary immunodeficiency cases.

General principles—live vaccines
- All live vaccines avoided when severe depression of cell-mediated immune response is likely.
- Live oral polio vaccine avoided additionally in all antibody deficiencies (including IgA deficiency).
- Live bacterial vaccines avoided additionally in neutrophil disorders such as chronic granulomatous disease.
- Live viral vaccines avoided in patients on immunoglobulin therapy (lack of efficacy).
- Live vaccines may sometimes be used in partial (and variable) combined immunodeficiencies
  - ? Decide on CD4 counts as for HIV.
  - ? Other criteria but little evidence base.

Some non-routine specific vaccines

Influenza
- Disease likely to be complicated in most immunocompromised states:
  - Poor viral handling
  - Risk of secondary bacterial infection.
- Non-live vaccine is safe (live inactivated vaccine not available in UK and little evidence for use of intranasal vaccine at present).
- Immunoglobulin replacement therapy may not provide protective antibodies against currently circulating antigenic variants.
- Annual influenza vaccination therefore indicated in all immunocompromised children regardless of cause.

Hepatitis B
- Potential risk through blood product or tissue exposure.
- Safe, non-live vaccine.
- Advise use for all cases capable of mounting an antibody response and in whom blood product or tissue treatment is likely.
- Where possible best given prior to commencement of immunosuppressive treatment or organ transplantation.

Table A3.1 Recommendations for immunization in specific forms of immunocompromise

	Recommendations for vaccinations
Primary immunodeficiencies	
Minor antibody deficiency, e.g. IgA deficiency	All vaccines given except live oral polio
Major antibody deficiency (usually on immunoglobulin treatment)	Non-live vaccines can be given as part of patient assessment. Avoid live oral polio. Avoid MMR and VZV if receiving immunoglobulin (lack of efficacy). BCG can be given in high-risk situations
Combined (T cell) immunodeficiencies	Non-live vaccines can be given as part of patient assessment. Avoid all live vaccines if CD4 count <200
Neutrophil disorders	In some circumstances patients with counts >200 can be given line vaccines. Seek specialist advice from an immunologist
	In 'pure' neutrophil disorders, e.g. chronic granulomatous disease and congenital neutropenia, all vaccines can be given except live bacterial vaccines, BCG and oral typhoid vaccine. Note: In some neutrophil disorders such as leucocyte adhesion deficiency or Chediak–Higashi syndrome there is also T cell dysfunction and live viral vaccines should be avoided
Complement disorders	All vaccines can be given. Particularly important to fully immunize against meningococcal disease including the quadrivalent ACWY vaccine
Other innate immune defects	Too variable to generalize—seek specialist advice from an immunologist
HIV infection	📖 see Further reading
	All vaccines should be used in those with mild or moderate depression of immunity (based on CD4 circulating counts). Avoid live viral vaccines in those with CD4 counts <200/mm³ (older children/adolescents) or <15% in children <5 years of age. BCG should be avoided in infants in whom HIV infection is confirmed
Standard chemotherapy (for leukaemia or solid tumours)	On treatment:
	Complete standard immunization programme with non-live vaccines if not completed before diagnosis made. Avoid live vaccines with possible exception of varicella vaccine which can be used in certain circumstances

Table A3.1 (*Contd.*)

	Recommendations for vaccinations
	After treatment:
	Re-immunize after 6 months with live and non-live vaccines Influenza for a minimum two seasons
Haemopoietic stem cell transplantation	📖 see Further reading, p. 802
	Early immunization with non-live vaccines (6–12 months) except conjugate pneumococcal vaccine (3–6 months)
	Live viral vaccines given at 24 months, provided immune recovery confirmed and off all immunosuppressive therapy
	In those with chronic GVHD avoid live vaccines but conjugate pneumococcal vaccine is particularly important
Solid organ transplantation	When possible immunize with live and non-live vaccines prior to transplantation and immunosuppression. Complete standard immunization programme with non-live vaccines if not completed before transplantation
Immunosuppression	Where possible vaccinations should be given before immunosuppression commences
Corticosteroids[a]	Complete standard immunization schedule with non-live vaccines
Anti-proliferatives, e.g. azathioprine, ciclosporin	Avoid live vaccines until 3 months have elapsed after cessation of therapy
Biologicals	After anti-CD20 avoid primary vaccinations until B cell count recovered
	Others (e.g. anti-TNF agents): all non-live vaccines can be given. Avoid live vaccines.
Hyposplenism including sickle cell diseases	All routine vaccines should be used. Particularly important to use bacterial vaccines against pneumococcal and meningococcal disease including ACWY vaccine

[a]Immunosuppressive dose is considered to be:

- Child 10kg or less: 2mg/kg/day for >2 weeks or 1mg/kg/day for >4 weeks.
- Child >10 kg: 20mg/day

Further reading

Ljungman P, Cordonnier C, Einsele H, et al. Vaccination of hemopoeitic cell transplant recipients. *Bone Marrow Transplant* 2009;**44**:521.

Mofenson LM, Brady MT, Danner SP, et al. Guidelines for the prevention and treatment of opportunistic infections among HIV-exposed and HIV-infected children: recommendations from CDC, the National Institutes of Health, the HIV Medicine Association of the Infectious Diseases Society of America, the Pediatric Infectious Diseases Society, and the American Academy of Pediatrics. *MMWR Recomm Rep* 2009;**58**:1–166.

Royal College of Paediatrics & Child Health. Best Practice Statement: Immunisation of the Immunocompromised Child. 2002. Available at: ℘ www.rcpch.ac.uk/ (accessed 23 September 2010).

The Children's HIV Association of the UK and Ireland. Guidelines on Immunisation of HIV-Infected Children. Available at: ℘ www.chiva.org.uk/health/guidelines/immunisation (accessed 23 September 2010).

Notification and surveillance of infectious diseases

Introduction

- Surveillance is the collection, collation, and analysis of data and dissemination to those who need to know so that an action can result.
- An ideal surveillance system should be simple, flexible, acceptable, complete, sensitive, specific, representative, and timely.
- The importance of the different criteria will depend on the particular infection and the objectives of surveillance programme.
- Surveillance of vaccine-preventable infections such as *Haemophilus influenzae* serotype b (Hib), meningococcal group C (MenC) and *Streptococcus pneumoniae* is particularly important because:
  - Surveillance prior to introduction of the vaccine into national immunization programmes allows for estimation of disease burden as well as selection of the most appropriate vaccine, vaccination strategy, and schedule.
  - Surveillance after vaccine introduction allows for monitoring of vaccine effectiveness and rare adverse events associated with vaccination, as well as emergence of non-vaccine preventable (replacement) disease.
  - Replacement disease may occur through a variety of mechanisms, such as development of mutations that allow the pathogen to cause disease even if the host is appropriately vaccinated (i.e. vaccine escape; e.g. hepatitis B), switching of capsular polysaccharide or a number of antigenic outer membrane proteins (e.g. *Neisseria meningitidis*), or an increase in invasive disease caused by previously uncommon serotypes after elimination of serotypes that are prevented by vaccination (e.g. *S. pneumoniae*).
- A range of different reporting systems may be used for surveillance, notably statutory notification by clinicians (see below), laboratory reporting of clinical isolates, death registrations, hospital admission episodes, and other clinical systems.
- Laboratory confirmations—through any combination of routine, reference laboratory or sentinel reporting—are useful because they provide accurate diagnosis and allow detailed testing such as serotyping and serogrouping, which play an important role in identifying clustering of cases that require public health action or identify the original source of infection (e.g. *Salmonella* gastroenteritis from abroad).

- Death registrations provide useful information because their completion by a clinician is a legal requirement; however, the coding of the information contained within death certificates may be variable and the information contained in death certificates may be incomplete, particularly if the clinician is not aware of all the results at time of completing the death certificate.
- Other clinical systems include computerized hospital admission episodes (HES), the general practice research databases, and the BPSU, each with their own strengths and weaknesses.
- Although all reporting systems are subject to underreporting, where underreporting is constant over time, secular trends can provide valuable insight into trends in disease incidence.

Statutory notifications

- In the UK and many EU countries, the notification of specific infectious diseases by a clinician making the diagnosis is a statutory requirement and has been crucial to health protection since the late nineteenth century.
- The aim of statutory notification of infectious diseases is to enable the prompt investigation, risk assessment, and response to cases. Statutory notification also allows collection of data for epidemiological surveillance of infection.
- Notifications should take place as soon as a clinician suspects the infection on clinical grounds, rather than wait for laboratory confirmation, so that health protection interventions and control measures can be initiated as soon as possible.
- On 6 April 2010, the Health Protection (Notification) Regulations 2010 came into force in England and replaced earlier legislation which applied only to specified infectious diseases.
- The new legislation is consistent with the **International Health Regulations** 2005 and uses an 'all hazards' approach, which encompasses infections and other contamination.
- Important changes in the new legislation include:
  - Extending the existing requirement on **registered medical practitioners** (RMPs) to notify the proper officer of a local authority of individual cases of specified infectious diseases (Table A4.1) as well as any infection or contamination (e.g. chemicals or radiation) that might present significant harm to human health.
  - A legal requirement (after 1 October 2010) for **diagnostic laboratories** to notify the HPA of specified infectious diseases identified in tests on human samples (Table A4.2)
  - Providing public authorities modernized powers and duties to prevent and control risks to human health from infection or contamination by chemicals and radiation.

- Medical practitioners are now required to notify the proper officer of the local authority in which the patient resides (Fig. A4.1) when they have 'reasonable grounds for suspecting' that the patient:
  - Has an infectious disease specified in Schedule 1 of the Notification Regulations (Table A4.1).
  - Has an infection not included in Schedule 1 which could present significant harm to human health (e.g. emerging or new infections, such as severe acute respiratory syndrome (SARS)).
  - Is contaminated (e.g. chemicals or radiation, such as polonium 210) in a manner which could present significant harm to human health.
  - Dies with (but not necessarily from) a notifiable disease or another relevant infection or contamination.
- Urgent notifications must be reported orally as soon as possible (always within 24 hours) after **clinical suspicion or clinical diagnosis** followed by written (paper, secure online reporting, secure email, or secure fax) notification which must be received by the proper officer within 3 days. Non-urgent notifications can be reported in writing only within 3 days of clinical suspicion.
- Guidance on which notifiable infectious diseases are likely to need urgent notification is provided by the Department of Health (🕮 see Further reading, p. 809). Clinicians should be aware that they are not required to de-notify a case if subsequent investigations exclude the diagnosis of a notifiable disease.

Table A4.1 List of infectious diseases to be notified by registered medical practitioners in the new 2010 Health Protection Legislation. Acute poliomyelitis, leptospirosis, ophthalmia neonatorum, and relapsing fever are no longer in the list of notifiable diseases

SCHEDULE 1: Notifiable diseases
Acute encephalitis
Acute meningitis
Acute poliomyelitis
Acute infectious hepatitis[a]
Anthrax
Botulism[b]
Brucellosis[b]
Cholera
Diphtheria
Enteric fever (typhoid or paratyphoid fever)
Food poisoning

(Continued)

Table A4.1 (Contd.)

SCHEDULE 1: Notifiable diseases

Haemolytic uraemic syndrome[b]

Infectious bloody diarrhoea[c]

Invasive group A streptococcal disease and scarlet fever[b]

Legionnaires' disease[b]

Leprosy

Malaria

Measles

Meningococcal septicaemia

Mumps

Plague

Rabies

Rubella

SARS[b]

Smallpox

Tetanus

Tuberculosis

Typhus

Viral haemorrhagic fever

Whooping cough

Yellow fever

[a]Modified in the new schedule from 'viral hepatitis' to 'acute infectious hepatitis'.

[b]Newly added notifiable infectious diseases.

[c]Modified in the new schedule from 'dysentery (amoebic or bacillary)' to 'infectious bloody diarrhoea'.

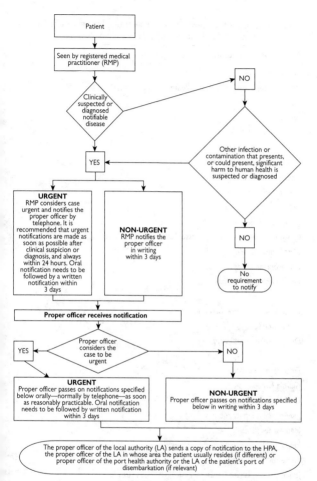

Fig. A4.1 Algorithm for clinicians to report a notifiable disease to the HPA.

Table A4.2 List of causative agents to be notified by diagnostic laboratories in the new 2010 Health Protection Legislation

SCHEDULE 2: Causative agents

Bacillus anthracis

Bacillus cereus (only if associated with food poisoning)[a]

Bordetella pertussis

Borrelia spp.[a1]

Brucella spp.

Burkholderia mallei[a]

Burkholderia pseudomallei[a]

Campylobacter spp.

Chikungunya virus[a]

Chlamydophila psittaci

Clostridium botulinum

Clostridium perfringens (only if associated with food poisoning)

Clostridium tetani[a]

Corynebacterium diphtheriae

Corynebacterium ulcerans

Coxiella burnetii

Crimean-Congo haemorrhagic fever virus

Cryptosporidium spp.

Dengue virus, Ebola virus

Entamoeba histolytica

Francisella tularensis

Giardia lamblia

Guanarito virus

Haemophilus influenzae (invasive)

Hantavirus

Hepatitis A, B, C, delta, and E viruses[a2]

Influenza virus[a3]

Junin virus, Kyasanur Forest disease virus, Lassa virus

Legionella spp.[a4]

Leptospira interrogans[a5]

Listeria monocytogenes

Machupo virus

Marburg virus

Measles virus

Mumps virus

Table A4.2 (*Contd.*)

SCHEDULE 2: Causative agents

Mycobacterium tuberculosis complex[a6]

Neisseria meningitidis

Omsk haemorrhagic fever virus

Plasmodium falciparum, P. vivax, P. ovale, P. malariae, P. knowlesi[a7]

Polio virus (wild or vaccine types)[a8]

Rabies virus (classical rabies and rabies-related lyssaviruses)

Rickettsia spp.[a]

Rift Valley fever virus

Rubella virus

Sabia virus

Salmonella spp.[a9]

SARS coronavirus

Shigella spp.

Streptococcus pneumoniae (invasive)

Streptococcus pyogenes (invasive)

Varicella zoster virus

Variola virus

Verocytotoxigenic *Escherichia coli* (including *E. coli* O157)

Vibrio cholerae

West Nile Virus

Yellow fever virus

Yersinia pestis

[a]Newly added notifiable infectious diseases.

[a1]Modified in the new schedule from "Borrelia burgdorferi" to Borrelia spp.

[a2]Added "delta" hepatitis in the new schedule.

[a3]Modified in the new schedule from "Influenza virus of a new subtype of influenza A" to Influenza virus.

[a4]Modified in the new schedule from "Legionella pneumophila" to "Legionella spp".

[a5]Modified in the new schedule from "L. interrogans spp" to "Leptospira interrogans".

[a6]Modified in the new schedule from "M. tuberculosis and M. bovis" to Mycobacterium tuberculosis complex.

[a7]Added "P. knowlesi" in the new schedule.

[a8]Modified in the new schedule from "polio virus wild/vaccine types" to "Polio virus".

[a9]Modified in the new schedule from "S. paratyphi and "S. typhi" to "Salmonella spp".

Further reading

Department of Health. *Health Protection Legislation Guidance* 2010. London: DH, 2010. ✆ www. dh.gov.uk/en/Publicationsandstatistics/Publications/PublicationsPolicyAndGuidance/DH_114510 (accessed 18 April 2010).

Blue Book Formulary

Introduction

This guidance aims to provide a quick reference for prescribing the antimicrobials discussed in the main text of the Blue Book. It is not a formulary of all available drugs and does not aim to replace Country Specific formularies. The general aim has been to simplify prescribing by using weight based dosing (where possible), rather than age bands or surface area; accepting that this might be a compromise. Doses are given as single individual doses followed by how often it is to be given, rather than total daily doses. Oral doses are stated as how many doses to give per day (e.g. four times a day), intravenous doses are stated as how many hours between doses (e.g. 8 hourly). The guide does not include side effects, drug interactions, and dosing in renal or hepatic impairment. Dosing guidance reflects where possible the licensed dose given in the manufacturer's Summary of Product Characteristics. Some of the guidance here involves the use of unlicensed medicines or of licensed medicines for unlicensed uses (off label use) and the drug and dose is then entirely used at the responsibility of the prescriber. Dosing guidance varies considerably across Europe, and clinicians need to be aware that this variation often reflects the limited evidence base for specific doses, particularly in neonates. Dosing of antibiotics may also vary depending on antimicrobial resistance patterns across Europe.

Leaflets for parents and children on some antibiotics can be found on www.medicinesforchildren.org.uk.

The editors are especially grateful to Steve Tomlin and other members of the Neonatal and Paediatric Pharmacists Group for their very considerable help with production of this dosing guide.

Approximate age, weight, and surface area conversion guide

Age	Mean weight for age kg	Mean surface area for age (m^2)	% of adult dose
New–born (full term)	3.5	0.23	12.5
2 months	4.5	0.27	15
3 months	6	0.34	20
1 year	10	0.5	25
3 years	15	0.65	33.3
7 years	24	0.9	50
10 years	32	1.1	60
12 years	40	1.3	75
14 years	50	1.50	80
16 years	58	1.65	90
Adult	68	1.73	100

1kg	=	1000 g
1g	=	1000 mg
1mg	=	1000 micrograms
1microgram	=	1000 nanograms

Medicines guide

Drug	Route	Neonatal dose	Paediatric dose	Comments
Abacavir	**By mouth**	Limited dosing information	≥3months: 8mg/kg/dose (max 300mg) given twice a day Can be given as 16mg/kg/dose (max 600mg) once a day when child over 3 years of age Tablet dosing: 14–21kg: 300mg/dose given once a day 21–30kg: 450mg/dose given once a day >30kg: 600mg/dose given once a day Adult ≥ 12 yrs 300mg/dose given twice a day or 600mg given once a day	HLA–B*5701 test before starting abacavir as if positive there is an increased risk of hypersensitivity reactions and should not be used. Hypersensitivity reactions usually within first 6 weeks of therapy–requires careful evaluation. If proven, abacavir not to be given again.
Abacavir + Lamivudine (Kivexa®)	**By mouth** *Tablets–one tablet contains abacavir 600mg + lamivudine 300mg*	Not applicable	≥40kg: 1 tablet given once a day	HLA–B*5701 test before starting Tablets can be cut

Drug	Route	Neonatal dose	Paediatric dose	Comments
Aciclovir	By mouth	No oral dosing information	1 month–18 years: 10mg/kg/dose given 4 times a day Double dose for Varicella Zoster, immunocompromised and CNS involvement	Doses highly dependent upon indication Maintain adequate hydration Dose adjustments required in renal failure
	Intravenous Infusion give over 60 minutes	0–28 days: 20mg/kg/dose given 8 hourly	1–3 months: 20mg/kg/dose given 8 hourly 3 months–12 years: 10mg/kg/dose given 8 hourly 12–18 years: 5mg/kg/dose given 8 hourly Double dose (max. 20mg/kg/dose) for Varicella Zoster, immunocompromised and CNS involvement	Use ideal body weight for dose calculation

(Continued)

Drug	Route	Neonatal dose	Paediatric dose	Comments
Albendazole	By mouth	No dosing information	2–18 years:	
			Hookworm, large roundworm and tapeworm: 400mg single dose repeated in 2–3 weeks for tapeworms.	
			Whipworms and Strongyloides: 400mg/dose given once a day for 3 days. Repeat after 3 weeks if necessary.	
			Trichinosis & cutaneous larva migrans: 400mg/dose given once a day for 5 days.	
			Neurocysticercosis: 7.5mg/kg/dose (max 400mg) given twice a day for 14–28 days.	
			Hydatid disease: 7.5mg/kg/dose (max 400mg) given twice a day for 28 days followed by a 14 day break and then repeat for up to 2–3 cycles.	
			Toxicariasis 10mg/kg/dose (max 400mg) given twice a day for 5 days	

Drug	Route	Neonatal dose	Paediatric dose	Comments
Amantadine	**By mouth**	No dosing information	1–18 years: 2–2.5mg/kg/dose (max 100mg) given twice a day	
Amikacin	**Intravenous** *Injection (over 3–30 mins)*	0–28 days: 15mg/kg/dose given 24 hourly	1 month–18 years: 15mg/kg/dose given 24 hourly	Pre-dose ('trough') plasma concentration should be less than 5mg/litre

Neonates, infants and those with renal impairment should have renal function monitored. |
| **Amoxicillin** | **By mouth** | Under 7 days: 30–50mg/kg/dose given twice daily

7–28 days: 30–50mg/kg/dose given 3 times daily (double in severe infection) | 1 month–18 years: 15mg/kg/dose given 3 times a day (max 500mg/dose)

Consider double dose in acute otitis media and severe infection (especially in areas of high pneumococcal resistance). | |
| | **Intravenous** *intravenous injection* | As for oral | 1 month–18 years: 30mg/kg/dose (max 4g daily) given 8 hourly. Double dose in severe infection e.g. *Listeria* meningitis | |

(Continued)

Drug	Route	Neonatal dose	Paediatric dose	Comments
Amphotericin B (Fungizone) Prescribe as brand i.e. Fungizone	**Intravenous** *Infusion over 2–6 hours*	0–28 days: 1mg/kg/dose given 24 hourly. After 7 days the dose can be reduced to 1mg/kg/dose given 48 hourly.	1 month–18 years: 1mg/kg/dose given 24 hourly. In very severe infection the dose can be increased to 1.5mg/kg/dose.	Avoid other nephrotoxic drugs if possible Saline pre-treatment reduces toxicity Consider giving a test dose of 0.1mg/kg prior to commencing treatment.
Amphotericin complex (Amphocil) Prescribe as brand i.e. Amphocil	**Intravenous** *Infusion at 1–2mg/kg/hour*	No dosing information	1 month–18 years: 3mg/kg/dose given 24 hourly Max dose 6mg/kg/dose given 24 hourly.	Avoid other nephrotoxic drugs if possible Consider giving a test dose of 0.1mg/kg prior to commencing treatment.
Amphotericin lipid complex (Abelcet) Prescribe as brand i.e. Abelcet	**Intravenous** *Infusion at 2.5mg/kg/hour*	No dosing information	1 month–18 years: 5mg/kg/dose given 24 hourly	Avoid other nephrotoxic drugs if possible Consider giving a test dose of 0.1mg/kg prior to commencing treatment.
Amphotericin liposomal (AmBisome) Prescribe as brand i.e. AmBisome	**Intravenous** *Infusion over 30–60 mins*	0–28 days: 3mg/kg/dose given 24 hourly Max dose 5mg/kg/dose given 24 hourly	1 month–18 years: 3mg/kg/dose given 24 hourly Usual max dose 5mg/kg/dose given 24 hourly	Avoid other nephrotoxic drugs if possible Consider giving a test dose of 0.1mg/kg prior to commencing treatment.

Drug	Route	Neonatal dose	Paediatric dose	Comments
Ampicillin	**By mouth**	under 7 days: 30mg/kg/dose given twice daily 7–21 days: 30mg/kg/dose given 3 times daily 21–28 days: 30mg/kg/dose given 4 times daily (max 62.5mg per dose) Doses may be doubled in severe infection	1 month–18 year: 10–15mg/kg/dose (max 500mg) given 4 times daily	Oral–to be taken on an empty stomach.
	Intravenous *intravenous injection*	under 7 days: 30–50mg/kg/dose given 12 hourly 7–21 days: 30–50mg/kg/dose given 8 hourly 21–28 days: 30–50mg/kg/dose given 6 hourly	1 month–18 years: 25mg/kg/dose (max 1g) given 6 hourly; may be doubled in severe infection For listerial meningitis 50mg/kg/dose (max 2g) given 4 hourly.	

(Continued)

Drug	Route	Neonatal dose	Paediatric dose	Comments
Artemether with Lumefantrine (Riamet®)	By mouth	No dosing information	5–15kg: 1 tablet initially followed by 5 further doses of 1 tablet given at 8, 14, 36, 48 and 60 hours after first dose 15–25kg: 2 tablets initially followed by 5 further doses of 2 tablets given at 8, 14, 36, 48 and 60 hours 25–35kg: 3 tablets initially followed by 5 further doses of 3 tablets given at 8, 14, 36, 48 and 60 hours Child 12–18 years and over 35kg: 4 tablets initially followed by 5 further doses of 4 tablets given at 8, 14, 36, 48 and 60 hours	Give with food
Atazanavir	By mouth	No dosing information	15–20kg: 150mg once a day with Ritonavir 100mg once a day 20–40kg: 200mg once a day with Ritonavir 100mg once a day ≥40kg: 300mg once a day with Ritonavir 100mg once a day	Avoid indigestion remedies and gastric acid suppressant Always check potential drug interactions between antiretrovirals and antiretrovirals and other medicines–see www.hiv-druginteractions.org

Drug	Route	Neonatal dose	Paediatric dose	Comments
Atripla® Tenofovir + Emtricitabine + Efavirenz	**By mouth** Tablets—one tablet contains tenofovir 300mg + emtricitabine 200mg + efavirenz 600mg	Not applicable	Child Individual tenofovir, emtricitabine and efavirenz—max dose as for adults Adult >18 years 1 tablet once a day	Give on empty stomach (2 hrs after food) Do not cut Always check potential drug interactions between antiretrovirals and other antiretrovirals and other medicines—see www.hiv-druginteractions.org
Atovaquone	**By mouth**	No dosing information	1–3 months: 15mg/kg/dose given twice a day 2–24 months: 22.5mg/kg/dose given twice a day > 24 months: 15mg/kg/dose given twice a day	Administer with food
Atovaquone/ Proguanil (Malarone)	**By mouth** Tablets: PAEDIATRIC tablet proguanil 25mg + atovaquone 62.5mg STANDARD tablet proguanil 100mg + atovaquone 250mg		*Treatment of malaria* 5–9kg: 2 paediatric tablets given once a day for 3 days 9–11kg: 3 paediatric tablets given once a day for 3 days 11–21kg: 1 standard tablet given once a day for 3 days 21–31kg: 2 standard tablets given once a day for 3 days 31–40kg: 3 standard tablets given once a day for 3 days >40kg: 4 standard tablets given once a day for 3 days	Reduce dose in renal impairment

(Continued)

Drug	Route	Neonatal dose	Paediatric dose	Comments
Azithromycin	By mouth	No dosing information	*Respiratory tract infections, otitis media, skin and soft tissue infections* 1 month–18 years: 10mg/kg/dose given once a day (max 500mg/dose) for 3 days *Uncomplicated genital chlamydial infection and non-gonococcal urethritis* 12–18 years: 1g as a single dose *Lyme disease, mild to moderate typhoid* 6 months–18 years: 10–15mg/kg/dose given once daily (max 500mg/dose) for 7–10 days	
Aztreonam	Intravenous	0–7 days: 30mg/kg/dose given 12 hourly 7–28 days: 30mg/kg/dose given 6 to 8 hourly	1 month–2 years: 30mg/kg/dose given 6 to 8 hourly 2–18 years: 30mg/kg/dose given 8 hourly (increase to 50mg/kg/dose 6 hourly in severe infection and cystic fibrosis. Max 2g/dose)	
Benzathine penicillin	Intramuscular	> 1200g: 50,000 units/kg/dose given once per week	1 month–18 years: 50,000 units/kg/dose given once per week	

Drug	Route	Neonatal dose	Paediatric dose	Comments
Benzylpenicillin	**Intravenous** *intravenous injection or infusion*	under 7 days: 25mg/kg/dose given 12 hourly	1 month–18 years: 25mg/kg/dose given 6 hourly	
		7–28 days: 25mg/kg/dose given 8 hourly	Double dose in severe infection to 50mg/kg/dose up to 4–6 hourly.	For doses of >50mg/kg consider giving over longer administration (e.g. 30 mins) times to avoid CNS toxicity.
		Double dose in severe infections		
		Neonatal meningitis– 75mg/kg/dose given 8 hourly		
Carbenicillin	**By mouth**	No dosing information	1 month–18 years: 7.5–12.5mg/kg/dose given 4 times a day (max 750mg/dose given 4 times a day)	
Caspofungin	**Intravenous** *Infusion over 60 mins*	0–28 days: 25mg/m²/dose given 24 hourly	1–3 months: 25mg/m²/dose given 24 hourly	Incompatible with glucose solutions.
			3–12 months: 50mg/m²/dose given 24 hourly	
			1–18 years: 70mg/m²/dose given 24 hourly on day 1, followed by 50mg/m²/dose given 24 hourly on subsequent days	
			Max dose 70mg/dose	
Cefaclor	**By mouth**	7–28 days: 15mg/kg/dose given twice daily	1 month–18 years: 7mg/kg/dose given 3 times daily, dose doubled in severe infection	

(Continued)

Drug	Route	Neonatal dose	Paediatric dose	Comments
Cefadroxil	By mouth	No dosing information	1 month–18 years: 12.5mg/kg/dose given twice daily, dose doubled in severe infection (max 1g/dose given twice daily)	
Cefalexin	By mouth	<7 days: 25mg/kg/dose given twice daily 7–21 days: 25mg/kg/dose given 3 times daily 21–28 days: 25mg/kg/dose given 4 times daily Max dose 125mg/dose.	1 month–18 years: 12.5mg/kg/dose given twice daily, dose doubled in severe infection, max 25mg/kg/dose (max 1.5g) given 4 times daily	
Cefixime	By mouth	No dosing information	6 months–18 years: 5–8mg/kg/dose given once daily (max 400mg/dose given once a day) Gonorrhoea 12–18 years: 400mg as a single dose	

Drug	Route	Neonatal dose	Paediatric dose	Comments
Cefotaxime	**Intravenous** intravenous injection or *infusion*	<7 days: 25mg/kg/dose given 12 hourly 7–21 days: 25mg/kg/dose given 8 hourly 21–28 days: 25mg/kg/dose given 6 hourly Doses may be doubled in severe infection	1 month–18 years: 50mg/kg/dose given 8 hourly. Increase dose to 6 hourly in very severe infection (max 4g/dose given 8 hourly) Gonorrhoea 12–18 years: 500mg as single dose	
Cefpodoxime	**By mouth**	15–28 days: 4mg/kg/dose given twice daily	1 months–18 years: 4mg/kg/dose given twice daily (up to 100mg/dose given twice daily) Increased to 200mg/dose given twice daily in sinusitis, skin and soft tissue infections, uncomplicated upper urinary tract infections, and if necessary lower respiratory tract infections	
Cefradine	**By mouth**	No dosing information	7–18 years: 12.5–25mg/kg/dose given twice daily up to 1g/dose given 4 times daily in severe infections)	

(Continued)

Drug	Route	Neonatal dose	Paediatric dose	Comments
Ceftazidime	**Intravenous** *Intravenous injection or infusion*	under 7 days: 50mg/kg/dose given 24 hourly 7–21 days: 50mg/kg/dose given 12 hourly 21–28 days: 50mg/kg/dose given 8 hourly All above, doses may be doubled in severe infection	1 month–18 years: 25–50mg/kg/dose (max 2g) given 8 hourly	
	By inhalation *Nebulised solution: dilute injection in 3ml water for injection*		1 month–18 years: 1g twice daily	
Ceftriaxone	**Intravenous or intramuscular** *Intravenous injection or infusion*	0–28 days: 50mg/kg/dose given once daily (infused over 60 minutes)	1 month–18 years: 50mg/kg/dose given once daily; 80mg/kg/dose given once daily in meningitis and severe infections (max 80mg/kg daily or 4g daily)	Ceftriaxone is not recommended in premature neonates. Doses over 50mg/kg should be infused over 60 minutes Do not give with calcium containing salts as risk of precipitation.

Cefuroxime	By mouth	No oral dosing	3 month–18 years: 10–15mg/kg/dose given twice daily (max 500mg/dose given twice daily)	Oral–to be taken with food.
			1 month–18 years: 30mg/kg/dose given 8 hourly up to 60mg/kg/dose (max 1.5g) given 6 hourly	
	Intravenous *Intravenous injection or infusion*	Under 7 days: 25mg/kg/dose given 12 hourly		
		7–21 days: 25mg/kg/dose given 8 hourly		
		21–28 days: 25mg/kg/dose given 6 hourly		
		Doses may be doubled in severe infection		
Cidofovir	**Intravenous**		1 month–18 years: 5mg/kg/dose given once a week	*With probenecid and hydration*
Ciprofloxacin	By mouth	0–28 days: 10–15mg/kg/dose given twice daily	1 month to 18 years: 10–15mg/kg/dose given twice daily (max 750mg/dose given twice daily)	Oral –not to be used with preparations containing zinc, iron, milk or indigestion remedies
	Intravenous *Infusion over 60 minutes*	0–28 days: 10–15mg/kg/dose given 12 hourly	1 month to 18 years: 10–15mg/kg/dose (max 400mg/dose) 8–12 hourly	Use with caution in children with epilepsy, G6PD deficiency, myasthenia gravis.

(Continued)

Drug	Route	Neonatal dose	Paediatric dose	Comments
Chloramphenicol	Intravenous	0–14 days: 12.5mg/kg/dose given 12 hourly 14–28 days: 12.5mg/kg/dose given 6–8 hourly	1 month–18 years: 12.5mg/kg/dose 6 hourly (Dose may be doubled in severe infections)	Consider monitoring plasma chloramphenicol levels when using double doses and in neonates
Chloroquine	By mouth	No dosing information	1 month to 18 years: 10mg/kg loading dose (max 620mg) then 6–8 hours later give a single dose of 5mg/kg (max 310mg) then 5mg/kg/dose (max 310mg) given once daily for 2 days	Doses are expressed as chloroquine base
Clarithromycin	By mouth	Birth–28 days: 7.5mg/kg/dose given twice daily	1 month–18 years: 7.5–15mg/kg/dose (max 500mg) given twice a day	
	Intravenous	Birth–28 days: 7.5mg/kg/dose given 12 hourly	1 month–18 years: 7.5mg/kg/dose (max 500mg) given 12 hourly	
Clindamycin	By mouth	0–14 days: 6mg/kg 3 times daily 14–28 days: 6mg/kg 4 times daily	1 month–18 years: 6mg/kg/dose given 4 times daily	
	Intravenous *Infusion*	No information	1 month–18 years: 6mg/kg/dose given 6 hourly (severe infections 10mg/kg/dose (max 1.2g) given 6 hourly)	

Drug	Route	Neonatal dose	Paediatric dose	Comments
Co-amoxiclav	**By mouth** *Expressed as amoxicillin/clavulanic acid*	0–28 days: 0.25ml/kg of 125/31 suspension three times a day	1 month–18 years: 15mg/kg/dose (of amoxicillin component) given 3 times a day	
	Augmentin Duo Suspension		2 months–2 years: 0.15–0.2ml/kg/dose given twice a day 2–6 years: 2.5–5ml/dose given twice a day >6 years: 5–10ml/dose given twice a day	
	Intravenous *Expressed as amoxicillin/clavulanic acid*	<7 days: 30mg/kg/dose given 12 hourly	1–3 months: 30mg/kg/dose given 8 hourly 3 months–18 years: 30mg/kg/dose given 8 hourly (increased to 6 hourly in severe infections).	
	Injection	7–28 days: 30mg/kg/dose given 8 hourly		
Colchicine	**By mouth**	No dosing information	1 month–18 years: 20–30 microgram/kg/dose (max 2mg/dose) given once a day	Avoid in patients with blood dyscrasias. Use in caution in patients with reduced renal function to avoid neuromuscular toxicity and bone marrow dysplasia.

(Continued)

Drug	Route	Neonatal dose	Paediatric dose	Comments
Colistin	**Intravenous** *Injection*	No dosing information	1 month–18 years: <60kg: 16,666–25,000 units/kg/dose given 8 hourly >60kg: 1–2 million units/dose given 8 hourly	
	Nebulized		1 month–2 years: 500,000–1 million units/dose given twice daily 2–18 years: 1–2 million units/dose twice daily	
Co-trimoxazole	**By mouth**	Avoid in infants under 6 weeks (except for treatment or prophylaxis of pneumocystis pneumonia	6 weeks–12 years: 24mg/kg/dose given twice daily 12–18 years: 960mg/dose given twice daily *Treatment of Pneumocystis jiroveci (P. carinii)* 1 month–18 years: 60mg/kg/dose given twice daily for 14 days; total daily dose may alternatively be given in 3–4 divided doses *Prophylaxis of Pneumocystis jiroveci (P. carinii)* 1 month–18 years: 30mg/kg/dose given once a day	480mg of co-trimoxazole consists of sulfamethoxazole 400mg and trimethoprim 80mg Monitor blood counts on prolonged treatment and discontinue if blood disorders or rash develop
	Intravenous *Infuse over 60–90 mins*		6 weeks–18 years: 18mg/kg/dose given 12 hourly; increased in severe infection to 27mg/kg/dose given 12 hourly *Treatment of Pneumocystis jiroveci (P. carinii)* infections: as oral dose above	

Drug	Route	Neonatal dose	Paediatric dose	Comments
Cycloserine	By mouth	No dosing information	2–18 years: 5mg/kg/dose (max 250mg) given twice a day.	Adjust dose based on blood concentration and response Peak concentration (at 3–4 hours post dose) should not exceed 30mg/L
Dapsone	By mouth	No dosing information	1 month–18 years: 2mg/kg/dose (max 100mg) given once a day	Possible haemolysis in G6PD deficient patients. Avoid in acute porphyria.
Darunavir	By mouth	No dosing information	20–30kg: 375mg/dose given twice a day with Ritonavir 50mg/dose given twice a day 30–40kg: 450mg/dose given twice a day with Ritonavir 60mg/dose given twice a day >40kg: 600mg/dose given twice a day with Ritonavir 100mg/dose given twice a day	Taken with or after food
Didanosine	By mouth	14–28 days: 50–100mg/m²/dose given twice a day	1 month–3 months: 50–100mg/m²/dose given twice a day >3 months: 200mg/m²/dose given once a day (range 180–240mg/m² once a day) (max <60kg = 250mg given once a day; max >60kg = 400mg given once a day)	Give on empty stomach (2 hrs after and 1 hr before food or milk) Caps can be opened and sprinkled on a spoonful of food eg yoghurt but decrease in AUC Do not co-administer with tenofovir

(Continued)

Drug	Route	Neonatal dose	Paediatric dose	Comments
Diethyl-carbamazine	By mouth	No dosing information	1 month–18 years: 0.3mg/kg/dose given 3 times a day Increase dose gradually over 3 days to 2mg/kg/dose given 3 times a day (Children under 10 years should only receive a maintenance dose of 1mg/kg/dose given 3 times a day)	Febrile reactions are possible in heavy infections. Encephalopathy is possible in *Loa loa* infection.
Diloxanide	By mouth	No dosing information	1 month–18 years: 6–7mg/kg/dose (max 500mg/dose) given 3 times a day	Treat for 10 days and repeat course if necessary.
Doxycycline	By mouth	No dosing information	12–18 years: 100mg/dose given once or twice daily according to clinical indication. 200mg loading dose may be given in certain infections	Antacids and products containing aluminium, calcium, iron, magnesium and zinc salts and milk may reduce the absorption of doxycycline. Do not give to children under 8–12 years, or pregnant or breast-feeding women, as deposits in growing bones and teeth

Drug	Route	Neonatal dose	Paediatric dose	Comments
Efavirenz	By mouth	No dosing information	*Child (3–5 years liquid only)* 13–15kg: 360mg given once a day 15–20kg: 390mg given once a day 20–25kg: 450mg given once a day 25–32.5kg: 510mg given once a day ≥5 years–tablet (or liquid) dosing 13–15kg: 200mg given once a day (liquid 270mg) 15–20kg: 250mg given once a day (liquid 300mg) 20–25kg: 300mg given once a day (liquid 360mg) 25–32.5kg: 350mg given once a day (liquid 450mg) 32.5–40kg: 400mg given once a day (liquid 510mg) >40kg: 600mg given once a day (liquid 720mg)	Preferably given before bedtime Liquid is not bioequivalent to tablets or capsules Always check potential drug interactions between antiretrovirals and antiretrovirals and other medicines–see www.hiv-druginteractions.org
Emtricitabine	By mouth	No dosing information	≥4 months: 6mg/kg/dose given once a day of the oral solution (max dose 240mg once a day) ≥33kg: 200mg given once a day as capsule; 240mg once a day of the oral solution	Can be administered with food Liquid is not bioequivalent to capsules

(Continued)

Drug	Route	Neonatal dose	Paediatric dose	Comments
Enfuvirtide	**Subcutaneous** *Injection*	No dosing information	6–18 years: 2mg/kg/dose twice a day subcutaneously (max dose 90mg/dose given twice a day)	Subcutaneous injection–upper arm, thigh, abdomen
Ertapenem	**Intravenous** *Infusion*	No dosing information	3 month–18 years: 15mg/kg/dose (max 500mg/dose) given 12 hourly	Incompatible with glucose solutions
Erythromycin	**By mouth**	0–28 days: 12.5mg/kg/dose given 4 times a day	1 month–18 years: 12.5–25mg/kg/dose (max 1g) given 4 times a day	Check for drug interactions Use with caution in impaired liver function and severe renal impairment
	Intravenous *Infusion*	0–28 days: 10–12.5mg/kg/dose given 6 hourly	1 month–18 years: 12.5mg/kg/dose (max 1g) given 6 hourly	Intravenous doses to be diluted to 1–5mg/ml with sodium chloride 0.9% and infused over 20–60 minutes. Concentrations of up to 10mg/ml may be used via central administration. Do not dilute with glucose solutions unless buffered with sodium bicarbonate.
Ethambutol	**By mouth**	0–28 days: 15mg/kg/dose given once daily for 2 months during the initial phase of TB treatment (used in combination with other antibiotics).	1 month–18 years: 15mg/kg/dose given once daily (for 2-month initial phase) OR 30mg/kg/dose given 3 times a week (for 2-month initial phase)	Toxic effects including visual disturbances more common where excessive dosage is used or if renal function impaired

Drug	Route	Neonatal dose	Paediatric dose	Comments
Ethionamide	By mouth	No dosing information	Treatment of tuberculosis 1 month–18 years 15–20mg/kg/dose (max 1g) given once a day Leprosy 1 month–18 years 5–8mg/kg/dose (max 375mg) given once a day	Administer with food to reduce GI distress Neurotoxic effects may be relieved by administration of pyridoxine
Etravirine	By mouth	No dosing information available	Adult: 200mg/dose given twice a day	Take with food (AUC decreased by 50% if taken on empty stomach) Tablet disperses in water Always check potential drug interactions between antiretrovirals and antiretrovirals and other medicines—see www.hiv-druginteractions.org
Famciclovir	By mouth	No dosing information	6 years–18 years: 5mg/kg/dose (max 250mg) given 3 times a day Double dose in the immunocompromised	

(Continued)

Drug	Route	Neonatal dose	Paediatric dose	Comments
Flucloxacillin	By mouth	under 7 days: 25mg/kg/dose given twice daily 7–21 days: 25mg/kg/dose given 3 times daily 21–28 days: 25mg/kg/dose given 4 times daily	1 month–18 years 12.5–25mg/kg/dose (max 500mg) given 4 times daily	Very rarely cholestatis jaundice and hepatitis may occur up to several weeks after treatment with flucloxacillin has stopped. Risk is increased with prolonged courses. Rash, fever, neutropenia occur with higher doses and prolonged treatment.
	Intravenous *injection*	As above Severe infection use 50mg/kg/dose	1 month–18 years 12.5–25mg/kg/dose (max 1g) given 6 hourly; may be doubled in very severe infection)	
Fluconazole	By mouth	0–28 days: 12mg/kg/dose given once a day. Consider giving a loading dose of 25mg/kg as the first dose.	1 month–18 years: 12mg/kg/dose (max 400mg) given every 24 hours	Caution when used alongside hepatotoxic drugs–increased risk of hepatotoxicity. Consider increasing the dosing intervals in renal impairment. For prophylaxis give 6mg/kg/dose daily for paediatrics and 72 hourly for neonates.
	Intravenous *Infuse over 10–30 mins*	0–28 days: 12mg/kg/dose given every 24 hours. Consider giving a loading dose of 25mg/kg as the first dose.	1 month–18 years: 12mg/kg/dose (max 400mg) given every 24 hours	

Drug	Route	Neonatal dose	Paediatric dose	Comments
Flucytosine	**Intravenous** Infuse over 20–40 minutes	0–28 days: 50mg/kg/dose given 12 hourly	Systemic yeast and fungal infections 1 month–18 years: 50mg/kg/dose given 6 hourly Cryptococcal meningitis 1 month–18 years: 25mg/kg/dose given 6 hourly for 2 weeks	Monitor renal and liver function and blood counts
Fosamprenavir	**By mouth**	No dosing information	25–32kg: 18mg/kg/dose given twice a day with Ritonavir 3mg/kg/dose given twice a day 33–38kg: (tablet or oral suspension) 18mg/kg/dose given twice a day with Ritonavir 100mg/dose given twice a day ≥39kg: (tablet or oral suspension) 700mg/dose given twice a day with Ritonavir 100mg/dose given twice a day	Give with or after food to aid palatability of liquid
Foscarnet	**Intravenous** Infuse over at least 60 mins	No dosing information	1 month–18 years: 60mg/kg/dose given 8 hourly for 2–3 weeks then 60mg/kg/dose given once a day as maintenance. (Can increase maintenance to 90–120mg/kg/dose given once a day if tolerated)	Repeat induction regimen for CMV retinitis if retinitis progresses whilst on maintenance dose. Monitor electrolytes, especially calcium and magnesium. Monitor renal function regularly and adjust dose in renal impairment.

(Continued)

Drug	Route	Neonatal dose	Paediatric dose	Comments
Fusidic acid	**By mouth** Suspension	0–28 days: 15mg/kg/dose given 3 times daily	1 month–18 years: 15mg/kg/dose (max 750mg) given 3 times daily	Fusidic acid is incompletely absorbed and doses recommended for suspension are proportionally higher than for sodium fusidate tablets
	By mouth (as sodium fusidate) Tablets	No dosing information	12–18 years: 500mg/dose given 3 times a day (dose doubled in sever infections)	
	Intravenous (as sodium fusidate)	0–28 days: 10mg/kg/dose given 12 hourly	1 month–18 years: 6–7mg/kg/dose (max 500mg) given 8 hourly	
Ganciclovir	**Intravenous** Infuse over 60 minutes	0–28 days: 6mg/kg/dose given 12 hourly	1 month to 18 years: 5mg/kg/dose given 12 hourly	Close full blood count monitoring required–significant risk of neutropenia Ensure adequate hydration
Gentamicin	**Intravenous** Injection over 3–30 mins	Less than 32 weeks gestation: 4–5mg/kg/dose given 36 hourly > 32 weeks gestation: 4–5mg/kg/dose given 24 hourly	1 month–18 years: 7mg/kg/dose given once a day Adjusted according to serum gentamicin concentrations	Intravenous administration–pre–dose (trough) plasma concentrations should be: <1mg/litre for children >1 month <2mg/litre for neonates. Neonates, infants and those with renal impairment should have renal function monitored together with serum gentamicin concentrations
Griseofulvin	**By mouth**	No dosing information	1 month–18 years: 10mg/kg/dose (max. 500mg) given once a day. In severe infection double dose and then reduce when response occurs.	Avoid in acute porphyria, patients with severe liver disease, and those with systemic lupus erythematosus.

Drug	Route	Neonatal dose	Paediatric dose	Comments
Halofantrine	By mouth	No dosing information	1 month–18 years: 10mg/kg/dose (max 500mg) given every 6 hours (3 doses)	3 doses only
Imipenem	**Intravenous** *Infuse over 20–60 mins*	<7 days: 20mg/kg/dose given 12 hourly, increase to 8 hourly if poor response 7–21 days: 20mg/kg/dose given 8 hourly 21–28 days: 20mg/kg/dose given 6 hourly	1–3 months: 20mg/kg/dose given 8 hourly 3 months–18 years: 15mg/kg/dose (max 500mg) given 6 hourly In children <12 years the maximum dose is 500mg. In children >12 years the dose may be doubled in severe infection to 1g.	Avoid in CNS disorders (e.g. epilepsy) Avoid in patients taking MAOIs
Isoniazid	**By mouth**	0–28 days: 10mg/kg/dose given once daily	Treatment of tuberculosis 1 month–18 years: 10mg/kg/dose (max. 300mg) given once daily OR 15mg/kg/dose given 3 times a week	Increased risk of side–effects in patients with slow acetylator status Possible peripheral neuritis with high doses and in breast feeding infants– consider pyridoxine prophylaxis
	Intravenous	0–28 days: 10mg/kg/dose given 24 hourly	1 month–18 years: 5–10mg/kg/dose (max. 300mg) given once daily	Seek immediate medical attention if symptoms of liver toxicity such as persistent nausea, vomiting, malaise or jaundice develop

(Continued)

Drug	Route	Neonatal dose	Paediatric dose	Comments
Itraconazole	By mouth	No dosing information	1 month–18 years: 3–5mg/kg/dose (max 200mg) given once a day	Capsules have extremely poor bioavailability, use liquid in preference as oral preparation. Avoid in hepatic impairment if possible and discontinue if signs of hepatitis develop.
	Intravenous *Infuse over 60 minutes*	No dosing information	1 month–18 years: 2.5mg/kg/dose (max 200mg) given 12 hourly for 2 days then 2.5mg/kg/dose (max 200mg) given 24 hourly for max of 12 days.	
Ivermectin	By mouth	No dosing information	*Strongyloides stercoralis* 5–18 years: 200 microgram/kg/dose (=0.2mg/kg/dose) given once daily for 2 days Prolong or repeat treatment in the immunocompromised *Onchocerciasis* 5–18 years: 150 microgram/kg/dose (=0.15mg/kg/dose) given as a single dose Repeat every 6–12 months for 10 years	Do not eat food 2 hours either side of the dose. Avoid in CNS disorders (e.g epilepsy) Monitor for ophthalmic and other hypersensitivity reactions when onchocerciasis is being treated.
Ketoconazole	By mouth	No dosing information	15–30kg: 100mg/dose given once daily >30kg: 200mg/dose given once daily (increase to 400mg if necessary)	Risk of hepatotoxicity increased if used for more than 10 days. Monitor liver function pre-treatment and at week 2 and 4 of treatment, then monthly

Drug	Route	Neonatal dose	Paediatric dose	Comments
Lamivudine	By mouth	0–28 days: 2mg/kg/dose given twice a day for 4 weeks	1 month–18 years: 4mg/kg/dose (max 150mg) given twice a day Can be given as 8mg/kg/dose (max 300mg) once a day when child over 3 years of age	
Levamisole	By mouth	No dosing information	1 month–18 years: 2.5mg/kg/dose (max 150mg) given as a single dose for roundworm or hookworm.	For hookworm the dose can be repeated after 7 days if necessary.
Linezolid	By mouth	< 7 days: 10mg/kg/dose given twice a day (increase to 3 times a day if poor response) 7–28 days: 10mg/kg/dose given 3 times a day	1 month to 12 years: 10mg/kg/dose (max 600mg) given three times a day 12–18 years: 600mg/dose given twice a day	Full blood count should be monitored weekly for patients receiving treatment for greater than 10 days, who have pre-existing myelosuppression, severe renal impairment or receiving concomitant drugs that have adverse effects on blood count, haemoglobin or platelet function. Visual function should be monitored regularly if treatment is required for longer than 28 days.
	Intravenous *Infusion over 30 to 120 minutes*	< 7 days: 10mg/kg/dose given 12 hourly (increase to 8 hourly if poor response) 7–28 days: 10mg/kg/dose given 8 hourly	1 month to 12 years: 10mg/kg/dose (max 600mg) given 8 hourly 12–18 years: 600mg/dose given 12 hourly	

(Continued)

Drug	Route	Neonatal dose	Paediatric dose	Comments
Lopinavir (LPV/r)	By mouth	14–28 days: 300mg/m^2/dose given twice a day	1 month–6 months: 300mg/m^2/dose given twice a day ≥6 months: 230–300mg/m^2/dose (max 400mg) given twice a day	Liquid give with or after food. Only available in combination with ritonavir (doses based on Lopinavir)
Maraviroc	By mouth	No dosing information available	Child: Insufficient data–seek specialist advice Adult: Recommended dose is 150mg, 300mg or 600mg twice daily depending on interactions with co-administered therapy **Caution major drug interactions**	Trofile assay for co-receptor tropism With or without food Pharmacy advice on dosing with potentially interacting drugs Always check potential drug interactions between antiretrovirals and antiretrovirals and other medicines—see www.hiv-druginteractions.org
Mebendazole	By mouth	No dosing information	*Threadworms* 6 months–18 years: 100mg given as a single dose *Whipworms, roundworms & hookworms* 1–18 years: 100mg/dose given twice a day for 3 days	For threadworms the dose can be repeated after 2 weeks if necessary.

Drug	Route	Neonatal dose	Paediatric dose	Comments
Mefloquine	By mouth	No dosing information	*Treatment* 3 months–18 years 15mg/kg/dose (max 750mg) given as a single dose, then 10mg/kg/dose (max 500mg) given as a single dose 6–8 hour later *Prophylaxis* 5–16kg: 62.5mg once weekly 16–25kg: 125mg once weekly 25–45kg: 187.5mg once weekly >45kg: 250mg once weekly	Prophylaxis can be taken for up to 1 year. Avoid in patients with cardiac conductive disorders, epilepsy and children under 3 months (5kg)
Meropenem	Intravenous *Infuse over 15–30 mins*	Under 7 days: 20mg/kg/dose given 12 hourly 7–28 days: 20mg/kg/dose given 8 hourly. Doses may be doubled in meningitis and other severe infections	1 month–12 years: 10mg/kg/dose (max 500mg) given 8 hourly Dose doubled in hospital-acquired pneumonia, peritonitis, septicaemia and infections in neutropenic patients *Meningitis* 1 month–12 years: 40mg/kg/dose (max 2g) given 8 hourly	Avoid if history of immediate hypersensitivity to beta-lactam antibacterials

(Continued)

Drug	Route	Neonatal dose	Paediatric dose	Comments
Metronidazole	By mouth	0–28 days: 15mg/kg/dose given as a stat dose, then 7.5mg/kg/dose given twice daily	1 month–18 years: 7.5mg/kg/dose (max 400mg) given three times a day Double dose in Amoebiasis and Giardiasis	Take tablets with or after food but suspension should be taken on an empty stomach Disulfiram-like reaction with alcohol
	Intravenous *Infusion over 20–30 minutes*	0–28 days: 15mg/kg as a single loading dose followed after 24 hours by 7.5mg/kg/dose given 12 hourly	1 month–18 years: 7.5mg/kg/dose (max 500mg) given 8 hourly	
	Rectal	Nil	1 month–18 years: 7.5mg/kg/dose (max 500mg) given 8 hourly (round to most suitable suppository)	
Micafungin	**Intravenous** *Infusion over 60 mins*	*Treatment* 0–28 days: 8mg/kg/dose given 24 hourly. *Prophylaxis* 0–28 days: 1mg/kg/dose given 24 hourly.	*Treatment* 1 month–18 years: 2–4mg/kg/dose (max 100mg) given 24 hourly. Double dose in severe infection *Prophylaxis* 1 month–18 years: 1mg/kg/dose (max 50mg) given 24 hourly	Monitor liver function and discontinue if significant and persistent abnormalities.

Drug	Route	Neonatal dose	Paediatric dose	Comments
Miconazole	**By mouth** *Oral Gel*	0–28 days: 1ml smeared around mouth 2–4 times a day.	1 month–2 years: 2.5ml smeared around mouth twice a day after food. 2–6 years: 5ml twice a day after 6–12 years: 5ml four times a day after food 12–18 years: 5–10ml four times a day after food (retain near lesions before swallowing)	
Minocycline	**By mouth**	No dosing information	Child 12–18 years: 100mg/dose given twice daily	Antacids and products containing aluminium, calcium, iron, magnesium and zinc salts and milk may reduce the absorption of minocycline. Do not give to children under 8–12 years, or pregnant or breast-feeding women, as deposits in growing bones and teeth
Nalidixic acid	**By mouth**	No dosing information	3 months–12 years: 12.5mg/kg/dose given 4 times a day for 7 days, reduced to 7.5mg/kg/dose given 4 times a day in prolonged therapy 12–18 years: 900mg/dose given 4 times daily for 7 days, reduced in chronic infections to 600mg/dose given 4 times daily	

(Continued)

Drug	Route	Neonatal dose	Paediatric dose	Comments
Nevirapine	By mouth	*Post-exposure prophylaxis for baby born to HIV positive mother* Refer to www.bhiva.org 0–14 days: 2mg/kg/dose given once a day for 1st week then 4mg/kg/dose given once a day for 2nd week then stop (if mother has received >3 days of Nevirapine therapy immediately before delivery, dose in neonate 4mg/kg/dose given once a day for 2 weeks then stop)	>14 days: 150–200mg/m²/dose given once a day for 14 days then 150–200mg/m²/dose given twice a day (max dose 200mg/dose twice a day) >12 years: 200mg/dose given once a day for 14 days then increase to 200mg/dose given twice a day if no rash or LFT abnormalities	Always check potential drug interactions between antiretrovirals and antiretrovirals and other medicines—see www.hiv-druginteractions.org

Drug	Route	Neonatal dose	Paediatric dose	Comments
Niclosamide	By mouth	No dosing information	*Pork, beef, fish tapeworms* 1 month–2 years: 500mg given as a single dose 2–7 years: 1g given as a single dose 7–18 years: 2g given as a single dose *Dwarf tapeworm* 1 month–2 years: 500mg given on day 1 then 250mg given daily for 6 days 2–7 years: 1g given on day 1 then 500mg given daily for 6 days 7–18 years: 2g given on day 1 then 1g given daily for 6 days	
Nitrofurantoin	By mouth	No dosing information	*Treatment* 3 months to 18 years: **1mg/kg/dose** (max 100mg) given 4 times a day *Prophylaxis* 3 months to 18 years: **1mg/kg/dose** (max 100mg) given once a day	Contraindicated in G6 PD deficiency

(Continued)

Drug	Route	Neonatal dose	Paediatric dose	Comments
Nystatin	**By mouth** 100,000 units/ml	0–28 days: 1ml given 4 times daily	1 month–12 years: 1ml given 4 times daily (immunocompromised children may require higher doses e.g. 5ml 4 times daily) 12–18 years: 5ml given 4 times daily (doubled in severe infections)	Give after feeds
Oseltamivir	**By mouth**	Limited data on use in children under 1 month of age–may be ineffective in first 2 weeks of life as they may be unable to metabolize oseltamivir to its active form. Premature and term neonates may be given 1–1.5mg/kg/dose twice daily	1–3 months: 2mg/kg/dose given twice daily 3–6 months: 2.5mg/kg/dose given twice daily 6–12 months: 3mg/kg/dose given twice daily 1–13 years: under 15kg: 30mg/dose given twice daily 15–23kg: 45mg/dose given twice daily 23–40kg: 60mg/dose given twice daily over 40kg: 75mg/dose given twice daily 13–18 years: 75mg/dose given twice daily * Treatment is for 5 days. Prophylaxis can be given for 10 days using the above doses once a day	If suspension not available, capsules can be opened and the contents mixed with a small amount of food, just before administration

Drug	Route	Neonatal dose	Paediatric dose	Comments
Oxytetracycline	By mouth	No dosing information	12–18 years: 250–500mg/dose given 4 times daily	Antacids and products containing aluminium, calcium, iron, magnesium and zinc salts and milk may reduce the absorption of oxytetracycline. Do not give to children under 8–12 years, or pregnant or breast–feeding women, as deposits in growing bones and teeth
Palivizumab	Intramuscular	0–28 days: 15mg/kg/dose given once a month during season of RSV risk	1 month–2 years: 15mg/kg/dose given once a month as prophylaxis only during season of RSV risk	Divide injection volumes over 1ml between 2 or more sites.
Paromomycin	By mouth	No dosing information	2–18 years: 8–12mg/kg/dose given 3 times a day for 5–10 days	
Pentamidine	Intravenous *Infuse over 60 mins*	No dosing information	1 month–18 year: 4mg/kg/dose given 24 hourly	Risk of severe hypotension following administration. Avoid concomitant use of other nephrotoxic drugs.
	Nebulized	No dosing information	1 month–18 years 600mg/dose given daily for 3 weeks treatment 300mg/dose given 4 weekly for prophylaxis	Use a nebulized bronchioldilator before nebulising pentamidine
Phenoxymeth-ylpenicillin (*Penicillin V*)	By mouth	No dosing information	1 month–18 years: 10–15mg/kg/dose (max 1g) given 4 times daily	

(Continued)

Drug	Route	Neonatal dose	Paediatric dose	Comments
Piperacillin with Tazobactam	**Intravenous** *Injection or infuse*	0–28 days: 90mg/kg/dose given 8 hourly	1 month to 18 years: 90mg/kg/dose (max 4.5g) given 6–8 hourly	Dose expressed as combination of piperacillin and tazobactam combined
Piperazine	**By mouth** *Oral Powder*	No dosing information available	3 month–1 year: 2.5ml given as a single dose 1–6 years: 5ml given as a single dose 6–18 years: Contents of one sachet given as a single dose	For threadworms repeat the dose after 14 days Take the dose in the morning.
Pivmecillinam	**By mouth**	No dosing information	*Acute uncomplicated cystitis* over 40kg: Initially 400mg as single dose, then 200mg/dose given 3 times a day for 3 days *Chronic or recurrent bacteriuria* under 40kg: 5–10mg/kg/dose given 4 times a day over 40kg: 400mg/dose given 3–4 times a day	
Posaconazole	**By mouth**	No dosing information	>12 years: 200mg/dose given 4 times a day	

Praziquantel	By mouth	No dosing information	*Tapeworm* Over 4 years: 5–10mg/kg/dose (up to 25mg/kg) as a single dose *Schistosomicides* Over 4 years: 20mg/kg/dose given for 2 doses 6 hours apart *S. Japonicum* Over 4 years: 20mg/kg/dose given for 3 doses 6 hours apart	Take doses after light breakfast
Primaquine	By mouth	No dosing information	*P. ovale* treatment 6 months–18 years: 250 microgram/kg/dose (=0.25mg/kg/dose) (max 15mg) given once a day. *P. vivax* treatment 6 months–18 years: 500 microgram/kg/dose (=0.5mg/kg/dose) (max 30mg) given once a day.	Treat for 14 days. For roundworms repeat the dose at monthly intervals for up to 3 months.
Procaine penicillin	Intramuscular injection	50,000 units/kg given once a day	50,000 units/kg given once a day (max 4.8 million units per day)	

(Continued)

Drug	Route	Neonatal dose	Paediatric dose	Comments
Proguanil with atovaquone (Malarone ®)	**By mouth** *Paediatric and standard tablets*	No dosing information	*Treatment of malaria* 5–8kg: 2 'paediatric tablets' given once a day 9–10kg: 3 'paediatric tablets' given once a day 11–20kg: 1 'standard tablets' given once a day 21–30kg: 2 'standard tablets' given once a day 31–40kg: 3 'standard tablets' given once a day over 40kg: 4 'standard tablets' given once a day *Treat for 3 days*	4 paediatric tablets are equivalent to 1 standard tablet
Pyrazinamide	**By mouth**	0–28 days: 35mg/kg/dose given once daily	1 month–18 years: 35mg/kg/dose (max 2g) given once daily	Seek immediate medical attention if symptoms such as persistent nausea, vomiting, malaise or jaundice develop
Pyrimethamine	**By mouth**	0–28 days: 1mg/kg/dose given twice a day for 2 days then 1mg/kg/dose given once a day for 6 months, then 1mg/kg/dose given three times a week for 6 months	1 month–18 years: 2mg/kg/dose once a day for 2 days then 1mg/kg/dose given once a day for 6 weeks.	Taken in combination with sulfadiazine and folinic acid. Check blood counts regularly.

Drug	Route	Neonatal dose	Paediatric dose	Comments
Quinine	By mouth	No dosing information	1 month–18 years: 10mg/kg/dose (max 600mg) given 3 times a day	
	Intravenous *Infusion over 4 hours*	0–28 days: 20mg/kg loading dose then 8 hours later 10mg/kg/dose 8 hourly	1 month–18 years: 20mg/kg (max 1.4g) loading dose then 8 hours later 10mg/kg/dose (max 700mg) given 8 hourly	
Raltegravir	By mouth	No dosing information available	16–18 years: 400mg/dose given twice a day	Avoid indigestion remedies
Ribavirin	By mouth	No dosing information available	*Chronic hepatitis C* 3–18 years: 7.5mg/kg/dose (max 600mg) given twice a day	Contraindicated in women who are or may become pregnant. Monitor FBC, platelets, electrolytes, creatinine, LFTs before and during treatment.
	Intravenous *Injection bolus*	0–28 days: 33mg/kg single dose then 16mg/kg/dose given 6 hourly for 4 days then 8mg/kg/dose given 8 hourly for 3 days.	*Life threatening viral infection in immunocompromised children* 1 month–18 years: 33mg/kg single dose then 16mg/kg/dose given 6 hourly for 4 days then 8mg/kg/dose given 8 hourly for 3 days.	
Rifabutin	By mouth	No dosing information	1–18 years: 5–7.5mg/kg/dose given once daily	May colour body secretions red

(Continued)

Drug	Route	Neonatal dose	Paediatric dose	Comments
Rifampicin	By mouth	0–28 days: 5–10mg/kg/dose given twice daily *Suspected congenital tuberculosis* 0–28 days: rifampicin 10mg/kg/dose given once daily for 6 months (used in combination with other antibiotics)	*Staphylococcal Infection* 1 month–18 years: 10mg/kg/dose (max 600mg) given twice a day *Treatment of tuberculosis* 1 month–18 years: 10mg/kg/dose (max 600mg) given once daily Or 15mg/kg/dose (max. 900mg) given 3 times a week	May colour urine red May colour contact lenses red Monitor liver function tests and blood counts in hepatic disorders, and on prolonged therapy
	Intravenous *Infuse over 2–3 hours*	0–28 days: 5–10mg/kg 12 hourly	1 month–18 years: 10mg/kg (max 600mg) 12 hourly	
Rimantidine	By mouth	No dosing information	1 month–18 years: 2.5mg/kg/dose (max 100mg) given twice a day	Not active against influenza B
Ritonavir	By mouth	No dosing information available	For boosting other PIs see specific drug. Not recommended as a single PI Adult: For boosting other PIs 100mg/dose given twice a day or 100mg once a day depending on drug (except with tipranavir 200mg/dose twice a day)	With or after food Can mask bitter taste with chocolate milk Always check potential drug interactions between antiretrovirals and antiretrovirals and other medicines—see www.hiv-druginteractions.org

Drug	Route	Neonatal dose	Paediatric dose	Comments
Saquinavir	**By mouth**	No dosing information available	Child: Insufficient data–seek specialist advice Adult: 1g/dose given twice a day with ritonavir 100mg/dose twice a day	Tablets can be cut Absorption significantly increased with food Always check potential drug interactions between antiretrovirals and antiretrovirals and other medicines—see www.hiv-druginteractions.org
Sodium Stibogluconate	**Intravenous** *Injection over 5 minutes*	No dosing information	1 month–18 years: 20mg/kg/dose (max. 850mg) given 24 hourly for at least 20 days	
Spiramycin	**By mouth**	0–28 days: 50mg/kg/dose given twice daily	12–18 years: 1.5g/dose given twice daily until delivery	3000 units = 1mg spiramycin May prolong QT interval
Stavudine	**By mouth**	≤13 days: 0.5mg/kg/dose given twice a day 13–28 days: 1mg/kg/dose given twice a daily	<30kg: 1mg/kg/dose given twice a day 30–60kg: 30mg/dose given twice a day >60kg: 40mg/dose given twice a day	Do not co-administer with zidovudine High risk of lipodystrophy

(Continued)

Drug	Route	Neonatal dose	Paediatric dose	Comments
Streptomycin	Intramuscular *Deep IM injection*	No dosing information	*Tuberculosis* 1 month–18 years: 15mg/kg/dose (max 1g) given 24 hourly *Adjunct to doxycycline in brucellosis* 1 month–18 years: 5–10mg/kg/dose given 6 hourly	Aim for 1 hour peak concentration of 15–40mg/L and pre-dose (trough) level of <5mg/L (<1mg/L in renal impairment) Change the injection site for each dose.
Sulfadiazine (Sulphadiazine)	By mouth	*Congenital toxoplasmosis* 0–28 days: 50mg/kg/dose given twice daily for 12 months	*Toxoplasmosis* 12–18 years: 50mg/kg/dose (max 1g) given twice daily for 12 months	To be given in combination with pyrimethamine and folinic acid
Sulfadoxine/ Pyrimethamine (Fansidar)	By mouth	No dosing information	*Treatment of P. falciparum (adjunct to Quinine)* 2 months–4 years: ½ tablet as single dose 5–6 years: 1 tablet as single dose 7–9 years: 1½ tablets as single dose 10–14 years: 2 tablets as single dose 14–18 years: 3 tablets as single dose	Avoid excessive exposure to the sun.

Drug	Route	Neonatal dose	Paediatric dose	Comments
Teicoplanin	**Intravenous** *Injection–bolus or infusion*	0–28 days: 16mg/kg for one dose followed 24 hours later by 8mg/kg/dose once daily	1 month–18 years: 10mg/kg/dose given 12 hourly for 3 doses then 6mg/kg/dose (max 200mg) given once daily In severe infections 10mg/kg/dose given 12 hourly for 3 doses the 10mg/kg/dose (max 400mg) given once daily	By intravenous infusion only in neonates
Tenofovir	By mouth	No dosing information available	2–8 years: 8mg/kg/dose given once a day >8 years: 210mg/m²/dose (max 300mg) given once a day	Do not co-administer with didanosine
Terbinafine	By mouth	No dosing information	1–18 years: 3–6mg/kg/dose (max 250mg) given once a day	Oral treatment is usually 4 weeks for tinea capitis; 2–6 weeks in tinea pedis; 2–4 weeks in tinea cruris; 4 weeks in tinea corporis; 6 weeks–3 months in nail infections.
Tetracycline	By mouth	No dosing information	12–18 years: 250–500mg/dose given 4 times daily	Antacids and products containing aluminium, calcium, iron, magnesium and zinc salts and milk may reduce the absorption of tetracycline. Do not give to children under 8–12 years, or pregnant or breast-feeding women, as deposits in growing bones and teeth.

(Continued)

Drug	Route	Neonatal dose	Paediatric dose	Comments
Tiabendazole	By mouth	No dosing information	1 month–18 years: 25mg/kg/dose (max 1.5g) given twice a day	
Ticarcillin (Ticarcillin/ Clavulanic acid)	Intravenous *Infuse over 30–40 mins*	under 2kg: 80mg/kg/dose given 12 hourly >2kg: 80mg/kg/dose given 8 hourly (increased to 6 hourly in severe infection)	1 month–18 years (<40kg): 80mg/kg/dose given 8 hourly (increased to 6 hourly in severe infection) Child <18 years and >40kg: 80mg/kg/dose (max 3.2g) given 6–8 hourly (increased to 4 hourly in severe infection)	Dose expressed as a combination of ticarcillin and clavulanic acid
Tinidazole	By mouth	No dosing information	*Intestinal amoebiasis & amoebic involvement of the liver* 1 month–18 years: 50mg/kg/dose (max 2g) given once a day *Urogenital trichomoniasis and giardiasis* 1 month–18 years: 50–75mg/kg/dose (max 2g) given as a single dose	For intestinal amoebisasis treat for 3 days. For amoebic involvement of the liver treat for 5 days. For urogenital trichomoniasis and giardiasis the dose can be repeated if necessary.
Tipranavir	By mouth	No dosing information	2–18 years: 14mg/kg/dose (max 500mg) given twice a day with ritonavir 6mg/kg/dose (max 200mg) twice a day or 375mg/m²/dose given twice a day with ritonavir 150mg/m²/dose twice a day	Complex interactions, reduced levels with abacavir and zidovudine. Give with or after food.

Drug	Route	Neonatal dose	Paediatric dose	Comments
Tobramycin	**Intravenous** *Injection–bolus or infuse over 30 mins*	Neonate <32 weeks corrected gestational age: 4–5mg/kg/dose given 36 hourly Neonate ≥32 weeks corrected gestational age: 4–5mg/kg/dose given 24 hourly	1 month–18 years: 7mg/kg/dose given 24 hourly	For IV therapy aim for pre-dose trough level of <1mg/L (<2mg/L for neonate). For IV therapy monitor renal function closely. Concurrent use with loop diuretics or other aminoglycosides increases the risk of nephrotoxicity and ototoxicity.
Triclabendazole	**By mouth**	No dosing information	6–18 years: 10mg/kg stat dose Repeat dose 12 hours later in severe infection	
Trimethoprim	**By mouth**	*Treatment* 0–28 days: 3mg/kg as a single dose then 1–2mg/kg/dose given twice daily. *Prophylaxis of urinary tract infections* 0–28 days: 2mg/kg/dose given at night	*Treatment* 1 month–18 years: 4mg/kg/dose (max. 200mg) given twice daily *Prophylaxis of urinary tract infections* 1 month–18 years: 2mg/kg/dose (max. 100mg) given at night	On long-term treatment, patients and their carers should be told how to recognise signs of blood disorders and advised to seek immediate medical attention if they occur

(Continued)

Drug	Route	Neonatal dose	Paediatric dose	Comments
Truvada® Tenofovir + Emtricitabine	**By mouth** Tablets—one tablet contains tenofovir 300mg + emtricitabine 200mg	Not applicable	Child: Individual tenofovir and emtricitabine—max dose as for adults Adult >18 years: 1 tablet once a day	Can be given with or without food Can be cut Can be dispersed in water Always check potential drug interactions between antiretrovirals and antiretrovirals and other medicines—see www.hiv-druginteractions.org
Valaciclovir	**By mouth**	No dosing information	12–18 years: 15–20mg/kg/dose (max 1g/dose) given three times a day (Use the higher dose for H. Zoster)	Doses highly dependent upon indication Maintain adequate hydration Dose adjustments required in renal failure
Valganciclovir	**By mouth**	0–28 days: 16mg/kg/dose given twice daily	1 month–18 years: 520mg/m²/dose (max 900mg) given once daily for long term suppression and twice daily for treatment	Take with or after food Decrease dose in renal impairment Full blood count monitoring required—significant risk of cytopenias

Drug	Route	Neonatal dose	Paediatric dose	Comments
Vancomycin	**Intravenous** *Infusion over 60 mins*	Neonate less than 29 weeks postmenstrual age 15mg/kg/dose given 24 hourly Neonate 29–35 weeks postmenstrual age 15mg/kg/dose given 12 hourly Neonate greater than 35 weeks postmenstrual age 15mg/kg/dose given 8 hourly	1 month–18 years: 15mg/kg/dose given 8 hourly	Doses to be adjusted according to plasma concentration Injection may be used orally
	By mouth		*Clostridium difficile infection* 1 month–18 years: 5mg/kg 4 times daily for 10–14 days (increased to 10mg/kg (max 500mg) if infection fails to respond or is life-threatening)	

(Continued)

Drug	Route	Neonatal dose	Paediatric dose	Comments
Voriconazole	By mouth	No dosing information	Child 2 years–18 years: 10mg/kg/dose (max 400mg) given 12 hourly for 24 hours, then 7mg/kg/dose (max 200mg) given twice a day	In mild to moderate hepatic impairment use initial dose and then halve subsequent doses.
	Intravenous Infuse at 3mg/kg/hour	No dosing information	Child 2 years–12 years: 7mg/kg/dose given 12 hourly (reduced to 4mg/kg/dose given 12 hourly if not tolerated) Child 12 years–18 years: 6mg/kg/dose given 12 hourly for 2 doses, then 4mg/kg/dose given 12 hourly (reduced to 3mg/kg/dose given 12 hourly if not tolerated).	
Zanamivir	Inhaled Dry powder inhaler	No dosing information	5–18 years: 10mg/dose given twice a day for 5 days (for post–exposure prophylaxis use 10mg/dose given once a day for 10 days).	Risk of bronchospasm in asthma. Use other inhaled drugs prior to zanamivir

Drug	Route	Neonatal dose	Paediatric dose	Comments
Zidovudine	By mouth	*Post-exposure prophylaxis for baby born to HIV positive mother* **Oral** Term (>34 weeks): 4mg/kg/dose given twice a day for 4 weeks Prem (30–34 weeks): 2mg/kg/dose given twice a day for 2 weeks then 2mg/kg/dose given three times a day for 2 weeks Prem (<30 weeks): 2mg/kg/dose given twice a day for 4 weeks	Child: 180mg/m²/dose twice a day (max dose 300mg per dose twice a day) OR ≥4kg to <9kg: 12mg/kg/dose twice a day (max 300mg per dose twice a day) ≥9kg to <30kg: 9mg/kg/dose twice a day (max 300mg per dose twice a day) Adult: 250mg per dose twice a day (300mg per dose twice a day for combivir or trizivir combinations) Combivir tablets—one tablet contains zidovudine 300mg + lamivudine 150mg Adult: Give one tablet twice daily Trizivir tablets—contains abacavir 300mg + lamivudine 150mg + zidovudine 300mg Adult: Give one tablet twice daily	Do not co-administer with stavudine

(Continued)

Drug	Route	Neonatal dose	Paediatric dose	Comments
	Intravenous *Infusion*	**Intravenous** Term: 1.5mg/kg/dose given four times a day Prem (< 34 weeks) 1.5mg/kg/dose given twice a day		

Index